Essentials of Computers for Nurses

Informatics for the New Millennium

?OOKFIELD

Notice

Essentials of Computers for Nurses
Informatics for the New Millennium

THIRD EDITION

Editors:

Virginia K. Saba, EdD, RN, FAAN, FACMI

Distinguished Scholar
Nursing Informatics Center
School of Nursing
Georgetown University
Washington, District of Columbia

Professor and Advisor, Educational Technologies and Distant Learning
Research Department
Graduate School of Nursing (GSN)
Uniformed Services University of the Health Sciences
Bethesda, Maryland

Kathleen A. McCormick, PhD, RN, FAAN, FACMI, FRCNA

Senior Principal
Health Division
SRA International, Inc.
Rockville, Maryland

Graduate School of Nursing (GSN)
Uniformed Services University of the Health Sciences
Bethesda, Maryland

with 44 contributors

McGraw-Hill
New York • San Francisco • Washington, DC • Auckland • Bogotá
Caracas • Lisbon • London • Madrid • Mexico City • Milan
Montreal • New Delhi • San Juan • Singapore
Sydney • Tokyo • Toronto

McGraw-Hill

A Division of The McGraw·Hill Companies

Essentials of Computers for Nurses: Informatics for the New Millennium, Third Edition

1234567890 DOC DOC 09876543210

ISBN 0-07-134900-6

This book was set in Sabon by V&M Graphics, Inc.
The editors were Sally J. Barhydt and Catherine Wenz.
The production supervisor was Minal Bopaiah.
The project was managed by Hockett Editorial Service.
The cover designer was Janice Bielawa.
The index was prepared by Emerald Editorial Services.
R. R. Donnelley & Sons was printer and binder.

This book is printed on acid-free paper.

Library of Congress Cataloging-in-Publication Data

Essentials of computers for nurses : informatics for the new millennium / [edited by] Virginia K. Saba, Kathleen A. McCormick ; with 44 contributors. — 3rd ed.
   p. ; cm.
  Rev. ed. of: Essentials of computers for nurses / Virginia K. Saba, Kathleen A. McCormick. 2nd ed. c1996.
  Includes bibliographical references and index.
  ISBN 0-07-134900-6
   1. Nursing—Data processing. 2. Computers. 3. Information storage and retrieval systems—Nursing. I. Saba, Virginia K. II. McCormick, Kathleen Ann. III. Saba, Virginia K. Essentials of computers for nurses.
   [DNLM: 1. Computers—Nurses' Instruction. 2. Automatic Data Processing—Nurses' Instruction. 3. Internet—Nurses' Instruction. 4. Medical Informatics Applications—Nurses' Instruction. 5. Nursing—trends—Nurses' Instruction. WY 26.5 E78 2000]
  RT50.5 .S23 2000
  610.73′0285—dc21

                             00-020237

Disclaimer: This book was written by Kathleen A. McCormick in her private capacity. No official support or endorsement by SRA International, Inc., or USUHS is intended or should be inferred.

CONTENTS

CONTRIBUTORS

Patricia A. Abbott, PhD, RNC
Assistant Professor and Coordinator of Graduate Program
in Nursing Informatics
Department of Education, Administration, Health Policy,
and Informatics
University of Maryland School of Nursing
Baltimore, Maryland
Chapter 20, "Challenges for Data Management in Long-Term Care"

Myrna L. Armstrong, EdD, RN, FAAN
Professor
School of Nursing
Texas Tech University Health Sciences Center
Lubbock, Texas
Chapter 24, "Distance Education: Using Technology to Learn"

Suzanne Bakken, RN, DNSc, FAAN, FACMI
Professor
School of Nursing and Department of Medical Informatics
Columbia University
New York, New York
Chapter 12, "Concept-Oriented Terminological Systems"

Amy J. Barton, PhD, RN
Assistant Professor and Associate Dean for Practice
Director, Integrative Center for Caring Practice
School of Nursing
University of Colorado Health Sciences Center
Denver, Colorado
Chapter 25, "Innovations in Telehealth"

Molly Billingsley, EdD, RN
Administrative Director
Patient Care Services
Washington Hospital Center
Washington, District of Columbia
Chapter 14, "Practice Applications"

Patricia Flatley Brennan, PhD, RN, FAAN, FACMI
Moehlman Bascom Professor
School of Nursing and College of Engineering
University of Wisconsin-Madison
Madison, Wisconsin
        Chapter 22, *"Health-Related Decision-Making by Patients"*

David Brocht, MS, RN
Independent Consultant
Brocht Associates
Haggerstown, Maryland
        Chapter 20, *"Challenges for Data Management in Long-Term Care"*

Suzy Ann Buckovich, JD, MPH
Associate
Department of Health Policy and Management
Johns Hopkins School of Hygiene and Public Health
Washington, District of Columbia
        Chapter 9, *"Privacy, Confidentiality, and Security"*

Caroline Campbell, MS, CCE
Director, Materials and Biomedical Technology Management
Department of Biomedical Engineering
Washington Hospital Center
Washington, District of Columbia
        Chapter 15, *"Critical Care Applications"*

Robyn Carr, RGON
Hospital Applications Manager
Information Services, Auckland Healthcare Services Limited
Auckland, New Zealand
        Chapter 30, *"Pacific Rim"*

Barbara Carty, EdD, RN
Clinical Associate Professor
Coordinator, Nursing Informatics Program
School of Education
New York University
New York, New York
        Chapter 23, *"The Nursing Curriculum in the Information Age"*

Betty L. Chang, DNSc, RN, FNP-C, FAAN
Professor
School of Nursing
University of California, Los Angeles
Los Angeles, California
        Chapter 26, *"Computer Use in Nursing Research"*

Marina Douglas, MS, RN
Clinical Practice Director
Science Applications International Corporation
Falls Church, Virginia
> Chapter 13, *"Implementing and Upgrading Clinical Information Systems"*

Susan Eckert, MSN, RN
Administrative Director
Surgical Nursing
Washington Hospital Center
Washington, District of Columbia
> Chapter 15, *"Critical Care Applications"*

Carole A. Gassert, PhD, RN
Informatics Nurse Consultant
Division of Nursing, Bureau of Health Professions
Senior Advisor, Distance Learning Methodologies
Office for the Advancement of Telehealth
Health Resources and Services Administration
Department of Health and Human Services
Rockville, Maryland
> Chapter 8, *"Nursing Informatics and Health Care Policy"*

Ulla Gerdin, RN
Senior Project Manager
Swedish Institute for Health Services Development
Stockholm, Sweden
> Chapter 29, *"Europe"*

William T. F. Goossen, BSN, RN, Certified Educator
Senior Researcher and Consultant
Acquest Consultancy, BV
Koudekerk aan den Rijn, The Netherlands
> Chapter 29, *"Europe"*

Kathryn Hannah, PhD, RN, FACMI
Professor (Adjunct)
Department of Community Health Sciences
Faculty of Medicine
The University of Calgary
Calgary, Canada
> Chapter 28, *"Canada"*

Nicholas R. Hardiker, RGN, MSc
Research Fellow
Medical Informatics Group
Department of Computer Science
University of Manchester
Manchester, United Kingdom
Chapter 12, "Concept-Oriented Terminological Systems"

Michelle Honey, RGON, Mphil(Nursing)
Information Systems Project Manager
Royal New Zealand Plunket Society, Inc.
Auckland, New Zealand
Chapter 30, "Pacific Rim"

Evelyn J. S. Hovenga, PhD, RN, FCHSE
Program Director, Health Informatics
School of Mathematical and Decision Sciences
Faculty of Informatics and Communication
Central Queensland University
Rockhampton, Queensland, Australia
Chapter 30, "Pacific Rim"

Kathleen Milholland Hunter, PhD, RN
Independent Practice in Informatics
President, Hunter Associates
Lithia, Florida
Chapter 11, "Nursing Informatics Theory"
Chapter 15, "Critical Care Applications"

Joyce E. Johnson, DNSc, RN, FAAN
Senior Vice President
Nursing and Patient Care Services
Washington Hospital Center
Washington, District of Columbia
Chief Operating Officer
Georgetown University Hospital
Washington, District of Columbia
Chapter 14, "Practice Applications"

June Levy, MLS
Managing Director
Cinahl Information Systems
Glendale, California
Chapter 27, "Computerized Information Resources"

Heimar F. Marin, MS, PhD, RN
Associate Professor in Nursing Informatics
Coordinator of the Nursing Informatics Group
Universidade Federal de São Paulo
Nucleo de Informática em Enfermagem
São Paulo, Brazil
    Chapter 31, "South America"

Robert Mayes, MS, RN
Director, Information Systems Group
Office of Clinical Standards and Quality
Health Care Financing Administration
Baltimore, Maryland
    Chapter 10, "Data Standards"

Patricia McCargar, MGA, RN, CPHQ
Administrative Manager
School of Nursing
University of Michigan
Ann Arbor, Michigan
    Chapter 14, "Practice Applications"

Kathleen A. McCormick, PhD, RN, FAAN, FACMI, FRCNA
Senior Principal
Health Division
SRA International, Inc.
Rockville, Maryland
Graduate School of Nursing (GSN)
Uniformed Services University of the Health Sciences
Bethesda, Maryland
    Chapter 1, "Overview of Computers and Nursing"
    Chapter 18, "Administrative Applications of Information
        Technology for Nursing Managers"
    Chapter 19, "Translating Evidence Into Practice: Guidelines
        and Automated Implementation Tools"
    Chapter 32, "Future Directions"

Mary L. McHugh, PhD, RN, C, ARNP
Associate Professor of Nursing
Department of Nursing Informatics
School of Nursing
University of Colorado Health Science Center
Denver, Colorado
    Chapter 3, "Computer Hardware"
    Chapter 4, "Software"
    Chapter 6, "Computer Systems"

Lynn McQueen, DrPH, RN
Associate Director, Health Services Research and Development Service
Quality Enhancement Research Initiative
Department of Veterans Affairs
Washington, District of Columbia
> Chapter 19, *"Translating Evidence into Practice: Guidelines
> and Automated Implementation Tools"*

Charles N. Mead, MD, MSc
Assistant Adjunct Professor
School of Nursing and Graduate Group in Medical Information Science
University of California, San Francisco
San Francisco, California
Chief Scientist
Simione Central Holdings, Inc.
Atlanta, Georgia
> Chapter 12, *"Concept-Oriented Terminological Systems"*

Shirley M. Moore, PhD, RN
Associate Professor
Frances Payne Bolton School of Nursing
Case Western Reserve University
Cleveland, Ohio
> Chapter 22, *"Health-Related Decision-Making by Patients"*

Ramona Nelson, PhD, RN, C
Professor and Co-Director
Health Care Informatics
Slippery Rock University
Slippery Rock, Pennsylvania
> Chapter 5, *"Data Processing"*

Susan K. Newbold, MS, RN, C
Doctoral Candidate and Instructor
University of Maryland, Baltimore School of Nursing
Baltimore, Maryland
> Chapter 17, *"Ambulatory Care Systems"*

Donna Ambler Peters, PhD, RN, FAAN
Health Care Consultant
Memphis, Tennessee
> Chapter 16, *"Community Health Applications"*

Elizabeth Phillip, MSN, RN
Instructor
St. Luke's Hospital School of Nursing
Bethlehem, Pennsylvania
> Chapter 23, *"The Nursing Curriculum in the Information Age"*

Diane S. Pravikoff, PhD, RN
Director of Research
Cinahl Information Systems
Glendale, California
> Chapter 27, *"Computerized Information Resources"*

Helga E. Rippen, MD, PhD, MPH
Director of Medical Informatics
Pfizer Health Solutions
Santa Monica, California
> Chapter 21, *"Consumers in Health Care"*

Virginia K. Saba, EdD, RN, FAAN, FACMI
Distinguished Scholar
Nursing Informatics Center
School of Nursing
Georgetown University
Washington, District of Columbia
Professor and Advisor, Educational Technologies and Distant Learning
Research Department
Graduate School of Nursing (GSN)
Uniformed Services University of the Health Sciences
Bethesda, Maryland
> Chapter 1, *"Overview of Computers and Nursing"*
> Chapter 2, *"Historical Perspectives of Nursing and Computers"*
> Chapter 16, *"Community Health Applications"*

Daniel Sigulem, MD, PhD
Associate Professor
Coordinator of the Health Informatics Department
Universidade Federal de São Paulo
São Paulo, Brazil
> Chapter 31, *"South America"*

Roy L. Simpson, RN, C, CMAC, FNAP, FAAN
Vice President, Nursing Informatics
Cerner Corporation
Kansas City, Missouri and Atlanta, Georgia
Chapter 18, *"Administrative Applications of Information
Technology for Nursing Managers"*

Diane J. Skiba, PhD
Associate Dean for Informatics
Director Academic Innovations
Office of Informatics
School of Nursing
University of Colorado Health Sciences Center
Denver, Colorado
Chapter 25, *"Innovations in Telehealth"*

Marianne Tallberg, PhD, RN
Associate Professor
Kuopio University
Kupoio, Finland
Chapter 29, *"Europe"*

Linda Q. Thede, PhD, RN, C
Consultant
Nursing Informatics Education
Aurora, Ohio
Adjunct Professor
Department of Nursing
St. Joseph College
Standish, Maine
Chapter 7, *"The Internet: A Nursing Resource"*

Elly Pluyter-Wenting, RN
Research Development
HISCOM bv
AX Leiden, The Netherlands
Chapter 29, *"Europe"*

Lucy Westbrooke, RCpN
Implementation Analyst, Information Services
Auckland Healthcare Services Limited
Auckland, New Zealand
Chapter 30, *"Pacific Rim"*

PREFACE

This new edition turns out to be a new book with csontributions from 46 authors who are specialists in the areas of their chapters. This is a book for the new millennium, and the editors and authors have tried to look into the year 2010 to determine the way that we must be prepared as nurses in the health profession to understand, use, and apply computer applications. Unlike previous editions, this edition brings to readers and students the perspectives on many new areas in health care and computers to influence the nursing profession. Whereas 20 years ago, a few persons had knowledge sufficient to write a book, now, with graduate programs preparing nurses at the masters and doctoral level, there is a critical mass of nurse informaticians. They are teaching, using computers for research, implementing computers in diverse practice arenas, and working within industry creating the new technologies for our future. Whereas 20 years ago, chapters were developed on only two desktop computers, now with laptops, electronic communications such as E-mail and other forms of multimedia distance communication, the chapters of this book were developed by persons who have taught, conducted research, and developed and implemented computer systems across the globe.

Some of the authors of this text were the students of the first edition of *Essentials of Computers for Nurses*. This book is a transition to another new and emerging way of learning, e.g., through the Internet. There are chapters devoted to the Internet for the history and technology, for the consumer on the Net, and as a new resource for health professionals. Unlike in previous editions, readers and students will notice a definite change in the numbers of URL addresses in the text and references. This text also includes many national and international citations.

This book is also international in scope. Contributors from most major continents have had the opportunity to describe the state of the science of nursing informatics in their continents. It is amazing to have witnessed that since the first edition in 1986, when we described the International Medical Informatics Association (IMIA) Nursing Section meetings in several countries, those networks have begun to foster and facilitate the advancement of nursing informatics in those countries. The international leaders describe the educational, research, practice, administration, and standards activities on those continents.

The new millennium is seeing new technologies in nursing that the first edition of *Essentials of Computers* did not even predict or foresee. This book doubles the previous book's chapters to include some of these new concepts. There is much new information on standards, legislation regarding privacy and confidentiality, the Health Insurance Portability and Accountability Act (HIPAA), and the Internet. One can see throughout this new edition the influence that managed care principles are having on nursing administration and practice.

This new edition also expands concepts that were just mentioned as paragraphs in the previous edition. For example, decision supports of consumers and health professions were just beginning technologies in the 1996 edition. Now, the experts have devoted entire chapters to these concepts. One can envision that the future will require entire books about incorporating evidence into information systems, decision support, knowledge discovery or data mining, vocabulary, or standards in nursing informatics. Books in specialty areas of nursing informatics are just now emerging.

As students and other readers use this book, we hope that they enjoy peeking into the new millennium as much as we have enjoyed reviewing the chapters prior to publication. We reflect that, as the chapter authors point out, distance education and multimedia forms of communicating with students, patients, and consumers are new forms of education and learning that will be used in the 21st century.

We had hoped that our contributions in nursing informatics would have assured that all nurses were computer-literate at the turn of the century. We began our quest for that goal 20 years before the turn of the century. We have witnessed great improvements in the volume, the quality, and the usage of computers in nursing, and this book serves as yet another contribution to our quest for the unification of nursing through its vocabulary and literacy of nurses internationally. The vision of "education without walls" has become an innovative trend and reality, demonstrating the vast changes seen in informatics and hinting at now unknown developments in education. Two forces that will shape nursing informatics in the next millennium are the Internet and its influence on the health care user and the consumer.

Acknowledgments

This is the first time we have invited experts to participate in this book. We believe that these contributors are best qualified to write in specific areas of nursing and new areas of informatics. We thank our contributors for their quick response and willingness to participate and prepare a chapter. We thank our editors, Rachel Youngman of Hockett Editorial Service, and John Dolan and Catherine Wenz of McGraw-Hill, for their support in the preparation of the book. We especially thank our families for giving us the extra time to prepare this book. With each new edition, the McCormick boys have also grown and experienced the changes in technology that have gone into producing the book. From their experience, hopefully, they will accept the challenge to write their own one day.

Virginia K. Saba
Kathleen A. McCormick

PART 1

Computers and Nursing

1

Overview of Computers and Nursing

Virginia K. Saba
Kathleen A. McCormick

OBJECTIVES

1. Introduce nursing informatics (NI) and nursing information systems (NISs).
2. Introduce nursing administration, nursing practice, community health, nursing research, and nursing education and other computer-based applications.
3. Introduce each chapter by author in this textbook.

KEY WORDS

information systems
computer science
computer-assisted decision-making
Internet
curriculum
distance education
practice management
medical informatics applications

As we enter the new millennium, computers and nursing informatics are becoming an integral part of the nursing profession and nursing information systems (NISs). Nurses are becoming computer literate and the nursing profession is implementing practice standards for its clinical care and data standards for its NISs.

Nursing informatics represents the processing of nursing information by the computer and other forms of technology. The NISs represent the nursing practice, administration, community health, nursing education, and nursing research applications. Nursing informatics also addresses other new applications, such as international aspects, or applications peripheral to the field such as legal, consumer, or theoretical issues.

■ Overview

Nursing represents the largest body of workers in the health care field, the largest group of professionals that provide clinical care to patients. Nurses also serve as administrators, researchers, educators, and community health care professionals. This textbook brings to the

nursing field and others interested in nursing an overview of nursing informatics and NISs that are applicable for this new century. This textbook provides the updated, revised, or newest NISs in computer-based health care industry, including the computer itself.

Nursing informatics is defined as the integration of computer science (hardware), information science (software), and nursing science (theory). The computer is used to process the nursing data into information and knowledge. The NISs are generally described by their purpose, focus, use, and services they provide. They are also being included in computer-based clinical information systems that include other professionals. However, the NISs applications can be generally identified by their nomenclatures and/or vocabularies or by their nurse providers.

In the past 25 years, nursing informatics was recognized as a new specialty by the American Nurses Association. In 1981, there were approximately 15 nurses who identified this new specialty as their area of interest and expertise; by 1990 this number had increased 500 percent to approximately 5,000 nurses; and by the year 2000 it had increased at least another 500 percent. By the year 2010, it is anticipated that the majority of nurses entering the profession will be computer-literate. It is also anticipated that every health care setting—acute care hospital, academic school of nursing, large community health agency, or health care setting where nurses function—will employ at least one nursing informatics specialist and will implement some type of a computer-based NIS.

The increased interest in nursing informatics occurred because of the concerted efforts of several groups that promoted nursing as an integral part of the computer-based medical record (CPR) systems being implemented in the changing health care field. The national and international professional nursing organizations began to endorse and approve data standards for the NIS systems as separate systems or as an integral component of the CPR systems. Individual nurses began to demand NIS systems to document their care, regardless of where they worked. Also, the vendors of the CPR systems began to include nursing care components in their systems.

Further, it was determined that the existing data standards and CPR systems primarily utilized medical, disease, and diagnostic assessment vocabularies and omitted the patient care aspects for an episode of illness. Thus, the users determined that nursing care data, NISs, should be included as an integral component of their systems. Such a strategy has made the goal of nursing care an integral part of CPR systems.

A description of each chapter by author follows.

Author Overviews

Dr. Saba, the co-editor of this book, provides an historical overview of the events, activities, and initiatives related to nursing informatics. Since she has been involved in many of the earlier events, she was able to include those events that impacted on the growth of this new nursing specialty. She describes the major milestones that influenced the introduction of computers into the nursing profession by five time periods and five nursing components. She highlights major computer-based nursing applications that have led to today's uses, including national events and international ones that have been critical to the field. The milestone table she provides is an excellent history for the NI field. This chapter includes an extensive list of references and bibliography that highlight the field of nursing informatics.

Dr. Mary McHugh has written two interrelated chapters that address hardware and software. It is critical for a user to understand the concepts of hardware: "what is a computer and/or a computer system." Further, she describes the concepts of software: "what makes the computer run and/or a computer system run." In each of her two chapters, she describes the historic landmarks and pioneers in their respective fields of computer technology. She also provides a detailed overview as to what constitutes hardware and software. In her chapter on hardware, she covers the components of the computer and describes the peripheral devices and media used to communicate, store, and process data. She also includes the major concepts, classes, and types of computers, components, and computer communications. In her chapter on software, she differentiates computer software from hardware and the reasons why they are both needed. She describes the differences between a software program, package, and language. She also describes how a software program is stored, processed, and used in the computer. Finally, she includes the key requirements for software to support nursing practice.

Dr. Nelson's chapter on data processing includes how it interfaces with hardware and software. She describes and explains the concepts of data, databases, information, and information systems. She explains how data are processed to create information and how information is processed to create knowledge. She also describes how data are stored by explaining the file structures and database models. She describes the purpose, structures, and functions of database management systems (DBMSs) and how a DBMS differentiates from other software systems. She outlines the life cycle of a database system, which is critical for the design and development of any NIS. Finally, she offers and explains the concept of data warehouses and how they are used in nursing and health care.

Dr. McHugh highlights the concepts of computer systems. She outlines each of the components and how they interrelate with each other in a computer system. She describes the different types of computer systems and how they are networked to each other. These systems set the stage for the remainder of the book.

Dr. Thede, in her chapter, describes the Internet and how it has become a resource for nursing in the new century. She discusses the history of the Internet and how it evolved into a worldwide network of networks. She describes the five major protocols that make up the Internet, namely, E-mail, File Transfer Protocol, the World Wide Web, Telnet, and Gopher. She also describes the functions for which one can use the Internet and how it has become a major component of any computer system. She explores the customs or strategies used with Internet communications and how they are used to communicate nursing information. She outlines the steps and criteria that one should use to evaluate the information obtained from the Internet since there is a great deal of "junk mail" on the Net. Finally, she discusses and outlines the steps for using the Internet, since it is has become an integral application of all computer systems in this new millennium.

Dr. Gassert serves as a nursing representative on major health committees within the Department of Health and Human Services (DHHS). In that capacity, she is involved in shaping the research support and agendas for nursing informatics in the new millennium. She differentiates the role of nursing in the health care arena and the policies that require support of that role in her chapter. From a public policy perspective, she stresses the importance of complete and accurate data sets for monitoring patient status in shaping health. She stresses the need to continue to pursue the literacy of nurses in informatics. She describes some of the newest of the DHHS trends in outcomes management, the Consumer Bill of Rights, telehealth initiatives, and the next generation Internet.

The chapter by Suzy Buckovich on privacy, confidentiality, and security expands these topics to a whole chapter. As a lawyer, she has been involved in health care issues in the private sector and therefore is able, from a legal point of view, to discuss the three interrelated topics. Her goal in preparing this chapter was to provide us with an understanding of these three areas—privacy, confidentiality, and security of health information. She defines each of these three topics in detail. She also identifies the federal laws that provide legal federal protection for health information as well as other laws related to the federal protection for each of these three areas. She also describes the technical mechanisms available to protect health care data that are critical to the users of the data. She describes in depth the need for an organizational policy for protecting the privacy, confidentiality, and security of health data. Further, she outlines the key issues involved in the federal privacy and confidentiality debate. This chapter provides a "stepping stone" to new legislation that will be enacted in the new century.

Robert Mayes has been leading many initiatives within the Health Care Financing Administration (HCFA). He represents HCFA on the Health Insurance Portability and Accountability Act (HIPAA) legislation which will be implemented by the time this book is published. He describes in this book the major legislative mandates that HIPAA legislation requires. In addition, Mr. Mayes represents HCFA on the American National Standards Institute (ANSI) Health Implementation System Board (HISB), which coordinates all of the national health standards. He presents the major accomplishments of

these standards organizations and described the importance of them to the nursing profession.

Dr. Milholland's chapter on nursing informatics theory provides a theoretical overview of the new nursing specialty. This chapter sets the stage for the remainder of the book. She discusses the relationship between healthcare informatics and nursing informatics. She also discusses the different definitions, models, and core concepts of nursing informatics. Further, she describes why nursing informatics is a new distinct nursing specialty. In this chapter, she describes the key aspects of nursing informatics as it relates to the electronic health record (EHR), or the CPR. She identifies the national and international informatics organizations and how they impact on this field. Further, she outlines the vocabularies "recognized" by the American Nurses Association that are complete and presents data that are indexed for an EHR. She then describes the opportunities for nursing informatics in relation to education and research. This includes what academic preparation nurses need to become a nursing informatics specialist. She also addresses the opportunities in research and the priorities outlined by national organizations and federal agencies.

Dr. Henry's chapter on concept-oriented terminological systems is thought-provoking and contributes a new approach to nursing nomenclatures, vocabularies, and classification systems. She describes that characteristics of concept-oriented terminological systems and highlights why such systems are needed to support the data needs of nursing. She also identifies the components of a concept-oriented terminological system. Further she provides the background necessary to understand the various approaches put forth in order to solve the nursing vocabulary dilemma. Additionally, she compares and contrasts two approaches for representing nursing concepts within a concept-oriented terminological system. To demonstrate the approaches, she includes several examples from the nursing field.

Chapter 13, "Implementing and Upgrading Clinical Information Systems," was revised by Marina Douglas, who has been involved in developing and implementing systems for several years in her role in the private sector and is well-qualified to prepare this chapter on this topic. She expands the six to eight phases in developing, implementing, or upgrading a clinical information system (CIS) including the nursing requirements (NIS). To develop such a system, she describes the personnel requirements and identifies the various tools of the trade used in developing, implementing, and upgrading a CIS including the NIS requirements. She also describes the roles and responsibilities of nursing for implementing and upgrading a CIS including the nursing requirements. She goes on to describe the methods of evaluating a CIS and concludes the chapter by describing the future challenges in implementing and upgrading a CIS including the nursing requirements.

The new practice applications chapter by McCarger, Johnson, and Billingsley, nurses who are front line administrators and practitioners in a busy and successful metropolitan hospital, brings refreshing new insight into the subject. They describe the historic changes in the field. But these authors have expanded on the execution of nursing process into information systems and integration of these principles with case management and decision supports. They combed the literature for new concepts that are guiding the administrator today with merging financial, administrative, and clinical practice content information. These authors have given us their benefit/risk analysis of the future.

Chapter 15, "Critical Care Applications," was revised by Carolyn Campbell. Although many of the principles have remained on how the monitoring systems function, she has done a scholarly update on the content. She stresses the need for integrated systems within the critical care environment and the connections between the critical care environment and other areas of nursing practice, as the patient moves through ambulatory, critical care, and medical/surgical units. New thoughts about the role of clinical pathways and outcomes management in critical care demonstrate how the discipline of critical care has broadened to include these concepts. As the patient moves from location to location, the need for a common vocabulary is required in nursing. This need is identified by Campbell. New technologies predicted for this area include the development of neural networks and computer simulations to manage the complex decisions in critical care.

Chapter 16, "Community Health Applications," has been updated by Donna Peters, who has been in the field as a developer of a community health system, a researcher and developer of a community health intensity rating scale, and as senior vice-president of a multiagency community health network organization. She discusses the development of community health computer applications. Also, she describes the management and practice applications for community and home health computer systems, i.e., what HHAs must be implemented to meet federal legislation requirements such as the Outcome and Assessment Informaton Set (OASIS); as well as applications designed to streamline document systems, such as the Home Health Care Classification (HHCC) system by Saba. She discusses the use of classification/

acuity schemes as tools for assessing care requirements of patients. Further, she describes the requirements for the major special purpose computer systems for: (1) outcomes management, (2) registration systems, (3) management information systems, (4) school health, (5) scheduling, (6) telehealth, (7) alternative care, and (8) home technologies. She provides a discussion of state and local health departments and their role in community health systems.

Chapter 17, "Ambulatory Care Systems," is a new chapter prepared by Susan Newbold that provides visibility to this growing health care service. Ambulatory care has been growing with the expansion of health maintenance organizations, walk-in clinics, store-front services, and other places where health care is provided. Issues concerning the professionals including nurses who staff these new facilities are not clear-cut; as a result, many are staffed with nonregistered employees who are not accountable for their care. The need for continuous and documented service improvements and information systems to measure and evaluate services provided and care outcomes are paramount.

Mr. Roy Simpson reinforces the point that the theoretical foundations of administrative applications have undergone little change in the past five years. He has added significant points related to administering individual patient care and monitoring organizational performance, staff productivity, governance, management, and support services. He provides a valuable table of emerging technologies that nurse administrators at the turn of the century are using to manage patient care.

Dr. Lynn McQueen worked as a guideline expert in the formative years when the Agency for Health Care Policy and Research was developing the first clinical practice guidelines. She was responsible for such guidelines as: *Benign Prostatic Hypertrophy.* She completed her doctoral degree in health policy at the University of North Carolina and conducted her doctoral dissertation on the politics of clinical practice guidelines. In her current position, she develops the clinical practice guidelines implementation program at the Department of Veterans Affairs in Washington, D.C. She and Dr. McCormick have written a comprehensive chapter on the science behind clinical practice guidelines, which are now known as evidence. Their backgrounds in the implementation of guidelines are extensive and so is the literature review that they provide. This should serve as background to the reader and students to help in the implementation of evidence. The second part of their chapter describes the history behind implementing guidelines into computer systems. The key to incorporating evidence into the information system is to measure a quality improvement in patient outcomes. They also describes a framework of multiple implementation tools to integrate guidelines into computerized systems. Most current research demonstrates that improved quality of evidence results in decreased costs of care.

Dr. Abbott has been involved in studying and implementing computers in hospital systems for long-term care. In her recent doctoral dissertation, she asked the question if the extensive data collected by nurses for the Medical Data System (MDS) in nursing homes could be used to predict patients' use of care in the acute care environment. She used a technology called Knowledge Discovery in Large Datasets (KDD), which included components of data mining in her studies. This chapter describes the science of KDD and data mining, how algorithms are developed to test data to determine if clusters or patterns are emerging from the data. These same technologies are described in Dr. McCormick's chapter, "Future Directions," and related to the new genomic discoveries. Dr. Abbott has conducted the most thorough literature review on this subject and referenced other nurse leaders who are also developing KDD tools to analyze nursing's potential contributions to predicting outcomes of high-risk pregnancies in complicated obstetrical cases.

Dr. Rippen has nationally coordinated the role of standards and code of ethics for the consumer on the Internet. She is a national expert for the consumer on the Net and has contributed theory and content to this book on the use of the Net for consumers and some policy issues that remain unresolved. She points out that the nursing profession has a major responsibility in developing, implementing, and recommending content on the Internet for consumers. We are all consumers of health information in this century, since the volume of information is so massive. Consumers are on the Internet, and they are asking for information about their health care. Dr. Rippen provides valuable sites on the Internet to monitor the standards, the usage, and the issues that patients are discussing with each other and with health care professionals. Her chapter complements the work of Drs. Brennan and Moore, since they focus more on how the patient is entering into the decision-making for health care.

Drs. Brennan and Moore provides an excellent theoretical framework and description of consumer decision-making. They have co-directed research on the patient at home with Alzheimer's and from their collective experience have described the major contributions that the nursing profession and informatics can make for consumer decision-making. They have reviewed the most important and significant literature in this area and provided a template for nurses to begin to become active in designing and implementing decision supports for consumers. This chapter also identifies the major contributions of research on the value of consumer decision-making. The outcomes on patient preference, outcomes, patient satisfaction, and quality of care are new discoveries of the 1990s to be utilized in the 21st century. Dr. Brennan will be the first nurse president of the American Medical Informatics Association in 2000. It is a new beginning for nurses to assume such leadership to develop the roles and responsibilities of all health professions in informatics to assure better patient care. Through her leadership, the use of decision supports and the Internet to benefit the consumer will be shaped and advanced. This chapter articulates some of the vision of Drs. Brennan and Moore.

Dr. Carty, in her chapter, "The Nursing Curriculum in the Information Age," has updated the educational applications to include curriculum design. She attempts to help us understand the paradigm shift from computer applications to information management and technology applications in nursing education. She indicates that information technology in education will cut across departments and disciplines and will facilitate interactions and connectivity. She describes the strategies needed to integrate information and computer technology into the nursing curriculum. Curriculum implications, including faculty development, interactive learning, cognition, electronic communication, and informatics, are summarized. They are also described as they relate to the nursing informatics curriculum. Additionally, Dr. Carty presents models and strategies for meeting educational challenges of the information age.

Dr. Armstrong expands upon the educational applications in her chapter, "Distance Learning: Using Technology to Learn." She has been involved in distance education for several years and has first-hand knowledge of this emerging nursing education application. Programs for distance learning are flourishing, especially Internet courses. She defines distance education and describes the historical and current development of this redesigned educational approach. She also discusses the important strategies and support needed for learning at a distance as well as the essential support needed for developing course content. She explores the associated research needed to assist future trends in nursing education.

Drs. Skiba and Barton describe those final educational applications in their chapter, "Innovations in Telehealth." They indicate that with the new advances in computing and communications, technologies will impact on where we live, work, and interact with each other. They indicate that these technologies not only will affect the practice of health care, but also education. Their chapter describes in detail the new technological telehealth advances. They define "telehealth" and address data communication applications available for the user. They include electronic communication, electronic bulletin boards, electronic networks, and forms of video media. They describe the tools used for integrating telehealth into care plans. They further describe how telehealth is used for learning and for consumer education. This broad overview of how telehealth links nursing practice, nursing education, and nursing research will prepare us for the new millennium.

Dr. Chang in her chapter, "Computer Use in Nursing Research," provides an update and a new approach to research applications. She identifies the general goals of quantitative and qualitative research. She describes how computer technology is applied for each of these research types. She further identifies the most appropriate tasks for the use of computer applications in quantitative and qualitative research. She also discusses the uses of computer programs and describes how they can be used for the four major steps of the research process: data collection, data coding, data analysis, and dissemination of data results. She identifies the precautions needed for the selection of software for data analysis. The evaluation of the existing software programs is critical for the different types of research being conducted. This new research chapter widens the horizons of nursing research for nurse researchers.

Dr. Pravikoff and June Levy provide the chapter on computerized information resources, including the MEDLARS databases. As two officers of Cinahl Information Systems, they are qualified to discuss the online bibliographic retrieval systems and other information resources used and needed by the nurses and other health professionals. They describe the content of a retrieval system as a database and identify the steps for choosing the appropriate database. They highlight what computer technology (what computer and modem) are required to conduct a search of the existing databases of nursing literature. They further discuss the searching of the Internet for similar nursing literature databases. They also describe and identify the steps for planning a computer search for information, including Boolean logic. They include the rationale for identifying the sources of information for practicing nurses. Finally, they identify the differences between essential and supportive computerized resources for the professional nurse searcher/user.

Each of the international chapters is especially insightful on the state of the science on other continents. The Canadian perspective was written by Dr. Kathryn Hannah, a nurse who has shaped nursing informatics in Canada. Through her insights, the advances in the Minimum Data Set in Canada are described. The chapter by Gerdin, Pluyter-Wenting, Gossen, and Dr. Tallberg describes the impressive initiatives on the European Continent. They describe the importance of projects that have obtained funding in Europe from the European Commission. These four authors represent four different countries in Europe. They have each been personally involved in the major developments advancing nursing and informatics in their respective countries in Europe and internationally. The Pan-Pacific chapter written by Dr. Hovenga representing Australia, and Ms. Carr, Honey, and Westbrook from New Zealand describes the unique government situation and the resulting information infrastructure that has developed to support health care and nursing. Because of the National Health Care environment, the use of information systems for acuity and rostering as well as workload are described. Their role in standards development also allows the reader to appreciate the unique contributions the nursing profession is making in the Pacific Rim, represented by the broader Asia innovations that are also taking place in Hong Kong. The chapter that Drs. Marin and Sigulem wrote on South America describes the extensive work on the development and use of information systems in South America. They identify the use of information technology in nursing practice. They also describe educational and distance learning initiatives in South America. They have begun impressive standard-setting activities that are also described in this chapter.

Dr. McCormick has given us a vision of three types of technologies that may play a prominent role in the future. She defines the science behind voice technologies or speech recognition systems. She predicts that these innovations that are just now emerging will become a predominant way that data are entered into computer systems in health care. This will bridge the final issues of computer literacy when the health care professional speaks into the computer. Computer warehouses and repositories are next described as the new areas that clinicians will access to find the integration of information in highly technical areas. The third is the concept of the changing genomic environment in health care is just now unraveling. The support of new diagnostic and treatment strategies for health care will emerge from data mining of the genomic databases.

CHAPTER 2

Historical Perspectives of Nursing and the Computer

Virginia K. Saba

OBJECTIVES

1. Describe the historical perspectives of nursing and computers.
2. Describe early computer-based nursing applications in hospitals, community health, education, and research.
3. List the milestones of computers and nursing (nursing informatics).

KEY WORDS

computer literacy
computer systems
information systems
Internet
nursing informatics
standards

The computer is the most powerful technological tool that has transformed the nursing profession in readiness for the new century. The computer has transformed the nursing paper-based records to computer-based records. Today and tomorrow, the computer and the Internet are essential for all settings where nurses function—hospitals, ambulatory care centers, health maintenance organizations, community health agencies, academic institutions, research centers, and schools of nursing.

"Computer" is an all encompassing term that refers to computer technology and computer systems and, when used for computer systems in nursing, refers to nursing information systems (NISs) and access to the Internet. "Nursing informatics" has emerged as a new term that encompasses the computer technologies that enable nurses to manage health care and patient care more efficiently and effectively and, at the same time, makes nurses more accountable.

Computers in nursing are used to manage information in patient care, monitor the quality of care, and evaluate the outcomes of care. Computers are being used for communicating (sending/receiving) data and messages via the Internet and accessing resources on the World Wide Web (WWW). The NISs are also used for planning, budgeting, and policy-making for patient care services. They are used for enhancing nursing education and distance learning with new media modalities. Computers are being used to support nursing research, test new systems, design new knowledge databases, and change the role of nursing in the health care industry for the new millennium.

This chapter provides an overview of the history of the computer, since its introduction into the field of nursing. This history is described by five time periods and five nursing components. This chapter also highlights computer-based nursing applications that have led to today's and tomorrow's uses. It describes the major milestones that influenced the introduction of computers into the nursing profession. The chapter is divided into three major sections:

■ Historical Perspectives of Nursing and Computers
■ Early Computer-Based Nursing Applications
■ Landmark Events in Nursing and Computers

9

Historical Perspectives of Nursing and Computers

Computer technology emerged in nursing in response to the changing and developing technologies in the health care industry and in nursing practice. It is analyzed according to: (1) five time periods (prior to the 1960s, the 1960s, the 1970s, the 1980s, and the 1990s), (2) four major nursing areas (nursing administration, nursing practice, nursing education, and nursing research), and (3) standards initiatives addressing nursing practice standards, nursing data standards, health care data standards, and federal legislation that has impacted the nursing profession and its need for technology.

As nursing focused on the computer age in readiness for the new millennium, nurses updated their practice standards, adapted computer-based materials, tested computer systems, and structured classification schemes for documenting the nursing process and patient care. They created the nursing minimum data set (NMDS), standardized nursing vocabularies, and nursing care planning protocols. Also, they designed several computer tools to support the use of the new technology for the field.

Five Time Periods

Five historical perspectives of nursing and computers follow:

Prior to the 1960s   Starting in the 1950s, as the computer industry grew, the use of computers in the health care industry also grew. During this time, there were only a few experts who formed a cadre of pioneers that attempted to adapt computers to health care and nursing. Also, during this time the nursing profession was undergoing major changes. The image of nursing was improving, nursing practices and services were expanding in scope and complexity, and the number of nurses was increasing. These events provided the impetus for the profession to embrace computers.

Computers were initially used in health care facilities for basic business office functions. The early computers used punch cards to store data and card readers to read computer programs, sort, and prepare data for processing. They were linked together and operated by paper tape and used teletypewriters to print their output. As the technology advanced, the health care equipment improved.

1960s   During the 1960s, the uses of computer technology in health care settings began to be questioned. Questions such as "Why computers?" and "What should be computerized?" were discussed. Nursing practice standards were reviewed, and nursing resources were analyzed. Studies were conducted to determine how computer technology could be utilized effectively in the health care industry and what areas of nursing should be automated. Was the nurses station, the area in the hospital viewed as the hub of information exchange, the most appropriate center for the development of the computer applications?

During this period, computers and technology advanced, while health care facilities increased. The introduction of cathode ray tube (CRT) terminals, online data communication, and real-time processing added other dimensions to the computer systems, making them more accessible and "user-friendly." The hospital information systems (HISs) that were developed primarily processed financial transactions and served as billing and accounting systems. Also, a few HISs emerged that documented and processed a limited number of medical orders and nursing care activities. Vendors were beginning to enter the health care field and market software applications for various hospital functions; however, because of the limitations of the technology, the lack of standardization, and the diversity of paper-based patient care records, progress was slow.

1970s   In the 1970s, the introduction of computers into nursing was inevitable. Nurses began to recognize the value of the computer for their profession. During this decade, giant steps were taken in both dimensions: nursing and computers. The nurses recognized the computer's potential for improving the documentation of nursing practice, the quality of patient care, and the repetitive aspects of managing patient care. They assisted in the design and development of nursing applications for the HISs and other settings where nurses function. Computer applications for the financial and management functions of patient care systems were seen as cost-saving technologies. Further, several mainframe HISs were designed and developed, a few of which became the forerunners of today's systems. Many of the early systems were funded by contracts or grants from federal agencies (National Center for Health Services Research, 1980).

During this period, several states and large community health agencies developed or contracted for their own computerized management information systems

(MISs). Generally, the public health MISs provided statistical information required by local, state, and federal agencies for specific program funds, whereas home health agencies provided billing and other financial information required for the reimbursement for patient services by Medicare, Medicaid, and other third-party payers.

1980s   During the 1980s, the field of informatics emerged in the health care industry and in nursing. Nursing informatics became an accepted specialty, and many nursing experts entered the field. Technology challenged creative professionals, and the use of computers in nursing became revolutionary. As computer systems were being implemented, the needs of nursing took on a cause-and-effect modality; that is, as new computer technologies emerged and as computer architecture advanced, the need for nursing software evolved. It became apparent that the nursing profession needed not only to update its practice standards, but also to determine its data standards, taxonomies, and classification schemes that could be coded for the computer-based patient record systems (CPRSs).

During this period, many mainframe HISs emerged with NIS subsystems. These systems documented several aspects of the patient record; namely, order entry that emulated the Kardex, results reporting, vital signs, and other systems that documented narrative nursing notes using word-processing packages. Discharge planning systems were developed and used as referrals to health care facilities in the continuum of care.

In the 1980s, the microcomputer or personal computer (PC) emerged. This invention made computers more accessible, affordable, and usable by nurses and other health care providers. PCs brought computing power to the workplace and point of care. PCs could serve not only as terminals linked to the mainframe computers, but also as stand-alone computers that allowed the nurses to create their own applications. This innovation made NISs more user-friendly, and they served as workstations as the technology advanced.

1990s   Beginning in the 1990s, computer technology became an integral part of health care settings, nursing practice, and the nursing profession. The professional organizations identified initiatives that addressed informatics. Policies and legislation were adopted that promoted computer technology in health care including nursing.

The nursing profession became actively involved in the promotion of nursing informatics. In 1992, nursing

informatics was approved by the American Nurses Association (ANA) as a new nursing specialty. The demand for nursing informatics expertise increased greatly in the workplace and other settings where nurses function. The technology revolution continued to impact the profession.

The need for computer-based nursing practice standards, data standards, nursing minimum data sets, and national databases emerged as well as the need for a unified nursing language, including nomenclatures, vocabularies, taxonomies, and classification schemes. Also, nurse administrators demanded that computer systems include nursing care protocols. Still, nurse educators required the use of innovative technologies for all levels and types of nursing and patient education. The nurse researchers also required knowledge representation, decision support, and expert systems based on aggregated data.

The 1990s brought smaller and faster computers to the bedside and to all of the point-of-care settings where nurses practice. Workstations and local area networks (LANs) were developed for hospital nursing units, wide area networks (WANs) were developed for linking care across health care facilities, and the Internet was used for linking across the different systems. Information and knowledge databases were integrated into the bedside systems. Laptops, notebooks, and other types of portable wireless PCs made it possible for professionals to record care at the point of care.

In the 1990s, the Internet brought new cyberspace tools that formed the building blocks for more sophisticated applications. By 1995, the Internet had moved into the mainstream, its electronic mail (E-mail), file transfer protocol (FTP), Gopher, Telnet, and WWW protocols greatly enhancing its usability and friendliness (Saba, 1996; Sparks, 1996). The Internet began to be used for High Performance Computing and Communication (HPCC), the "information superhighway." Also, it was used to exchange data between the computer-based patient record (CPR) systems across facilities and settings and over time. It became the means for communicating on-line services and resources to the nursing community. The Internet has become an integral component of all computer systems, and the WWW is used to link and map information (Nicoll, 1998; Saba, 1995b).

By the year 2008, it is predicted that clinical information systems that integrate hospital, patient, and nursing information will become the information systems (technological tools) used to process an ever-increasing amount of complex patient data via the Internet. Further, clinical HISs will be individualized, and patient-specific systems will be stored on a "smart card" and considered a patient's life-long health record (Collen, 1999).

Four Major Nursing Areas

This second section addresses the historical perspectives of nursing that influenced the need for computers. It focuses on the four major nursing areas: nursing practice, nursing administration, nursing education, and nursing research.

Nursing Practice   The need for computers in nursing arose as nursing practice increased in scope and complexity. Over 100 years ago, nursing theory began with Florence Nightingale's six cannons. Her *Notes on Nursing: What It Is, and What It Is Not* alluded to the need for a computing device. Nightingale described the need for nurses to record manually "the proper use of fresh air, light, warmth, cleanliness, quiet, and the proper selection and administration of diet" (Nightingale, 1946, p. 6). She stated that the purpose of documenting such observations was to collect, store, and retrieve data so that patient care could be managed intelligently (Seymer, 1954).

Until the 1930s, nursing notes on patient care generally focused on the medical diagnosis and medical record. In 1937, Henderson recommended that nurses should write nursing care plans as a tool for planning, providing, and communicating patient care (Harmer and Henderson, 1939; Henderson, 1964). By 1960, a century after Florence Nightingale wrote on the six canons of nursing, assessment of nursing practice had become part of the patient's record. Three schemes were primarily available for documenting patient care: "21 nursing problems" for assessing patient needs developed by Abdellah and associates (1960), "14 major activities" for categorizing nursing care identified by Henderson (1964), and Orem's "7 components" of universal self-care (1971).

Between the 1960s and the 1970s, hospital staffing began to change as nursing practice models were being introduced. Workload studies, based on resource use, produced patient classification/acuity methods for determining staffing requirements. Generally, they characterized a patient in terms of acuity of illness or self-care activities. Other studies were conducted that attempted to measure the quality and outcomes of care. Computer-based instruments were developed, such as questionnaires, that measured the degree of patient satisfaction.

Beginning in the 1970s, computer technology started to become an integral part of the profession. Nurses developed theories, methods, and frameworks to assess patients' needs, determine care requirements, and document plans of care. Also, professional nursing became a science and clinical practice standards changed, providing new directions for the patient record. The early developers of computer systems conducted "studies of the nursing unit" to determine which aspects of nursing care should be computerized in a hospital setting. Nursing practice standards were reviewed, nursing resources were analyzed, and nursing cost studies were conducted to determine how computer technology could be utilized effectively.

The early systems were designed to support the patient care activities performed by the nursing staff. Primarily, they included census status (admission, discharge, and transfer (ADT)), order entry and results reporting, medication administration, intake and output, vital signs, and discharge planning. However, the documentation and care planning nursing subsystems took a great deal of resources to develop and were difficult to program. These subsystems were rarely implemented because the nursing profession did not provide the tools—neither a standardized nursing language nor a standardized method on how to document the care process. These needs became a challenge to the nursing profession starting in the 1980s.

Nursing Administration   Nursing administration in hospitals emerged with the introduction of nursing departments, expansion of critical patient care services, and requirements for care resources. They required complex computations that prompted the use of the computer. In the early 1920s, studies were performed on the ratio of nurses to patients (Roberts, 1954). From the 1930s through the 1960s, the staffing studies were based on time and motion. Such studies determined that nurse staffing was based not only on the ratio of patients to personnel, but also the number of nursing care hours needed per patient per day (Aydelotte, 1973). As nursing care of patients became more complex, complex computations were required, prompting the use of the computer.

Nursing administration as a specialty also advanced as nurses became qualified. In the 1950s, federal funds became available for graduate nursing education with a major in nursing administration. The educational programs focused on the nursing administrator's role in health care facilities. Funding also became available for nurses to conduct studies that focused on the need to evaluate administration activities such as personnel management, nurse staffing, quality assurance, and an array of other functions, all of which required computer-based applications.

In the 1980s, funding was extended to NISs and nursing informatics. In 1992, when federal legislation eliminated the funding for nursing administration programs, including nursing informatics, the emphasis on this specialty declined in the academic programs (National Advisory Council on Nurse Education and Practice, 1997). However, the specialty organization of nurse executives that emerged in the 1980s began to take the lead in defining a minimum data set and other activities pertaining to nursing administration.

Nursing Education   The introduction of computers into nursing education developed as the schools of nursing grew. Formal education was suggested by Florence Nightingale, and her concepts have influenced nursing education over the years (Nightingale, 1946). In the early 1900s, as the number of hospitals increased, schools of nursing were established, since nursing students were viewed as an economical way of staffing the hospitals (Lysault, 1973).

During and after the 1950s, federal funds supported the introduction of new types of educational nursing programs. Two-year community college programs were introduced, replacing many of the 3-year hospital schools of nursing (Montag, 1954). Funding was also available for graduate education leading to a masters and/or doctoral degree, with specialization in education, research, administration, supervision, or advanced clinical practice.

As schools of nursing expanded in the 1970s and 1980s and the number of student nurses increased, there was an urgent need for computers to assist in the management of schools and student records, such as on-line access to student information. Studies were conducted to determine the extent of nursing informatics in the nursing curricula (Carty and Rosenfeld, 1997; Gassert, 1995). By the 1990s, computer laboratories were also installed in schools of nursing to assist students in the educational process, using computer-assisted instruction (CAI), interactive video (IAV), and CD-ROM programs. These new multimedia technologies enhanced the courses by offering tutorials, drill and practice, case studies, and decision-making software programs (Rizzolo, 1994).

By late 1990s, campus-wide computers were available to students to access the Internet. Students were able to communicate via E-mail, transfer data files, and access resources stored on millions of Internet Web sites. The development of Internet courses via the WWW

began to change the way material was taught. Web courses started to be directed to outside the classroom setting, requiring distance education/learning technologies. The Web courses also supported a full array of multimedia educational strategies, making them user-friendly and stimulating to the student, such as the "chat rooms" that allowed for open discussion between students and faculty. Further, interactive teleconferencing courses began to bring live classroom lectures via digital telephone lines or satellite communication to remote sites that could receive the transmissions. This "face-to-face" medium made it possible for students to stay at home and work while attending classes in their own environments. Time, distance, and cost were no longer barriers to the educational programs (Joos and Nelson, 1992; Saba, 2000).

Nursing Research   Nursing research provided the impetus to use the computer not only for analyzing nursing data, but also for on-line searching of the literature. Statistical analysis was first performed by Florence Nightingale, who conducted studies on nursing education, nursing practice, and health services research (Werley, 1981). She manually collected and analyzed pertinent information because she recognized the need for solid nursing data to improve the health care delivery system of her day.

The emphasis on nursing research emerged in 1955, when the Public Health Service Act was passed. That legislation provided funds for nursing research through grants to schools of nursing, health care institutions, and individuals. As a result of federal funding, nurses started to conduct research to investigate nursing problems to improve nursing practice, determine the supply and requirements of nurses, highlight staffing needs, develop educational standards, and determine the direction of nursing education (Gortner and Nahm, 1977; Vreeland, 1964). Different types of staffing studies were conducted using innovative engineering methods that focused on four major techniques: (1) time and task frequency, (2) work sampling, (3) observation, and (4) self-reporting of nursing activities.

During the 1980s, the use of computer-based statistical programs for processing nursing research study data provided new correlations and interpretations that changed the practice of nursing. Statistical programs that ran only on mainframe computers were now able to run on desktop PCs. Because the statistical programs could process more complex problems, researchers were able to develop decision support systems designed to improve patient care and advance the science of nursing.

As the technology advanced in the 1990s, databases supporting nursing research emerged, namely bibliographic retrieval systems for nursing literature and other literature that contained relevant content, such as drug data. These large databases were used for meta-analysis to develop evidenced-based practice guidelines. Further, the electronic libraries that were developed employed technological advances in the management and on-line searching and retrieval of bibliographic information (Saba et al., 1989). They used the Internet to expand their on-line capabilities, in the academic centers, to the WWW for on-line literature, journals, and books. The Internet also provided on-line access to the millions of WWW resources and computer networks around the world. These expanded capabilities influenced the field of nursing research.

Standards Initiatives

The third perspective that is significant concerns the standards initiatives focusing on nursing practice standards, nursing data standards, health care data standards, and federal legislation that influenced the introduction of the computer into nursing. They influenced the nursing profession and its need for computer systems and nomenclatures to gain acceptance among the health care policy makers.

Nursing Practice Standards   In 1951, the nursing standards for nursing practice were formally imposed by the Joint Commission on Accreditation of Hospitals (JCAH), which was newly established. The JCAH stressed the need for adequate records on patients in hospitals and set practice standards for the documentation of medical records by nurses (Namdi and Hutelmyer, 1970).

Joint Commission on Accreditation of Hospitals Nursing Standards   In the 1970s, the JCAH, who considered nursing notes to be legal documents, recommended that the nursing process be used as the framework for documenting nursing care. In 1981, they also recommended that hospitals classify patients by using a reliable method for allocating nursing staffing. This requirement led to computer systems designed to improve the efficiency of patient care and the accuracy of resource use. The computer was needed to process acuity schemes, analyze workload data, and measure quality indicators. As a result, many computerized patient classification systems were developed that determined nursing resources. Even though the systems varied, they met the JCAH

accreditation standards (Alward, 1983; Joint Commission on Accreditation of Hospitals, 1970, 1981).

In 1990, the **Joint Commission on Accreditation of Hospital Organizations** (JCAHO, new name) advocated the continuation of acuity systems to determine resource use but also recommended that care plans be developed for documenting nursing care (Joint Commission on Accreditation of Hospital Organizations, 1994). They also introduced in 1994 the JCAHO *Accreditation Manual for Hospitals*, which contained many changes. It included a new chapter, "The Management of Information," that addressed information management processes for meeting the needs of a health care facility. New standards were outlined on what a patient record should contain, what data should be collected, and how the information in the database should be organized (Corum, 1993). It also included standards for determining "what is done" and "how it is done." These new standards affected what CPR systems were used and what data were collected.

American Nurses Association Nursing Practice Standards   The ANA also has been involved in establishing nursing practice standards. In 1980, the ANA defined the nature and scope of nursing practice in *Nursing: A Social Policy Statement*, using the "nursing process" as the framework for documenting nursing care. The ANA also recommended the development of a patient classification/acuity system for nurse staffing (American Nurses Association, 1980).

In 1982, the ANA formed the Steering Committee on Classification of Nursing Practice, which began to develop strategies to identify and classify the phenomena of nursing practice. In 1991, the ANA revised its *Standards for Clinical Nursing Practice* and continued to use the "nursing process" as its conceptual framework for documenting patient care (American Nurses Association, 1991).

Nursing Data Standards
American Nurses Association Nursing Data Standards
In 1973, the first recognized nursing data standard, a list of "37 nursing diagnoses" critical for assessing health conditions that required nursing interventions, appeared (Gebbie, 1975). This list of nursing diagnoses labels was expanded to "50 nursing diagnoses" in 1982, "114 diagnostic categories" in 1992, and "135 diagnostic categories" in 1998. This **North American Nursing Diagnosis Association** (NANDA) list was classified by nine patterns of human responses to health and illnesses; however, it was also coded for computer pro-

cessing by *Taxonomy I–Revised* (Kim et al., 1984; North American Nursing Diagnosis Association, 1990, 1992).

Another vocabulary was initiated in 1976 by the Omaha Visiting Nurse Association (VNA). It consisted of a list of 49 nursing problems describing "conditions" addressed by community health nurses. This list was expanded and finalized in 1986, resulting in the *Omaha System* that now consists of 44 client problems, 63 intervention labels, and a five-point Likert-type scale for rating outcomes (Martin and Sheets, 1992, 1995; Visiting Nurse Association of Omaha, 1986).

A HHCC system of two interrelating vocabularies emerged in 1991—the **Home Health Care Classification (HHCC) of Nursing Diagnoses and HHCC of Nursing Interventions**. They were developed by Saba and colleagues to document the nursing care process in home health and ambulatory care settings. The two HHCC vocabularies are structured and classified according to "20 Care Components." Specifically, the HHCC of Nursing Diagnoses consists of 145 nursing diagnoses with three expected outcomes/goals (axes) used as modifiers; the HHCC of Nursing Interventions consists of 160 nursing interventions with four types of actions (axes) used as modifiers representing 640 nursing actions (Saba, 1992, 1995a, 1997; Appendix A). The HHCC vocabularies are coded for computer processing that allows the two schemes to be linked to each other and to other care schemes. (See detailed description in Chap. 16.)

In 1992, another scheme for documenting nursing practice in hospitals was introduced called the **Nursing Intervention Classification** (NIC). It consists of 433 nursing interventions with definitions and related activities that describe what a nurse does (McCloskey and Bulechek, 1992; Bulechek and McClosky, 1994).

During the 1990s, several other vocabularies were created and recognized by the ANA as the data standards for nursing practice. They included the **Nursing-Sensitive Outcome Classification** (NOC) developed at the University of Iowa (Johnson and Maas, 1994), the **Patient Care Data Set** (PCDS) developed by Ozbolt (1996), and the **Perioperative Nursing Data Set** by the Association of Operating Room Nurses, Inc. which is described on the ANA Web pages. Other vocabularies were also being developed by nursing specialty groups.

American Nurses Association Steering Committee on Databases to Support Nursing Practice In 1989, the ANA was mandated to develop nursing databases designed to measure and determine the cost and quality of nursing services. This activity was assigned to the ANA Cabinet on Nursing Practice, which formed in 1990 the ANA Steering Committee on Databases to Support Nursing Practice to carry out this charge. The Database Steering Committee was mandated to (1) support activities related to nursing classification schemes, uniform data elements, data sets, and databases; (2) develop standardized national data sets for clinical nursing practice, and (3) coordinate efforts related to the development of computer-based databases for nursing practice standards, data standards, and payment reform.

In 1990, the ANA House of Delegates recognized the NMDS as the minimum data elements that should be included in any paper-based or computer-based patient record. This event led the Database Steering Committee to make the NMDS the umbrella for four classification vocabularies/schemes that the committee recognized, in 1992 (McCormick et al., 1994). The Database Steering Committee determined that the four schemes not only were the most complete and mature classification systems available for nursing practice, but also met its criteria for a Unified Nursing Language System (UNLS). They in turn were included in the National Library of Medicine (NLM) Unified Medical Language Systems (UMLS). Other nomenclatures were being developed (described elsewhere) and submitted to the ANA; once recognized they would also be submitted to the NLM for inclusion in the UMLS (American Nurses Association, 1994). In 1997, the Database Steering Committee was renamed the Committee for Nursing Practice Information Infrastructure.

Other Nursing Data Standards Activities In the late 1990s, the recognized nursing nomenclatures described above were studied and analyzed to determine how effective they are in documenting nursing care (Henry and Mead, 1996). In 1999 and 2000, the Vanderbilt Nursing Vocabulary Summit Conferences were held. These summits brought all of the developers together to determine if and how the nomenclatures could remain intact while serving as components of categorical structures for a concept-oriented reference terminology (Bakken et al., 2000). Further, in the fall of 1999, SNOMED International held a similar meeting of the major developers of the nursing nomenclatures (Convergent Terminology Group for Nurses) to determine if they could participate in the modeling and mapping of their works by SNOMED International (College of American Pathologists and American Veterinary Medical Association, 1998).

Heath Care Data Standards
American Society for Testing and Materials The ASTM is the oldest standards organization in the United

States. The ASTM is a charter member of ANSI and is the largest nongovernment standards body, with over 30,000 members from 90 countries. The ASTM E-31 Committee on Healthcare Informatics, established in 1970, became an accredited committee that develops standards for health information and health information systems designed to assist vendors, users, and anyone interested in systematizing health information. It supports several subcommittees that address architecture, content, portability, format, privacy, and communications. The Committee coordinates its efforts with those of other developers. The ASTM Committee E-31 is responsible for the development of medical information standards (Cendrowska, 1999; Hammond, 1994).

In 1987, **Health Level Seven** (HL7) was created to develop standards for the electronic interchange of clinical, financial, and administrative information among independent health care-oriented computer systems. It grew out of efforts to involve multiple vendors to initiate open hospital information systems (Agency for Health Care Policy and Research, 1999; Fitzmaurice, 1995; Hammond, 1994; Van Bemmel, 1997). The Health Level Seven (1999) created the most broadly defined standard for the transmission of patient clinical data. The HL7 is accredited by the American National Standards Institute (ANSI).

In 1991, the Institute of Medicine's report on the computer-based patient record recommended that a **computer-based patient record** (CPR) and a CPR system (CPRS), be developed using health care standards and nomenclatures (Amatayakul, 1998; Dick and Steen, 1991). Several organizations became involved at the national and international levels to implement the recommendations. Thus, in 1992, the **Computer-Based Patient Record Institute** (CPRI) was created and became a leading voice for the implementation of electronic patient records in the U.S.

The CPRI, since its inception, has held annual conferences on the topic and took the leadership, produced several documents, and co-hosted several meetings on specific topics related to the CPR. In 1995, it also started to hold an annual CPRI-sponsored Nicholas E. Davies CPR Recognition Award of Excellence Symposium. This award was designed to recognize excellence in the use of CPR systems to improve health care delivery. The applicants are judged by a panel of industry experts who evaluated whether a provider organization has successfully implemented computer-based patient records in their system (Teich, 1997).

In the U.S., the **American National Standards Institute** (ANSI), a private nonprofit membership organiza-

tion, was instituted to coordinate and approve voluntary standards efforts in the U.S. It was also combined with the **Health Care Informatics Standards Board** (HISB), founded in 1992, to fulfill a request by the European standards coordinating organization (CEN TC/251) to represent the U.S. standards effort. Thus, the **ANSI-HISB** organization acts as one and links to the two major organizations in Europe, the **European Standardization Committee** (CEN) and **International Standards Organization** (ISO).

Another organization, **SNOMED International**, serves as an umbrella of the structured nomenclatures, and its merger with the **READ Codes** from the National Health Service in the United Kingdom in 1999 is also being submitted for approval. Since the existing medical and disease conditions nomenclatures are already indexed, they serve as the coding strategies and therefore the standards for CPRSs. The nursing standards that have been put forth are those nomenclatures recognized by the American Nurses Association.

The **National Commission on Vital and Health Statistics (NCVHS) Workgroup on Computer-based Patient Records** was established in 1997 to help the Department of Health and Human Services investigate and approve of a set of nomenclatures for the federal government. That committee evaluated the recognized medical, nursing, and other health profession nomenclatures for the DHHS (National Commission on Vital and Health Statistics, 1996). An *Inventory of Health Care Standards* (1997), pertaining to the implementation of the Health Insurance Portability and Accountability Act (HIPAA) of 1996 legislation was developed. The NCVHS Work Group on CPRSs has also prepared a report for the Congress on HIPAA-mandated standards for the patient medical record information and its electronic transmission, focusing primarily on privacy and security. The HIPAA legislation has mandated that it be implemented by the end of 2002. At this time, no one health care standard has been developed and/or submitted to this committee, but rather a list of approximately 28 vocabularies.

Federal Legislation   At the federal level, several pieces of legislation have been enacted during the past 50 years that have significantly influenced the introduction of the computer into nursing. These acts stimulated the growth and advancement of the nursing profession using computer technology. Also, NISs were developed to measure quality care and determine reimbursement for patient care services. Other legislation has also influenced this trend; however, the following acts are probably the most significant.

Nurse Training Act of 1943   The initial Nurse Training Act of 1943 (PL 74-78) established the U.S. Cadet Nurse Corps. Enactment was delegated to the United States Public Health Service (US PHS) and was designed to ensure an adequate supply of nurses during World War II not only for the military, but also for civilian hospitals on the home front. This legislation began the trend toward expanding schools of nursing and increasing the number of nurses.

Health Amendments Act of 1956   The Health Amendments Act of 1956 (PL-911) established traineeships for professional nurses. Title II of this act provided additional funds for professional nurses, including public health nurses, to obtain graduate education (advanced training) in the areas of teaching, administration, and supervision. This act increased the supply and expanded the managerial skills of nurse administrators and supervisors and increased the number of graduate programs in schools of nursing.

Nurse Training Act of 1964   The Nurse Training Act of 1964 (PL 88-581), Title VIII Nurse Training Amendment to the Public Health Service Act, was also responsible for the increase in the number of schools of nursing and number of nurses. This legislation, administered by the Division of Nursing (DN), US PHS, Department of Health and Human Services was funded for 3-year intervals, is periodically revised, and is still being enacted by Congress (most recent passage in 1998). It provided extensive financial support to both institutions and students for nursing education. It also mandated various projects for determining requirements and projections on the supply of nurses.

Social Security Amendments of 1965   The Social Security Amendments of 1965, Medicare and Medicaid (PL 89-97), were enacted to improve and increase health services to the aged and indigent. These amendments provided reimbursement for the cost of health care services for eligible persons over age 65 (Medicare) and for certain low-income persons (Medicaid). This legislation promoted the development of community health information systems designed to document billable care.

Quality Assurance Program of 1972   Another important piece of legislation was the Quality Assurance Program of 1972 (PL 92-603), which established Professional Standards Review Organizations (PSROs) to evaluate and monitor health care services. The first step for implementing this legislation was the collection and analysis of data on quality of care.

National Health Planning and Resources Development Act of 1974   The National Health Planning and Resources Development Act of 1974 (PL 93-641) established health planning agencies throughout the nation with authorization to establish planning methods and criteria. It mandated the creation of the National Health Planning Information Center (NHPIC), which contained a nursing component (Saba and Skapik, 1979). NHPIC housed a reference collection and a computerized database of health planning literature. The NHPIC database is now part of the MEDLARS (MEDical Literature and Analysis Retrieval System) as the Health Planning and Admin (Health Planning and Administration) on-line database.

Health Services Research, Health Statistics, and Medical Libraries Act of 1974   In 1974, the Health Services Research, Health Statistics, and Medical Libraries Act (PL 93-353) was passed. This law mandated that the National Center for Health Services Research (NCHSR) undertake research activities covering all aspects of health services in the country. NCHSR supported numerous grants and contracts that focused on technological solutions to health care problems facing the nation.

Social Security Amendments of 1983   In 1983, the passage of the Social Security Amendments (PL98-21) mandated under Medicare Part A a prospective payment system (PPS) commonly known as diagnosis-related groups (DRGs). This new system of payment for in-hospital Medicare and Medicaid patient services was based on 467 DRGs. The PPS required that patients' diagnoses and charges for services, including nursing, be integrated with medical record data for billing, general ledger, and cost accounting requirements.

Omnibus Budget Reconciliation Act of 1987   The Omnibus Budget Reconciliation Act of 1987 (PL 100-203) contained many provisions that affected the Medicare program. This law mandated that plans of care be included as part of the clinical record. The Omnibus Budget Reconciliation Act of 1989 (PL 101-239) required that the DHHS conduct research on outcomes of health care services and procedures. This led, in December 1989, to the establishment of Agency for Health Care Policy and Research (AHCPR) now known as the Agency for Healthcare Research and Quality (AHRQ).

The AHRQ is the federal organization that is the focal point for research on medical effectiveness and health services. The purpose of the agency is to enhance the quality, appropriateness, and effectiveness of health care services and to improve access to that care. The agency was also mandated to carry out not only its original activities but also a broad program of scientific research and information dissemination. It was mandated to develop standards for clinical databases, clinical practice guidelines, and quality outcomes that can improve the quality, appropriateness, and effectiveness of health care services (Agency for Health Care Policy and Research, 1990, 1992).

Health Insurance Portability and Accountability Act of 1996 HIPAA (PL104-191) was enacted to streamline health care transactions and reduce costs. This legislation mandates that standards be implemented for the electronic collection and transmission of all federally required data. HIPPA mandates that a concerted effort be employed at the local level to evaluate security measures for the protection of data in the electronic transmission of transactions. This legislation also recommends that health care providers use a Provider Identification Number (PIN) to maintain privacy and security of patient information. The HIPAA deadline for implementing this act is the end of year 2002 (Appavu, 1999).

Other relevant legislation has been passed by Congress to improve health care and health services. These laws all require accurate data collection and analyses, making the computer an essential tool for their implementation. The relevant legislation that influenced computer use in nursing is listed in Table 2.1.

Early Computer-Based Nursing Applications

Several computer-based nursing applications were developed before the mid-1970s as part of larger HISs, and many of them still exist. Each in its own way developed different nursing applications to improve documentation of nursing practice and manage patient care. The applications were designed for hospitals, ambulatory care settings, and community health agencies. Additionally, several significant nursing projects were conducted to improve nursing care documentation methodologies that in turn could be computerized. The major nursing applications that influenced the industry are subsystems or components of early HISs, described below. Special projects that influenced the design of nursing information systems are also highlighted.

- Early hospital information systems
- Early ambulatory care information systems
- Early community health nursing information management systems
- Early computer-focused nursing projects

Table 2.1   Legislation that Influenced Computer Use in Nursing

Legislation and Year	Public Law
Nurse Training Act of 1943	74–78
Health Amendments Act of 1956	84–911
Nurse Training Act of 1964	88–581
Social Security Amendments of 1965 Medicare and Medicaid	89–97
Quality Assurance Program of 1972 Professional Standards Review Organizations (PSROs)	92–603
National Health Planning and Resources Development Act of 1974	93–641
Health Services Research, Health Statistics, and Medical Libraries Act of 1974	93–353
Social Security Amendments of 1983 Prospective Payment System (PPS) & Diagnosis Related Groups (DRGs)	98–21
Omnibus Budget Reconciliation Act of 1987	100–203
Omnibus Budget Reconciliation Act of 1989	101–239
High Performance Computing Act of 1991	102–194
Health Insurance Portability and Accountability Act of 1996	104–191

Early Hospital Information Systems

The early HISs were primarily designed for mainframe computers that could support hundreds of CRTs located in nursing units and other departments where data were processed. The CRTs were "dumb terminals" that provided communication with the mainframe. Data were input either on a keyboard or via video screen activated by a light pen. Many of the systems were developed and tested on one nursing unit before being implemented throughout a hospital. Most of the early systems have, over time, been renamed because their developers were purchased by other vendors.

Technicon Medical Information System In 1973, the Technicon Medical Information System (TMIS), also known as TDS by Health Care Systems Corp., was developed at El Camino Hospital, in Mountain View, California. The TMIS, now called Ecylypsis, is now almost 30 years old and is considered the oldest hospital/patient information system that has the most advanced user functions at the nurses' station. This hospital-wide computer system was initiated in 1965 by the Lockheed Missiles and Space Company to make its communication technology available to health care (Hodge, 1990).

The original TMIS managed all patient information during a hospital stay. It consisted of nursing care protocols generated from patients' medical diagnoses and predicted outcome measures that were used as guides to record patients' problems and care plans. Thousands of nursing care protocols were developed for the original system. The early system was housed in a mainframe computer that supported a large number of CRTs located throughout the hospital. The CRTs were dumb terminals that could be activated by a light pen and were connected to the mainframe (Cook and Mayers, 1981; Cook and McDowell, 1975; Mayers, 1974).

In 1975, the TDS was installed at the Clinical Center, National Institutes of Health (NIH), in Bethesda, Maryland, where the patient care functions were expanded to encompass extensive research protocols. The revised system, called the Clinical Center Medical Information System (CCMIS), contains nursing care protocols designed to document plans of care using the nursing process and the nursing diagnosis. The CCMIS follows the nursing process by using 13 patient care needs, based on Maslow's Hierarchy of Needs to assess patients from which diagnoses were identified. The nursing diagnoses were further branched into expected outcomes and nursing actions with data points to determine the progress or time of expected achievement (McNeely, 1983; Romano, 1982).

At NIH, the original CRTs have been upgraded to high-speed multipurpose workstations that are Macintosh or DOS-based computers (National Institutes of Health, 1994). It has revised its hardware architecture and upgraded its software to support patient care. The NIH is also planning to install new wireless point-of-care notebooks for health care professionals to carry.

Burroughs/Medi-Data Hospital Information System
Another early hospital information system was the Burroughs/Medi-Data HIS, which was developed in the 1970s, specifically for the Charlotte Memorial Hospital in Charlotte, North Carolina. This system was designed to provide accurate information, faster communication, and standardized patient care documentation. The initial system consisted of the diagnosis and other pertinent information on the patient with a care plan containing physicians' and nurses' orders. The nursing portion of the system consisted of a database of 200 symptoms or conditions requiring nursing action called "initiators of care" that were activated through a CRT. As a result, it was possible to devise a standardized care plan to document patient care and generate summary reports for each shift (Smith, 1974; Somers, 1971).

Problem-Oriented Medical Information System
The Problem-Oriented Medical Information System (PROMIS) was in the forefront of patient care data handling. PROMIS was developed at the Medical Center Hospital of Vermont in Burlington as early as 1968. Its goal was to create a computerized problem-oriented medical record (POMR) system to collect, store, and process all relevant medical information on a patient and provide feedback to evaluate care. PROMIS incorporated the four phases of POMR: (1) collection of information (database), (2) development of a problem list, (3) development of a plan of action, and (4) follow-up for each problem (progress notes) (Giebnik and Hurst, 1975; Lindberg, 1977; Weed, 1969).

The PROMIS also incorporated video displays for nursing, called "frames," that consisted of nursing care protocols for a patient's specific disease or medical condition. The frames, activated by a light pen, were used to formulate SOAP (subjective symptoms, objective signs, assessment, and plans) plans for patient care. Thus, a computer-based system was designed to plan and document patient care using the POMR structure with SOAP notes. The PROMIS was developed and tested for nearly 4 years on a gynecology ward and for

3 years on a medical ward. Federal funding was halted in 1981-1982, and the research and development of the PROMIS system ceased (Gane, 1972; McNeill, 1979; Pryor et al.,1985). However, the concepts have reappeared in the new Windows-based point-of-care information tools called the Problem Knowledge Couplers. These new tools can be used to identify patient problems and risk factors, elicit and record patient findings, and refine diagnostic management strategies (Problem Knowledge Couplers 1996).

Health Evaluation Logical Processing System   The Health Evaluation Logical Processing (HELP) system developed at the Latter Day Saints (LDS) Hospital in Salt Lake City, Utah, is another system that originated in the late 1960s. It was under development for over 30 years. The basic goal was to create an integrated computer-based patient care record system and a knowledge base. The HELP system was designed to meet the medical, clinical, administrative, decision-making, teaching, and research goals of the hospital based on the acquisition of critical care data including nursing (Pryor, 1992). Parallel with the development of HELP in the LDS Hospital, the Intermountain Health Care system was also being developed, creating two interrelated systems that still exist today (Teich, 1997).

Decentralized Hospital Computer Program   Another pioneer in the field of HISs was the Department of Veterans Affairs (DVA). In the 1970s, the DVA began to develop a clinical computing system known as the Decentralized Hospital Computer Program (DHCP). The DVA developed the DHCP system over the course of a decade, and it was implemented in more than 170 medical centers by the late 1980s. This system consisted of three modules that focused on (1) system/database management, (2) administrative management, and (3) clinical management. As part of the clinical management module, the DVA launched the Clinical Record Project, which includes a nursing subsystem (Andrews and Beauchamp, 1989; Dayhoff et al., 1990).

By 1990, the DVA had upgraded the computer capacity at all medical centers and implemented software on a national scale that supported integrated health care. In 1996–1997, the system was replaced by the Veterans Health Information System and Technology Architecture (VISTA). VISTA was configured as a rich automated environment that supported day-to-day operations at the local DVA health care facilities. VISTA was envisioned to support the development of a CPR as its long-term goal. Nursing became a major component of VISTA, which was comprised of multiple modules that consisted of administrative, educational, clinical, quality assurance, and management applications (Chief Information Officer, Veterans Affairs, 1996–1997, 1997–1998; Technical Services, Veterans Affairs, 1998).

Tri-Service Medical Information System   The U.S. Department of Defense (DoD) began contracting for the development of a clinical information system in the mid-1970s. It took over a decade to complete and was originally named the Tri-Service Medical Information System (TRIMIS). In the mid-1980s, the DoD completed the design specifications and renamed it the Composite Health Care System (CHCS). In the early 1990s, CHCS began to be tested in military health care facilities and settings around the country (Committee on Armed Services, 1990). The design of nursing activities was also an integral part of the CHCS; the system was designed to support nursing care with the goal of improving patient care. Nursing identified the design specifications for nursing patient care unit management as well as the nursing administration of inpatient, outpatient, and operating room areas (Rieder and Norton, 1984).

In the late 1990s, the Military Healthcare System introduced CHCSII as the next step in providing a CPR. The major goal of a CPR was to have an interactive and virtual longitudinal comprehensive record of an individual's health status and health care. The CHCSII provided a seamless repository of health data that could support the health care delivery processes and clinical business functions. It could facilitate current and future management of health information requirements for the DoD and health care personnel during peacetime and wartime (CHCSII Program, 1999). By 2000, the DoD planned to have a system interface and link with other systems around the world in the military health care network.

Early Ambulatory Care Information Systems

Regenstrief Medical Record System   In 1972, the Regenstrief Institute, Wishard Memorial Hospital Institute in Indianapolis, Indiana instituted the Regenstrief Medical Record (RMRS), which was considered to be one of the earliest ambulatory care systems designed to include most of the information needed for patient care in the ambulatory care clinics. The record consists of comprehensive clinical data, providing most of the information needed for patient care and also coded in a form

appropriate for decision support, research, and other applications. Data are collected on the clinics using a computer-tailored encounter form. Since this system has evolved over time, it is "home-grown" and difficult to export to other environments. RMRS exemplifies a continuously evolving system in an ever-changing environment (Collen, 1995; McDonald et al., 1997).

Computer-Stored Ambulatory Record System.

Another early computerized ambulatory care information system, the Computer-Stored Ambulatory Record System (COSTAR), was developed over a 10-year period (1968–1978) at the Massachusetts General Hospital (MGH) Laboratory of Computer Science for the ambulatory patients served by the prepaid Harvard Community Health Plan. The purpose of COSTAR was to computerize the medical record so that patient care encounter data could be integrated to meet providers' medical, financial, and administrative needs. A standardized dictionary was developed to provide uniform documentation including nursing terms (Barnett, 1976).

COSTAR has been upgraded to an on-line system allowing interaction between the users (nurses) and a mainframe computer located at the MGH Computer Laboratory. The on-line system allowed for retrieval of patient information via the CRT. COSTAR is still available and has been adapted to run on minicomputers and/or PCs using a unique programming language originally called MUMPS (Massachusetts General Utility Multi-Programming System).

The Medical Record System

The Medical Record (TMR) system began in 1968 at the Duke University Medical Center Department of Community Health Services in Durham, North Carolina. The goal was to replace paper charts with computerized records for the practicing physician. TMR initially focused on capturing patient histories and physical examinations in a prenatal clinic and was later designed to meet the needs of the ambulatory care practice and the clinical requirements for a primary care record. The TMR system was finally designed to cover all of the activities of an HIS in order to satisfy managerial, patient care, and research needs in inpatient and outpatient settings. It was designed to permit nurses and other health providers to enter data directly into the database during the process of patient care (Pryor, 1992).

Indian Health Service Health Information System

Another pioneering system was the Indian Health Service Health Information System designed by Bell Aerospace Company for the Papagoe Indian Reservation in Tucson, Arizona. This system was designed to provide a centralized life-long surveillance, documentation, and communication of the health care services, status, and conditions of all Papagoe reservation residents. The system contained a centralized database of patients that all health care providers, including nurses, could access via an on-line computer terminal. For example, a nurse could obtain the latest health care information via a modem before visiting a patient in the home. This system still exists; however, the software continues to be revised and the hardware upgraded (Brown et al., 1971; Giebnik and Hurst, 1975).

Other Early Health Care Information Systems

Several other early systems were developed to capture nursing data. The Texas Institute for Rehabilitation and Research (Houston, Texas) hospital data management system focused on the individual patient care process and used CRTs connected to the hospital's computer (Cornell and Carrick, 1973; Giebnik and Hurst, 1975; Valbona and Spencer, 1974). The Institute of Living, in Hartford, Connecticut, developed the first real-time computerized psychiatric information system designed to facilitate patient care. The system provided an integrated patient record that included nurses' progress notes and other pertinent information (Lindberg, 1977).

Still other hospital and ambulatory health care facilities have successfully implemented computer-based patient records (CPRs) in their systems. Several facilities have been selected to receive the Nicholas E. Davies Recognition Award of Excellence. Since 1995, they have been awarded annually at the CPR Recognition Program sponsored by the Computer-based Patient Record Institute (CPRI) (Teich, 1997). The 11 most widely recognized Davies recipients are: in 1995: (1) Department of Veterans Affairs, (2) Columbia Presbyterian Medical Center—New York, and (3) Intermountain Health Care—Salt Lake City, Utah; in 1996: (4) Brigham & Women's Hospital, Boston, Massachusetts; in 1997: (5) Kaiser-Permanente of Ohio, (6) North Mississippi Health Services, and (7) Regenstrief Institute for Health Care, Indianapolis, Indiana; in 1998: (8) Northwestern Memorial Hospital, Chicago, Illinois; and (9) Kaiser-Permanente Northwest, Portland Oregon; and in 1999: (10) The Queens's Medical Center, Honolulu, Hawaii; and (11) Kaiser Permanente Rock Mountain Region, Nevada.

Early Community Health Nursing Information Management Systems

Statewide Systems   One of the nation's first statewide computer-based community health information system was begun in 1970 by the **New Jersey State Department of Health**. This agency developed, tested, and implemented a home health MIS for community nursing service agencies. The major goal of the system was to help community health care agencies make more effective use of their limited resources and assist community health nursing directors in managing their agencies. The system consisted of precoded paper forms that were batch-processed by computer and produced reports designed to facilitate state reporting requirements. Because the processing of forms was slow, tedious, costly, and could not be done on-line, the system was abandoned in the late 1970s (Saba and Levine, 1981).

In 1973, another statewide system, Nursing Information System for Public Health Nursing, was initiated by the **Florida Department of Health and Rehabilitative Services**. The goal was to produce accurate, timely, and comprehensive information about the work performed by public health nurses. The system was designed to create a statistical database that could provide information to improve management, report cost, and justify public health activities. The system went through several revisions beginning with a batch-processing paper system and moving to an on-line transmission of data that is conceptually used today.

Early Computer-Focused Nursing Projects

Several computer-focused nursing projects and other activities were funded by the DN, US PHS, Department of Health, Education and Welfare (DHEW) to help community health nursing (CHN) agencies develop computer-based information systems. Each of these projects advanced the documentation requirements for different health care settings and influenced the development of today's NISs (Saba, 1981b; Saba, 1982).

Early Community Health Nursing Projects

In 1971, the **Rockland County Project** was conducted by the Rockland County Health Department in New York. It attempted to computerize patients' progress by using an innovative methodology designed for the public health setting. The project represented one of the first attempts to computerize patient care in that type of setting (Rockland County Health Department, 1971).

The **Buffalo Project** was another attempt to computerize patient care needs. The project, "Systematic Nursing Assessment," attempted to develop a standardized tool that could be computerized to assist nurses in their assessment of patients' needs and then be used for making decisions about patient care (Taylor and Johnson, 1974). In the early 1970s, the **Philadelphia Project** attempted to develop an information system that could be used to plan and evaluate CHN services (Community Nursing Services of Philadelphia, 1976).

Another **CHN Project** was initiated in 1975 by the VNA of Omaha, Nebraska, to develop a problem classification scheme for community health/public health nursing. Its goal was to design a system for documenting nursing services and develop a methodology for its computerization. The project produced a problem classification scheme consisting of 49 problem labels categorized into four domains that were potentially amenable to nursing interventions. Each problem was identified by a cluster of signs and symptoms. The project was continued and enhanced over the next 25 years and is still in operation today (Simmons, 1982; Visiting Nurse Association of Omaha, 1986; Martin and Sheet, 1992, 1995).

In the late 1980s and early 1990s, the **Home Care Classification Project** was conducted at the Georgetown University School of Nursing by Saba and Associates. This project, funded by the Health Care Financing Administration (HCFA), was designed to develop a method for assessing and classifying home health Medicare patients in order to predict their need for nursing and other home care services including their outcomes of care. A national sample of almost 10,000 cases was collected from which data were abstracted on an entire episode of illness. This study amassed the largest database ever collected providing descriptive information on home health care services in the U.S. One aspect of the database was the collection of 40,000 nursing diagnostic statements and almost 80,000 nursing intervention and action statements. These statements were computer-processed and used to develop the HHCC of Nursing Diagnoses and HHCC of Nursing Interventions (Saba, 1992, 1995a, 1997).

Hospital Nursing Projects   In 1977, another project was initiated by the DN, US PHS, DHEW, to determine the **Effects of the Computerized Problem-Oriented Record** on the nursing components of patient care. This project was conducted by the Department of Nursing, Medical Center Hospital of Vermont, in Burlington. It identified the differences in recording nursing care under the computerized system and under the manual problem-oriented system. No conclusions could be drawn because of the short time during which the system was operational. Nevertheless, the project's three data collection instruments—record review, time sampling, and nurse satisfaction—were used by other researchers to evaluate other HISs (Hanchett, 1981).

Early Educational Applications

During the 1960s, special-purpose computerized information systems were also being developed in educational institutions. Computer-based education (CBE) programs were designed to computerize and individualize student instruction while serving a large number of students simultaneously on-line in a classroom.

Programmed Logic for Automatic Teaching Operation

The PLATO was the first on-line CBE system to be developed. It was designed so that students could use a CRT to interact with the computer in a distant classroom. Many nursing courses were adapted for PLATO, which became an excellent tool for teaching drill and practice courses. PLATO individualized the learning process, provided instant feedback on student progress, and tracked student progress for the faculty (Bitzer and Boudreaux, 1968). With the introduction of desktop PCs and the creation of CAI, IVD, and CD-ROM programs, PLATO was no longer in demand. However, by 2000, PLATO's basic skills courseware resurfaced and began to be offered in a joint run venture by TRO Learning and Sylvan Learning Centers for distance education.

Multimedia Software

In the 1980s, with the introduction of the PC, CAI programs were developed as applications for individual PCs. They were less expensive and easier to implement, and they allowed students to access the system on their own time. Schools of nursing could purchase their own CAI programs and subsequently IAV programs and then CD-ROM programs as stand-alone PC applications (Rizzalo, 1994).

The CAI and IAV software programs provide students with the tools to support the teaching process. The CAI programs primarily consist of narrative text prepared for the student to interact with, whereas the IAV programs combine motion, sound, and graphics stored on a laser videodisc and are designed to allow students to interact with the sequences either by action or text. The newest PC technology, CD-ROM, replaced CAI and IAV programs. The CD-ROM allows for entire books and educational courses to be programmed for student use.

Internet   In 1991, the Internet, the "network of networks" became the newest media for the electronic communication of information. The Internet requires that a user links, via a modem, to a file server, which links to other networks around the world. By 1995, the major Internet protocols being used were E-mail, FTP, Telnet, Gopher, and the WWW browser. E-mail and the WWW have become the most popular uses of the Internet. The WWW supports a full range of multimedia (sound, images, video graphics), and E-mail provides free communication with anyone anytime and anywhere in the world (Information Technology Center, 1996; Edwards, 1996).

The Internet and the WWW radically changed the education of nurses. The Internet made it possible to network the PCs in the learning resource centers in schools of nursing to each other, to the faculty and students, and to other internal and external departments. The Internet also made it possible to perform on-line searching of the nursing literature in the library and the literature in other locations such as MEDLINE at the NLM. The Internet makes it possible for students and faculty to use E-mail to communicate on and off the campus via its free electronic communication network. The Internet can be used by students to search the Web resources around the world for information to support their education (Ellett et al., 1999).

Internet Education   Internet education generally uses software specific for structuring the interaction between students and teachers, students and students, and students and resources. The Internet made possible distance education, which allows students in remote sites to interact with faculty and other students via educational technologies in the classroom. Internet software structures the Internet course in such a way that the course syllabus can be disseminated on a school's "home page," "chat rooms" can be set up for discussions among students, and electronic bulletin boards or E-mail can be used by teachers as a forum for communicating with students (Armstrong, 1998).

In the 1990s, another form of distance education emerged through interactive teleconferencing, which uses digital telephone lines or satellites to link the school to the remote locations. In such an environment, the students can interact with the teacher in the classroom and the other students in the different locations.

Education in the 21st century will be conducted at home through the Internet connected to the university.

It is predicted that the "universities without walls" will enroll the largest number of students, and "virtual graduations" will be attended by the largest number of graduating students (Armstrong, 1998).

In May 1999, a virtual graduation of the inaugural post-masters adult nurse practitioner certificate program class of approximately 30 students was held at the Uniformed Services University of the Health Sciences (USUHS). They used the interactive teleconferencing equipment to link eight Veterans Affairs Medical Centers sites with the Graduate School of Nursing at USUHS for the formal ceremony (Saba, 2000).

Early Research Applications

The earliest computer system that supported nursing research was the on-line searching of the medical and nursing literature in MEDLINE as early as 1972. MEDLINE evolved from the MEDLARS bibliographic retrieval system that was developed by the NLM in the late 1950s and early 1960s. In 1972, MEDLARS advanced to an on-line system, MEDLINE, that became the first of several MEDLARS databases to became available nationwide (National Library of Medicine, 1986). In 1965, the "Special List Nursing," a special file for nursing literature in the MEDLARS database, was established. This file was also used to index the nursing periodical literature and to prepare the *International Nursing Index* for publication by the American Journal of Nursing Company (1998) (Saba, 1981a).

During this period, several other indexes of relevant nursing literature were being computerized as bibliographic retrieval systems. The major ones include (1) the Cumulative Index to Nursing and Allied Health Literature (CINAHL), developed by the Seventh Day Adventist Association in Glendale, California; (2) the Educational Resources Information Center (ERIC) of nursing education literature; (3) the SOCIAL SCI for Social SciSearch Citation Index; and (4) the Dissertation Abstracts (Saba et al., 1989; Verhey et al., 1998).

During the late 1980s and early 1990s researchers began to gain access to on-line "public use" federal databases consisting of aggregated data. Databases that were maintained by the HCFA, such as the Medicare and Medicaid claims database and the Uniform Clinical Data Set (UCDS), became available to the public. Even though nursing information was not an integral part of these databases, some inferences about nursing care could be made from the patient data contained in them.

Knowledge databases were also being developed that could be used for research. They focused on a specific topic or disease condition and could be remotely accessed on-line, such as a drug database, a clinical condition cancer database such as the PDQ (Physician Data Query) diagnostic, and clinical care protocol systems such as DxPlain and RECONSIDER.

 ## Landmark Events in Nursing and Computers

Computers were introduced into the nursing profession almost 30 years ago. The major milestones of nursing are interwoven with the advancement of computer technology, the increased need for nursing data, development of nursing applications, and changes that made the nursing profession an autonomous discipline. The major developments in the use of computers and nursing and in the introduction of nursing informatics are described below chronologically, by program effort, or by organizational initiative. The major efforts are categorized as follows and outlined in Table 2.2:

- Early Conferences and Meetings
- Early Academic Initiatives
- Initial American Nurses Association initiatives
- Initial National League for Nursing initiatives
- Early International Initiatives
- Initial Educational Resources
- Significant Collaborative Events

Early Conferences and Meetings

The early conferences on computers and nursing occurred as computer-based systems were being introduced into the health care industry. These conferences were primarily designed to teach nurses about computer systems, computer data, and nursing requirements. They were conducted so that nurses could learn about state-of-the-art NISs.

Invitational Conferences　　In 1973, the first invitational conference was held on **Computerized Management Information Systems for Public Health/Community Health Agencies.** It was designed to help agency administrators address their reporting requirements for the reimbursement for Medicare and Medicaid home health services. This initial national conference was followed by five workshops held around the country, culminating in a national conference on **State of the Art in Management Information Systems for Public Health/**

Table 2.2   Landmark Events in Computers and Nursing

Year	Title	Sponsor	Site
1973	First invitational conference on management information systems for public/community health agencies	National League for Nursing and Division of Nursing, U.S. Public Health Service	Fairfax, VA
1974–1975	Five workshops on management information systems for public/community health agencies	National League for Nursing and Division of Nursing, U.S. Public Health Service	Nationwide
1976	State-of-the-art conference in management for public/community health agencies	National League for Nursing and Division of Nursing, U.S. Public Health Service	Washington, DC
1977	First research: state-of-the-art conference on nursing information systems	University of Illinois College of Nursing	Chicago, IL
1977	First undergraduate academic course on computers and nursing	The State University of New York at Buffalo	Buffalo, NY
1979	First military conference on computers in nursing	TRIMIS Army Nurse Consultant Team, Walter Reed Hospital	Washington, DC
1980	First workshop on computer usage in health care	University of Akron School of Nursing, Continuing Education Department	Akron, OH
1981	Special interest group: computers in nursing (SIG-CIN)	SCAMC event	Washington, DC
1981	First national conference on computer technology and nursing	NIH Clinical Center and TRIMIS Army Nurse Consultant Team, and Division of Nursing, US PHS	Bethesda, MD
1981	First nursing session at Fifth Annual Symposium on Computer Applications in Medical Care	SCAMC, Inc.	Washington, DC
1982	Study group on nursing information systems	University Hospitals of Cleveland, Case Western Reserve University and National Center for Health Services Research, US PHS	Cleveland, OH
1982	First Annual National Nursing Computer Technology Conference	Rutgers, State University of New Jersey, College of Nursing	Newark, NJ
1982	First international meeting: Working Conference on Nursing Uses and Computers in Nursing	Working Group, International Medical Informatics Association	London and Harrogate Yorkshire, England
1982	Second national conference on computer technology and nursing	National Institutes of Health Clinical Center and TRIMIS Army Nurse Consultant Team, and Division of Nursing, US PHS	Bethesda, MD
1982	First newsletter: *Computers in Nursing*	School of Nursing, University of Texas at Austin	Austin, TX
1982	1st workshop on computers and nursing	Boston University School of Nursing	Boston, MA
1983	First nursing participation at MEDINFO '83: Fourth World Congress on Medical Informatics	American Medical Informatics Association (AMIA)	Amsterdam, Holland
1983	Third national conference on computer technology and nursing	National Institutes of Health Clinical Center and TRIMIS Army Nurse Consultant Team, and Division of Nursing US PHS	Bethesda, MD
1983	Second annual joint congress and conference	International Association of Medical Informatics	San Francisco, CA, and Baltimore, MD
1983	Newsletter: *Computers in Nursing*	Lippincott	Philadelphia, PA
1983	MEDINFO '83	International Medical Informatics Association (IMIA)	Amsterdam, The Netherlands
1983	First hospital workshop on computers in nursing practice	St. Agnes Hospital and HEC	Baltimore, MD

Table 2.2   Landmark Events in Computers and Nursing (*continued*)

Year	Title	Sponsor	Site
1984	Fourth national conference on computer technology and nursing	National Institutes of Health Clinical Center, TRIMIS Army Nurse Consultant Team, and Division of Nursing, US PHS	Bethesda, MD
1984	First microcomputer seminar	University of California at San Francisco	San Francisco, CA
1984	First nursing computer journal: *Computers in Nursing*	Lippincott	Philadelphia, PA
1984	Council on Computer Applications in Nursing (CCAN) Formed	American Nursing Association	Kansas City, MO
1984–1995	*Directory of Educational Software for Nursing*	Christine Bolwell and National League for Nursing	New York, NY
1984	2nd workshop on computers and nursing	Boston University School of Nursing	Boston, MA
1985	Council on Nursing Informatics Formed	National League for Nursing	New York, NY
1985	Annual seminar on computers and nursing practice	New York University Medical Center	New York, NY
1985	First invitational nursing minimum data set conference	University of Illinois School of Nursing	Chicago, IL
1985	Essentials of Computer Elective: Initiated, Undergraduate/Graduate Programs	Georgetown University School of Nursing	Washington, DC
1985/1990	Continuing Nursing Education in Computer Technology Project	Southern Regional Education Board	Atlanta, GA
1985	Second Nursing Informatics '85: international conference	IMIA/Nursing Informatics— Working Group Eight	Calgary, Alberta, Canada
1986	Microcomputer Institute for Nurses	Georgetown University and University of Southwest Louisiana	Washington DC and Lafayette, LA
1986	Nurse Educators *Micro World* Newsletter	Christine Bolwell and Stewart Publishing	Alexandria, VA
1986	MEDINFO '86	IMIA/SCAMC	Washington, DC
1987	Working group and task force on education	IMIA Working Group 8	Stockholm, SW
1987	Initiated interactive videodisc software programs	American Journal of Nursing Grants	New York, NY
1987	Video Disk for Health Conference/Interactive Healthcare Conference	Stewart Publishing	Alexandria, VA
1988	Recommendation No. 3: Support automated information systems	Secretary's Commission on Nursing Shortage	Washington, DC
1988	Priority Expert Panel E: Nursing Informatics Task Force	National Center for Nursing Research	Bethesda, MD
1988	Third Nursing Informatics '88: International Conference	IMIA/NI Working Group Eight	Dublin, Ireland
1989	First Nurse Scholars Program	HBO and HealthQuest Corp.	Atlanta, GA
1989	MEDINFO '89	IMIA	Singapore, Malaysia
1989	Invitational Conference on Nursing Information Systems	National Commission on Nursing Implementation Project (NCNIP), ANA, NLN, and NIS Industry	Orlando, FL
1990	Invitational conference on state-of-the-art of information systems	National Commission of Nursing Implementation Project	Orlando, FL
1990	ANA Steering Committee on Databases to Support Nursing Practice	American Nurses Association	Washington, DC
1990	1st Annual European Summer Institute	International Nursing Informatics Experts	Amsterdam, Netherlands
1990	Task Force on Nursing Information Systems	NCNIP, ANA, NLN, NIS Industry Task Force	Project Hope, VA
1991	Annual Nursing Informatics Working Group	AMIA/SCAMC event	Washington, DC

Table 2.2   Landmark Events in Computers and Nursing (*continued*)

Year	Title	Sponsor	Site
1991	International classification of nursing practice (ICNP) initiated	International Council of Nurses	Geneva, Switzerland
1991	WHO workshop on nursing informatics	World Health Organization	Washington, DC
1991	First summer institute in nursing and healthcare informatics	University of Maryland School of Nursing	Baltimore, MD
1991	First doctoral specialty in nursing informatics	University of Maryland School of Nursing	Baltimore, MD
1991	Fourth Nursing Informatics '91: International Conference	IMIA/NI Working Group Eight	Melbourne, Australia
1992	WHO Workshop on Nursing Management Information Systems	World Health Organization	Geneva, Switzerland
1992	MEDINFO '92	IMIA	Geneva, Switzerland
1992	ANA nursing informatics specialty	American Nurses Association	Washington, DC
1992	Virginia Henderson International Nursing Library (INL)	Sigma Theta Tau International Honor Society	Indianapolis, IN
1992	ANA recognized four nursing taxonomies: HHCC, OMAHA, NANDA, NIC	American Nurses Association Database Steering Committee	Washington, DC
1992	Clinical thesaurus added nursing terms	Read Codes Clinical Terms Version 3	London, UK
1993	Unified nursing languages system (UNLS): Four nursing vocabularies for UMLS	ANA and National Library of Medicine	Washington, DC
1993	Electronic library on-line	Sigma Theta Tau International Honor Society	Indianapolis, IN
1993	AJN network on-line via the Internet	American Journal of Nursing Company	New York, NY
1993	ANC postgraduate course: Computer Applications for Nursing	Army Nurse Corps	Washington, DC
1993	Nursing informatics fellow program	Partners Healthcare Systems	Boston, MA
1993	Alpha version of ICNP	International Council of Nurses	Geneva, Switzerland
1993	Denver Free-Net	University of Colorado Health Sciences Center	Denver, CO
1994	ANA*NET on-line	American Nurses Association	Washington, DC
1994	NCLEX-RN on-line	National Council Licensure Examination for Registered Nurses	New York, NY
1994	Nursing educators' workshops	University of Maryland and Southern Council on Collegiate Regional Education	Baltimore, MD and Atlanta and Augusta, GA
1994	Next generation clinical information systems conference	Tri-Council for Nursing and Kellogg Foundation	Washington, DC
1994	Fifth Nursing Informatics '94: International Conference	IMIA/NI Working Group Eight	San Antonio, TX
1995	MEDINFO '95	IMIA	Vancouver, British Columbia, Canada
1995	First International NI TeleConference*	HIS-AU; NI-NZ; NI Experts—US	Melbourne, AU Aukland, NZ and Bethesda, MD
1995	Nursing Informatics Conference: A Clinical Focus	NY University and NY Hospitals Center	New York, NY
1996	Nursing Information and Data Set Evaluation Center (NISDEC) established	American Nurses Association	Washington, DC

Table 2.2   Landmark Events in Computers and Nursing (*continued*)

Year	Title	Sponsor	Site
1996	Nightingale Project initiated	University of Athens/European Union	Athens, Greece
1996	TELENURSE Project initiated	Danish Institute for Health and Nursing Research and European Union	Copenhagen, Denmark
1996	First Harriet Werley Award—best nursing informatics paper	AMIA-NI Working Group	Washington, DC
1997	National nursing informatics work group	National Advisory Council on Nurse Education and Practice and Division of Nursing US PHS	Washington, DC
1997	NISDEC standards and scoring guidelines published	ANA	Washington, DC
1997	Sixth Nursing Informatics '97: International Conference	IMIA/Nursing Informatics-Special Interest Group (NI-SIG)	Stockholm, Sweden
1998	NursingCenter.com Websites	Lippincott	New York, NY
1998	MEDINFO '98	IMIA	Seoul, South Korea
1999	Beta version of ICNP	International Council of Nurses	Geneva, Switzerland
1999	ICNP Program Office established	International Council of Nurses	Geneva, Switzerland
1999	Nursing vocabulary summit conference	Vanderbilt University	Vanderbilt, TN
1999	Convergent Terminology Group for Nursing	SNOMED International	Northbrook, IL
1999	Inaugural virtual graduation—postmasters adult nurse practitioner certificate program	Graduate School of Nursing, Uniformed Services University of the Health Sciences TeleConference to VA Medical Centers (MCs)	Bethesda, MD; and 8 VA MCs Atlanta, GA, Baltimore, MD Bronx, NY Charleston, SC Fayetteville, NC Leavenworth, KS San Diego, CA Los Angeles, CA
2000	Seventh Nursing Informatics '2000: International Congress	IMIA/Nursing Informatics Special Interest Group (IMIA/NI-SIG)	Auckland, New Zealand
2000	Eighteenth Annual International Nursing Computer and Technology Conference	Rutgers, State University of New Jersey, College of Nursing	Arlington, VA
2000	Tenth annual summer institute in nursing informatics	University of Maryland, School of Nursing	Baltimore, MD
2000	AMIA 2000 annual symposium	AMIA	Los Angeles, CA
2000	CPRI 2000 conference	CPRI	Los Angeles, CA
2000	Davies CPR Recognition Award of Excellence Symposium	CPRI	Los Angeles, CA

AMIA/SCAMC conducted an annual symposium on computer applications in medical care in cooperation with numerous professional societies, governmental units, universities, and health care organizations, including the ANA and NLN.
*Videotape on file at Medical History Department, NLM.

Community Health Agencies held in 1976. The workshops and conferences were designed to teach public and community health nurses how to investigate, initiate, and implement computerized MISs. They demonstrated how computer systems could be used for statistical reporting, cost analysis, and agency administration. This effort was funded by the DN, US PHS, DHEW under the auspices of the National League for Nursing (NLN) (National League for Nursing, 1974, 1975, 1976, 1978).

In 1977, the first Invitational Research Conference focused on **NISs** and the use of computer technology in the delivery of patient care, including care plans, elements of the nursing process, and nursing notes. The conference also provided information on computer applications that were being developed not only in hospitals but also in other health care settings. This conference was sponsored by the University of Illinois College of Nursing in Chicago (Werley and Grier, 1981).

The first **Computer Conference for Military Nurses** was held in 1979, when a TRIMIS conference was held to introduce military nurses to the emerging role of computers in health care and nursing. It was conducted by the TRIMIS Army Nurse Consultant Team at Walter Reed Hospital, in Washington, D.C. The Army Nurse Corps was committed to educating nurses about computers and conducted several workshops in the United States and abroad on this topic. In 1993, they held a similar conference, when the Army Nurse Corps conducted the **Postgraduate Short Course on Computer Applications in Nursing.**

As interest in computers increased, in 1981, the **First National Conference: Computer Technology and Nursing** was conducted by National Institutes of Health (NIH). This one-day conference was considered a critical event in the field that focused on state-of-the-art computers and nursing. It was attended by more than 700 nurse administrators, practitioners, clinicians, researchers, and educators from around the country. The Nursing Department of the Clinical Center, NIH, hosted this conference in collaboration with the DN, US PHS, and the TRIMIS Army Nurse Consultant Team. The NIH held its **Second National Conference: Computer Technology and Nursing** in 1982, a third in 1984, and a fourth and fifth in subsequent years (National Institutes of Health, 1983, 1984).

Symposium on Computer Applications in Medical Care/American Medical Informatics Association

A focus on nursing was introduced in the **Fifth Annual Symposium on Computer Applications in Medical Care** (SCAMC) in 1981. Papers that dealt with NISs and the nursing aspects of computer technology were presented in four nursing sessions by pioneers in the field. The symposium offered technical sessions, demonstrations, workshops, tutorials, hands-on experience, poster sessions, and exhibits of systems for the health care industry. SCAMC gave nurses an opportunity to learn how computer applications could affect patient care (Heffernan, 1981).

The SCAMC, sponsored by the **American Medical Informatics Association** (AMIA), formed in 1991, continues to include nursing papers and presentations in its annual SCAMC symposia. AMIA continues to offer nursing tutorials and workshops for the novice and advanced nursing informaticians. Nursing experts and nursing informatics specialists are now an integral part of the AMIA organization and can be found on the AMIA board, committees, and working groups. In 2000, a doctorally prepared nurse presides over the AMIA as president.

Healthcare Information and Management System Society

The **Healthcare Information and Management System Society** (HIMSS), was formed in the mid-1990s and is serving as a resource to health care professionals including nurses. This organization hosts annual conferences and exhibits focusing on the management of clinical systems, information systems, and telecommunication systems. In the late 1990s, the annual meeting increased its attendance, and it attracted practicing nurses in the health care computer technology field.

Special Interest Groups

In 1981 the first **Special Interest Group—Computers in Nursing** (SIG-CIN) was formed. It convened at the fifth annual SCAMC, held the first nursing sessions, and became an informal group that met at the annual SCAMC/AMIA meetings. The group had an executive board, published an annual newsletter, and provided mailing lists of members for local groups. The SIG-CIN was responsible for designing the nursing tract for SCAMC/AMIA. The group was dissolved in 1991 with the formation of the AMIA's Nursing Informatics Working Group. This group had essentially the same mission as the SIG-CIN, to promote the advancement of nursing informatics within the larger multidisciplinary context of health informatics, and has a newsletter and international Internet listserv.

Local special interest groups also emerged in the United States and in other countries. In 1983, the **Capital Area Roundtable on Informatics in Nursing** (CARING) was formed for those nurses residing in Maryland, Virginia, and Washington, D.C. interested and involved in this new field. This group grew to approximately 500 members by 2000. Similar groups were created in cities or regions, such as Boston, Massachusetts or Puget Sound for Northwest Washington State; in states, such as California, Delaware, Florida, New Jersey, etc.; and in countries, such as Brazil, Canada, the United Kingdom, etc. A list of the special interest groups is available from the University of Maryland Web site. *http://nursing.umaryland.edu/students/-snewbol/skngroup.html.*

Study Group

In 1982, a **Nursing Information Systems—Study Group** was convened at the University Hospitals of Cleveland, Ohio, to discuss issues and describe categories of data needed for the NISs. It identified the functions, structures, and components needed for the NISs and the specific applications that had to be developed, such as resource allocation and patient care management. The meeting was funded by the NCHSR (Kiley et al., 1983; Study Group on Nursing Information Systems, 1983).

Early Academic Initiatives

In the 1970s, several educational strategies were initiated to educate nurses about computer technology. Several universities held conferences as part of their continuing education programs. Hospitals and national associations initiated workshops as forums for teaching the state of the art, and computer conferences provided other forums for learning. As nurses became computer-literate, they began to present papers, conduct workshops, demonstrate applications, and describe their research. In the 1980s, formal academic courses were introduced into schools of nursing, and in the 1990s, graduate programs at the master's and doctoral levels were established.

Workshops and Institutes In 1980, the first university-based workshop, titled "Computer Usage in Health Care," was conducted by the University of Akron School of Nursing in Ohio. It was a one-week course designed to orient nurses to all aspects of computer applications in nursing. Several nurses with expertise in computer technology served as the faculty who lectured on computer applications in nursing. In the early 1980s, other workshops on computers and nursing were conducted by selected universities. Boston University conducted two such workshops, one in in 1982 and another in 1984; the University of Texas at Austin conducted one in 1983. By the 1990s, almost every academic medical center held similar conferences for the medical and nursing faculties.

University Conferences In 1982, a series of annual conferences was initiated at the New Jersey State University College of Nursing at Rutgers. The major focus of its annual national computer conference was to educate nurses on computer applications and nursing informatics in education. Nurses presented papers and demonstrations on the uses of existing software, shared experiences, and tried to prevent "reinventing the wheel." Since then, Rutgers has continued to conduct an annual computer conference. Rutgers also compiled key papers presented at these conferences and published a book,

Computer Applications in Nursing Education and Practice (Arnold and Pearson, 1992).

In 1985, New York University Medical Center started an annual seminar that focused on computers and nursing practice. It targeted nurses who wanted to learn state-of-the-art applications for clinical nursing practice. The seminars also included exhibits by vendors of hospital and nursing information systems. Since 1995, the New York Hospital Center in collaboration with the New York University Center for Continuing Education in Nursing has continued to conduct conferences on nursing informatics with a clinical focus.

Microcomputer Seminars The first microcomputer/PC seminar was convened in 1984 by the **University of California at San Francisco**. It was a one-week microcomputer seminar that included hands-on experience using generic microcomputer software applications. Other universities conducted similar workshops. In 1986, a one-week Microcomputer Institute for Nurses was conducted and co-sponsored at two university schools of nursing: Georgetown University in Washington, D.C., and University of Southwestern Louisiana in Lafayette.

Between 1985 and 1990, the **Southern Regional Education Board** (SREB) administered by the Southern Council on Collegiate Regional Education (SCCREN) was awarded a grant by the DN, US PHS, to conduct the SREB Continuing Nursing Education in Computer Technology Project. During a 5-year period, SREB conducted over 40 basic workshops, 3 regional conferences, and 12 seminars for nurse educators in 15 states. The workshops were conducted at universities in the South to help nurse educators become competent in the use of computers. SREB also promoted the integration of computers into the nursing curriculum (Aiken, 1990; Mikan, 1992). In 1994, the DN, Health Research and Services Agency (HRSA), awarded another grant to SCCREN, who in partnership with the University of Maryland School of Nursing, conducted four workshops for nurse educators who had an interest in understanding information management and information technology in the Southern region. Two were held in Baltimore and two in Georgia (Augusta and Atlanta).

In 1989, the **Nurse Scholars Program**, sponsored by the HBO and HealthQuest Company (now renamed McKesson HBOC) in Atlanta was initiated and was conducted annually until 1995. They conducted a one-week program designed to help nurses evaluate, select, and use health care information systems. This program gave nurse educators the opportunity to gain a comprehensive understanding of automated health care information systems and the hospital technology expected in the new century (Skiba et al., 1992).

In 1991, the annual **Summer Institute in Nursing and Health Care Informatics** by the University of Maryland School of Nursing in Baltimore was first conducted. It is a one-week program focusing on nursing informatics, the effect of information technology on nursing practice, the selection and evaluation of information systems, and strategies for implementing a system. The attendees are also given the opportunity to visit hospitals to view NISs first-hand. This summer institute continues to be conducted annually.

In 1993, **Partners Healthcare Systems** in Boston initiated a one-year NI fellowship open to nurses who have completed a graduate informatics program of study. The program is designed to provide hands-on informatics experience and mentorship with experts in the field who are developing hospital information systems applications.

Academic Courses and Programs   Several university schools of nursing initiated computer technology courses at the graduate and undergraduate levels. In 1977, the first university to offer an undergraduate elective course was The State University of New York at Buffalo. In the early 1980s, a 3-credit course was offered at the NIH, in Bethesda, Maryland, as part of its educational program. In 1985, the School of Nursing at Georgetown University in Washington, D.C., initiated elective courses at the undergraduate and graduate levels on the essentials of computers for nurses. Since 1995, the elective courses have been combined and offered to all students on campus.

During the 1980s, many literacy programs were sponsored by continuing education departments in colleges and universities nationwide. Special courses, workshops, and meetings were offered to introduce nurses to computers and computing.

In the late 1980s and early 1990s, several universities began to educate nurses in computer applications in nursing, NISs, and nursing informatics at either the graduate or undergraduate levels. In 1988, the University of Maryland in Baltimore; in 1990, the University of Utah in Salt Lake City; and in 1995, New York University began to offer graduate degrees in nursing informatics. Further, in 1991, the University of Maryland initiated the first doctoral program and continues to offer a doctorate for nurses specializing in informatics (Gassert, 1992).

Many other universities also offer academic courses in computer applications in nursing. Some schools have made such a course a requirement for the graduate degree in nursing administration, others offer a course as an elective at the graduate level, and still others are integrating computer concepts into graduate level core nursing courses. Generally, these courses are offered at universities where nursing informatics pioneers and experts are faculty members, such as at Georgetown University; the University of New York at Buffalo; the University of California at San Francisco; Case Western Reserve in Cleveland; George Mason University in Fairfax, Virginia; the University of Texas at Austin; the University of Maryland in Baltimore; and New York University in New York City.

Today most schools of nursing offer computer courses in combination with other departments such as the business school and/or offer Health Policy as a double major. Other universities have started to offer informatics courses via distance learning technology such as Regents College, New York. Many universities have initiated a unique nursing informatics department and nursing informatics positions, such as an Endowed Chair for Nursing Informatics or an Associate Dean for Informatics.

Initial American Nurses Association Initiatives

During the 1980s, the ANA launched several initiatives on computer technology for nursing practice. In 1984, the ANA formed the Council on Computer Applications in Nursing (CCAN). In 1986, the ANA passed a resolution urging that the organization assume a leadership role and encourage the development and implementation of NISs to improve patient care and provide essential data to nurses and other professionals in the health care field.

In 1990, a resolution was passed advocating that the ANA establish national nursing databases to support clinical nursing practice, establish standards for NISs, and develop comprehensive payment systems for nursing practice. As a result of the resolution, the Steering Committee on Databases to Support Clinical Nursing Practice was formed. Also in that year, the ANA House of Delegates recognized the NMDS as the minimum data elements that should be included in any paper-based or computer-based patient record (CPR). In 1992, the ANA passed another resolution that supported the involvement of nursing in CPRSs.

American Nurses Association Council on Computer Applications in Nursing   The ANA CCAN was very active in promoting computer technology in nursing, including the development of computer-based nursing materials. It published between 1986 and 1992 a newsletter, *Input/Output*. Also, it spearheaded five monographs between 1988 and 1994: (1) *Computer Design Criteria* (Zielstorff et al., 1988), (2) *Computers in Nursing Education* (Grobe et al., 1987), (3) *Computers in Nursing Research: A Theoretical Perspective* (Abraham et al., 1992), (4) *Next-Generation Nursing Information Systems* (Zielstorff et al., 1993), and (5) *Computers in Nursing Management* (Saba et al., 1994). The CCAN prepared two *Computer Nurse Directories* identifying nurses in the field of Nursing Informatics in 1987 and 1991. Beginning in 1986 through 1994, the CCAN conducted a demonstration theater and software exchange at the biennial ANA conventions and, to further this emerging specialty, gave an award for excellence in the field.

American Nurses Association Steering Committee on Databases to Support Nursing Practice   In 1990, the ANA established the Steering Committee on Databases to Support Nursing Practice, and in 1997 it was renamed the Committee for Nursing Practice Information Infrastructure (see previous description under "Nursing Data Standards"). This committee was mandated by the Congress on Nursing Practice to propose policy and program initiatives regarding nursing classification schemes, uniform nursing data sets, and the inclusion of nursing data elements in national databases. It was also directed to build national data sets, coordinate initiatives in this regard, and provide advice on the process so that the profession could "recognize" vocabularies and taxonomies (Lang et al., 1995; McCormick et al., 1992).

In January 1992, the ANA designated Nursing Informatics as a nursing specialty and defined it. A subcommittee was established to develop the requirements for a certification program to credential new nursing specialists called "Informatics Nurses." The process also included the development of a scope of practice, guidelines, and standards as well as the actual questions for the credentialing examination, which was first offered in 1995 (American Nurses Association, 1994; Council on Computer Applications in Nursing, 1992).

In 1992, the Database Steering Committee recognized four vocabularies and/or classification schemes as meeting the criteria for creating a nursing language. The four schemes, listed earlier in this chapter, are also considered as having acceptable nursing data standards for documenting nursing care in NISs and CPRSs. By 1999, this committee had recognized four additional schemes that were previously listed.

American Nurses Association Nursing Information and Data Set Educational Center   The ANA Database Steering Committee also established in 1996–1997 the Nursing Information and Data Set Educational Center (NIDSEC). It was formed to provide approval of vendors that submitted NISs and met ANA NIDSEC standards (e.g. the NIS included one of the recognized nursing vocabularies) (Milholland, 1997; American Nurses Association Nursing Information and Data Set Educational Center Committee, 1997).

The new Database Steering Committee, renamed the Committee for Nursing Practice Information Infrastructure, continues to focus its activities on computer technology and its impact on the nursing profession. The committee participates in the major national and federal conferences, meetings, and organizations that address data standards and technology transfer in the health care industry.

Initial National League for Nurs\g Initiatives

The NLN promotes educational initiatives for nursing informatics. In 1985, it formed the National Forum on Computers in Health Care and Nursing, which in 1989 was renamed the Council on Nursing Informatics. The NLN also passed resolutions supporting computer technology in nursing. In 1987, the NLN passed a resolution recommending the inclusion of computer technology in nursing education. In 1991, it passed another resolution recommending that computer technology in nursing become a part of the educational accreditation criteria for schools of nursing.

The NLN hosts the NLN Council for Nursing Informatics at its biennial conferences and at several other educational conferences they hold. The Council generally conducts panels and presents papers at all NLN conferences to bring attention to the needs of technology in education. The Council for Nursing Informatics has published several documents that focus on the educational criteria for integrating nursing informatics into nursing curricula and into books and education materials. In 1987, the NLN published its first document on nursing and computers: *Guidelines for Basic Computer Education in Nursing* (Ronald and Skiba, 1987). The NLN continues to support computer technology in nursing education.

Other Significant Organization Initiatives

Several of the other national and international nursing and other health-related organizations also conducted conferences on nursing informatics and/or health care informatics with sessions on NISs. From 1987 to 1995, the Stewart Publishing Co. conducted an annual Interactive Healthcare Conference in Alexandria, Virginia. At those meetings, nurses and other informatics experts presented and demonstrated cutting edge technologies including interactive video programs, CD-ROM applications, Internet applications, etc.

Sigma Theta Tau International held one-day conferences on nursing informatics and/or computer technology in nursing as an optional part of their national conferences. The Electronic Medical Records Institute in Boston included nursing informatics sessions specific for nurses as part of its annual national and international conferences. Today, almost all nursing conferences include sessions on technology and informatics.

Initial International Initiatives

Working Groups   In 1981, the International Medical Informatics Association (IMIA) formed Working Group 8 on Nursing Informatics. It consisted of representatives from 25 countries, including the United States. This working group met at the IMIA MEDINFO meetings that were held every 3 years and in 1985 began to sponsor its own international symposia that are titled Nursing Uses of Computers and Information Sciences.

In 1982, Working Group 8, which had become the Nursing Informatics Special Interest Group (IMIA/NI-SIG), conducted its first international meeting, in London, for nurses and professionals interested in this field. This meeting was designed to assist worldwide development of computers in nursing. The event started with an open forum in London, followed by a postconference working group in Harrogate, Yorkshire. The working group held intensive discussions to describe the state of the art in computers in nursing and attempted to predict future needs. The group's postconference deliberations were published later (Scholes et al., 1983).

International Conferences
International Medical Informatics Association Working Group 8 Nursing Informatics Special Interest Group
The IMIA Working Group 8 on NI, recently renamed as the IMIA/NI-SIG, following the London meeting, has held subsequent meetings: (1) 1985 in Calgary, Alberta, Canada (Hannah et al., 1985); (2) 1988 in Dublin, Ireland (Daly and Hannah, 1988); (3) 1991 in Mel-

bourne, Australia (Hovenga et al.,1991); (4) 1994 in San Antonio, Texas (Grobe and Pluyter-Wenting, 1994); (5) 1997 in Stockholm, Sweden (Gerdin et al.,1997); and (6) 2000 in Auckland, New Zealand (Saba et al., 2000).

The renamed IMIA/NI-SIG meetings follow a similar format, an open meeting followed by an invitational workshop with a working group selected to address a specific critical issue and to prepare a publication on the topic. These publications have been published primarily as separate documents or articles in a journal (Ehnfors et al., 1998; Henry et al., 1994).

Special Meeting   In 1987, the IMIA Working Group 8: Task Force on Education convened in Sweden under the auspices of the Stockholm County Council. The group defined the critical competencies needed to guide the education of nurses for their roles in informatics. Nursing computer competency, defined as "having sufficient knowledge, judgement, skill, or strength," was identified as the major criterion for the skills that should be taught and emphasized in an educational program designed to teach computer technology in nursing (Peterson and Gerdin-Jelger, 1988).

MEDINFO   In 1983, for the first time, a large international group of nurses participated in two one-day nursing sessions at the *Fourth World Congress on Medical Informatics, MEDINFO 1983*, held in Amsterdam. They presented scientific papers on computer applications in nursing and conducted seminars focusing on nursing systems. Nursing experts have continued to participate at the conferences, which are sponsored by IMIA every 3 years (Fokkens, 1983; Van Bemmel et al.,1983). The subsequent international conferences sponsored by IMIA continue to include a nursing tract and several nursing functions. They were held as follows: MEDINFO 1986 in Washington, D.C. (Salamon et al., 1986), MEDINFO 1989 in Singapore (Barber et al., 1989), MEDINFO 1992 in Geneva, Switzerland (Lun et al., 1992), MEDINFO 1995, in Vancouver, British Columbia, Canada (Greenes et al., 1995), and MEDINFO 1998, in Seoul, Korea (Cesnik et al., 1998).

World Health Organization   The World Health Organization (WHO) is involved in the promotion of informatics around the world. In 1989, the ANA submitted to the WHO an "International Classification of Nursing Diagnosis" for inclusion into the *10th Revision of the International Classification of Diseases and Health-Related Conditions* (ICD-10). This classification was a coded version of *NANDA Taxonomy I: Revised*

(Fitzpatrick et al., 1989; World Health Organization, 1992a). However, because the classification had not been approved by the international nursing community, it was not put up for a vote at the general assembly. Instead, in 1989, it was presented at the ICN Quadrennial Congress in Seoul, Korea, for review by its member organizations at their regional meetings. The WHO plans to present the nursing classification for approval by the WHO General Assembly when it is certain that it has the support of the international nursing community.

During the interval, the WHO World Health Assembly (WHA) has passed a resolution (WHA 42-27) recommending strengthening nursing and midwifery in support of strategies for Health for ALL (HFA). The resolution included several recommendations, one of which requested the Director-General to "promote and support the training of nursing/ midwifery in . . . the development of information systems" (World Health Organization, 1992b, p. 1).

As a result of this resolution, a WHO Workshop on Nursing Informatics was held in 1991, at the WHO Regional Offices for the Americas/Pan American Sanitary Bureau, in Washington, D.C. The major purpose of the workshop was to highlight the status of nursing informatics at various levels around the world—national, regional, and global. The workshop was also designed to educate participants on the principals, development, and uses of nursing management information systems focusing on system, design, hardware, and software requirements.

In September 1992, as a follow-up to the WHO workshop, a Work Group on Nursing Management Information Systems was convened in Geneva. The Work Group focused on WHO activities related to health information systems. They identified the major constraints inhibiting the collection of data needed for human resource management. The Work Group also believed that nurses, the chief providers of primary health care, have the professional responsibility to ensure that basic health care needs in the community are met and are responsible for monitoring the quality and effectiveness of care. They stated that "management information is necessary to ensure the right persons for the right jobs and in the right places at the right times, all within budgetary constraints" (World Health Organization, 1993). The participants in these two WHO workshops included representatives from professional nursing organizations, representatives from four WHO regions, and other experts in nursing informatics, midwifery, and human resource planning.

International Council of Nurses   At the ICN Council of Representatives 1989 Quadrennial meeting in Seoul, Korea, the Professional Services Committee agreed that it would develop a common language and classification for the international nursing community. In 1991, the ICN initiated a project to develop the International Classification of Nursing Practice (ICNP). Its major purpose was to establish a common language and classification for nursing practice to improve communication among nurses and between nurses and other health care providers.

The alpha version of the ICNP was presented at the 1993 ICN Congress in Madrid, Spain and distributed to its member countries for review. The alpha version consisted of three alphabetized lists of existing nomenclatures for (1) nursing diagnoses/problems, (2) nursing interventions, and (3) outcomes, collected from the United States, Canada, and several European countries. As of 1999, the ICNP had been translated into 16 different languages. A beta version has been developed consisting of computer-based care linkages designed for computer processing. This version is also being translated and tested by many of the ICN member countries around the world (Affara, 1995; International Council of Nursing, 1996; Mortensen, 1996; Nielson 1995). It was followed by the beta version, which was developed for computer processing and presented at the 1999 ICN Congress in London. At the London meeting, the Council of Representatives voted to assign a staff member and provide funding to continue the work required to enhance the ICNP, test it, and get endorsement from its member countries around the world.

TELENURSE Project   The TELENURSE is a European Union (EU)-funded project designed to support the promotion of the ICNP in Europe. The ICN agreed with the EU to allow the funding of the TELENURSE consortium to field test the alpha version of the ICNP. The major purpose of this field testing is to evaluate the ICNP alpha version when translated into the different European languages. The funding also included conferences as well as financing the electronic programming of the scheme (Mortensen, 1996).

Nightingale Project   In 1996, the 3-year Nightingale Project was initiated by the University of Athens and funded by the European Union. It major focus was to implement a strategy for training the nursing profession in health care information systems including nursing. The Nightingale Project contributed to the Telematics infrastructure in Europe by developing an educational strategy for introducing nursing informatics. To accomplish their objectives, the project sponsored several European conferences and workshops and developed educational materials such as a CD-ROM, computer-based graphical presentations, articles, and textbooks (Mantas, 1998).

Initial Educational Resources

In 1984, the first nursing journal in the field, *Computers in Nursing*, was published. This journal began as a newsletter in 1982 at the School of Nursing at the University of Texas at Austin. It continues and now has an editorial staff of eight experts in the field of computers and nursing. It is the only nursing journal that focuses on nursing informatics and computer applications in nursing.

The *Directory of Educational Software for Nursing* was first introduced as a handout at one of the many workshops at Computers in Health Care 84: A Symposium and Exhibition held in Sacramento, California (Bolwell, 1984–1995). The original directory contained brief descriptions of 52 CAI programs from a collection of software demonstrated at the symposium. The directory was updated and published annually and provided information on the majority of microcomputer programs, including CAI and IAV programs, that were available for the nursing community. The fifth and final edition of the *Directory*, published in 1995, was organized into 50 sections with over 320 programs. It included over 100 CAI programs and 50 interactive videodisc (IVD) programs.

In 1986, the *Nurse Educator's Microworld* newsletter was also introduced by Bolwell to provide nurse educators using or planning to use a microcomputer a comprehensive source of information on software programs. This newsletter, which was published by Stewart Publishing in Alexandria, Virginia, provided periodic information in the field of nursing and was also terminated in 1995.

Information from numerous journal articles, books, trade journals, and papers on the proceedings from computer conferences also provide state-of-the-art information for this specialty. Books on computers in health care did not appear until 1977. From 1977 to 1983 only six books were published in this area (Pocklington and Guttman, 1984). Since then, many textbooks have been published that offer comprehensive information about computers and nursing, nursing informatics, and nursing

applications. In the future, journals and books will be offered on-line or as CD-ROMs instead of as paper copy.

Learning Resource Centers As schools of nursing introduced computer technology in their educational programs, they established learning resource centers (LRCs). Many of these LRCs have been established through start-up grant funds from the Helene Fuld Institute. The LRC is a computer laboratory with PCs configured for teaching students hands-on generic software packages and other software applications specific for nursing. The Helene Fuld Institute also supported interactive video equipment for running both CAI and IAV software. More recently, the microcomputer laboratories have installed LANs that link the desktop PCs together in order to share software programs. Additionally, they have installed modems that access the Internet as well as an Intranet, which allows on-line access to/from remote faculty offices, student rooms, and classrooms. The Internet with its cybernet tools, including the WWW, has changed the format of student and faculty use of educational resources.

Educational Software Initially, individual nurses created CAI and IAV programs; however, as the industry grew, several commercial organizations and publishing companies took on this function. These organizations were also involved in the development and dissemination of multimedia educational technologies, which included CAI and IAV software programs and, more recently CD-ROM. In the 21st century, courses will be digitized and installed on dedicated computer file servers that link the student to the LRC. The "digital streaming" of lectures will make it possible for students to hear (audio) and see (video) the lecturer while reading his/her lecture notes on the video screen. The Internet courses will be developed and transmitted to off-campus sites and via the Internet to other remote sites as distance education programs. Further, software programs will be developed that emulate the CPR and are used by students for the different courses in their academic program to document their care electronically.

Educational Library In 1992 and 1993, the Sigma Theta Tau International Honor Society of Nursing, Virginia Henderson International Nursing Library (INL), initiated an electronic library. The library consists of a collection of electronic databases and knowledge resources, including an on-line network. This on-line communication network was created not only to transmit its on-line journal but also to share its research information with the nursing community (Graves, 1994; Hudgings, 1992).

Educational Networks   Educational networks have been formed by professional groups. The AJN Network was an on-line service created by the American Journal of Nursing Company (AJN) to provide information and offer formal and informal continuing educational services to nurses. In 1998, this network was purchased by a publishing company and renamed Nursing Center.com (1999), and it has emerged as an Internet Web site for nursing professionals and students worldwide. This Web site provides expanded features for nurses to access such as continuing education, full text delivery of nursing journals, newsletters, etc.

Other on-line electronic systems have been created such as the electronic accreditation software program developed by NLN. This on-line nationwide NLN accreditation database is available to the nursing community. The computer-based testing for the Registered Nurse Examination, NCLEX-RN, is also being administered on-line nationwide.

Web Sites   Another on-line network is ANA*NET, initiated by the ANA. It consists of public and private databases compiled to assist ANA staff and state ANAs by providing instant access to information that addresses their information needs. It also offers a bulletin board system that electronically links developers and users of interactive educational materials. In the year 2000, almost every nursing organization, government department, and private resource of nursing interest has a "home page" on the WWW. They include:

- American Nurses Association (*http://www.ana.org*)
- American Medical Informatics Association (*http://www.amia.org*)
- National League for Nursing (*http://www.nln.org*)
- International Council of Nurses (*http://www.icn.ch*)
- National Institutes of Health (*http://www.nih.gov*)

Significant Collaborative Events

Several collaborative events took place in the late 1980s and early 1990s that advanced the field of computers and nursing. These initiatives consisted of conferences and projects that recommended computer technology as a means of enhancing the nursing profession. Other events

continue to occur as technology becomes an integral part of nursing programs, conferences, and media.

First Invitational Nursing Minimum Data Set   In 1985, the First Invitational Nursing Minimum Data Set (NMDS) Conference was held in Chicago (Werley and Lang, 1988). It was a follow-up to the Nursing Information Systems Conference that met in 1986, which had recommended the creation of a NMDS. The NMDS provides the basis for the nursing component of the CPR. In 1990, the NMDS was approved by the ANA as the standard data set structure for automating nursing practice and developing a national database.

National Commission on Nursing Implementation Project   In 1986, the National Commission on Nursing Implementation Project (NCNIP) Work Group II, Research and Development, advocated that NISs track care. In 1989, NCNIP conducted an invitational conference in collaboration with the ANA CCAN and the NLN Nursing Informatics Forum and selected NIS vendors in Orlando, Florida. The major purpose was to outline for the industry the nursing perspectives on the state of the art of information systems. The conference was attended by developers and vendors, nurse purchasers, and users of NISs interested in planning collaborative efforts in the design and development of future NISs. In 1994, a second invitational conference was held in Washington, D.C., to critique and discuss the findings of a 1993 report on the next generation of NISs (Zielstorff et al., 1993).

Secretary's Commission on Nursing Shortage   The Secretary's Commission on Nursing Shortage in its 1988 final report stated that the federal government should sponsor further research and encourage health care delivery organizations to develop and use automated information systems and other new labor-saving technologies to better support nurses and other health professionals (Office of the Secretary, 1988).

Priority Expert Panel E: Nursing Informatics Task Force   The Priority Expert Panel E: Nursing Informatics Task Force initiated in 1988 by the National Center for Nursing Research (NCNR), now the National Institute for Nursing Research (NINR), was one of a series of expert panels established by the NCNR to develop a national nursing research agenda. This initiative began with a conference designed to develop broad priorities for the NCNR. This was followed by the establishment of the Priority Expert Panel E, which was charged with setting priorities for computer technology research topics (National Institutes of Health, 1992). The panel "was committed to maintaining the clinical perspective, assessing needs for research that would bear directly on improving patient care" (NCNR Priority Expert Panel, 1993, p. 12). The panel produced a report that outlined six program goals, each with a series of recommendations for research to support computers in nursing.

National Informatics Agenda for Nursing Practice and Education
In 1997, a collaborative event between the DN, PHS, DHHS and the National Advisory Council on Nurse Education and Practice was convened as an invitational conference designed to develop a National Informatics Agenda for Nursing Practice and Education. In attendance were a broad range of nursing informatics experts in informatics education and competencies. The National Nursing Informatics Work Group was convened for a 2-day meeting to identify initiatives that would help the nation's nursing workforce to utilize technology in education and practice as well as assist patients in accessing health care information (NACNEP, 1997).

The major landmark events of computers in nursing are shown in Table 2.2.

Summary

This chapter highlights the historical perspectives and changes in the nursing profession since Florence Nightingale's time. These changes have dealt primarily with redefining nursing practice, managing nursing services, advancing nursing education, and planning nursing research. Expansion in all health fields made it necessary for nurses and nursing to study and use the technological advances that affect the delivery of care.

Computers emerged during the past four decades in the health care industry. Hospitals began to use computers as tools to update their paper-based patient records. Computer systems in health care settings provided the information management capabilities needed to assess, document, process, and communicate patient care. As a result, the "man-machine" interaction of nursing and computers has become a new and lasting symbiotic relationship (Blum, 1990; Collen, 1994; Kemeny, 1972).

Computer applications in nursing and early computerized information systems were described. These systems are considered to be the forerunners of systems that are still used in hospitals. In community health, several projects were also described that have influenced today's systems. Additionally, computer applications that support nursing education and research were highlighted.

The last section focused on landmark events in nursing and computers, including major milestones in national and international conferences, symposia, workshops, and organizational initiatives that contributed to the computer literacy of nurses. The success of the conferences and the appearance of a nursing journal on this topic demonstrated the intense interest nurses had in learning more about computers. These advances confirmed the status of computers as a new specialty in the nursing profession and have helped to bring nursing into the 21st century.

References

Abdellah, F., Beland, I., Martin, A., and Matheney, R. (1960). *Patient-Centered Approaches to Nursing*. New York: Macmillan.

Abraham, I. L., Schroeder, M.A., and Schwirian, P. M. (1992). *Computers in Nursing Research*. Kansas City, MO: American Nurses Association.

Affara, F. A. (1995). Towards an international classification for nursing practice: The role of the International Council of Nurses. In R. A. Mortensen (Ed.), *Creating a European Platform: Proceedings of the First European Conference on Nursing Diagnoses* (pp.64–69). Copenhagen, Denmark: Danish Institute for Health and Nursing Research.

Agency for Health Care Policy and Research. (1999). *Current Activities of Selected Healthcare Informatics Standards Organizations: A Compilation*. Rockville MD: AHCPR, U.S. DHHS.

Agency for Health Care Policy and Research. (1990). *AHCPR: Purpose and Programs* (DHHS Publication No. OM90-0096). Rockville, MD: PHS, US DHHS.

Agency for Health Care Policy and Research. (1992). *AHCPR Fact Sheet*. Rockville, MD.

Aiken, E. (1990). *Continuing Nursing Education in Computer Technology: A Regional Experience* (Grant No. D10NU24198). Atlanta, GA: Southern Regional Education Board.

Alward, R. R. (1983). Patient classification systems: The ideal vs. reality. *Journal of Nursing Administration, 13*(2), 14–19.

Amatayakul, M. (1998). The state of the computer-based patient record. *Journal of AHIMA, 69*(9), 34–37.

American Journal of Nursing. (1975–1998). *International Nursing Index*. New York.

American Nurses Association. (1980). *Nursing: A Social Policy Statement*. Kansas City, MO.

American Nurses Association. (1991). *Standards for Clinical Nursing Practice*. Kansas City, MO.

American Nurses Association. (1994). *Scope of Practice for Nursing Informatics*. Washington, D.C.

American Nurses Association, NIDSEC Committee.
(1997). *NIDSEC: Standards and Scoring Guidelines: Nursing Information and Data Set Evaluation Center.* Washington, D.C.

Andrews, R. D. and Beauchamp, C. (1989). A clinical database management system for improved integration of the Veterans Affairs hospital information system. *Journal of Medical Systems, 13,* 309–320.

Appavu, S. I. (1999). Federal Administrative Simplification Law (PL 104-191/HIPAA) Toward standardization of healthcare information. In *Proceedings of the 1999 Annual HIMSS Conference: Volume 3* (pp. 339–347). Chicago, IL: HIMSS Publications.

Armstrong, M. L. (1998). *Telecommunications for Health Professionals: Providing Successful Distance Education and Telehealth.* New York: Springer Publishing.

Arnold, J. M.,and Pearson, G. A. (1992). *Computer Applications in Nursing Education and Practice.* New York: National League for Nursing (Publication No. 14-2406).

Aydelotte, M. (1973). *Nursing Staffing Methodology: A Review and Critique of Selected Literature* (DHEW Dec-NU [NIH] 73-433). Washington, D.C.: U.S. Government Printing Office.

Bakken, S., Cashen, M. S., Mendonca, E. A., O'Brien, A.O., and Zieniewicz, J. (2000). Representing nursing activities within a concept-oriented terminological system: Evaluation of a type definition. *Journal of the American Medical Informatics Association, 6*(1), 81–90.

Barber, B., Cao, N., Qin, D., and Wagner, G. (Eds.). (1989). *MEDINFO 89 (Vol. 1-2). Proceedings of the Sixth World Congress on Medical Informatics.* Amsterdam: North-Holland.

Barnett, O. G. (1976). *Computer-Stored Ambulatory Record (COSTAR)* (DHEW Publication No. HRA 76-3145). Rockville, MD: National Center for Health Services Research, PHS, US DHEW.

Bitzer, M. D. and Boudreaux, M. C. (1969). Using a computer to teach nursing. *Nursing Forum, 8*(3), 234–254.

Blum, B. I. (1990). Medical informatics in the United States, 1950–1975. In B. Blum,and K. Duncan (Eds.), *A History of Medical Informatics* (pp. xvii–xxx). Reading, MA: Addison-Wesley.

Bolwell, C. (1984–1995). *Directory of Educational Software for Nursing* (Pub. No. 41-2279). New York: National League for Nursing Press.

Bolwell, C. (Ed.). (1986). *Nurse Educator's Microworld.* Alexandria, VA: Stewart Publishing.

Brown, V. B., Mason, W. B., and Kaczmarski, M. (1971). A computerized health information service. *Nursing Outlook, 19*(3), 158–161.

Bulocheck, G. M. and McClosky, J. C. (1995). Nursing Intervention Classification (NIC): A language to describe nursing treatments. In ANA Database Committee, *Nursing Data Systems: The Emerging Framework* (pp. 9–32). Washington, D.C.: ANA.

Carty, B. and Rosenfield, P. (1997). *Technology as the Tool, Information as the Commodity: A Plan of Action for Nursing Education.* Paper presented at the Rutgers Fifteenth Annual International Nursing Informatics Conference. Atlantic City, NJ.

Cendrowska, T. J., Amatayakul, M., and Tessier, C. Standards in healthcare: Meeting industry's needs by using ASTM standards. In *Proceedings of the 1999 Annual HIMSS Conference: Volume 3* (pp. 433–442). Chicago, IL: HIMSS Publications.

Cesnik, B., McCray, A. T., and Sacherrer, J. R. (Eds.). (1998). *MEDINFO 98 (Vol 1-2). Proceedings of the Ninth World Congress on Medical Informatics.* Amsterdam: IOS Press.

CHCSII Program. (1999). *Composite Health Care System II.* Falls Church, VA: CHCSII Program.

Chief Information Office, Veterans Affairs. (1996–1997). *Veterans Health Information Systems and Technology Architecture (VISTA).* Washington, D.C.: Department of Veterans Affairs.

Chief Information Office, Veterans Affairs. (1997–1998). *Veterans Health Information Systems and Technology Architecture (VISTA).* Washington, D.C.: Department of Veterans Affairs.

Chute, C. G., Cohen, S. P., and Campbell, K. E. (1996). The content coverage of clinical classifications. *Journal of the American Medical Informatics Association, 3,* 224–233.

Collen, M. F. (1994). The origins of informatics. *Journal of the American Medical Informatics Association, 1*(2), 91–107.

Collen, M. F. (1995). *A history of medical informatics in the United States 1950 to 1990.* Bethesda, MD: American Medical Informatics Association.

Collen, M. F. (1999). A vision of health care and informatics in 2008. *Journal of the American Medical Informatics Association, 6*(1), 1–5.

College of American Pathologists, and American Veterinary Medical Association. (1998). *SNOMED International.* Northfield, IL.

Committee on Armed Services. (1990). *Defense's Acquisition of the Composite Health Care System.* Washington, D.C.: U.S. House of Representatives, GAO (T-IMTEC-90-04).

Community Nursing Services of Philadelphia. (1976). *Development of a Computerized Record System to Store and Summarize Information Relevant to Administration, Evaluation and Planning of Nursing Services* (Contract No. 1-NU-241271). Washington, D.C.: Division of Nursing, HRA, US DHEW.

Cook, M. and Mayers, M. (1981). Computer-assisted data base for nursing research. In H. Werley and M. Grier (Eds.), *Nursing Information Systems* (pp. 149–156). New York: Springer.

Cook, M. and McDowell, W. (1975). Changing to an automated information system. *American Journal of Nursing, 75*(1), 46–51.

Cornell, S. A. and Carrick, A. G. (1973). Computerized schedules and care plans. *Nursing Outlook, 21*(12), 781–789.

Corum, W. (1993). JCAHO's new information management standards. *Healthcare Informatics, 10*(8), 20–21.

Council on Computer Applications in Nursing. (1992). *Report on the Designation of Nursing Informatics as a Nursing Specialty.* Washington, D.C.

Daly, N. and Hannah, K. J. (Eds.). (1988). *Proceedings of Nursing and Computers: Third International Symposium on Nursing Use of Computers and Information Science.* Washington, D.C.: Mosby.

Dayhoff, R. E., Maloney, D. L., and Kuzman, P. M. (1990). Examination of architecture to allow integration of image data with hospital information systems. In R. A. Miller (Ed.), *Proceedings of the Fourteenth Symposium on Computer Applications in Medical Care* (pp. 694–698). Washington, D.C.: IEEE Computer Society Press.

Dick, R. S. and Steen, E. B. (1991). *The Computer-Based Patient Record: An Essential Technology for Health Care.* Washington, D.C.: National Academy Press.

Edwards, M. A. (1996). *The Internet for Nurses and Allied Health Professionals (2nd Ed.)* New York, NY: Springer.

Ehnfors, M. E., Grobe, S. J., and Tallberg, M. (1998). *Nursing Informatics: Combining Clinical Practices Guidelines and Patient Preferences Using Health Informatics.* Stockholm, Sweden: Spri.

Ellett, M. L., Ellett, S. G., and Ellett, L. D. (1999). Conducting nursing research via the internet. *Computers In Nursing PLUS, 2*(3), 4–5.

Fitzmaurice, M. J. (1995). Computer-based patient records. In J. Bronzino (Ed.), *Biomedical Engineering Handbook* (pp. 2623–2634). Boca Raton, FL: CRC Press, Inc.

Fitzpatrick, J. J., Kerr, M. E., Saba, V. K., et al. (1989). Translating nursing diagnosis into ICD code. *Nursing Outlook, 89*(4), 493–495.

Fokkens, O. (Ed.). (1983). *MEDINFO '83 Seminars.* Amsterdam: North-Holland.

Gane, D. (1972). The computer in nursing. In J. Hurst and H. Walker (Eds.), *The Problem-Oriented System* (pp. 251–257). New York: Medcom Press.

Gassert, C. A. (1995). Academic preparation in nursing informatics. In M. J. Ball, S. K. Hannah, S. K. Newbold, and J. V. Douglas. (Eds.), *Nursing Informatics: Where Caring and Technology Meet.* (2nd ed.) (pp. 333–349). New York: Spring-Verlag.

Gebbie K. M. (Ed.). (1975). *Summary of the Second National Conference: Classification of Nursing Diagnoses.* St. Louis, MO: National Group for Classification of Nursing Diagnoses.

Geibnik, G. A. and Hurst, L. L. (1975). *Computer Projects in Health Care.* Ann Arbor, MI: Health Administration Press.

Gerdin, U., Tallberg, M., and Wainwright, P. (1997). *Nursing Informatics: The Impact of Nursing Knowledge on Health Care Informatics.* Amsterdam, Holland: IOS Press.

Gortner, S. R. and Nahm, M. H. (1977). An overview of nursing research in the United States. *Nursing Research, 26*(1), 10–33.

Graves, J. R., (1994). Updates: Virginia Henderson International Nursing Library. *Reflections, 20*(3), 39.

Greenes, R. A., Peterson, H. E., and Protti, D. J. (1995). *MEDINFO 95: Proceedings of the Eighth World Congress on Medical Informatics.* Amsterdam: North-Holland.

Grobe, S. and Pluyter-Wenting, E. (1994). *Nursing Informatics: An International Overview for Nursing in a Technological Era.* Amsterdam: Elsevier.

Grobe, S., Ronald, J., and Tymchyshyn, P. (1987). *Computers in Nursing Education.* Kansas City, MO: American Nurses Association.

Hammond, W. E. (1994). The role of standards in creating a health information infrastructure. *International Journal of Bio-Medical Computing, 34,* 29–44.

Hanchett, E. S. (1981). Appropriateness of nursing care. In H. Werley and M. Grier (Eds.), *Nursing Information Systems* (pp. 235–242). New York: Springer.

Hannah, K. J., Guillemin, E. C., and Conklin, D. N. (Eds.). (1985). *Nursing Uses of Computers and Information Science. Proceeding of the IFIP-IMIA International Symposium on Nursing Uses of Computers and Information Science.* Amsterdam: North-Holland.

Harmer, B. and Henderson, V. (1939). *Textbook of the Principles and Practice of Nursing* (4th ed.). New York: Macmillan.

Health Level Seven. (1999). *Catalog of HL7 Resources.* Ann Arbor, MI: Health Level Inc.

Heffernan, S. (Ed.). (1981). *Proceedings: The Fifth Annual Symposium on Computer Applications on Medical Care.* New York: IEEE Computer Society Press.

Henderson, V. (1964). The nature of nursing. *American Journal of Nursing, 64*(8), 62–68.

Henry, S. B., Holzemer, W. L., Tallberg, M., and Grobe, S. J. (1994). *Informatics: The Infrastructure for Quality Assessment & Improvement in Nursing.* San Francisco, CA: UC Nursing Press.

Henry, S. B. and Mead, C. N. (1997 May/June). Nursing classifications systems: Necessary but not sufficient for representing "what nurses do" for inclusion in computer-based patient record systems. *Journal of the American Medical Informatics Association, 4,* 222–232.

Hodge, M. H., (1990). History of the TDS medical information system. In B. I. Blum and K. Duncan (Eds.), *A History of Medical Informatics* (pp. 328–344). Reading, MA: Addison-Wesley.

Hovenga, E. J. S., Hannah, K. J., McCormick, K. A., and Ronald, J. S. (1991). *Nursing Informatics '91: Proceedings of the Fourth International Conference on Nursing Use of Computers and Information Science.* Amsterdam: North-Holland.

Hudgings, C. (1992). The Virginia Henderson International Nursing Library: Improving access to nursing research databases. In J. M. Arnold and G. A. Pearson (Eds.), *Computer Applications in Nursing Education and Practice* (pp. 3–8). New York: National League for Nursing (Publication No. 14-2406).

Humphreys, B. L. and Lindberg, D. A. B. (1992). The unified medical language system project: A distributed experiment in improving access to biomedical information. In K. C. Lun, P. DeGoulet, T.E. Piemme, and O. Rienhoff (Eds.). *MEDINFO 92: Proceedings of the Seventh World Congress on Medical Informatics* (pp. 1496–1500). Amsterdam: North-Holland.

Information Technology Center. (1996). *Internet Starter Kit.* Washington, D.C.: Bureau of Transportation Statistics.

International Council of Nurses. (1996). *The Classification of Nursing Practice: A Unifying Framework: The Alpha Version.* Geneva Switzerland: ICN.

Johnson, M. and Maas, M. (1995). Classification of nursing-sensitive patient outcomes. In ANA Database Committee. *Nursing Data Systems: The Emerging Framework* (pp. 170–176). Washington, D.C.: ANA.

Joint Commission on Accreditation of Hospitals. (1970). *Accreditation Manual for Hospitals.* Chicago.

Joint Commission on Accreditation of Hospitals. (1981). *Accreditation Manual for Hospitals.* Chicago.

Joint Commission on Accreditation of Health Care Organizations (1994). *Accreditation Manual for Hospitals.* Oakbrook Terrace, IL.

Joos, I. and Nelson, R. (1992). Strategies and resources for self-education in nursing informatics. In J. Arnold and G. Pearson (Eds.), *Computer Applications in Nursing Education and Practice.* New York: National League for Nursing Press.

Kemeny, J. G. (1972). *Man and the Computer.* New York: Charles Scribner.

Kiley, M., Holleran, E. J., and Weston, J. L., et al. (1983). Computerized nursing information systems (NIS). *Nursing Management, 14*(7), 26–29.

Kim, M. J., McFarland, G. K., and McLane, A. M. (Eds.). (1984). *Classification and Nursing Diagnoses: Proceedings of the Fifth National Conference.* St. Louis: Mosby.

Lang, N. M, Hudgins, C., Jacox, A., et al. (1995). Toward a national database for nursing practice. In ANA Database Steering Committee, *An Emerging Framework for the Profession: Data System Advances for Clinical Nursing Practice.* Washington, D.C.: American Nurses Association.

Lindberg, D. (1977). *The Growth of Medical Information Systems in the United States.* Lexington, MA: The Lexington Books.

Lun, K. C., DeGoulet, P., Piemme, T. E., and Rienhoff, O. (Eds.). (1992). *MEDINFO 93: Proceedings of the Seventh World Congress on Medical Informatics.* Amsterdam: North-Holland.

Lysaught, J. P. (1973). *From Abstract into Action.* New York: McGraw-Hill.

Mantas, J. (1998). A new perspective in nursing informatics education in Europe. In J. Mantas (Ed.), *Advances in Health Telematics Education: A Nightingale Perspective* (pp. 102–113). Athens, Greece: IOS Press.

Martin, K. S. and Scheet, N. J. (1992). *The Omaha System, Applications for Community Health Nursing.* Philadelphia: W. B. Saunders.

Martin, K. S. and Sheet, N. J. (1995). The Omaha system: nursing diagnoses, interventions, and client outcomes. In ANA Database Committee, *Nursing Data Systems: The Emerging Framework* (pp. 105–113). Washington, D.C.: ANA.

Mayers, M. (1974). *Standard Nursing Care Plans.* Palo Alto, CA: K.P. Co. Medical Systems.

McCloskey, J. C. and Bulechek, G. M. (Eds.). (1992). *Nursing Interventions Classification (NIC): Iowa Intervention Project.* St. Louis: Mosby.

McCormick, K. A., Lang, N., Zirlstorff, R., et al. (1994). Toward standard classification schemes for nursing language: Recommendations of the American Nurses Association Database Steering Committee to Support Nursing Practice. *Journal of the American Medical Informatics Association, 1,* 422–427.

McDonald, C. J., Tierney, W. M., Overhage, J. M., Dexter, P., Takesue, B., and Abernathy, G. (1997). The three legged stool: Regenstief Institute for Health Care. In J. M. Tiech (Ed.), *Third Annual Nicholas E. Davies CPR Recognition Symposium Proceedings* (pp. 101–123). Schaumburg, IL: Computer-based Patient Record Institute.

McNeely, L. D. (1983). Preparation and data base development. In National Institutes of Health, *1st National Conference: Computer Technology and Nursing* (pp. 17–25) (NIH Pub. # 83-2142). Bethesda, MD: NIH, PHS, US DHHS.

McNeill, D. G. (1979). Developing the complete computer-based information system. *Journal of Nursing Administration, 9*(12), 34–46.

Milholland, D. K. (1992, July/August). Congress says informatics is nursing specialty. *American Nurse,* (24), 10.

Mikan, K. J. (1992). Implementation process for computer-supported education. In J. M. Arnold and G. A. Pearson (Eds.), *Computer Applications in Nursing Education and Practice* (pp. 191–199). New York: National League for Nursing (Publication No. 14-2406).

Montag, M. (1954). Experimental programs in nursing education. *Nursing Outlook, 2*(12), 620–621.

Mortensen, R. A. (Ed.). (1996). *The International Classification for Nursing Practice—ICNP with TELENURSE Introduction.* Copenhagen, Denmark: The Danish Institute for Health and Nursing Research.

Namdi, M. F. and Hutelmyer, C. M. (1970). A study of the effectiveness of an assessment tool in the identification of nursing care problems. *Nursing Research, 19*(4), 354–358.

National Advisory Council on Nurse Education and Practice. (1997). *A National Informatics Agenda for Nurse Education and Practice, December 1997.* Rockville, MD: Division of Nursing, BHP, HRSA, DHHS.

National Center for Health Services Research. (1980). *Computer Applications in Health Care* (NCHSR Research Report Series, DHHS Pub. No. 80–3251). Hyattsville, MD.

National Commission on Health and Vital Statistics. (1996). *Report: Core Health Care Data Elements.* Washington, D.C.: GPO (Pub No. 1996-1722-677/82345).

National Institutes of Health. (1983). *1st National Conference: Computer Technology and Nursing* (NIH Pub. # 83-2142). Bethesda, MD: NIH, PHS, US DHHS.

National Institutes of Health. (1984). *2nd National Conference: Computer Technology and Nursing* (NIH Pub. # 84-2623). Bethesda, MD: NIH, PHS, US DHHS.

National Institutes of Health. (1992). *Patient Outcomes Research: Examining the Effectiveness of Nursing Practice* (NIH Pub. No. 93-3411). Bethesda, MD: NIH, PHS, US DHHS.

National Institutes of Health. (1994). *The Clinical Center Medical Information System at the National Institutes of Health.* Bethesda, MD: Clinical Center Communications.

National League for Nursing. (1974). *Management Information Systems for Public Health/Community Health Agencies: Report of the Conference.* New York.

National League for Nursing. (1975). *Management Information Systems for Public Health/Community Health Agencies: Workshop Papers.* New York.

National League for Nursing. (1976). *State of the Art in Management Information Systems for Public Health/Community Health Agencies: Report of a Conference.* New York.

National League for Nursing. (1978). *Selected Management Information Systems for Public Health/Community Health Agencies.* New York.

National Library of Medicine. (1986). *Building and Organizing the Library's Collection: Report of Panel 1.* Bethesda, MD: NIH, PHS, US DHHS.

NCNR Priority Expert Panel on Nursing Informatics. (1993). *Nursing Informatics: Enhancing Patient Care* (NIH Publication No. 93-2419). Bethesda, MD: National Center for Nursing Research, NIH, PHS, US DHHS.

Nicoll, L. H. (1998). *Nurses Guide to the Internet,* 2nd Ed. New York: Lippincott.

Nielsen, G. H. (1995). Diagnostic labels in nursing and their semantics. In R. A. Mortensen (Ed.), *Creating a European Platform: Proceedings of the First European Conference on Nursing Diagnoses* (pp. 70–95). Copenhagen, Denmark: Danish Institute for Health and Nursing Research.

Nightingale, F. (1946). *Notes on Nursing, What It Is and What It Is Not* (facsimile of 1859 edition). Philadelphia: Lippincott.

North American Nursing Diagnosis Association. (1990). *Taxonomy I Revised–1990.* St. Louis.

North American Nursing Diagnosis Association. (1992). *NANDA: Nursing Diagnosis: Definitions and Classifications.* St. Louis.

NursingCenter.com (1999). *NursingCenter.com.* New York, NY: Lippincott.

Office of the Secretary. (1988). *Secretary's Commission on Nursing: Final Report* (Vol. 1). Washington, D.C.: US DHHS.

Orem, D. E. (1971). *Nursing: Concepts in Practice.* New York: McGraw-Hill.

Ozbolt, J.G. (1996). From minimum data to maximum impact: Using clinical data to strengthen patient care. *Advanced Practice Nursing Quarterly, 1*(4), 62–69.

Peterson, H. E. and Gerdin-Jelger, U. (Eds.). (1988). *Preparing Nurses for Using Information Systems Recommended Informatics Competencies.* (Pub. No. 14-2234) New York: National League for Nursing.

Pocklington, D. B. and Guttman, L. (1984). *Nursing Reference for Computer Literature.* Philadelphia: Lippincott.

Problem Knowledge Couplers. (1996). *Working with Problem Knowledge Couplers.* Burlington, VT: PKC Corp.

Pryor, A. T. (1992). Current state of computer-based record systems. In M. J. Ball and M. F. Collen (Eds.), *Aspects of the Computer-Based Patient Record* (pp. 67–82). New York: Springer-Verlag.

Pryor, T. A., Califf, R. M., Harrell, F. E., et al. (1985). Clinical data bases. *Medical Care, 23*(5), 623–647.

Rieder, K. A. and Norton, D. A. (1984). An integrated nursing information system: A planning model. *Computers in Nursing, 2*(3), 73–79).

Rizzolo, M. A. (Ed.). (1994). *Interactive Video: Expanding Horizons in Nursing.* New York, NY: American Journal of Nursing CO.

Roberts, M. (1954). *American Nursing: History and Interpretation.* New York: Macmillan.

Rockland County Health Department. (1971). *Rockland County Pilot Study: Nursing Care of the Sick* (Contract No. H 108-67-35). Washington, D.C.: Division of Nursing, HRA, US DHEW.

Romano, C., McCormick, K., and McNeely, L. (1982). Nursing documentation: A model for a computerized data base. *Advances in Nursing Science, 4*, 43–56.

Ronald, J. S. and Skiba, D. J. (1987). *Guidelines for Basic Computer Education in Nursing.* New York: National League for Nursing.

Saba, V. K. (1981b). How computers influence nursing activities in community health. In National Institutes of Health, *1st National Conference: Computer Technology and Nursing* (pp. 7–12). Bethesda, MD: National Institutes of Health, PHS, US DHEW.

Saba, V. K. (1981a). A comparative study of document retrieval system of nursing interest (Dissertation No. 8124656). *Dissertation Abstracts International, 42*(5), 1837 A.

Saba, V. K. (1981b). How computers influence nursing activities in community health. In National Institutes of Health, *1st National Conference: Computer Technology and Nursing* (pp. 7–12). Bethesda, MD: National Instiues of Health, PHS. US DHEW.

Saba, V. K. (1982). The computer in public health: Today and tomorrow. *Nursing Outlook, 30*(9), 510–514.

Saba, V. K., (1992). The classification of home health care nursing diagnoses and interventions. *CARING Magazine, 11*(3), 50–57.

Saba, V. K. (1995b). A new nursing vision: The information highway. *Nursing Leadership Forum, 1*(2), 44–51.

Saba, V.K. (1995a). Home Health Care Classifications (HHCCs): Nursing diagnoses and nursing interventions. In ANA Database Committee, *Nursing Data Systems: The Emerging Framework* (pp. 50–60). Washington, D.C.: ANA.

Saba, V. K. (1996). Developing a home page for the World Wide Web. *American Journal of Infection Control, 24*(6), 468–470.

Saba, V. K. (1997). Why the home health care classification is a recognized nursing nomenclature. *Computers in Nursing, 15*(2S), S69–S76.

Saba, V. K. (1998). Nursing information technology: Classifications and management. In J. Mantas (Ed.), *Advances in Health Education: A Nightingale Perspective.* Amsterdam: IOS Press.

Saba, V.K. (2000) *Distance Education Using Teleconferencing.* Bethesda, MD: Uniformed Services University of the Health Sciences.

Saba, V.K., Carr, R., Sermeus, W., and Rocha, P. (Eds.). (2000). *Nursing Informatics 2000: One Step Beyond: The Evolution of Technology and Nursing.* Auckland, NZ: Adis Inc.

Saba, V. K., Johnson, J. E., and Simpson, R. L. (1994). *Computers in Nursing Management.* Washington, DC: American Nurses Association.

Saba, V. K. and Levine, E. (1981). Patient care module in community health nursing. In H. Werley and M. Grier (Eds.), *Nursing Information Systems* (pp. 243–262). New York: Springer.

Saba, V. K., Oatway, D. M., and Rieder, K. A. (1989). How to use nursing information sources. *Nursing Outlook, 37*(4), pp. 189–195.

Saba, V. K. and Skapik, K. (1979). Nursing information center. *American Journal of Nursing, 79*(1), 86–87.

Salamon, R., Blum, B. I., and Jorgenses (Eds.). (1996). *MEDINFO 96* (Vols. 1-2). *Proceedings of the Fifth World Congress on Medical Informatics.* Amsterdam: North-Holland.

Scholes, M., Bryant, Y., and Barber, B. (Eds.). (1983). *The Impact of Computers on Nursing: An International Review.* Amsterdam: North-Holland.

Seymer, L. R. (1954). *Selected Writings of Florence Nightingale.* New York: Macmillan.

Simmons, D. A. (1982). Computer implementation in ambulatory care: A community health model. In NIH, *2nd National Conference: Computer Technology in Nursing* (pp. 19–23). Bethesda, MD: NIH, PHS, US DHEW.

Skiba, D. J., Ronald, J. S., and Simpson, R. L. (1992). HealthQuest/HBO Nurse Scholars Program: A corporate partnership with nursing education. In J. M. Arnold and G. A. Pearson (Eds.), *Computer Applications in Nursing Education and Practice* (pp. 227–235). New York: National League for Nursing (Publication No. 14-2406).

Smith, E. J. (1974). The computers and nursing practice. *Supervisor Nurse, 5*(9), 55–62.

Somers, J. (1971). A computerized nursing care system. *Hospitals, 45*(8), 93–100.

Sparks, S. (1996). Use of the Internet for infection control and epidemiology. *American Journal of Infection Control, 24*(6), 435–439.

Study Group on Nursing Information Systems. (1983). Special report: Computerized nursing information systems: An urgent need. *Research in Nursing and Health, 6*(3), 101–105.

Taylor, D. B. and Johnson, O. H. (1974). *Systematic Nursing Assessment: A Step Toward Automation* (DHEW Publication No. 7417). Washington, D.C.: U.S. Government Printing Office.

Technical Services, Veterans Affairs (1998, October). Veterans Health Information Systems Technology Architecture: VISTA. Clinical Applications. Chicago, IL: Department of Veterans Affairs.

Teich, J. M. (Ed.). (1997). *Third Annual Nicholas E. Davies CPR Recognition Symposium Proceeding.* Schaumburg, IL: Computer-based Patient Record Institute.

Valbona, C. and Spencer, W. A. (1974). Texas Institute for Research and Rehabilitation Hospital Computer System (Houston). In M. Collen (Ed.), *Hospital Computer Systems* (pp. 662–700). New York: John Wiley.

Van Bemmel, J. H., Ball, M. S., and Wigertz, O. (Eds.). (1983). *MEDINFO 83* (Vols. 1–2). Amsterdam: North-Holland.

Van Bemmel, J. H. and Musen, M. A. (Eds.). (1997). *Handbook of Medical Informatics*. The Netherlands: Springer-Verlag.

Verhey, M. P., Levy. J. R., and Schmidt, R. (1998). *RN Information: Searching for Lifelong Learning in Nursing*. Glendale, CA: Cinhal Information Systems.

Visiting Nurse Association of Omaha, (1986). *Client Management Information System for Community Health Nursing Agencies*. Rockville, MD: Division of Nursing, BHP, HRSA, PHS, US DHHS. (NTIS Pub. HRP–0907023).

Vreeland, E. M. (1964). Trends in nursing education reflected in the federal medical services. *Military Medicine, 129*(5), 415–422.

Weed, L. (1969). *Medical Records, Medical Education and Patient Care*. Cleveland: Case Western Reserve University Press.

Werley, H. (1981). Nursing data accumulation: Historical perspective. In H. Werley and M. Grier (Eds.), *Nursing Information Systems* (pp.1–10). New York: Springer.

Werley, H. and Grier, M. (Eds.). (1981). *Nursing Information Systems*. New York: Springer.

Werley, H. and Lang, N. M. (Eds.). (1988). *Identification of the Nursing Minimum Data Set*. New York: Springer.

White House Domestic Policy Council. (1993). *The Clinton Blueprint: The President's Health Security Plan*. Washington, D.C.: The White House.

World Health Organization (1992a). *International Statistical Classification of Diseases and Health Related Problems: Tenth Revision* (ICD-10). Geneva, Switzerland: WHO.

World Health Organization (1992b). *Report of a WHO Workshop on "Nursing Informatics."* Geneva, Switzerland: WHO.

World Health Organization (1993). *Report of a Nursing Management Information System*. Geneva, Switzerland: WHO.

Zielstorff, R. D., Hudgings, C. I., and Grobe, S. J. (1993). *Nursing Information Systems: Essential Characteristics for Professional Practice*. Washington, D.C.: American Nurses Association.

Zielstorff, R. D., McHugh, M. L., and Clinton, J. (1988). *Computer Design Criteria: For Systems That Support the Nursing Process*. Kansas City, MO: American Nurses Association.

Selected Reading

Abu-Saad, H. H. (1995). Nursing diagnosis in nursing education. In R. A. Mortensen (Ed.)., *Creating a European Platform: Proceedings of the First European Conference on Nursing Diagnoses* (pp. 244–248). Copenhagen: Danish Institute for Health and Nursing Research.

Amatayakul, M. (1999). Modeling CPR outcomes. In *Proceedings of the 1999 Annual HIMSS Conference: Volume 4* (pp. 1–7). Chicago: HIMSS Publications.

Austin, C. J. (1979). *Information Systems for Hospital Administration*. Ann Arbor, MI: Health Administration Press.

Boisvert, C. (1995). The nursing diagnosis: Revolution or evolution. In R. A. Mortensen (Ed.), *Creating a European Platform: Proceedings of the First European Conference on Nursing Diagnoses* (pp. 249–253). Copenhagen: Danish Institute for Health and Nursing Research.

Ball, M. (1973). Fifteen hospital information systems available. In M. Ball (Ed.), *How to Select a Computerized Hospital Information System* (pp. 10–27). Basel, Switzerland: S. Karger.

Ball, M. (1974). Medical data processing in the United States. *Hospital Finance Management, 28*(1), 10–30.

Ball, M. J. and Hannah, K. J. (1984). *Using Computers in Nursing*. Reston, VA: Reston Publishing.

Blum, B. I. (Ed.). (1982). *Computers and Medicine: Information Systems for Patient Care*. New York: Springer-Verlag.

Blum, B. (1982). *Proceedings: The Sixth Annual Symposium on Computer Applications in Medical Care*. New York: IEEE Computer Society Press.

Bridgman, M. (1953). *Collegiate Education for Nursing*. New York: Russell Sage Foundation.

Bronzino, J. D. (1982). *Computer Applications for Patient Care*. Reading, MA: Addison-Wesley.

Brown, E. L. (1948). *Nursing for the Future*. New York: Russell Sage Foundation.

Bullough, B. and Bullough, V. (1966). *Issues on Nursing*. New York: Springer.

Campbell, K. E., Oliver, D. E., Spackman, K. A., and Shortliffe, E. H. (1998). Representing thoughts, words, and things in UMLS. *Journal of the American Medical Informatics Association, 5*(5), 421–431.

Carty, B. (2000). *Nursing Informatics: Education for Practice*. New York: Springer.

Casey, A. (1995). Standard terminology for nursing: Results of the nursing midwifery and health visiting terms project. *Health Informatics, 1*, 41–43.

Cohen, G. (Ed.). (1984). *Proceedings: The Eighth Annual Symposium on Computer Applications in Medical Care*. New York: IEEE Computer Society Press.

Collen, M. F. (1983). General requirements for clinical departmental systems. In J. H. Van Bemmel, M. J. Ball, and O. Wigertz (Eds.), *MEDINFO 83* (pp. 736–739). Amsterdam: North-Holland.

Collen, M. F. (Ed.). (1974). *Hospital Computer Systems*. New York: John Wiley.

Cornell, S. and Bush, F. (1971). Systems approach to nursing care plans. *American Journal of Nursing, 71*(7), 1376–1378.

Cote, R. A., Rothwell, D. J., Beckett, R. S., and Palotay, J. L.(Eds.). (1993). *SNOMED International: The*

Systematized Nomenclature of Human and Veterinary Medicine. Northfield, IL: College of American Pathologists.

Dayhoff, R. E. (Ed.). (1983). *Proceedings: The Seventh Annual Symposium on Computer Applications in Medical Care*. New York: IEEE Computer Society Press.

Donnelley, G. F., Mangel, A., and Sutterley, D. C. (1980). *The Nursing System: Issues, Ethics, and Politics*. New York: John Wiley.

Edmunds, L. (1983). Making the most of a message function for nursing services. In R. Dayhoff (Ed.), *Proceedings: The Seventh Annual Symposium on Computer Applications in Medical Care* (pp. 511–513). New York: IEEE Computer Society Press.

Ehnfors, M. (1995). Documentation of nursing diagnosis and patient problems in nursing records in Sweden. In R. A. Mortensen (Ed.). *Creating A European Platform: Proceedings of the First European Conference on Nursing Diagnoses* (pp. 148–156). Copenhagen: Danish Institute for Health and Nursing Research.

Federal Security Agency. (1950). *The United States Cadet Nurse Corps*. Washington, D.C.: U.S. Government Printing Office.

Fedorowicz, J. (1983). Will your computer meet your case-mix information needs? *Nursing and Health Care, 4*(9), 493–497.

Fiddleman, R. H. and Kerlin, B. D. (1980). *Preliminary Assessment of COSTAR V at the North (San Diego) County Health Services Project* (Grant No. CS-D-000001-03-0). McLean, VA: The MITRE Corporation.

Flynn, J. B., Foerst, H., and Heffron, P. B. (1984). Nursing: Past and present. In J. B. McCann/Flynn and P. B. Heffron (Eds.), *Nursing: From Concept to Practice* (pp. 237–258). Bowie, MD: Robert J. Brady.

Fordyce, E. M. (1984). Theorists in nursing. In J. B. McCann/Flynn and P. B. Heffron (Eds.), *Nursing: From Concept to Practice* (pp. 237–258). Bowie, MD: Robert J. Brady.

Gebbie, K. M. (Ed.). (1976). *Summary of the Second National Conference: Classification of Nursing Diagnoses*. St. Louis: National Group for Classification of Nursing Diagnoses.

Goldmark, J. (1923). *Nursing and Nursing Education in the United States*. New York: Macmillan.

Gordon, M. (1981). Identifying data through the nursing diagnosis approach. In H. Werley and M. Grier (Eds.), *Nursing Information Systems* (pp. 32–35). New York: Springer.

Grobe, S. J. (1984). *Computer Primer and Resource Guide for Nurses*. Philadelphia: Lippincott.

Hannah, K. J. (1976). The computer and nursing practice. *Nursing Outlook, 24*(9), 555–558.

Health Care Financing Administration (HCFA). (1983). *HCFA Legislative Summary: Prospective Payment Revision: Title VI of the Social Security Amendment* (PL 98-21, No. 381-858:343). Washington, D.C.: U.S. Government Printing Office.

Henderson, V. (1966). *The Nature of Nursing*. New York: Macmillan.

Henderson, V. (1973). On nursing care plans and their history. *Nursing Outlook, 21*(6), 378–379.

Henderson, V. and Nite, G. (1978). *Principles and Practice of Nursing* (6th ed.). New York: Macmillan.

Hope, G. S. (1984). Delivery system and nursing in the 21st century. In J. M. Virgo (Ed.), *Health Care: An International Perspective* (pp. 215–224). Edwardsville, IL: International Health Economics and Management Institute.

Hudgings, C. (1991). An international nursing library: Worldwide access to nursing research databases. In E. S. Hovenga, K. J. Hannah, K. A. McCormick, and J. S. Ronald (Eds.), *Nursing Informatics '91* (pp. 780–784). New York: Springer-Verlag.

International Council of Nurses. (1993). *Nursing's Next Advance: An International Classification for Nursing Practice (ICNP). A Working Paper*. Geneva, Switzerland.

Kalish, P. A. and Kalish, B. J. (1977). *Federal Influence and Impact on Nursing* (NTIS Publication No. HRP-0900636). Annandale, VA: National Technical Information Service.

Kerlin, B. and Greene, P. (1981). *COSTAR: An Overview and Annotated Bibliography* (Contract No. 233-79-3201). McLean, VA: The MITRE Corporation.

Mayers, M. G. (1972). *A Systematic Approach to the Nursing Care Plan*. New York: Appleton-Century Crofts.

McCann/Flynn, J. B. and Heffron, P. B. (Eds.). (1984). *Nursing: From Concept to Practice*. Bowie, MD: Robert J. Brady.

McCloskey, J. (1981). Nursing care plans and problem-oriented health records. In H. Werley and M. Grier (Eds.), *Nursing Information Systems* (pp. 119–126). New York: Springer.

McCormack, C. and Jones, D. (1998). *Building a Web-Based Education System*. New York, NY: Wiley Computer Publications.

McCormick, K. A. (1996). *Nursing in the 21st Century Guideposts in an Information Age*. Paper delivered at the Royal College of Nursing Australia, Annual Meeting. Parliament House, Canberra, Australia.

McCormick, K.A. and Kover, C. (1997). The role of the Agency for Health Care Policy and Research in improving outcomes of care. *Nursing Clinics of North America, 32*(3), 521–521.

McDonald, C. J. and Barnett, G. O. (1990). Medical-record systems. In E. H. Shortliffe and L. E. Perreault (Eds.). *Medical Informatics: Computer Applications in Health Care* (pp. 181–218). Reading, MA: Addison-Wesley Publishing.

McFarland, G. K., Leonard, H. S., and Morris, M. M. (1984). *Nursing Leadership and Management: Contemporary Strategies.* New York: John Wiley.

Medical Information Resources Management Office. (1991). *Decentralized Hospital Computer Program.* Salt Lake City, UT: Department of Veterans Affairs, Veterans Health Administration.

Naisbitt, J. (1982). *Megatrends: Ten New Directions Transforming Our Lives.* New York: Warner Books.

National Center for Health Services Research. (1979). *Automation of the Problem-Oriented Medical Record* (NCHSR Research Summary Series, DHEW Publication No. HRA 77-31770). Rockville, MD.

National Center for Health Services Research. (1976). *The Program in Health Services Research* (DHEW Publication No. [HRA] 78-3136). Hyattsville, MD.

National Library of Medicine. (1981). *MEDLARS: The Computerized Literature Retrieval Services of the National Library of Medicine* (NIH Brochure Pub. No. 83-1286). Bethesda, MD.

National League for Nursing Education. (1937). *A Study of Nursing Services in Fifty Selected Hospitals.* New York.

National Library of Medicine. (December). *Report of Panel 4: Long Range Plan: Medical Informatics.* Rockville, MD: NIH, PHS, DHHS.

New Jersey State Department of Health. (1969). *Study of Home Health Agencies in New Jersey* (Contract No. 1-NU-04147). Hyattsville, MD: Division of Nursing, HRA, US DHEW.

Office of Technology Assessment. (1983). *Diagnoses Related Groups (DRGs) and the Medical Program: The Implications for Medical Technology* (Technical Memorandum OTA-TM-H-17). Washington, D.C.: U.S. Congress, Office of Technology Assessment.

Piemme, T. E. and Ricnhoff, O. (Eds.). *MEDINFO '92* (pp. 1496–1500), Amsterdam: North-Holland.

Pritchard, K. (1982). Computers 3: Possible applications in nursing. *Nursing Times, 78*(8), 465–466.

Pritchard, K. (1982). Computers 4: Implication of computerization. *Nursing Times, 78*(8), 491–492.

Randall, A. M. (1984). Surviving the 80s and beyond: Strategic planning for health care data processing. In J. M. Virgo (Ed.), *Health care: An International Perspective* (pp. 115–132). Edwardsville, IL: International Health Economics and Management Institute.

Rogers, M. E. (1970). *An Introduction to the Theoretical Basis of Nursing.* Philadelphia: Davis.

Rosenberg, M. and Carriker, D. (1966). Automating nurses' notes. *American Journal of Nursing, 66*(5), 1021–1023.

Roy, C. (1975). A diagnostic classification system for nursing. *Nursing Outlook, 23*(2), 90–94.

Saranto, K. (1997). *Outcomes of Education in Information Technology: Towards a Model of Nursing Informatics Education.* Turun, Yliopisto: University of Turku.

Sermeus, W. (1995). Nursing diagnosis in nursing management. In R. A. Mortensen (Ed.), *Creating A European Platform: Proceedings of the First European Conference on Nursing Diagnoses* (pp. 254–20). Copenhagen: Danish Institute for Health and Nursing Research.

Stewart, S. A. CD-ROM: 1995 *Interactive Healthcare Directory.* Alexandria, VA: Stewart Publishing.

Stewart, I. M. (1943). *The Education of Nurses: Historical Foundations and Modern Trends.* New York: Macmillan.

Stratman, W. C. (1979). *A Demonstration of PROMIS* (NCHSR Research Summary Series, DHEW Pub. No. [PHS] 79-3247). Hyattsville, MD: National Center for Health Services.

Sweeney, M. A. and Olivieri, P. (1981). *An Introduction to Nursing Research.* Philadelphia: Lippincott.

Thede, L. Q. (1999). *Computers in Nursing: Bridges to the Future.* New York: Lippincott.

Veazie, S. and Dankmyer, T. (1977). HISs, MISs and DBMSs: Sorting out the letters. *Hospitals, 51*(20), 80–84.

Virgo, J. M. (Ed.). (1984). *Health Care: An International Perspective.* Edwardsville, IL: International Health Economics and Management Institute.

Wesseling, E. (1972). Automating the nursing history and care plan. *Journal of Nursing Administration, 2*(3), 34–38.

Young, D. A. (1984). Prospective payment assessment commission: Mandate, structure and relationships. *Nursing Economics, 2,* 309–311.

Yura, H. and Walsh, M. B. (1973). *The Nursing Process: Assessing, Planning, Implementing, Evaluating* (2nd ed.). New York: Appleton-Century-Crofts.

Zielstorff, R. D. (Ed.). (1980). *Computers in Nursing.* Wakefield, MA: Nursing Resources.

PART 2

Computer Systems

CHAPTER 3

Computer Hardware

Mary L. McHugh

OBJECTIVES

1. List the key hardware components of a computer and their four basic operations of the CPU.
2. Describe how power is measured for computers.
3. Describe common computer input, output, and storage devices.
4. Discuss the history of computers.
5. Describe the three classes of computers and key functionality of each class.
6. Describe computer network/communications devices and functionality.

KEY WORDS

information systems
computer science
software
hardware

Computer technology has evolved from huge electronic calculators developed with military funding during World War II to desktop-sized information processing machines available to virtually everybody. Today, computer processors are encountered in most areas of people's lives. From the grocery store to the movie theater; from infusion pumps to physiologic monitors; from the kitchen to the high tech office in Silicon Valley, computer processors are employed so widely that the late 20th century can accurately be described as the beginning of the information age.

Computer hardware advances during the late 1900s have made possible many changes to the health care industry. The first operations to be modified were special administrative functions such as finance, payroll, billing, and nurse staffing and scheduling support. Later, the computer allowed fantastic changes in the practice of radiology and imaging, allowing noninvasive visualization of the human body that heretofore could only be performed in surgery (Karasov, 1982; Mariani, 1988). Computers are now pervasive throughout the health care industry. Their applications are expected to continue to expand and thereby improve the quality of health care while at the same time reducing some costs. Most important, the applications of computers to health

care will greatly expand the diagnostic and therapeutic abilities of practitioners and broaden the options available to recipients of health care. Additionally, telemedicine will be used to reduce the impact of distance and location on accessibility and availability of health care (Author Unknown [*Health Devices*], 1999; Chaffee, 1999; Wallace et al., 1998). None of these changes could have happened without tremendous advances in the machinery, the hardware, of computers.

This chapter covers various aspects of computer hardware: components and their functions, classes of computers, and their characteristics and types. It also highlights the functional components of the computer and describes the devices and media used to communicate, store, and process data. Major topics addressed include basic computer concepts and classes and types of computers, components, and computer communications.

A computer is a machine that uses electronic components and instructions to the components to perform calculations and repetitive and complex procedures, process text, and manipulate data and signals. The **hardware** of a computer is defined as all of the physical components of the machine. The basic hardware of a computer includes the electronic circuits, microchips, processors, input and output devices (peripherals)

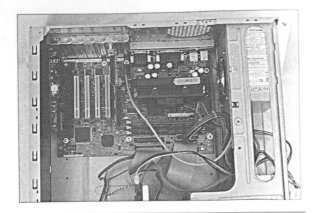

Figure 3.1
Computer box with components loaded.
(Reproduced, with permission, from Rosenthal M. *Build Your Own PC*. New York NY, McGraw-Hill, 1999:82.)

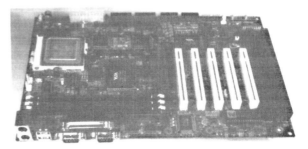

Figure 3.2
Motherboard with CPU, chips, and slots.
(Reproduced, with permission, from Pilgrim A. *Build Your Own Pentium III PC*. New York, NY, McGraw-Hill, 2000:34.)

attached to the computer, and storage components such as the hard drive, floppy drives, tape drives, etc. Typical computer systems consist of many different component parts, including external or peripheral devices that enable the computer to communicate with other computers and produce work. The group of required and optional hardware items that are linked together to make up a computer is called its configuration. When computers are sold, many of the key components are placed inside a rigid plastic case called the **box**. What can typically be seen from the outside is a box (Fig. 3.1) containing the internal components, a keyboard, a monitor, speakers, and a printer. To understand how a computer processes data, it is necessary to examine the component parts and devices that comprise computer hardware.

Computer Hardware Fundamentals

The box of any computer contains a **motherboard** (Fig. 3.2). The motherboard is a thin, flat sheet made of a firm, nonconducting material on which the internal components—printed circuits, chips, slots, etc.—of the computer are mounted. The motherboard is made of a **dielectric** or nonconducting plastic material, and the electric conductions are etched or soldered onto the bottom of the board. The motherboard has holes or perforations through which components can be affixed (Fig. 3.3). Typically, one side looks like a maze of soldered metal trails with sharp projections (which are the attach-

ments of the chips and other components affixed to the motherboard). On one side, can be seen the microchips, wiring, and slots for adding components. The specific design of the components—especially the CPU and other microprocessors—is called the computer's architecture.

A computer has four basic components, although most have many more added on components. At its most basic, a computer must consist of a central processing unit (CPU), input and output controllers, and storage media.

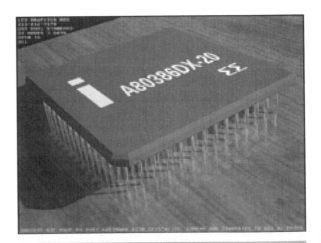

Figure 3.3
CPU chip attached to motherboard.
(Courtesy of James C. Miller)

Central Processing Unit

The CPU is the "brains" of the computer. It consists of at least one arithmetic and logic unit, a control unit, and memory. The arithmetic and logic units control mathematical functions such as addition and subtraction and functions that test logic (Boolean) conditions, such as, "Is this number being read equal to or greater than 4?" The control unit carries out the machine language functions called **fetch, execute, decode,** and **store.** For an extremely simplified example, when a command is given to add two numbers, the control unit "fetches" the instruction and numbers from their storage locations and decodes the instruction so that the proper operations can be performed. These are called the fetch and decode cycles. Then the control unit initiates the execute cycle, which sends the instruction to the arithmetic and logic unit. Finally, the control unit initiates the store cycle, which places the result of the instruction in a memory location. Memory includes the locations of the computer's internal or main working storage. Memory consists of registers (a small number of very high speed memory locations), random access memory (RAM), which is the main storage area in which the computer places the programs and data it is working upon, and cache (a small memory storage area holding recently accessed data).

Memory

There are two types of memory in the main memory of a computer. They are read only memory (ROM) and RAM.

Read Only Memory ROM is a form of permanent storage. This means that data and programs in ROM can only be read by the computer, and cannot be erased or altered. ROM generally contains the programs, called firmware, used by the control unit of the CPU to oversee computer functions. In microcomputers, this may also include the software programs used to translate the computer's high-level programming languages into machine language (binary code). ROM storage is not erased when the computer is turned off.

Random Access Memory RAM refers to working memory used for primary storage. It is volatile (changeable) and used as temporary storage. RAM can be accessed, used, changed, and written on repeatedly. It contains data and instructions that are stored and processed by computer programs called applications programs. RAM is the work area available to the CPU for all processing applications. The computer programs, which are stored on diskettes, on the hard drive, or on CD-ROM (compact disk, read only memory), are not permanent parts of the computer itself. They are loaded when needed, and they can be altered. The contents of RAM are lost whenever the power to the computer is turned off.

Input and Output

To do work, the computer must have a way of receiving commands and data from the outside and a way of reporting out its work. The motherboard has slots and circuit boards that allow the CPU to communicate with the outside world. Input and output devices are wired to a **controller** that is plugged into the slots or circuit boards of the computer. Many devices can serve as both input and output devices. Such devices as the hard drive upon which is stored most of the programs people use as well as their personal data, the disk drive upon which people store most of their personal data, and more recently, the compact disk drives serve to both receive and send information to the computer.

Input devices These allow the computer to receive information from the outside world. The most common input devices are the **keyboard** and **mouse.** Others commonly seen on nursing workstations include the **touch screen, light pen,** and **scanner.** A touch screen is actually both an input and output device combined. Electronics allow the computer to "sense" when a particular part of the screen is pressed. A light pen is a device attached to the computer that has special software that allows the computer to sense when the light pen is focused on a particular part of the screen. For both the touch screen and light pen, software interprets the meaning of that screen location to the program. Many other input devices exist. Some devices are used for security and can detect users' fingerprints, retinal prints, voiceprints, or other personally unique physical characteristics that identify users who have clearance to use the system. In health care computing, some medical devices serve as input devices. For example, the electrodes placed on a patient's body provide input into the computerized physiologic monitors.

Output Devices These allow the computer to report its results to the external world. Output can be in the form of text, data files, sound, graphics, or signals to other devices. The two most obvious output devices are the monitor (display screen) and printer.

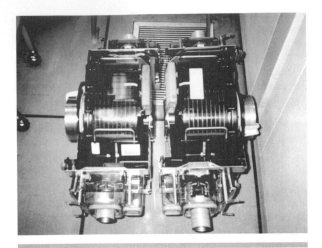

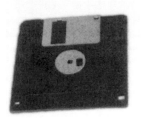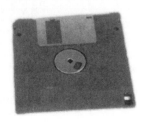

Figure 3.5
Diskette with write protect slot.
(Reproduced, with permission, from Pilgrim A. *Build Your Own Pentium III PC*. New York, NY, McGraw-Hill, 2000:165.)

Figure 3.4
Hard disk platters from an IBM mainframe computer.
(Courtesy of Akos Varga.)

Storage Media

Storage includes the main memory but also external devices on which programs and data are stored. The most common storage devices include the hard drive, diskettes, and CD-ROMs. The hard drive and diskettes are magnetic storage media. The CD-ROM is a form of optical storage. Optical media are read by a laser "eye" rather than a magnet (Hwan, 1988).

Hard Drive   The hard drive is a peripheral that has very high speed and high density. (Fig. 3.4). That is, it is a very fast means of storing and retrieving data as well as having a large storage capacity in comparison with the other types of storage.

Diskettes   The diskette drive allows input and output from a diskette, which is a round magnetic disk encased in a flexible or rigid case (Fig. 3.5). It allows the user to transport data and programs from one computer site to another.

CD-ROM   The CD-ROM is a rigid disk that holds a much higher density of information than a diskette and has a much higher speed (Fig. 3.6). Until the late 1990s, CD-ROMs were strictly input devices. However, new technology developed by Phillips Corporation permitted the development of a new type of compact disk that could be written upon by the user. These are called CD-RWs. Other output devices include magnetic tape drives

and Zip drives, which are primarily used for backing up information stored on the hard drive.

As computers became more standard in offices during the 1990s, more and more corporate and individual information was stored solely on computers. Even when paper back-up copies were kept, loss of information on the hard drive was usually inconvenient at the least and a disaster at worst. Diskettes could not store large amounts of data, so people began to search for economical and speedy ways to back up the information on their hard drives. Magnetic tape backup devices were the most commonly used media in the 1980s and 1990s. How-

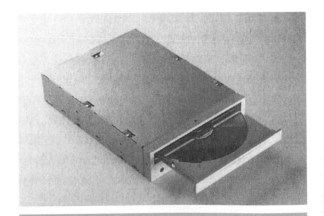

Figure 3.6
CD-ROM Drive.
(Reproduced, with permission, from Mitsumi.)

ever, they were relatively slow. In 1996, Iomega Corporation won the *Byte* Magazine's Readers' Hardware Choice Award for its development of a removable, 100-megabyte (100 million-byte) hard drive and disk product. This product, called a **Zip drive** greatly streamlined the backup process for personal computer users. Later, the company introduced its "Jaz" drive, which stores 1 gigabyte (1 billion bytes) of information.

Computer Power

The terms **bits** and **bytes** refer to how the machine stores information at the lowest, or "closest to machine registers and memory," level. Computers don't process information as words or numbers. They handle information in bytes. A byte is made up of eight bits.

Bits and Bytes

A "bit" (**b**inary dig**it**) is a unit of data in the binary numbering system. Binary means, two, so a bit can assume one of two positions. Effectively, a bit is an on/off switch—on equals the value of 1 and off equals 0. Bits are grouped into collections of eight, which then function as a unit. That unit describes a single character in the computer, such as the letter A or the number 3, and is called a "byte."

A byte looks something like this:

0	0	0	0	1	1	0	0

There are 255 different combinations of 0 and 1 in an 8-character (or 1-byte) unit. That forms the basic limit to the number of characters that can be directly expressed in the computer. Thus, the basic character set hardwired into most PCs contains 255 characters. In the early days of personal computers, this was a problem because it severely limited the images that could be produced. However, with the advent of graphics cards and additional character sets and graphics that the new technology allowed, virtually any image can be produced on a computer screen or printed on a printer. Even without graphics cards, additional character sets can be created by means of programming techniques. The size of a variety of computer functions and components is measured by how many bytes they can handle or store at one time (Table 3.1).

Main memory, which includes the ROM on the motherboard in today's computers, is very large as compared with that of even 10 years ago. Since the size of memory is an important factor in the amount of work a computer can handle, large main memory is another key measure in the power of a computer. In the early 1970s, the PCs on the market were typically sold with between 48 and 64 kilobytes of main memory. In the late 1990s, the size of main memory in computers sold to the public increased rapidly, and by the end of 1999, most computers were advertised with between 32 and 128 megabytes (MB) of main memory.

Another important selling point of a computer is the size of the hard drive that is installed in the box. The first drives sold for microcomputers in the 1970s were

Table 3.1 Meaning of Storage Size Terms

Number of Bytes	Term	Formula ($\approx$ means approximately)	Approximate Size in Typed Pages or Other Comparison
1,024	1 kilobyte (K)	$2^{10} \approx 1,000$	One-third of a single-spaced typed page
1,048,576	1 megabyte (M or MB)	$2^{20} \approx 1,024^2$	600-page paperback book
1,073,741,824	1 gigabyte (G or GB)	$2^{30} \approx 1,024^3$	Approximately 1 billion bytes or an encyclopedia
1,099,511,627,776	1 terabyte (T or TB)	$2^{40} \approx 1,024^4$	Approximately 1 trillion bytes
1,125,899,906,842,624	1 petabyte	$2^{50} \approx 1,024^5$	None available
1,152,921,504,606,846,976	1 exabyte	$2^{60} \approx 1,024^6$	About 10 to the 18th power bytes
1,180,591,620,717,411,303,424	1 zettabyte	$2^{70} \approx 1,024^7$	None available
1,208,925,819,614,629,174,706,176	1 yottabyte	$2^{80} \approx 1,024^8$	None available

external devices that stored about 1,500 Kilobytes (K). At that time, few home computers had internal hard drives. When the user turned on the computer, they had to be sure the operating system (see Chap. 4, "Software") diskette was in the disk drive, or the computer couldn't work. This architecture severely limited the size and functionality of programs. Therefore, consumer demand for hard drives was such that their size grew exponentially while at the same time cost of hard drive storage decreased exponentially. By late 1999, home computers typically sold with between 6 and 20 gigabytes of space on the hard drive. Applications programs have become so large that both the main memory and especially the hard drive storage space have had to increase exponentially. The typical hard drive sold with a microcomputer in 1990 was 80 to 100 megabytes while the hard drives advertised in 1999 typically ranged from 6 to 20 *giga*bytes.

Computer Speed

Earlier in the discussion about the CPU, it was noted that the basic operations of the CPU are called cycles (fetch, decode, execute, and store cycles). It takes time for the computer to perform each of these functions. The CPU speed is measured in cycles per second which are called the **clock speed** of the computer. One million cycles per second is called one **megahertz** (MHz). CPU speeds are very fast, and today's computers perform many millions of cycles per second. For example, the original IBM PC introduced in 1981 had a clock speed of 4.77 MHz (4.77 million cycles per second). In the late 1990s, Intel Corporation introduced its Pentium III processor, which had clock speeds of 550 MHz.

In general the more MHz possessed by the CPU, the faster and (in one dimension) the more powerful the computer. However, clock rate can be misleading, since different kinds of processors may perform a different amount of work in one cycle. For example, general purpose computers are known as complex instruction set computers (CISCs) and their processors are prepared to perform a large number of different instruction sets. Therefore, a cycle in a CISC computer may take longer than that for a specialized type of computer called a reduced instruction set computer (RISC). Nonetheless, clock speed is one important measure of the power of a computer.

Overview of Descriptive Terms Used in Computing

The computer is generally described in terms of several major characteristics that have been generally explained—

automatic, electronic, and general purpose—as well as in terms of speed, reliability, and storage capacity. The computer is **automatic** because it is self-instructed; that is, it automatically processes data using computer programs called software. The computer is **electronic** because it uses microelectronic components etched on silicon chips for its circuitry. This means that its basic building blocks are microminiaturized. The computers discussed so far are **general purpose** machines, because the user can program them to process all types of problems and can solve any problem that can be broken down into a set of logical sequential instructions. Special purpose machines designed to do only a very few different types of tasks have also been developed. An example of a special use computer is the RISC computer described above. The computer is also characterized by its **speed** and split-second processing of large amounts of data, its **reliability** due to the silicon circuitry, and its ability to **store** large amounts of data that can be retrieved quickly.

The computer is also described by its **architecture**, which refers to the design of the individual hardware components and to the microprocessor used. A key characteristic of a computer is its hardware platform, or simply, its platform. The two main types of platform in the commercial personal computer market are the IBM and Apple Macintosh platform. The two are not compatible, and without a translator, one computer cannot read the other's diskettes.

History of Computers

The first true digital computer, called the Collosus Mark I, was built in 1943 with funding from the U.S. military and used in airplane design and other complex engineering applications. At the same time, Bell Laboratories was working on development of a computer, as were two scientists at the University of Pennsylvania, J. Presper Eckert and John Mauchly, later founders of Eckert-Mauchly Corporation.

The prototype World War II military computers were very different from today's computers. First, they were big. A computer with much less power than an ordinary desktop computer of the 1990s took up an entire room. Second, there were relatively few operations they could perform as compared with today's computers. Essentially, they were giant and complex mathematical calculators. Third, they were difficult to program. In fact, they were programmed by the scientists getting to the back of the computer and changing the wires. This approach was slow, tedious, and impractical for a commercial machine.

After the war, Eckert and Mauchly produced the first vacuum tube computer, the Electronic Numerical Integrator and Computer, more commonly known as the ENIAC (Weik, 1961). In 1950, the Remington Rand Corporation bought Eckert and Mauchly's company (Unisys, date unknown) and one year later began to market the first large scale commercial computer system, called the UNIVAC-I (Watson, 1999). In 1955, the Sperry Corporation merged with Remington Rand, forming the giant Sperry Rand Corporation. That year, the very first commercial application was run when General Electric processed its payroll on a UNIVAC computer, and the age of business computing was born. The American business establishment recognized the value of this machine that could do thousands of repetitive, mathematical calculations. In response, companies such as Bell Labs, National Cash Register (NCR), Burroughs, and IBM began to develop their business computer products. Today, these early computers are called **first generation computers**.

The Univac and other first generation computers used vacuum tubes in their design. Those computers ran hot and thus required lots of cooling. Vacuum tubes got hot easily, and when they got hot, they failed regularly. Given that those computers used many vacuum tubes, and the high (and random) failure rate of vacuum tubes, the early computers were a real challenge to keep operational.

For the first generation of computers, the speed of the main processor was measured in access speeds (how fast the CPU could access commands entered through punched cards). Access speeds were measured in thousandths of a second (milliseconds). First generation computers were physically huge (one computer took up a large room), but their power was much less than that of the average desktop computer of the 1900s. Main memory was less than 10 kilobytes of storage.

Second generation computers were introduced in the late 1950s. They included the IBM 1401 and 1620. They used transistors instead of vacuum tubes. This meant less heat, improved reliability, and much greater speeds. Second generation CPU access speeds were measured in millionths rather than thousandths of a second (microseconds). They still were quite large, but transistors were smaller and more durable than vacuum tubes. They also allowed for the development of much more powerful computers.

Third generation computers were introduced in the mid-1960s. These used microminiature, solid state components. Third generation CPU access speeds were measured in billionths of a second (nanoseconds). The IBM 360 and 370 were the classic computers in this genera-

tion. They had about 110 K of main memory, and it was this generation in which hard disk drives were introduced. Those hard disks were not encased in protective plastic cases, so they were very vulnerable to dust. Any magnetic media is vulnerable to dirt, even the diskettes used today. However, today the hard drives are much better protected against dust than was the case in the 1960s. That is why pictures of computer rooms taken during the third generation era often show people in surgical type garb. They were trying to keep the failure rate down by keeping the computer room as clean as possible.

The Rise of the Modern Personal Computer

In November 1972, Intel Corporation introduced the first commercial microprocessor, called the Intel 8008 (Maxfield and Brown, 1997). This invention made the personal computer, or **microcomputer,** possible. Shortly thereafter, two teenaged boys named Steve Jobs and Steve Wozniak who shared an intense interest in electronics bought a microprocessor for $25 and built a very simple computer they called the "Apple" (MIT, 1996). Like Henry Ford's dream of bringing automobiles to everyone, Jobs had a passionate dream of bringing computers to everybody. They failed to interest Wozniak's employer, Hewlett-Packard Corporation (HP), in their idea to build a small computer that people could have and use in their homes (Mesa, 1997). At that time, according to legend, HP executives couldn't imagine why anyone would want such a machine in the home. They were focused on business computing, with its billing and payroll processing, and people's home finances simply didn't require such power. Not to be refused, the two Steves decided to pursue their dream anyway. They began building the machines in Steve Jobs' garage, and in May of 1976, they introduced their first computer at a meeting of the Homebrew Computer Club, at which Paul Terryl, president of the Byte Shop chain, ordered 50 computers (Mesa, 1997). At the time, Steve Jobs was 21 years old and Wozniak was 26. The Apple Computer Company and the first personal computer were born. (In 1999, Steve Jobs was Chairman and CEO of Pixar, the computer animation studio that won an Academy Award for its work on the motion picture, "Toy Story." The home page of Pixar may be found at *http://www.pixar.com* (Fig. 3.7).

At the same time that Jobs and Wozniak were working in the garage, IBM introduced the first **fourth generation** mainframe, the IBM 370 (Watson, 1999). This was the first mainframe family that had printed circuits. This computer was so fast that the old measurement of speed was deemed unsuitable. Since a CPU processes

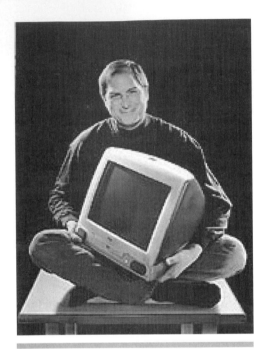

Figure 3.7
Stephen Jobs.
(Courtesy of Apple Computer, Inc.
Photographer: Moshe Brakha.)

7600, a computer 10 times more powerful than the CDC 6600, often called the first supercomputer.

Shortly thereafter, Cray and CDC parted ways over the development of a whole new concept in computer architecture that Cray wished to pursue. Unwilling to invest in this new concept, CDC did not agree to work with Cray to produce it. Therefore, in 1972, Cray decided to go into business for himself so that his dream could be realized (Breckenridge, 1996). The new company, Cray Research, in Minnesota was the result of this split. Cray Research's first product was the Cray-I supercomputer. Most consider the Cray-I to be the first true supercomputer, since its architecture was innovative and its power was orders of magnitude greater than anything that came before it. In 1989, history repeated itself, and Cray left Cray Research to open a new company in Colorado Springs. That company went bankrupt, some say due to a combination of reduced need for supercomputing due to the end of the Cold War and Cray's unwillingness to compromise speed for compatibility with other computer technology. Sadly, Cray was involved in a terrible accident and died on October 5, 1996, at the age of 71 from severe head injuries. At the time of his death, Cray was a vital, energetic, and creative man who had just founded yet another new company dedicated to the advancement of computer power and speed (Bell, 1997). Cray was truly a genius. Certainly the Father of Supercomputing, in many ways, Cray was instrumental in the development of the modern digital computer (Breckenridge, 1996; Bell, 1997), and it will never be known what further advances already in his mind were lost with him.

Classes of Computers

Three broad classes of computers exist: the analog computer, the digital computer, and the hybrid computer. Analog computers handle continuous input data, such as are found in the continuously changing electric patterns of the heartbeat. Digital computers handle input that comes in at discrete points in time, such as the workload measured at ten o'clock in the morning. The hybrid computer—as suggested by its name—is a computer that is able to process both kinds of signals.

Analog Computer

The analog computer operates on continuous physical or electrical magnitudes, measuring ongoing continuous analog quantities such as voltage, current, temperature, and pressure. Selected physiological monitoring equip-

instructions (which the CPU fetches, decodes, executes, and stores), the new CPU's speed was measured by the speed with which it could process instructions, rather than accesses. Fourth generation computer CPU speeds were (and still are today) measured by instructions per second that they can process. The IBM 370's CPU speed was measured in "millions of instructions per second" (MIPS). Today's mainframes are measured in billions of instructions per second (BIPS) or giga-instructions per second (GIPS).

Supercomputers

The first supercomputer was developed by a computer engineer named Seymour Cray (The Franklin Institute, 1999). Cray had been one of the architects of the UNIVAC (Bell, 1997). He left UNIVAC in 1957 to join in the development of a new company, Control Data Corporation (CDC), and continued his processor development work throughout the 1950s and 1960s. His work at CDC culminated in the production of the CDC ment, which accepts continuous input/output signals is in the analog class of computers. An example of these machines in the clinical setting include heart monitors and fetal monitors. An analog computer handles data in continuously variable quantities rather than breaking the data down into discrete digital representations.

Digital Computer

The digital computer, on the other hand, operates on discrete discontinuous numerical digits using the binary numbering system. It represents data using discrete values for all data. Its data are represented by numbers, letters, and symbols rather than by waveforms such as on a heart monitor. Most of the computers used in the health care industry for charting and decision support are digital computers.

Hybrid Computer

The hybrid computer, as its name implies, contains features of both the analog and the digital computer. It is used for specific applications, such as complex signal processing, and other engineering oriented applications. It is also found in some monitoring equipment that converts analog signals to digital ones for data processing. For example, physiologic monitors that are able to capture the heart waveform and also to measure the core body temperature at specific times of the shift are actually hybrid computers. Some physiological research projects can make use of hybrid computers that have analog ability to capture waveforms of physiological monitors (i.e., EKG, EEG, etc.) and convert them into digital format suitable for analysis.

Types of Computers

Today, three basic types of computers are generally recognized. Each type of computer was developed as the computer industry evolved, and each was developed for a different purpose. The basic types of computers include the supercomputer, the mainframe, and the microcomputer. They differ in size, composition, memory and storage capacity, processing time, and cost. They generally have had different applications and are found in many different locations in the health care industry.

Supercomputers

The largest type of computer is the supercomputer. A supercomputer is a computational-oriented computer

specially designed for scientific applications requiring gigantic amounts of calculations. The supercomputer is truly a world class "number cruncher." The supercomputer is designed primarily for analysis of scientific and engineering problems and for tasks requiring millions or billions of computational operations and calculations. It is found primarily in areas such as defense and weaponry, weather forecasting, and scientific research. The supercomputer is also providing a new source of power for the high-performance computing and communication (HPCC) environment.

Mainframes

The mainframe computer is the fastest, largest, and most expensive type of computer used in corporate America for processing, storing, and retrieving data. It is a large multiuser central computer that meets the computing needs—especially the large amount of repetitive calculations of bills, payroll, and the like—of a large organization. A mainframe is capable of processing billions of instructions per second and accessing billions (gigbytes) of characters of data (Figs. 3.8 and 3.9). Mainframes can serve a large number (hundreds) of users at the same time. In many settings, hundreds of terminals (input and output devices that may or may not have any processing power of their own) are wired directly onto the mainframe. Typically, there are also phone lines into the computer so that remote users can gain access to the main-

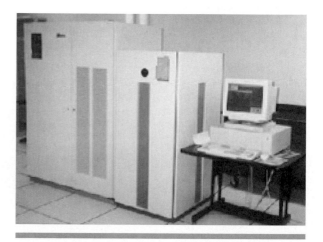

Figure 3.8
Hitachi 2 mainframe computer.
(Reproduced, with permission, from Wright State University, Dayton, OH.)

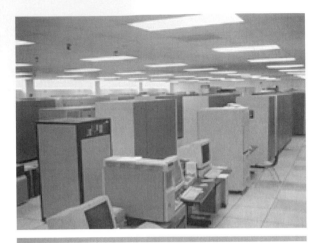

Figure 3.9
IBM mainframe computer room at Virginia Poly-
technic and State University, circa 1996.
(Reproduced, with permission, from Virginia Polytechnic and
State University, Blacksburg, VA. *http://black-ice.cc.vt.edu.*
Photographer: Valdis Kletnieks.)

frame. As compared with a desktop personal computer, a
mainframe has an extremely large memory capacity and
fast operating and processing time, and it can process a
large number of functions (multiprocessing) at one time.

Microcomputers (Personal Computers)

While mainframe computers provide critical service to
the health care industry, microcomputers are being used

for an increasing number of independent applications as
well as serving as a desktop link to the programs of the
mainframe (Fig. 3.10). Hospital nursing departments
are using PCs to process specific applications such as
patient classification, nurse staffing and scheduling, and
personnel management applications. Microcomputers
are also found in educational and research settings,
where they are used to conduct a multitude of special
educational and scientific functions. Desktops are
replacing many of the mainframe attributes. Desktops
can serve as stand-alone workstations and can be linked
to a network system to increase their capabilities. This
is advantageous, since software multiuser licensing fees
are usually less expensive per user than having each user
purchase his or her own copy.

Microcomputer Sizes   Microcomputers are also
available as portable, laptop, notebook, and hand-held
computers. The portable and laptop versions are smaller
than the standard desktop microcomputer. The notebook microcomputer is generally 8½ by 11 inches and
weighs approximately 4 pounds. Hand-held computers
are small, special function computers, although a few
"full function" hand held computers were introduced in
the late 1990s. Even though of smaller size than the
standard desktop microcomputer, some have the same
size memory, storage capacity, and processing capabilities
as the standard desktop microcomputer. However, they
are limited in their expansion possibilities, their ability to
serve as full participants in the office network, and the
peripherals they can support. They are invaluable to the
busy professional who must travel and wishes to con-

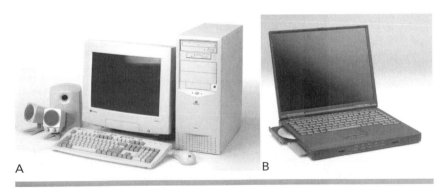

A   B

Figure 3.10
Gateway desktop (A) and notebook (B) computers.
(© 2000 Gateway, Inc. Photos courtesy of Gateway, Inc.)

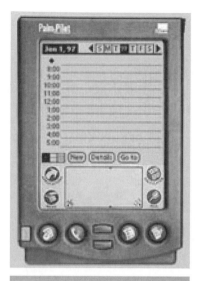

Figure 3.11
Palm Pilot.

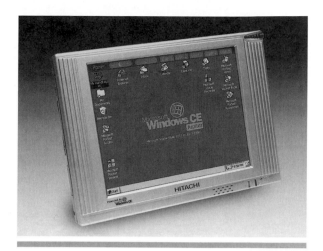

Figure 3.13
Hitachi hand-held PC.
(Reproduced, with permission, from Hitachi America, Ltd., *www.hitachi.com/.*)

duct some work at home or on the road (Figs. 3.11, 3.12, and 3.13). They can dowload the network to the office desktop and on the network system.

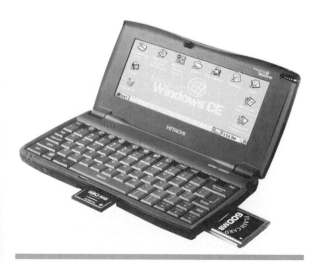

Figure 3.12
Hitachi hand-held computer.
(Reproduced, with permission, from Hitachi America, Ltd., *www.hitachi.com/.*)

Common Hardware Peripherals

Keyboard

The keyboard is the most common input device. It is similar to the keyboard of a typewriter and is connected to the box with a cord (Fig. 3.14). There are several different types of keyboards; however, regardless of type they all have similar sections of keys: (1) typewriter keys, (2) function keys, (3) numeric keypad, (4) cursor keys, (5) toggle keys, and (6) special operations keys. Carpal tunnel syndrome has been a severe problem for many people whose jobs require them to spend many hours a day typing on a keyboard. In response, several different styles designed to reduce the incidence of carpal tunnel have been introduced.

The **typewriter key** section is the largest and contains keys that follow the standard QWERTY arrangement of keys of a standard typewriter. (The term represents the first six letters in the first alphabetic row.) The **function keys** (F1–F12) are **software-specific**; that is, they are programmable, since their function is dependent upon the software program being processed. For example, the function key F10 is used to retrieve a file in one word processing package and to save in another. Generally, a template is provided for the function keys that defines how the keys are used for the specific software package. Three other keys on the key-

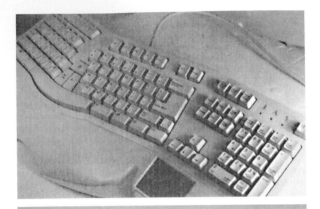

Figure 3.14
Ergonomic keyboard with touch pad.
(Reproduced, with permission, from Pilgrim A. *Build Your Own Pentium III*. New York, NY, McGraw-Hill, 2000:305.)

board labeled **Shift, Ctrl,** and **Alt** expand the function keys by being used in combination with them to carry out other commands.

The **numeric keypad** is a second set of numeric keys that are placed differently on the keyboard than the alphabetic keys. The numeric keypad is a separate rectangle-shaped calculator-type section that enables the user to enter numeric data more efficiently. This section of keys can be converted to represent other keys, including moving the cursor in four directions, just by turning on the **Num Lock key**. The four **cursor keys** are used to direct the position of the pointer on the display monitor. They control the movement: **up** (↑), **down** (↓), **right** (→), and **left** (←) over the display screen. The **toggle keys** are those that have a dual purpose. When a toggle key is pressed once, the function is **on**, and when pressed a second time it is **off**. The major toggle keys include: **Num Lock, Caps Lock, Scroll Lock,** and **Insert/Typeover.**

There are also **special operations keys** that are unique to the microcomputer and are used to make the keyboard easy to manipulate. The **Home** and **End** keys bring the cursor to the beginning or end of a line, **Print Screen** prints the screen display or saves it to the clipboard as a snapshot, **Esc** (escape) interrupts or cancels a function, a **Tab** (↔) key moves the cursor to predetermined set tabs, the **Del** key deletes text, and a **space bar** inserts blank spaces in a line. The **Enter** key performs a variety of functions depending upon the context of the program. It sends information to the computer, such as during sign-on procedures, in word processing it creates

a new paragraph, and it can be used to create a blank section in a document.

Monitor

The monitor is a display screen component of a terminal that allows the user to see images, programs, commands the user sends to the computer, and results of the computer's work (output). Similar to a television screen, the monitor can show colors, animation, text, and virtually anything that the computer can produce. Up to a point, larger screens are desirable on monitors, because people spend so much time looking at monitors that eye strain is common. Most PCs today come with monitors from 14″ to 21″, although larger screens are available. The resolution or clarity of the monitor screen is related to the number of dots, **pixels**, on the screen. Customers can order anything from a 14″ viewing screen with 1,024 × 768 pixels to 21″ screens with a resolution of 1,600 × 1,280 pixels. As pixel count rises, the sharpness and clarity of images and colors on the screen improve.

Mouse and Trackball

The mouse was introduced with the microcomputer as a new type of input device to replace moving the arrow keys on the keyboard. It is a hand-controlled mechanical device that electronically instructs the cursor to move across the video display screen. It resembles a bar of soap with a tail. As the user slides the mouse across a desktop pad, a ball on the bottom of the mouse senses the motion and transmits it to the the cursor (pointer) on the screen. The cursor moves in conjunction with the mouse. The mouse has at least two buttons and sometimes a roller at the top. The left button is used primarily to: (1) select the icon, (2) activate a process, and (3) implement a function to be performed. The right button is a special function button, and its function is dependent upon the program. A mouse requires a certain amount of space on a desk, and it is associated with carpal tunnel and wrist fatigue. Additionally, the mouse often "runs" off the pad and must be repositioned to work. The trackball was developed for people who prefer a stationary device. Similar to a mouse, the trackball has the ball on the top, and movement of the cursor is controlled by the fingers rolling the ball in place.

Floppy Disks/Diskettes

The floppy disk, commonly called a diskette, is another form of secondary storage or auxiliary memory. It serves as both input and output media. The floppy disk is largely used by microcomputers. Data are read and written, using disk drives, in the same manner as with magnetic tapes and magnetic disks. A floppy diskette turns a read/write head similar to a phonograph record to transfer electronic impulses between the diskette and memory. Each diskette has a disk window, which exposes the area on the magnetic surface where the data can be retrieved or stored. A write-protect slot is also cut near the top of the jacket. Covering the slot (or sliding the slot cover to the closed position) renders the diskette unavailable to the writing head. Thus, nothing can be erased or written onto the disk (see Fig. 3.7).

A floppy disk is a flexible mylar plastic oxide-coated disk thinly covered with magnetic spots. It is available in $3\frac{1}{2}''$ and $5\frac{1}{4}''$ sizes, though $5\frac{1}{4}''$ floppy disks are rarely seen these days. The $3\frac{1}{2}''$ diskette is encased in a hard plastic case that is sturdy and easier to store. The $5\frac{1}{4}''$ diskette can hold 360 K to 1 MB of data, and the $3\frac{1}{2}''$ diskette can hold 1.55 MB (double density) to 2.0 MB (high density). Each floppy disk is sectioned into concentric rings or tracks ranging from 9 to 15; and each track is divided into sectors ranging from 40 to 48 or from 80 to 96. Sectors store the smallest unit of data. Tracks and sectors are used to provide the addresses of fields of data. The procedure to mark the tracks and sectors is called formatting. Formatting is done at the factory, but when a user wishes to completely erase a diskette, it is wise to reformat the disk to ensure that no sectors are lost to hidden files.

Touch Pad and Mouse Button

The touch pad was developed by the makers of laptop computers for use in place of the mouse. A mouse is not practical for use in an airplane or other travel location. The touch pad is a flat, rectangular depression on the keyboard that senses pressure and movement of the user's finger. The user simply drags the finger around the touchpad to move the cursor on the screen. A slight tap on the touch pad works as double-clicking the left mouse button or pressing the "Enter" key on the keyboard.

Light Pen/Touch Screen

A light pen is a photosensitive device that responds to light images when placed against a monitor screen. When the pen comes in contact with the display screen it highlights the item and sends data to the computer. Touch screens involve the use of a special filter on a monitor screen that allows the screen to "sense" the pressure of the user's finger on a particular position of

the screen. That pressure can signal the computer to initiate an action (similar to a mouse click) or can function to let the user select a particular item on the screen, such as on a menu. Sensors on the screen pinpoint the X and Y axis location touched by a user.

Optical Character Recognition

Optical character recognition (OCR) is a specialized computer input medium that allows data to be read directly from a form or document. An electronic optical scanning device, a **wand reader**, or a bar code reader reads special marks, bar codes, numbers, letters, or characters. The scanner used in a grocery store uses a special type of OCR. Such a device converts the optical marks, characters, and bar codes into electrical signals that become computer input. OCR-readable codes include those outlined in areas on the answer sheet of the nursing state board examinations, which are filled in with pencil. The bar codes called universal product code symbols (zebra-striped bars) are another example. Ten bars, about $1''$ long, signify different numbers to code groceries or medical items. If read with a special scanning device, they can become input into some hospital inventory systems, similar to the way product codes read in the grocery check-out line become input into the store's inventory control system.

Magnetic-Ink Character Recognition

Magnetic-ink character recognition (MICR) is another medium for reading characters by computer. Here the characters are made of magnetized particles printed on paper. A MICR reader can examine the shape of the magnetic-ink characters and convert them into binary code for computer input. The most common example of a MICR is the magnetized characters imprinted on checks, which most banks use.

Voice Synthesizer

A voice synthesizer allows users to input data into the computer by speaking into a connected microphone. Also known as a speech synthesizer, it digitizes the sound for processing by the CPU. Although automatic recognition of the human voice is not yet perfected, voice input is used in situations requiring only a few spoken words, and it is becoming a common medium for all computer systems. The study of neural networks (many processors working in parallel in a single computer) offers one hope of improving the performance of voice recognition technology.

Imaging

The field of computer imaging exploded in the 1980s and 1990s with the enormous development of medical imaging. Many of the advanced imaging technologies, such as computerized axial tomography (CAT scans) and magnetic resonance imaging (MRI) are computer-enhanced imaging technologies. Several different types of image input devices are available that primarily transform images from various types of graphics into digital form, which the computer can accept, represent on the screen, and process. Many types of graphic images on paper such as x-rays can be scanned as computer input and/or digitized for computer use.

Digital Versatile Disk

While DVD began as "digital video disk," it is now commonly and more correctly referred to as "digital versatile disk" to better reflect its capabilities of playing audio and multimedia as well as video. A DVD looks and feels like a CD-ROM but holds much more information and contains many more multimedia features. DVD technology is in the process of replacing most CD-ROM technology. The technology was developed to support high resolution and dense applications such as placement of motion pictures on compact disks.

Printers

The printer, the most important output device, converts information produced by the computer system into printed form, rendering data in the binary code into readable English. The major types of printed output include printed hard copy (paper), microfilm (microfiche), photographs, and graphic copy. The printer's output, known as **hard copy**, is output produced on paper. Most printers sold today are laser printers or jet printers —either inkjet or bubble-jet printers. Laser printers offer a substantial increase in output quality and speed over the jet printers. The laser printer's engine is composed of an integrated system of electronic and chemical parts that work together with optical processes to produce the printed image. The laser printers generally use fonts or typefaces as their printing elements, making documents look like they were typeset. They are also used for printing graphical images and illustrations. The inkjet and bubble-jet printers fire small bursts of ink on the paper. The principal difference between bubble-jet printers and other inkjet printers is that bubble-jet printers use special heating elements to prepare the ink, whereas inkjet printers use piezoelectric crystals to ionize the ink.

Modems

The modem is a communication device used to connect a terminal with a mainframe or another computer. A modem (**mo**dulating and **dem**odulating device) translates digital data into waves (analog) for transmission over the communication lines to the computer system and converts the waves back to their original digital form for input into the computer. Modems connect the user with a remote computer's CPU, enabling communication through telephone lines. By dialing the remote computer's modem, data can be both sent and received from outside sources. Modems, therefore, facilitate the function of both input and output devices and link remote computers to networks of computers. Modems are described by the rate of communication transmission or line transfer called the bits per second (bps) rate. 57K is a common modem speed in late 1990s models. Most modems sold for PCs are actually **fax-modems,** which can send documents over the phone or network lines to be downloaded via fax machine at a distant site. The computer programs for fax-modem communication can save the fax as a data file for editing and storage. They also can save the graphics/images using OCR technology and convert them into text files for storage.

Basics of Computer Network Hardware

A network is a set of cooperative interconnected computers for the purpose of information interchange. The networks of greatest interest include local area networks (LANs), wide area networks (WANs), and the Internet, which is a network of networks. A LAN usually supports the interconnected computer needs of a single company or agency. The computers are physically located close to each other, and generally, only members of the company or agency have legitimate access to the information on the network. WANs support geographically dispersed facilities, such as the individual grocery stores in a national chain. A subset of WANs include the metropolitan area networks (MANs) that support and connect the many buildings of local governmental agencies or university campuses.

The most important components of network hardware are the **adapter or interface card, cabling,** and **server**. The most important concepts in network hardware are **architecture** and **topology**. Note that much of the information in this section was generated with the assistance of on-line computer dictionaries and encyclopedias such as those offered by the following.

1. Infostreet.com, 18345 Ventura Blvd., Tarzana, CA 91356 and their "Information Please" on-line resource, which is located at *http://www.Instant Web.com/foldoc/index.html.*

2. The "Whatis" resource, located at *http://www. whatis.com/.*

3. The on-line dictionary, encyclopedia, and thesaurus information provided through the Dictionary.com Company located at *http://www.dictionary.com/.*

Network Hardware

The role of hardware in a network is to provide an interconnection between computers. For a computer to participate on a network, it must have at least two pieces of hardware:

1. **Network adapter, or network interface card**   A network interface card (NIC) is a computer circuit board or card that is installed in a computer so that it can be connected to a network. Personal computers and workstations on LANs typically contain a network interface card specifically designed for the LAN transmission technology, such as Ethernet. Network interface cards provide a dedicated, full-time connection to a network. Most home and portable computers connect to the Internet through modems on an as-needed dial-up connection. The modem provides the connection interface to the Internet service provider.

   The oldest and still most commonly used "network interface" (or "adapter card") is an Ethernet card. But there exist other options such as arcnet, serial-port boards, etc. Most of the time, the choice of NIC depends on the communication medium.

2. **Communication medium (cabling)**   The "communication medium" is the means by which actual transfer of data from one site to another takes place. Commonly used communication media include twisted pair cable, co-axial cable, fiber-optics, telephone lines, satellites, and compressed video. Most of the time, the choice of a communication medium is based on the following.

   (a) *Distance.* Relatively short distances are required for compressed video and coaxial cables. For much longer distances, fiber-optics, telephone lines, and satellite transmission are used. For shorter distances where video is needed, co-axial cable and compressed video are used.

   (b) *Amount of data transfer.* Large amounts of data (especially video) are best handled with co-axial cables and compressed video and through satellite communications (satellite and compressed video are very expensive). Smaller amounts of data, or serial (non-video) streams are best handled through the other wire types, such as twisted pair copper wire and optical fiber, and are less expensive.

   (c) *How often the transfer is needed.* Co-axial works best for locally wired networks that are used constantly by a very limited number of users. Telephone wires work well for the relatively high usage public networks (like the Internet) but are more likely to get overloaded when many users try to use the system at the same time. Consider, for example, the busy Internet or phone lines getting clogged up when a tornado or hurricane has struck a community.

   (d) *Availability.* Availability depends upon cost, transmission speed, number of users (who might clog up the system), weather conditions (satellites), etc.

Telephone Line Communications

Specialized phone lines called integrated services digital network (ISDN) lines are used to carry communications across phone lines. ISDN is a set of communication standards for optical fibers that carry voice, digital, and video signals across phone lines. There are a variety of types of ISDN connections, each having a different bandwidth. The bandwidth controls how fast the signals can be transmitted across the phone lines. The first was DS0, which stands for "digital service—zeroth level," that transmitted at 64 kilobytes per second. Today, those have been replaced with **T-Lines**, which are used to handle the high speed transmissions needed for network communications. The American Bell Telephone Company introduced the T-carrier system in the 1960s because increasing phone usage was overloading the DS lines. There are four bandwidths available for T-lines, ranging from the 1.54 megabytes per second (Mbps) speed and 24 channels of the T-1 line to the 274.1 Mbps speed and 4,032 channels of a T-4 line. Many Internet service providers still pass information through T-1 lines. However, with the increasing use of the Internet, more and more problems with slow transmission have created demand for even faster lines. The T-3 line has a transmission speed of 447.36 Mbps, and most large ISPs have had to move their customers to T-3 lines in order to provide adequate customer service. Some users, dissatisfied with the speed limitations of their own home phone line have purchased fractional T-1 line service. Fractional T-1 line service involves the rental of some portion of the 24 channels in a T-1 line.

Server

The concept of a server is very important when networks are discussed today. For a network to exist, there must be a server. Most networks today use the client/server approach. In a pure client/server approach, one computer is the core or server computer that receives requests from the client (user) computer and fulfills those requests. For example, when the user requests a site on the Internet, the server receives the request, decodes it, and sends the link on to the correct Internet address.

1. In general, a server is a computer program that provides services to other computer programs in the same computer **or in other computers on a network**.

2. The computer that runs the server program is also frequently referred to as "the server" (although the server computer may contain a number of server and client programs).

3. In the client/server programming model, a server is a program that awaits and fulfills requests from client programs in the same or other computers. A given application in a computer may function as a client with requests for services from other programs and a server or requests from other programs.

Architecture

In informatics, "architecture" refers to overall physical structure, peripherals, interconnections within the computer, and its system software, especially the operating system. Computer architecture can be divided into five fundamental components: input/output, storage, communication, control, and processing. These are also called the computer's subsystems. When networks are discussed, "architecture" refers to how communication among the various computers in the network is accomplished. Broadly speaking, there are two types of network architectures.

1. **Broadcast.**   Here the communication is done by transmitting the same information to all the computers in the network that are expected to respond to it. This is typically used in local area networks.

2. **Point-to-point.**   The computer for which information is intended is identified first, and the communication is only to that particular computer. This is typically used in "dial-up" networking, such as an individual who dials up the network through his/her internet service provider.

Topology

Topology defines how the network computers in a LAN are interconnected within a physical area and describes their physical interconnection. Several possible topologies are the following.

1. **Bus.**   A bus is a network topology or circuit arrangement in which all the node computers are directly attached to a line. Therefore, all communications travel through each of the node computers. Each computer has a unique identity and can recognize the transmissions sent to it. In this fashion all computers are connected in parallel to each other. The big advantage of this topology is that if one computer fails, other computers still can access the information. This structure is decentralized. (Note: the term "bus" is also used in computer hardware. In that context, it usually refers to an expansion slot on the motherboard of the computer.)

2. **Star.**   This is a centralized structure where all computers are connected through a central computer, called the server. If this central computer fails, information cannot be sent or received by any of the computers connected to this server.

3. **Ring.**   Originally, all LAN computers were connected in a ring fashion with wires or cables that directly connected all the computers together. If one computer failed, none of the computers could communicate and share the resources. That topology has been replaced by the **token ring** network protocol. Token rings work by having the server pass a marker, or "token," to the computer that is next in line to communicate. No computer can send or receive data unless it is the target of the token. In this way, collisions between two workstations that wish to transmit information at the same time are avoided. It should be noted that, generally, the token is passed so rapidly that the LAN users may never know they had to wait. A token ring structure can support networks in which the computers are up to 124 miles apart.

   (a) **Hub: A form of ring topology.** A hub consists of a "backbone," or main circuit, attached to a number of outgoing lines. Each of the outgoing lines can support a number of ports to which devices can be attached. Generally, HUB LANs are used for a relatively small number of connected workstations. In the hub, all computers are connected to a central hub processor that contains the networking software and provides for communication among the various computers on the network. For a computer to talk to one or more of the other computers on the network, it must first go through the hub.

(b) **Arcnet.** Another type of ring technology used for local area networks is arcnet. It uses what is called a "token-bus" system for managing line sharing among all the users on the network. It works well for LANs in which all the links are physically near each other (each cable can go only 2,000 feet, but the total span can be up to 20,000 feet). While not as powerful as some other topologies, it is by far the least expensive.

Summary

This chapter described computer hardware, including both internal and peripheral hardware. It explained the fundamental components of a computer and provided a simple overview of how computers function at the machine level. It offered a brief history of the development of computer hardware and of some of the people who played major roles in the computer industry. It also described computer classes, characteristics, and types. It outlined the four major functions of a computer: input, output, processing, and storage. The most common peripheral hardware was introduced and described. Finally, it presented basic concepts of computer networks and the hardware necessary to support networks.

References

Author Unknown. (1999). Telemedicine: An overview. *Health Devices, 28*(3), 88–103.

Bell, G. (1997). The Seymour Cray Lecture Series. University of Minnesota. *http://research.microsoft.com/users/gbell/craytalk/sld001.htm*

Breckenridge, C. (1996). A Tribute to Seymour Cray. Keynote Presentation at Supercomputing '96, November 19, 1996. *http://www.cgl.ucsf.edu/home/tef/cray/tribute.html*

Brocht, D., Abbott, P., Smith, C. et al. (1999). A clinic on wheels: A paradigm shift in the provision of care and the challenges of information infrastructure. *Computers in Nursing, 17*(3), 109–113.

Chaffee, M. (1999). A telehealth odyssey. *American Journal of Nursing, 99*(7), 27–32.

Dermer, M. (1999). Voice-recognition software: Transforming record keeping. *Canadian Family Physician, 7*(45), 1650.

Hwan, K. (1988). *Modern Optical Disk Technology.* Pusan National University Parallel Multimedia Lab. *http://apple.cs.pusan.ac.kr/~ihkim/tr/index.htm*

Karasov, C. (1982). The potential for computerization of ultrasound images. *Applied Radiology, 11*(4), 91–93.

Koerner, S. and Becker F. (1999). Advances in Navy pharmacy information technology: accessing Micromedex via the Composite Healthcare Computer System and local area networks. *Military Medicine, 164*(7), 481–484.

Jefferies, P. R. (1999). Learning how to perform a 12 lead ECG using virtual reality. *Progess in Cardiovascular Nursing, 14*(1), 7–13.

Mariani, G. (1988). Evolution of functional imaging in nuclear medicine. *Journal of Nuclear Medicine and Allied Science, 32*(4), 223–225.

Massachusetts Institute of Technology. (1996). *The Lemelson-MIT Awards: Invention Dimension. http://web.mit.edu/invent/www/inventorsI-Q/apple.html*

Maxfield, C. and Brown, B. (1997). *Bebop Bytes Back.* Madison, Alabama: Doone Publications.

McDonald, C., Overhage, J., Tierney, W., et al. (1999). The Regenstrief Medical Record System: A quarter century experience. *International Journal of Medical Informatics, 54*(3), 225–253.

Mesa, A. (1997). Apple history timeline. *The Apple Museum. http://www.applemuseum.seastar.net/*

Targowski, A. (1990). *The Architecture and Planning of Enterprise-Wide Information Management Systems.* Harrisburg, PA: Idea Group Publishers.

The Franklin Institute. (1999). Seymour Cray. *http://sln.fi.edu/tfi/exhibits/cray.html*

Unisys Corporation. (Date Unknown). A Brief Historical Overview. *http://www.unisys.se/presentation/nyckelh.htm*

Wallace, S., Wyatt, J., and Taylor, P. (1998). Telemedicine in the NHS for the millennium and beyond. *Postgraduate Medicine Journal, 74*(878), 721–728.

Watson, B. (1999). Dead computational platforms, dead mainframes, and their dates. *The Dead Media Project. http://www.islandnet.com/~ianc/dm/0/006.html*

Weik, M. (1961). The ENIAC Story. Washington, D.C. Reprinted from the January–February 1961 issue of O R D N A N C E. The Journal of the American Ordnance Association, 708 Mills Building. *http://ftp.arl.mil/~mike/comphist/eniac-story.html*

Software

Mary L. McHugh

OBJECTIVES

1. Define the difference between computer software and computer hardware.
2. Discuss the origin of computer programming.
3. Identify the two categories of software, and discriminate between the two for purpose and functionality.
4. List the categories of programming languages, and identify at least one example of each.
5. Identify key requirements for software designed to support nursing practice.

KEY WORDS

information systems
computer science
software

A computer program is a set of stored instructions that tells the computer what to do. Software allows the user to communicate with the computer, so it can perform a desired action, function, or procedure. A software program can be viewed as a sort of algorithm—a clearly defined procedure for obtaining the solution to a general type of problem (Dunne, 1994). Software consists of logically organized statements, or commands, presented to the computer in a proper sequence of steps that direct the execution of a task.

Software is the general term applied to the instructions that direct the computer's hardware to perform work. It is distinguished from hardware by its conceptual rather than physical nature. Hardware consists of physical components, whereas software consists of instructions communicated electronically to the hardware. Software is needed for two purposes. First, computers do not understand human language, and software is needed to translate instructions created in human language into machine language. (As explained in Chap. 2, at the machine level, computers can understand only binary, not English or any other human language.) Second, packaged or stored software is needed to make the computer an economical work tool. Users could create their own software every time they needed to use the computer. However, writing software instructions (programming) is extremely difficult, time-consuming, and, for most people, tedious. It is much more practical and economical for one highly skilled person or programming team to develop programs that many other people can buy and use to do common tasks. Software is supplied as organized instruction sets called "programs" (or as a set of related programs called a "package").

A program is a single instruction set or unit that consists of a group of instructions designed to perform a particular sort of job, such as a game or a simple math calculator on the computer. Most commonly, computer programs are sold in packages. A software package is usually a group of interrelated programs that support a particular complex job function or group of related functions. For example, several prominent software companies sell their own version of a package of programs that are typically needed to support an office computer, including a word processor, a spread sheet, a graphics program, and sometimes a database manager.

Programs translate operations the user needs into language and instructions that the computer can understand. By itself, computer hardware is merely a collection of printed circuits, plastic, metal, and wires. Without software, hardware is nonfunctional.

History of Computer Programming and Software

The idea of having computer programs stored on a hard drive and brought into memory at the user's command has its roots in the 1800s, long before the first true computer was invented. Augusta Ada Byron, Countess of Lovelace (1816–1852), a mathematician and co-researcher with Charles Babbage (1791–1871), first described the concept of a stored computer program (Toole, 1992). Babbage was a late nineteenth century mathematician and inventor (Keller, 1996). He "invented" (but never built) a device that he named the "analytical machine." Babbage's son finally built his machine in 1910 but was never able to make it work reliably (Fig. 4.1). However, the concept of a machine that could perform mathematical functions stimulated the thinking of other scientists and mathematicians about how to build such a machine and how instructions could be communicated to the machine. In her writings about Babbage's concept of an analytical engine, Countess Lovelace theorized the use of automatic repetitious arithmetic steps that the analytical engine would follow to solve a problem, namely the "loop concept" (Keller, 1996). This concept gave her the title of the "first programmer" in computer history. However, it was Robert Von Newmann (1888–1976) who proposed that both data and instructions could be stored in the computer and that the instructions could be automatically carried out. The stored program concept was subsequently implemented as a major concept in the evolution of the computer.

Programs often require data as input. Today, people take for granted that computers will process huge amounts of data. However, it was not always feasible to handle large datasets. In the case of management of very large collections of data, necessity was truly the mother of invention. As part of the development of the new nation, America's founders decreed that a census of the population be taken every 10 years, the first of which commenced on August 2, 1790. The order was more difficult to carry out than anticipated. It took over 9 months to gather and process the 1790 census information, and there were only about 3.8 million people in the United States at the time. There were simply no machines to help with data collection or collation—they hadn't been invented yet! By the 1860 census, it was apparent that the manual methods of processing the census were inadequate. Unless the number of questions was severely limited, it would take more than 10 years to process the 10-year census data (Dunne, 1996). Some type of machine was needed if the constitutional requirement for a census was to be fulfilled successfully.

Ultimately, the development of data processing machines was taken from the field of textiles. Jacquard blouses so popular in women's better clothing stores were made possible by an invention of a weaver from France, Joseph Jacquard (Evan, 1979). Jacquard invented the Jacquard loom, a device that used blocks of wood with holes drilled in such a way that the threads to be woven into cloth could form a "program," or set of machine instructions, to the loom (Fig. 4.2). The instructions varied the way the cloth was worked by the loom so that a particular design (such as flowers or birds) would be produced in the fabric; that is, the weave produced images without changing the thread color or type.

In 1881, Herman Hollerith (1860–1929), a 19-year-old graduate of the Columbia School of Mines, was employed as a special agent by the U.S. Census Bureau (Austrian, 1982; Dunne, 1994). Recognizing the problem with trying to process such massive amounts of data, Hollerith used Jacquard's idea but developed a machine that could read punched cards and tabulate the results. In 1884, Hollerith patented his machine and punched card system (Austrian, 1982) (Fig. 4.3). Hollerith's ideas were so successful that he formed a company called Tabulating Machine. Eventually, after several changes of ownership and name changes, the company became International Business Machines, more popularly known as

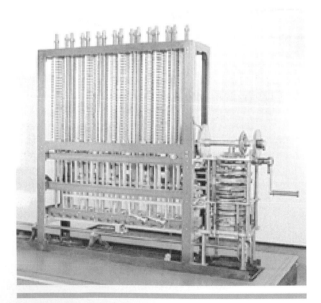

Figure 4.1
Babbage's analytic machine.

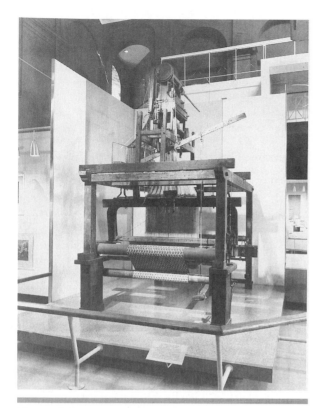

Figure 4.2
The Jacquard loom.
(Smithsonian Institution Photo No. 45599.)

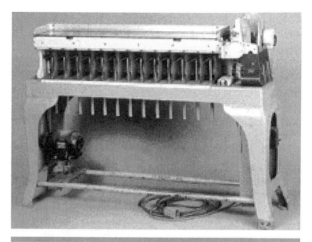

Figure 4.3
Holleriths counting machine.

gramming and program languages (Fig. 4.4). She is said to have written the third program ever on the Mark I, which was the first large-scale, digital computer in history. In 1946, the Navy returned Hopper to inactive duty, but they recalled her to active duty in 1967 during the Vietnam War. Her brilliance with computers was considered irreplaceable by the military, and she continued to serve her country until she retired a second time in 1986 at the age of 79. Throughout her career, she developed many of the concepts and mathematical foundations of computer programming science.

IBM. The punched card method of entering programs (software) and data into computers continued to exist until the late 1960s (Dunne, 1994).

In any history of computer programming, a remarkable woman known as "The Mother of Computing" should be acknowledged (Women's International Center, undated). Rear Admiral Grace Murray Hopper was born in New York in 1906 (Lee, 1987). She obtained a degree in mathematics and physics, Phi Beta Kappa from Vassar in 1928, and her Ph.D. in mathematics in 1934. In 1941, she offered her services to her country by enlisting in the U.S. Naval Reserve. On active duty throughout World War II, she was assigned to the Bureau of Ordinance Computation at Harvard University, where she worked with the first digital computer, the Mark I, and its successor, the Mark II. Dr. Hopper was perhaps the world's most expert programmer of early computers. During her long career, she greatly advanced the power of computers through her innovations in computer pro-

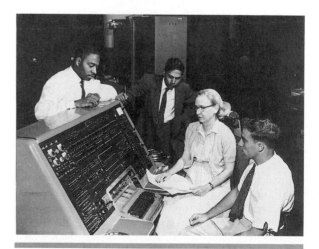

Figure 4.4
Rear Admiral Grace Hopper, Ph.D., and colleagues.
(Smithsonian Institution Photo No. 83.4878.)

A major activity in program testing is **debugging**, which means checking the program to ensure that it is free of error. This term was coined by Grace Hopper. In 1945, when working at Harvard on the MARK II computer, her program crashed. Upon examination of the computer, she discovered that a moth caught in the machine had caused the crash. To correct the problem and get the system working again, she "debugged "the computer. As a result, the term was used to refer to any correction of a computer problem.

Admiral Hopper was widely known not only for her accomplishments in computer programming language development but also for her extraordinary vision and wit. She was the early force behind the idea that computer programming languages should become more English-like. She recognized that obscure assembly and machine-like programming languages limited access to the computer and therefore the utility of the machines. Her work on programming languages in the early 1950s formed the foundation for the first truly English-like language, the <u>Co</u>mmon <u>B</u>usiness-<u>O</u>riented <u>L</u>anguage (COBOL). COBOL was considered the first "universal" programming language and is still widely used in business applications. In an age when the focus was on bigger rather than on more friendly computers, she quipped, "In pioneer days they used oxen for heavy pulling, and when one ox couldn't budge a log, they didn't try to grow a larger ox. We shouldn't be trying for bigger computers, but for more systems of computers." (Schieber, 1987). She recognized that a better approach would be to have many computers working independently and together so that more work could be accomplished. Today, the Internet, the network of networks, might be viewed as the realization of Grace Hopper's early vision of computing.

It is appropriate that this section be closed with another of her quotes: "Life was simple before World War II. After that, we had systems." (Schieber, 1987).

History of Operating Systems

Operating systems did not exist for the early computers. Human operators were needed for those machines. They manually loaded the punched cards that contained the computer programs into card readers and performed other manual tasks involved in scheduling computer time among the various projects, handling the printed output, etc. Each programmer was responsible not only for producing code for the work the computer was to do, but also for managing the computer's storage during the run (Ettinger, 1999). This was inefficient. Every programmer makes typographical errors, and every program requires more or less extensive editing and corrections (debugging). Since many of the same operations (called "housekeeping tasks" by programmers) had to be performed exactly the same way for every program, it made sense to automate as much of the routine process of computer operation as possible. The program that performs the housekeeping tasks on a computer is called the "operating system."

Mainframe Operating Systems   The first true operating systems were developed for mainframe computers in the early 1960s—the most famous was IBM's OS/360. The original operating systems were primarily designed to handle the storage management operations and offered programs to run very common program components such as sorting data. Automating these operations greatly improved programmer efficiency. Also, since the operating system was the product of expert programmers and was made standard across users, it improved the operating efficiency of the computer itself.

However, another problem plagued the first computers. Computers were enormously expensive, and as fast as they worked, their productive use was seriously hampered by the slowness of the input and output portion of their operation. At that time, input consisted of IBM punched cards being run through a mechanical card reader machine. Output consisted of operations like page printing, graphical plotters drawing graphs, or files being written onto a magnetic tape via a tape drive. These operations all involve mechanical moving parts. Mechanical parts are very slow in comparison with CPU speeds. (That is why a file that takes two seconds for your PC to load into a word processor takes ten minutes to print.) While the slow mechanical component of the system was working, the CPU—the most expensive component of the system—sat idle.

The one-user computer model is called a single-processor, and originally, all computers were single-processors. Since only one user's work could run at a time, no other user's job could start until the final printing of the previous job was complete. The reality of computer processing, however, was that programs actually could be broken down into "chunks" of work. Once a processor finished a processing chunk, it might have to wait while the operating system executed a store or print function. As demand for computer time increased, the inefficiencies of a single-user strategy became less and less tolerable in the industry. Part of the solution was to add smaller, inexpensive processors for handling the slow input and output operations. This required new operating systems that could receive from a front-end processor and send the slow output operations to a back-end processor.

Even freeing the CPU from the input/output (I/O) operations left the CPU idle much of the time when a user's project had multiple iterations of input/processing/output work to perform. The CPU could perform chunks of work from one user while the auxiliary processors handled the work of other users. This breaking of each user's work into chunks and allocation of the CPU time as necessary was so complex that a human operator could never manage it. However, mathematical algorithms already in existence could be easily applied to the problem and programmed into a scheduler program. That is what IBM's programmers did when they developed the first true multi-user operating system for the IBM-360 mainframe computer in the early 1960s.

With the advent of the first multi-user operating systems, the power of the mainframe CPU could be used far more productively, and the demand for programmers and new applications for the computers grew exponentially. The importance of these advances cannot be overemphasized. Without the operating system power of the multi-user mainframe computer, life as it is known in 21st century America could not exist. There would be no real space program. Man would not have walked on the moon. Health care would have no computerized diagnostics such as CAT scans and MRIs. Large, multinational corporations as we know them today could never exist. The bookkeeping and billing operations needed could not be performed manually. Modern food production and distribution systems are dependent upon agricultural, inventory control, and trucking operations that could not be managed manually. Utility companies could not provide services at a reasonable cost to the large, distributed populations that exist. For better or worse, the modern computer operating systems and application programs are the foundations of modern society.

PC Operating Systems It may be logically concluded that without the development of operating systems, the personal computer might never have been developed. Certainly it could never have become the pervasive technology in our daily home and work lives that it is today. The first microcomputer, the Apple I, had no hard drive. The company supplied a basic operating system on a single diskette. The diskette had to be in the floppy disk drive when the computer was turned on. A Ph.D. named Gary Kindall developed one of the first and most popular operating systems for PCs and called his product CP/M. When IBM decided to get into the PC market as a direct competitor to Apple, they asked Kindall to consider customizing his OS for their product. Unfortunately, IBM's time constraints required an immediate response, and Kindall had plans. When Kindall did not meet IBM's requirements, they asked a young programmer whose fledgling company was focused on development of a programming language to work with them. The programmer's name was Bill Gates, and the company was Microsoft. Microsoft didn't have an operating system to put on the table, but Gates, recognizing the opportunity was not to be lost, contacted a programmer named Tim Patterson who had developed an OS similar to CP/M, named QDOS. Patterson did not own the rights to the program since he had developed it as an employee of Seattle Computer Products. Gates bought the rights to QDOS from that company, and MS-DOS (Microsoft Disk Operating System) was launched.

Later, IBM decided to try to launch their own operating system called OS/2. It was a considerable improvement over DOS (it was actually written by Microsoft under contract to IBM). Unfortunately, OS/2 was introduced at about the same time that the computing public began to take notice of the radically new operating system on the Macintosh, and OS/2 was made obsolete before it really had a chance to get started.

It will be noticed that the discussion of operating systems (OSs) for PCs has been clearly separated into the Apple versus the IBM type PC. Operating systems differ for the various types of computers and sometimes even for different brands of computers. The operating system used in one type of mainframe is very different from the operating system used in a different brand of mainframe and is more different still from that of a desktop computer. Even within the desktop computer market, there are several very different—and incompatible—types of CPU. The two main CPU types in personal computers are the Apple platform and the IBM type of platform. The operating systems for each were developed specifically for their respective equipment and cannot be used for the other's brands. This is the reason that diskettes from an Apple machine will not work on an IBM (or IBM clone) computer.

The Apple Corporation initially developed its own disk operating system, AppleWorks for the Apple PCs developed by Steve Jobs and Steve Wozniac. However, users could also buy a version of CP/M and install it on their Apple computer. Microsoft called the first operating system for the IBM machine platform MS-DOS, and it was released along with the first IBM PC in 1981. However, the world of PC operating systems was truly revolutionized by Apple in the early 1980s.

History of Graphical User Interface Operating Systems   The first graphical user interface (GUI) was developed in the early 1970s by a research team from Xerox Corporation (see below for a detailed description of how GUIs function). It was written in a computer language called Smalltalk. This OS was not carried forward into modern GUI systems. In 1984, Apple Computer Corporation introduced its first Apple Macintosh (Mac) OS, a GUI that made the Macintosh one of the most highly regarded, user-friendly computers on the market. Bill Gates happened to be at the press conference where Apple introduced its first GUI and immediately recognized GUI operating systems as the future of personal computing. Shortly thereafter, Microsoft Corporation began work on its own GUI, which was called Windows 1.0 when it was introduced in 1987.

Windows   The Windows program was originally more of a utility than an operating system. Users had to load the MS-DOS operating system, and then Windows was loaded on top of DOS. Windows 1.0 was not a very successful program. Its performance was far inferior to the Mac GUI, and most IBM users continued to use DOS. Later versions of Windows were greatly improved. First, the operating system was incorporated into the Windows program itself and no longer had to be separately loaded. Windows 95 and higher versions load directly into random access memory (RAM) and include both the operating system commands and the GUI interface. The later versions offered many highly popular innovations, such as the ability to have several programs open at the same time, the ability to move blocks of text back and forth among the open programs, support for networking, and a variety of different applications programs that all had a similar look and feel. Computer packages developed for this operating system all used the same basic menu and used the same menu format and wording for the same operations; these innovations greatly lessened the time users spent in the initial learning process. MS-Windows eliminated the need for memorizing different commands for different software packages and made entire groups of applications programs more user-friendly.

One problem with early versions of Microsoft Windows was a lack of compatibility between the PC OS and network systems. In response, Microsoft developed a network-friendly version of the Windows operating system, MS-Windows/NT. Windows/NT enhances the microcomputer in a multi-user and multitasking network environment. Further, it has a graphical interface and can run applications developed for different operating systems such as those used to run the Apple Macintosh.

It also has a built-in networking capability, making it possible to share processing resources and facilitate communication in and between local area networks (LANs). Similar advances are also offered by Version 2 of the IBM OS/2 operating systems, the Solaris Unix workstations offered by Sun Microsystems, and several other advanced operating systems. However, the popularity of Windows had made it the overwhelmingly dominant force in PC operating systems at the end of the 1990s.

Categories of Software

As the short history of software implies, there are two categories of software: systems software and applications software. Systems software "boots up" (starts up and initializes) the computer system; controls input, output, and storage; and controls the operations of the application software. Applications software includes the various programs that users require to perform day-to-day tasks. They are the programs that support the actual work of the user.

System Software

System software consists of a variety of programs that control the individual computer and make the user's application programs work well with the hardware. System software consists of a variety of utilities that initialize, or boot up, the computer when it is first turned on and thereafter control all the functions of the computer hardware and applications software. System software helps speed up the computer's processing, expands the power of the computer by creating cache memory, reduces the amount of confusion when multiple programs are running together, "cleans up" the hard drive so that storage is managed efficiently, and performs other such system management tasks.

Basic Input Output System

The first level of system control is handled by the basic input output system (BIOS) stored on a read only memory (ROM) chip on the motherboard. The software on the BIOS chip is the first part of the computer to function when the system is turned on. It first searches for an operating system and loads it into the RAM. Given that the BIOS consists of a set of instructions permanently burned onto a computer chip, it is truly a combination of hardware and software. Programs on chips are often called "firmware," because they straddle the line between hardware and software. For this reason, many computer engineers make a distinction between firmware and software. From that perspective, the operating system is actually the first level of system software.

Operating Systems

OSs are actual software, loaded from the hard drive into RAM as soon as the computer is turned on. While the firmware cannot be upgraded without changing the hardware chip, the operating system can be upgraded or entirely changed through software. The user simply deletes OS files from the hard drive and installs a new OS from a CD-ROM or floppy diskettes. Most users purchase a computer with the operating system already installed on the hard drive. However, the OS can be purchased separately and installed by the user. Operating systems handle the connection between the CPU and peripherals. (The connection between the CPU and a peripheral or a user is called an "interface.") The OS manages the interfaces to peripheral hardware, schedules tasks, allocates storage in memory and on disks, and provides an interface between the machine and the user.

One of the most critical tasks (from the user's perspective) performed by the operating system involves the management of storage. In the early computers, there were no operating systems. Every program had to explicitly tell the CPU exactly where in RAM to locate the lines of program code and data to be used during processing. That meant the user had to keep track of thousands of memory locations, and be sure to avoid writing one line of code over another active line of code. Also, the programmer had to be careful that output of one part of processing did not accidentally get written over output from another part of processing. As can be imagined, the need for management of storage consumed a great deal of time and programming code, and it produced many errors in programs. Since those errors had to be discovered and corrected before the program would run correctly, the lack of an operating system made programming enormously time-consuming and tedious. In comparison, programming today—while still a difficult and time-consuming task—is much more efficient.

User Interfaces

Disk Operating System   The operating system also provides a basic interface between the user and the hardware and software. There are two types of OS user interface: the interface provided by DOS and a GUI pro-

vided by operating systems such as Microsoft Windows. Essentially, the DOS operating systems present a blank screen to the user, and the user submits typed commands.

DOS operating systems were first designed for mainframe computers and replicated the procedures programmers used under the manual operating systems. They were an extension of the move away from dependency upon human operators and tedious memory allocation programming requirements. When operating systems were first developed for mainframes, they permitted tremendous advances in productivity in the computer department. However, just about everybody associated with the computer department at that time was a programmer. They all knew the syntax (wording and sequencing of commands). Thus, the need to type in long, non-English-like commands wasn't viewed as a great burden.

As computers became more popular and their applications became more useful to the general population, the need to learn DOS's obscure syntax became a real issue in office and home computing. Businesspeople, office support personnel, and home users may have wanted to use computers for document preparation, financial management tasks, games, and other personal applications; however, they very much did not want to learn programming. Unfortunately, some programming skills had to be acquired to use the DOS interface effectively. During the late 1970s and early 1980s, a great proportion of the potential market for PCs was lost because of people's extreme resistance to using systems with such a poor user interface.

Graphical User Interface   In 1979, Steve Jobs of the Apple Computer Company made a strategic decision to abandon the DOS interface and move to a GUI system for a new product to be called the Macintosh. The idea came as a result of his visit to the Xerox laboratory, where he saw the GUI that had been developed for a system that never really succeeded in the popular computer market. In 1984, the Macintosh with the first commercially available GUI was introduced. This was the "computer for everybody," and the PC market exploded. While the GUI did not eliminate the need for users to spend time learning new programs, it did bring closer to reality the ideal that computers could become "self-teaching" devices. People could begin to use computers with minimal training, using built-in tutorials and online answers to common questions. Bill Gates, founder and CEO of the Microsoft Corporation, quickly recognized the need to provide a GUI product and immediately began development of Windows, the GUI for the IBM PC platform. The popularity of GUIs is a function of their use of pictures rather than typed narrative commands.

A GUI operating system supports use of graphic images called "icons" to represent commands to the computer. Each icon image is designed to look like the physical representation of the operation the user wishes to employ. For example, a small image of a printer is used to symbolize the command to print a page or document. Rather than typing in commands such as "PRINT FILE," the user simply clicks the mouse button on the printer icon, and the print command is executed.

There are far too many commands needed for running most applications programs for all commands to be represented by icons. Therefore, GUI operating systems also support the operation of **menus**. Similar to menus in restaurants, the GUI menu provides a narrative list of common commands, or operations that the computer can execute. Rather than typing out a command, the user simply clicks the mouse button on the menu item desired, and the command represented by that menu word is executed. In complex programs that have hundreds or thousands of commands, the GUI supports **nested menus.**

Nested menus are submenus and sub-submenus; that is, the user clicks on a menu item, and instead of executing a command, the computer presents another menu of choices. (The submenu is fit, or nested, inside the main menu.) Clicking on a menu choice on a submenu might bring forth yet another menu. The process proceeds until the actual operation to be executed is listed. The nested menu format permits a virtually unlimited number of command options to be presented to the user, who never needs to remember the proper wording and order of a command in order to execute it.

Utility Programs

In addition to the operation system, there are a variety of other system programs available to the user. Some are called **utility** programs, and are designed to enhance the functions of the OS or perhaps to add facilities that the basic OS does not offer. These include programs that provide algorithms (formulae) for efficiently sorting a large set of numbers or character-based items, copying utilities, security programs, and the like.

Language Translation Utilities   As noted in Chapter 2, the computer only understands binary. However, human beings don't speak binary. Consequently, it is very difficult to write a program in the machine's language. Translation programs are needed to convert instructions written

in an English-like language into binary. These types of translation programs are called **assemblers, compilers,** or **interpreters**. Originally, they were all machine-dependent; that is, a compiler written for an IBM 360 mainframe computer could not work on a Hitachi mainframe computer. Even worse, a program written to work with one compiler could not work on a computer with a different compiler, even if the programming language was the same. With the advent of portable translators, that limitation has been at least partially overcome. Translation programs today are often 90% or more portable among different computer platforms. However, when buying a compiler, one still needs to purchase the version that has been customized to the user's computer platform.

The World Wide Web   The World Wide Web (WWW) is a sort of network system utility program for the Internet. It provides a protocol for document transfer across the Internet. Prior to the advent of the World Wide Web, commands to access and transfer documents throughout the Internet required users to know the command syntax of the Unix operating system. While Unix is still the operating system of the Internet, its command language is about as obscure to the average reader as assembly language.

The Internet is a system of data and voice lines routed through dedicated servers to create a network of networks; that is, it consists of linkages that allow users from one computer network to access the documents and files available on another network. The trick in developing a network is figuring out how to make documents stored on one platform available to networks that use entirely different platforms. Early in the development of computer communications, utility programs called file transfer protocols (FTPs) were developed to allow files to be ported from one computer to another and from one network to another.

While the original Internet was an extremely useful system to programmers and scientists who could construct commands in the Unix syntax, it was time-consuming to use. In 1989, Tim Berners-Lee, a scientist at Cern, Switzerland's laboratory for particle physics, originated the idea of having a protocol that would be standard for all documents and sites on the Internet (Berners-Lee and Fischetti, 1999) (Fig. 4.5). In this way, use of the Internet would be greatly facilitated not only for programmers, but for just about everybody who might want to use it. In August of 1991, Cern released the first WWW software.

Berners-Lee conceived the WWW as a system utility program that requires all users to adhere to a standard set

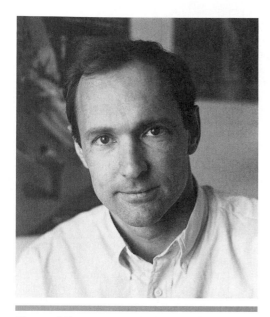

Figure 4.5
Tim Berners-Lee.
(Courtesey Donna Coveney/MIT.)

of text retrieval protocols (i.e., a standard command syntax for transfer of text from one computer to another). This set of protocols is called the <u>H</u>ypertext <u>T</u>ransfer <u>P</u>rotocol (HTTP). "Hypertext" refers to the facility that permits a standard text-linking command to be incorporated into documents. Text linking occurs when content in one document refers to another document, and the user can click on the linking text and have the protocol automatically move the user from the first document to the linked document (Berners-Lee and Fischetti, 1999). The WWW also needed to have a standard addressing system, so that every document would have one and only one address. This addressing system is called the <u>U</u>niversal <u>R</u>esource <u>L</u>ocator. Finally, it needed a way to have documents formatted so that colors, fonts, spacing, tables, and images could be created and transmitted across the Internet. The language developed for the Internet is called HTML, which stands for <u>H</u>ypertext <u>M</u>arkup <u>L</u>anguage. HTML allows document creators to format their text.

Although the WWW was an enormous advance, it still lacked one utility necessary to making the Web a household tool for everyone; it lacked a user-friendly graphical user interface. This problem was addressed through the release of Mosaic, a GUI interface for the Web developed by the National Center for Supercomputing Applications (NCSA) at the University of Illinois, Champaign-Urbana

campus. Mosaic was largely developed by Marc Anderson who later founded Netscape, one of the two most popular Web browsers.

Application Software

Application software includes the various programs people use to do work, process data, play games, communicate with others, or watch multimedia programs on a computer. Unlike system programs, they are written by or for system users. When the user orders the OS to run an application program, the OS transfers the program from the hard drive, diskette, or CD-ROM into RAM and executes it.

Application programs are written in a particular programming language. Then the program is "compiled" (or translated) into machine language so the computer can understand the instructions and execute the program. Originally, programs were written for a specific computer and could only run on that machine. However, the science of programming languages and their translation eventually advanced to the point that programs today can generally be "ported" (or transferred) across many machines. This advance permitted programmers to develop programs that could be used on any of a class of machines, such as the IBM type or Macintosh (the two are still generally incompatible). This advance opened a whole new industry, since programs could be marketed as off-the-shelf software packages.

Programming Languages

A programming language is a means of communicating with the computer. Actually, of course, the only language a CPU can understand is binary, or machine language. While it is certainly possible for programmers to learn to use binary—some highly sensitive defense applications are still written in machine language—the language is painfully tedious and inefficient of human resources, and its programs are virtually impossible to update and debug. Since the invention of computers, users have longed for a machine that could accept instructions in everyday human language. While that goal largely escapes the industry, a variety of English-like languages have been developed.

Generations and Levels of Programming Languages

Programming languages are divided into five generations, or sometimes into three levels. The term "level" refers to how close the language is to the actual machine. The first level includes the first two generations of programming languages: machine language and assembly language. The second level includes the next two generations: high-level procedural and nonprocedural languages. The third level (and fifth generation) is natural language.

The low-level languages are machine-like. Machine language is, of course, binary. It consists of strings of zeros and ones and can be directly understood by the computer. However, it is difficult to use and to edit.

Machine Language   Machine language is the true language of the computer. Any program must be translated into machine language before the computer can execute it. The machine language consists only of the binary numbers 1 and 0, representing the **on** and **off** electrical impulses. All data—numbers, letters, and symbols—are represented by combinations of binary digits. For example, the number 3 is represented by eight binary numbers (00000011), and 6 is represented by 00000110. Traditionally, machine languages are machine-dependent, which means that each model of computer has its own unique machine language.

Assembly Language   Assembly language is far more English-like, but it is still very close to machine language. One command in machine language is a single instruction to the processor. Assembly language instructions have a one-to-one correspondence with a machine language instruction. Assembly language is still used a great deal by systems programmers and whenever applications programmers wish to manipulate functions at the machine level. As can be seen from Fig. 4.6, assembly language, while more English-like than machine language, is extremely obscure to the nonprogrammer.

```
PRINT_ASCII PROC
        MOV DL, 00h
        DL MOV CX, 255
PRINT_LOOP:
        CALL WRITE_CHAR
        INC DL
        LOOP PRINT_LOOP
        MOV AH,4Ch
        INT 21h ;21h
PRINT ASCII     ENDP
```

Figure 4.6
Assembly language lines of code.

Third Generation Languages   Third generation languages include the procedural languages and were the beginning of the second level in programming languages. Procedural languages require the programmer to specify both what the computer is to do and the procedure for how to do it. These languages are far more English-like than assembly and machine language. However, a great deal of study is required to learn to use these languages. The programmer must learn the words the language recognizes, and must use those words in a rigid style and sequence. A single comma or letter out of place will cause the program to fail, or "crash." The style and sequence of a language are called its "syntax." FORTRAN and COBOL are examples of early third generation languages.

A third generation language written specifically for use in health care settings was MUMPS (Massachusetts General Hospital Utility Multi-Programming System). MUMPS was originally developed to support Medical Records applications at Massachusetts General. MUMPS offers powerful tools to support database management systems; this is particularly useful in any setting in which many users have to access the same databases at the same time. Therefore, MUMPS is now found in many different industries such as banks, travel agencies, the stock exchange, and of course, other hospitals. Originally, MUMPS was both a language and a full operating system. However, today most installations load MUMPS on top of their own computer's operating system.

Today, the most popular computer language for writing new operating systems and other systems programs is called C. (It was named after an earlier prototype program called simply B.)

Two important late third generation languages are increasing in importance as the importance of the Internet grows (see Chap. 6, "Computer Systems"). They include the visual programming languages and Java. Java was developed by Sun Microsystems to be a relatively simple language that would provide the portability across differing computer platforms and the security needed for use on a huge, public network like the Internet. The world community of software developers and Internet content providers has warmly received Java. Java programming skills are critical for any serious Web developer.

Visual Programming Languages   As the popularity of graphical user interface technology grew, several languages were developed to facilitate program development in graphics-based environments. Microsoft Corporation has marketed two very popular such programs:

Visual BASIC and Visual C++. These programs and their "cousins" marketed by other companies have been used for a variety of applications, especially those that allow users to interact with electronic companies through the Internet.

Fourth Generation Languages Fourth generation languages are specialized applications programs that require more involvement of the user in directing the program to do the necessary work. Some people in the computer industry do not consider these to be programming languages. Procedural languages include programs such as spreadsheets, statistical analysis programs, and database query languages. The difference between these languages and the earlier generation languages is that the user specifies **what** the program is to do, but not **how** the program is to perform the task. The "how" is already programmed by the manufacturer of the "language" program. For example, to perform a chi-square calculation in FORTRAN, the user must specify each step involved in carrying out the formula for a chi-square and the data upon which the operations are to be performed. In SPSS, a statistical analysis program, the user enters a command (from a menu of commands) that tells the computer to compute a chi-square statistic on a particular datasheet. The formula for chi-square is already part of the SPSS program; the user does not have to tell SPSS how to calculate the chi-square.

Fifth Generation Languages Fifth generation or third level languages are called natural language. In these types of programs, the user tells the machine what to do in the user's own natural language or through use of a set of very English-like commands. Ideally, voice recognition technology is integrated with the language so that voice commands are recognized and executed. True fifth generation languages are emerging. True natural language recognition, in which any user could give understandable commands to the computer in his or her own word style and accent is being performed at the beginning of the 21st century. However, natural language systems are clearly in the future of personal computing. The great difficulty is, of course, how to reliably translate natural, spoken human language into a language the computer can understand.

To prepare a translation program for a natural language requires several levels of analysis. First, the sentences need to be broken down to identify the subject's words and relate them to the underlying constituents of speech (i.e., parsed). The next level is called semantic analysis, whereby the grammar of each word in the sentence is analyzed. It attempts to recognize the action described and the object of the action. There are several computer programs that translate natural languages based on basic rules of English. They generally are specially written programs designed to interact with databases on a specific topic. By limiting the programs to querying the database, it is possible to process the natural language terms.

Software Packages

Software packages are application programs that are prepared sets of computer programs developed for a specific function and designed to fit the common computing needs of many different microcomputer users. For example, any user preparing a document can use a word-processing software package. Generally written for compatibility with the Windows or Macintosh GUI operating systems, they require little or no programming knowledge and are ready to use when purchased from a computer supply store and installed on the user's hard drive.

Software packages are sometimes developed and sold by computer manufacturers. However, more commonly they are developed by companies whose entire business is devoted to software development. The most powerful such company in the world is the Microsoft Corporation, founded by Bill Gates. Until the early 1990s, the number of software developers for PCs rapidly expanded each year. However, during the 1990s, market consolidation took place, and Microsoft's corporate strategy of making applications programs that were fully compatible—in some cases integrated with—the operating system was so successful that other companies' products began to disappear from the market. So much consolidation took place that the U.S. government began to file antitrust suits against Microsoft. The philosophy of seamless integration across a wide variety of programs has become firmly established in the market.

Common Packages in Health Care Institutions

The most common package sold with computers is a standard office package. The standard office package includes a word-processing program, a spreadsheet, a presentation graphics program, and some form of database management system. Most programs have to be written in two versions: one for the IBM PC platform and one for the Macintosh. Typically, software packages are sold on CD-ROM, although some are still available on floppy disks.

Software Package Ownership Rights

Protecting ownership rights in software has presented a challenge to the computer software industry. A program sold to one customer can be installed on a very large number of machines. This practice obviously seriously harms the profitability of software development. If programs were sold outright, users would have every right to distribute them as they wished. However, the industry could not survive in such market conditions. As a result, the software industry has followed an ownership model more similar to that of the book publishing industry than to the model used by vendors of most commercial products.

When a commercial product is sold, the buyer cannot use the product or resell it or loan it to a friend if so desired. The product sold is a physical product that can be used only by one customer at a time. Copying the product is not feasible. However, intellectual property is quite a different proposition; what is sold is the idea. The medium on which the idea is stored is not the product. However, when the PC industry was new, people buying software viewed their purchase as the physical diskette on which the intellectual property was stored. Software was expensive, but the diskettes were cheap. Therefore, groups of friends would often pool money to purchase one copy of the software and make copies for everyone in the group. This, of course, enraged the software vendors.

As a result, copyright laws were extended to software so that only the original purchaser was legally empowered to install the program on his or her computer. Any other installations were considered illegal copies, and such copies were called pirate copies. Purchasers of software do not buy full rights to the software. They purchase only a license to use the software. Individually purchased software is licensed to one and only one computer. An exception can be made if the individual has both a desktop and a laptop. Fair use allows the purchaser to install the software on all the machines he or she personally owns—so long as the computers are for that user's personal use only. Companies that have multiple computers that are used by many employees must purchase a separate copy for each machine, or in some cases they may purchase a "site license." A site license is a way of buying in bulk, so to speak. The company and software vendor agree on how many machines the software may be used on, and a special fee is paid for the number of copies to be used. Additional machines over

the number agreed upon require either an increase in the allowable sites—and payment of the higher site-license fee, or separate copies of the software may be purchased. What is not permitted, and is, in fact, a form of theft, is to install more copies of the software than were paid for.

The common software packages that are being used by health professionals include the following:

- Word-processing packages
- Desktop publishing packages
- Spreadsheet packages
- Database management packages
- Graphic packages
- Communication packages
- Statistical packages

Word-Processing Packages

A word-processing software program is the most common application used by microcomputer users. They have almost entirely replaced typewriters in American homes and offices. They still require typing skills, but many typists find they can work much faster on a word processor than on a typewriter—both for physical and psychological reasons. A word processor is physically easier to use. Setting margins, tabs, tables, and other special formatting tasks is far easier on a word processor than on a typewriter. The word processor also relieves the typist of worry about typing errors.

Everybody makes typing errors. On an old manual typewriter, error corrections were visible at best and messy at worst. It took an inordinate amount of time to take the paper out of the typewriter, erase or cover up the error, and then try to fit the page back into the typewriter so that the correction would not be off center. Later models offered correction tapes right on the machine, but even then corrections were often visible. Word processing packages are designed to let the user do all the work and editing on the screen and then print the document only after everything is done to his or her satisfaction. The user can print drafts and make changes and then print out another draft. Multiple drafts in a manual typewriter required fully or partially retyping the document.

Word processors have revolutionized the office. Document preparation is far more efficient. Many people find that their creative processes are enhanced when they work on the computer. Changes do not require tedious rewriting of the same text. Deletions are instant. Ideas can be typed as they occur, and organized later without tedium. Conference and symposia managers have greatly benefited from the change. Office computers are nearly universally available. Due to the dominance of Microsoft's word processor (MS Word), other word processor companies have had to offer some compatibility with that product. Therefore, it is no longer unreasonable to require users to prepare their conference paper on MS Word or its nearest competitor, Corel WordPerfect, and submit the paper electronically through E-mail. The symposia organizers merely need to compile and perform minor editing before submitting the proceedings to the publisher (although I'm sure, the process does not seem simple to the conference organizers!).

Word processors have caused a revolution in the work place—but everyone has not welcomed the changes. When management began to provide word processors to virtually all office workers, the trade-off was often a reduction in the secretarial staff. Office workers and educators have, by and large, lost the option to give handwritten work to secretaries. They are expected to construct their work on their own machine and then print it out themselves or perhaps send it electronically to the secretary for final edits and printing.

Desktop Publishing Packages

For more formal documents, such as newsletters, advertisements, journals, and the like, desktop publishing packages are available. Given the power of word processing programs, the distinction between word processors and desktop publishers is not as sharp as it was in the 1980s. However, when high quality print, color, and photographs are needed in a document, desktop publisher programs are still more versatile than word processing programs. They can manipulate words, add headlines, include pictures, and do a better job of arranging words into columns and fitting text around images so that the paper looks professionally prepared.

Spreadsheet Packages

Spreadsheet packages, also called electronic spreadsheets, are used to help customers with a variety of business and personal tasks that require mathematical operations on columns of numbers. The first spreadsheet package was a little program called VisiCalc developed by Dan Bricklin and Bob Frankston in Massachusetts in 1978. Dan Bricklin, a Harvard MBA student got the idea while working on a Texas Instruments Business calculator (Bricklin, 1999).

Bricklin, a bit annoyed at the tedium of using a calculator formed the idea that it would be much easier to perform business calculations if his calculator (or computer) would let him scroll up and down the column of figures. Having seen a demonstration by Douglas Engelbart, the inventor of the mouse, Bricklin developed the idea of a computer program that would support management and calculations of columns of numbers and let the user easily scroll up and down through the worksheet. He joined with an MIT engineer named Bob Frankston, and together they programmed the first spreadsheet, and named it VisiCalc. In 1979 when the product first went to market, the law had not yet caught up with the computer industry. Bricklin and Frankston consulted an attorney in an effort to patent their idea. However, at that time the courts were quite reluctant to permit patents on software products. The 1978 courts generally viewed software ideas as mathematical algorithms, which are ineligible for patent protection. In 1981, the Supreme Court radically changed software inventors' right to patent their ideas. But by that time it was too late; VisiCalc had already been copied by another company. Therefore, when the Lotus Company took Bricklin and Frankston's idea and produced a competing product, Lotus 1-2-3, the inventors had no royalty rights and no recourse.

Electronic spreadsheet packages are widely used for the preparation of financial statements, budgets, cash projections, etc. They are used to perform mathematical calculations, including addition, subtraction, multiplication, and division. Calculations are prepared by formulas that allow automatic recalculation of the calculated values when one value used in the formula is altered.

Database Management System Packages

Database management system (DBMS) packages are designed to help with storage and retrieval of data. They allow the user to treat stored data as a renewable resource. This concept is a true paradigm shift in the way data are viewed. For example, when data are stored in a paper chart, they can be viewed only in the same way as they were stored. If a report different from the original chart form is desired, the data must be copied from the original paper chart to another format. With a DBMS, the data are stored in electronic files. The screen formats used for data collection are merely windows and do not reflect the structure of the database. The power of this approach is that when data are wanted for a purpose different from that for which they were originally collected, the user merely enters a query to the database, and a command to format the output in a new format. Subsets of th can be quickly extracted. The power and economy approach are immense. Data truly become a r resource like energy from the sun, rather than a restricted asset, which, like money, can be used only in one way.

Presentation Graphics Packages

Graphic packages communicate ideas via pictures. They are used to display visual representation of ideas in the form of graphics, colored slides, images, and tables. These programs make it easy for the user to produce professional looking visuals for professional presentations or to enhance documents with colored images and graphics. The packages allow the user to enter data and have those data presented in various types of graphs. For example, line graphs, bar graphs, scatter plots, pie graphs, contour plots, and the like can all be generated in minutes with programs such as Microsoft Power Point or Corel Presentations. Users can also create text "slides" such as title slides, tables, and bulleted item presentations with these programs. Other widely available graphics programs such as Corel Draw and Microsoft Paint allow users to manipulate images and create their own drawings.

Some of these programs can also perform some of the tasks that were formerly available only through special computer-aided design (CAD) support programs. CAD programs were designed to help the work of engineers. CAD programs support preparation of product drawings and flow diagrams, and today they provide a wide variety of other applications that support the work of engineering. However, many people want to prepare flow charts and organizational charts. Therefore, the major producers of presentation graphics programs have included facilities to help users produce flow charts and organizational charts and a variety of other special graphics.

Internet Communication Packages

The Internet has offered new means of electronic communication—including electronic conferencing—that are rapid and inexpensive. Distance ceases to be a factor in communication when everybody has access to the Internet. Language incompatibility may be a problem, but the Internet is rapidly making English a sort of world standard for language communication. Some of the means by which people communicate across the Internet are E-mail, chat rooms, video conferencing, bulletin boards (including listserv technology), and electronic forum.

Electronic Mailbox Packages   Electronic mailboxes are used to transmit messages (letters, memos, and reports) from one person to another person or group. E-mail messages can be stored and forwarded without the receiver having to be present to receive it. They can

be used to upload (send) work from a home office to an office computer or download (receive) files. E-mail is used to transmit letters and other messages via data communications channels and combines the features of both telephone calls and conventional mail. E-mail is so fast that regular mail sent through the post office is now often called "snail mail."

E-mail involves a one-to-one or one-to-many relationship. However, sometimes messages need to be placed in a conferencing medium that allows a many-to-many relationship. Just as E-mail is analogous to postal mail, several types of technology allow communication that is analogous to group meetings or conferences.

Chat Rooms   Chat rooms are like electronic conference calls. Multiple users can send and receive messages at the same time. Some chat rooms are private and require a password to enter. Others are open to the public. All members of the chat room can see all the messages posted, just as all people at a party can hear all the conversations near them. The strengths of chat room technology include the ability of many people to "meet" without having to leave their homes. Distance doesn't matter with a chat room. The person the user is "chatting" with can be at another computer in the same room, or halfway around the world. Chat room technology is real-time technology; that is, messages disappear once they scroll off the screen unless they are printed or otherwise explicitly saved. Chat rooms have their dangers. Users can remain anonymous, and anybody can participate in a public chat room. There have been cases where pedophiles have used chat rooms to become acquainted with children and to entice them into face-to-face meetings. The general rule in a public chat room is, "Let the buyer beware."

Electronic Bulletin Boards

An early form of computer conferencing involved electronic bulletin boards. Even today this form of communication is very popular. As with chat rooms, some are public and some private. However, most are private. They are called by different names, depending upon the terminology used by the software creator. They may be called discussion boards, listservs, or electronic forums. However, they all work in similar ways. This technology creates space where users can post a message. In the better software, the messages can be posted according to user-defined or system administrator-defined categories. For example, there may be a discussion on CPU technology and problems, another discussion about peripherals, and so forth.

The least powerful version of an electronic bulletin board is a listserv. This program functions more like an electronic mailing list than a true discussion board. When a user posts a message to the board, it is merely E-mailed to all members of the conference. The software may or may not store all the messages in an accessible archive so users can review all the entries at one time. A user can respond to an item on the listserv by posting a new item. Some users find the listserv technology inconvenient because E-mailboxes can get filled up with messages the user does not need to view immediately. Limiting one's own access to the messages on a listserv to the times that are personally convenient is not possible. The messages arrive whenever other members send them.

Electronic discussion boards or forums are more powerful and are an important technology in distance courses offered through the Internet. These programs are accessed entirely at the user's convenience. Most such programs let the user define a new topic of discussion, add a new item to an existing topic, or respond to an item placed by another user. The strengths of this technology are that the items are organized according to topic, and they remain available until the conference organizer explicitly removes them. Unlike chat rooms, users access the board at their own convenience and can take time to formulate a response.

Computer Programming

Computer programming refers to the process of writing a computer program, which is a series of instructions written in proper sequence to solve a specific problem. A program primarily encompasses the program instructions and is generally written by a computer programmer.

The five major steps in writing any computer program are as follows:

- Problem definition (functional specifications)
- Program design
- Writing the code and program documentation
- Alpha testing
- Beta testing and program documentation

Problem or Functions Specification

Defining the problem to be solved or the functions to be performed by the program is the most critical step in programming. It requires that the problem or task be very precisely defined and the procedures to be performed by the program to be perfectly understood. In essence, the problem definition must analyze and outline in detail the scope of the problem and all the elements needed to solve

it. For example, a very simple problem definition for the cost of a nursing visit might read as follows: "Calculate the cost of nursing visit 'C' by totaling cost of nurse 'A' and cost of supplies 'B.'"

Program Design Specifications

Once the problem/task is precisely specified, the process for solving the problem must be designed. There are generally two types of specifications involved in program creating. The first is the set of functional specifications that identifies all the functions the program is to perform. This should include a narrative description of the functions of the system and a graphical representation of the system's process flow. This is used to ensure that both the system designer and the people who have contracted for the designer's services share the same understanding of the planned system. The second set of specifications (called "specs") is the design specifications. The design specs are the instructions given to the programmer. Design specs may be highly technical and are not typically viewed by the customers. They are prepared by the systems analyst after consultation with the customer about the functional specs. The systems analyst, an expert in both analysis and design, is typically a person with expertise in programming. It is the analyst's job to ensure that the programmer's instructions not only fully meet the functional specs, but also help the programmer prepare a program that runs smoothly and consumes no more of the computer's processing power than necessary.

Program Preparation

Program preparation, the actual writing (or coding) of the program, entails translating the design specifications into the programming language to be used. The program instructions (algorithms) must be coded in detail and in logical sequence so that the program can process data correctly. The programming language selected must not only be appropriate for processing the problem but must be translated by the computer for which it is written. The language rules must be followed precisely, because a single coding error can stop the program from running or cause program malfunction. The process of error correction so that the program runs is called "debugging."

Documentation

Two types of documentation must be produced during programming. First, the program itself should be designed in a highly structured, top-down manner, and the lines of code should be liberally sprinkled with explanatory statements. These statements are not part of the program itself. However, they clearly identify what program modules or individual lines of code do in the program. Program documentation also includes a narrative manual of instructions to system administrators who will have to maintain the program after the initial programming is completed. A well-documented program is easier to edit, easier for other programmers to support, and easier to debug. The second type of documentation that must be produced is the user's manual. The user's manual provides clear directions and examples of how to make the program work as intended. It should also provide suggestions for how to proceed when users cannot get the program to function as they expect. The process of manual development proceeds throughout several stages of the programming process, including code preparation, program testing, and program implementation.

Program Testing

Alpha Testing   Program testing occurs during and after coding. Two types of testing are performed. First, the programming team and system analysts carefully desk check the program in a process called "alpha testing." This process is also called "desk checking." The purpose of alpha testing is to see if all the processes appear to be functioning as specified in the flow charts, functional specifications, and design specs.

Beta Testing   The second level of testing is called "beta testing." In beta testing, the program is installed in the actual user environment, and further programming of screen formats and other user interface functions is performed. Documentation adequacy is examined. Some users are trained to use the system. Users begin the final testing phase by entering real data and checking that the system products are accurate and complete. During initial beta testing, the system implementation process is begun. Usually, only one unit or workstation is brought on-line and only for the purpose of system testing. During beta testing, users should actually perform both the old manual procedures and the new computer program. In that way, when the new program fails to perform exactly as required (and virtually all new programs need further debugging during beta testing), the work of the organization is not compromised.

Program Implementation

Program implementation is the final step in programming. In this phase, the program is implemented through-

out the beta site. All the users are trained, and the full day-to-day data load is imposed upon the system. At this point, there will still be bugs, but the problems should be relatively minor. However, sometimes when the large amounts of data that the system must handle on a daily basis are entered, and the full range of program functions is called, new problems arise. Programmers must be readily available to solve these problems at any time of the day or night. This step is where user-related problems are most likely to be discovered. When users who are perhaps not favorable to making a system change—and are perhaps not naturally talented in the use of computers—begin to use the system on a daily basis, new problems will arise. When these problems are solved and the beta site is up and running smoothly, then—and only then—is the program ready to be sold on the consumer market.

A final caution for users of software packages. Users may design screens and report formats, but they must be aware that all copyrights remain with the software package creators. Any plans to distribute designed screens or report formats must first be cleared with the vendor of the program.

■ Summary

This chapter highlighted computer software, which includes the computer programs, the programming languages in which they are written, and major software programs available on the market. It provided a bit of history related to software development and described the process by which new programs are developed.

Computer programs are sets of instructions stored in computer memory that are used to make the computer perform work. Computer languages are divided into five generations, or three levels. The lower level languages (encompassing the first two generations) are machine language and assembly language. The second level (encompassing the second two generations) includes all the procedural and nonprocedural computer languages. The third level (and fifth generation) languages are natural human language processors. The fifth generation computer languages are still evolving but are clearly the future of computing. Several of the commonly used computer languages are described.

The most commonly used software packages for the personal computer were described. These packages include word processors, spreadsheets, graphics packages, and communication packages. Communication packages include E-mail, chat room software, and computer conferencing programs such as listservs and forums or discussion boards.

Finally, an overview of the key steps in the computer system development process was provided. Those steps are problem definition, development of functional and design specifications, code development, program and system documentation, system alpha and beta testing, and final system implementation.

 # References

Austrian, G. (1982). *Herman Hollerith: Forgotten Giant of Information Processing*. New York: Columbia University Press.

Berners-Lee, T. and Fischetti, M. (1999). *Weaving the Web: The Origin, Design and Ultimate Destiny of the World Wide Web by Its Inventor*. San Francisco, CA: Harper Books.

Bricklin, B. (1999). The idea. VisiCalc: Information from its creators, Dan Bricklin and Bob Frankston. *http://www.bricklin.com/visicalc.htm*

Dunne, P. E. (1994). Mechanical Aids to Computation and the Development of Algorithms. *http://www.csc.liv.ac.uk/~ped/teachadmin/histsci/htmlform/lect1.html*

Evan, C. (1979). *The Micro Millennium*. New York: Viking Press.

Ettinger, J. (1999). *A Brief History of Operating Systems*. United Kingdom: Department of Software Engineering, Cavendish School of Computer Science. *http://www.wmin.ac.uk/~ettingj/se101/Lect06.html*

Keller, K.H. 1996. Charles Babbage. *http://www.ualr.edu/~klheller/babbage.html*

Lee, J. (1987). Grace Murray Hopper. *Annals of the History of Computing, 9(3)*, 273.

Schieber, P. (1987). The wit and wisdom of Grace Hopper. *OCLC Newsletter*, No. 167, March/April. *http://www.cs.yale.edu/~tap/Files/hopper-wit.html*

Toole, B.A. (1992). *Ada: The Enchantress of Numbers*. Sausalito, CA: Strawberry Press.

Women's International Center. (Undated). Grace Hopper: Mother of the Computer. *WIC Biography Series*. *http://www.wic.org/bio/ghopper.htm*

5

Data Processing

Ramona Nelson

OBJECTIVES

1. Explain data, databases, information, and information systems
2. Explain file structures and database models
3. Describe the purpose, structures, and functions of database management systems
4. Outline the life cycle of a database system
5. Explain concepts and issues related to data warehouses in health care

KEY WORDS

information systems
computer science
data processing

Nurses are knowledge workers providing care to individuals, families, and communities in the information-intensive environment of modern health care. They are continually collecting data about their clients and their clients' environment. The data are organized and processed, producing information about client needs and potential interventions. Using an extensive nursing knowledge database, the information is interpreted to develop a plan. The plan may apply to an individual, a family, or a whole community. Nurses then use these plans as well as their judgement and wisdom in providing caring cost-effective quality care.

In the information-intensive environment of modern health care, automated database systems are a major resource for meeting these wide ranging client needs. This chapter introduces the nurse to concepts, theories, models, and issues necessary to understand the effective use of automated database systems.

Defining Data, Databases, Information, and Information Systems

Data are raw uninterpreted facts that are without meaning. For example, a patient's weight is recorded as 140 lbs. Without additional information, this fact or datum cannot be interpreted. The patient could be a young child who is very overweight or an adult who is several pounds underweight. When data are interpreted, information is

produced. While data are meaningless, information by definition is meaningful. For data to be interpreted and information produced, the data must be processed. This means that the data are organized so that patterns and relationships between the data can be identified. There are several approaches to organizing data.

Some common approaches include sorting, classifying, summarizing, and calculating. For example, students will often take all of their notes and handouts from their nursing classes and organize these into folders. Each folder is used for a different topic. The data in the folders can be organized by nursing problems, interventions, medical diseases, cell biology, or drugs, to name but a few classifications for the information. Sometimes it is difficult to decide which folder the notes should be stored in. The student may make a copy of the notes and store it in both folders or may put the notes in one folder and a cross-reference note in the other folder. The folders are then placed in a box, file cabinet, or some other storage media, and a database has been created.

Another common example of a database is a checkbook used to store everyday financial data. Each number by itself means nothing. However, if the owner of the checkbook is careful to capture each entry and correctly calculates as money moves in and out of the account, the final number will summarize the current status of the checking account. This information can be very meaningful to the owner of the checkbook.

A database is an organized collection of related data. Placing notes in folders and folders in file cabinets is one example of creating a database. However, a database can be organized and stored in many different formats. A common paper example is the phone book. A much more complex example can be a patient's medical record. Each of these databases can be used to store data and to search for information. The possibility of finding information in these databases depends on several factors. Three of the most important are how the data are organized, the size and complexity of the database, and the type of data within the database.

The systematic approach used to organize and store data in a database has a major impact on how easy it is to find information in the database. The phone book is organized alphabetically by name. This makes it very easy to find a phone number if you know the person's name and very difficult to find a person's name if you start with the phone number. A large database can be more difficult to search than a small database. The size of a database is determined not only by the amount of data in the database, but also by the number and complexity of the relationships between the data. For example, the phone book may be for a large city and require two volumes, while the patient's chart may reflect an overnight observational visit at the hospital. While the phone book may be larger, there is a minimum number of relationships between the data. Those data in the patient's chart can be organized in an infinite number of ways. A wide range of caregivers will see different relationships and reach different conclusions from reading the same chart.

Information systems are used to process data and produce information. The term "information system" is often used to refer to computer systems, but this is only one type of information system. There are manual information systems as well as human information systems. The most effective and complex information system is the human brain. People are constantly taking in data and processing that data to produce meaning. At the beginning of this chapter, there was a reference to a patient weighing 140 lbs. Most people when they read that sentence begin to fill in the "missing data" or start to list their additional questions. This piece of datum is being structured and organized to produce meaning. However, each person starts with a different conceptual framework. As a result, no two people will process the data in exactly the same way. While computers offer more consistency, they cannot deal with the wide range of complex data that the human mind can interpret. In health care, you are working with a combination of manual, automated, and human information processing systems. This offers both the advantages and disadvantages of each of these systems as well as a multitude of interface problems.

Types of Data

When developing automated database systems, each data element is defined. As part of this process, the data are classified. There are two primary approaches to classifying data in a database system. First, they are classified in terms of how these data will be used by the user. This is sometimes referred to as the conceptual view of the data. For example, the data may be classified as financial data, patient data, or human resource data. The conceptual view of the data has a major impact on how the data are indexed. Second, data are classified by their computerized data type. For example, data can be numbers or letters or a combination of both. This classification is used to build the physical database within the computer system. It identifies the number of spaces needed to capture each data element and the specific functions that can be performed on these data.

Computer-Based Data Types   Alphanumeric data include letters and numbers in any combination. However, the numbers in an alphanumeric field cannot perform numeric function. For example, an address is alphanumeric data that may include both numbers and letters. A social security number is an example of alphanumeric data made up of numbers. It makes no logical sense to add or perform any other numerical functions on either addresses or social security numbers. The number of spaces that can be used for an alphanumeric field must be identified for the computer system. Memo is a specific type of alphanumeric data with increased spaces and decreased indexing options.

Numeric data are used to perform numeric functions including adding, subtracting, multiplying, and dividing. There are several different formats as well as types of numeric data. The number of digits after the decimal or the presence of commas in a number are examples of format options. Numeric data can be long integer, currency, or scientific.

Date and time are special types of numeric data with which certain numeric functions are appropriate. For example, two dates could be subtracted to determine how many days, months, and/or years are between the two dates. However, it would not make sense to add together several different dates.

Logic data are data limited to two options. Some examples include YES or NO, TRUE or FALSE, 1 or 2, and ON or OFF.

Conceptual Data Types Conceptual data types reflect how users view the data. These can be based on the source of the data. For example, the lab produces lab data, and the x-ray department produces image data. Conceptual data can also be based on the event that the data are attempting to capture. Assessment data, intervention data, and outcome data are examples of data that reflect event capturing. One of the major advantages of an automated information system is that each of these data elements can be captured once and used many times by different users for different purposes. For example, a patient with diabetes mellitus has an elevated blood sugar level. This datum may be used by the physician to adjust the patient's insulin dose and used by the nurse in a patient education program. These basic data elements can also

be aggregated and summarized to produce new data and information that may be used by a different set of users. This is referred to as "data collected once, used many times." Figure 5.1 gives an excellent example of this concept.

Database Management Systems

Database management systems (DBMSs) are computer programs used to input, store, modify, process, and access data in a database. Before a DBMS can be used, the DBM software must first be configured to manage the data specific to the project. This process of configuring the database software is called database system design. Once the software is configured for the project, the database software is used to enter the project data into the computer. A functioning DBMS consists of three interacting parts. These are the data, the DBMS configured software program, and the query language used to

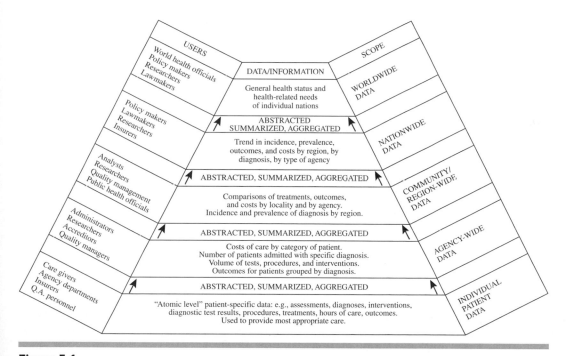

Figure 5.1

Examples of uses of atomic-level patient data collected once, used many times.

(Reprinted, with permission, from Rita D. Zielstorff, Carole I. Hudgings, Susan J. Grobe, and The National Commission on Nursing Implementation Project Task Force on Nursing Information Systems. Next-generation nursing information systems. © 1993 American Nurses Publishing, American Nurses Foundation/American Nurses Association, Washington, D.C.)

access the data. Some examples of DBMS in everyday life include computerized library systems, automated teller machines, and flight reservation systems. When these systems are being used, the data, the DBMS, and the query language interact together. As a result, it is easy to confuse one with the other. Earlier in this chapter, a database was created for class notes. The notes and handouts are the data. The folders and file cabinet are the DBMS. The labels on the folders and the file cabinet are the database system design. It is possible to remove all the notes and to put new data that are unrelated to course work in the DBMS or to put the notes into a new set of folders and files. In either case, the folders and files would need to be relabeled.

The user knows how the data are organized and how to look for specific pieces of information. This makes it possible for the user to find information in the files. With a manual system, the index and query language are usually in the user's head. However, there are problems storing and finding data with a manual system. Putting the data in sometimes requires duplicate copies. Once data have been stored, it is not unusual to forget where it is stored or to forget about the data completely. Automated DBMSs deal with many of these problems.

Advantages of Automated Database Management Systems   Automated DBMSs decrease data redundancy, increase data consistency, and improve access to all data. These advantages result from the fact that in automated systems all data exist in only one place. The data are never repeated.

Data redundancy occurs when the same data are stored in the database more than once. Making a copy of class notes to store the same notes in two different folders is an example of data redundancy. In health care, there are many examples of data redundancy. Patients, as they are assessed by different health care providers, will complain that they have answered the same questions over and over. Often nurses will need to chart the same data on different forms in a patient's medical record. In an automated DBMS, the data are recorded once and accessed from this single location each time it is needed.

When the same data are stored in different manual or automated databases, a second problem emerges. The data become inconsistent. As different users working with different databases update or change data, they do not always consistently record it in the same format. Once the data are inconsistent, it can be impossible to know the correct data. Two examples from education and health care may make this clearer. Most universities

maintain several different databases with the student's address. Some of the databases are manual, and some are automated. When the student changes addresses, it is not unusual for the student to receive mail at both the old and new address. The person or department sending the letter has no way of knowing which is the correct address. When a patient is admitted to a hospital, different caregivers will ask the patient to identify all medication he or she was taking at home. Sometimes the patient will list only prescription medications; other times the patient will include over-the-counter drugs taken on a routine basis. Sometimes the patient will forget to include a medication. As these different lists are recorded in different sections of the medical record, inconsistency occurs. In an automated DBMS, each caregiver is working with the same list each time the data are reviewed.

With an automated DBMS, access to data becomes much easier. The database management software program uses a structured approach to organize and store data. The same software uses a query language, making it possible for the computer to do the work of searching for the data. This structured approach for storing data uses fields, records, and files.

Fields, Records, and Files

Figure 5.2 demonstrates the terms field, record, and file. Each of the blocks or cells in the table is a field. The top row lists the field names. The field name for the third column is L-NAME. Field names usually reflect the type of data that will be recorded in the related fields. For example, L-NAME refers to last name. In rows 2 through 5, each cell includes a field attribute. A field attribute is the specific datum for that field for that record. Each row represents a record. For example, row 2 is the record for Betty Smith. Each row is assigned a primary identifier. A primary identifier is unique to that record. No other record in the database will have that identifier. In this table, the field name for the unique identifier is ID. The ID datum for each of these records is a unique number.

All the records in the table constitute a file. In a DBMS, there are several tables or files. A file is defined as a set of related records that have the same data fields. A database consists of several files. The DBMS can then search across the tables or files to find data related to any one entity in the database. The unique identifier is in each record in each file. It is the unique identifier that is used to tie the files together when searching across tables. In summary, a database is made up of files, files are made up of records, records are made up of fields, and fields contain data.

ID	F-NAME	L-NAME	ADDRESS-1	ADDRESS-2	CITY	ST
01	Mike	Smith	SRU, School of Nursing	20 North St	Pgh	PA
02	Leslie	Brown	DBMS Institute	408 Same St	NY	NY
03	Dori	Jones	Party Place	5093 Butler St	Any	VA
04	Glenn	Clark	Univ of Study	987 Carriage Rd	Field	PA

Figure 5.2
Examples of files, records, and fields.

There are several different types of data, as discussed earlier, that can be inserted in each field. The key datum used to tie the tables together and make it possible to search the total database is the unique identifier.

Types of Files

Within a DBMS, there are two basic types of files. These are the data files, as described in the previous section, and the processing files that direct the computer activities. On a personal computer, it is easy to see a list of the files that are stored on the computer. For example, on a computer using one of the Windows operating systems, click on MY COMPUTER. Then click on any of the disk drives. At this point, a list of files and folders will usually be displayed. If folders are displayed, simply open the folders by clicking on them. The name for each file will be displayed. Depending on the way the computer has been configured to display the files, there may also be additional information including the size, type, and date the file was created. Each of these files serves one of two basic purposes. There are files that direct the computer on how data are to be processed, and there are files that store data.

Processing files

Executable files consist of a computer program or set of instructions that, when executed, causes the computer to open or start a specific computer program or function. These are the files that tell a computer what actions the computer should perform when running a program. For example, running a SET-UP.EXE file will tell the computer to begin installing the related computer program on the computer. On a personal computer, most executable files end with the extension EXE

Command files are a set of instructions that perform a set of functions as opposed to running a whole program. For example, command files are used to boot or start the operating system when a computer is turned

on. On a personal computer, some of the key command files include AUTOEXEC.BAT and CONFIG.SYS The extension BAT indicates that the file is a specific type of command file called a batch file. A batch file contains a set of operating system commands. For example, a batch file may tell the computer to open or start a virus-checking program when the computer is booted.

Data files

Data files contain data that have been captured and stored on a computer using a software program. Many times the extension for the file identifies the software program used to create the file. For example, a document created in Microsoft Word will have the extension DOC. Sometimes the extension indicates the format, especially if it is a standard format used across several computer programs. For example, a word processing document can be saved as "text only." This means that all the formatting such as bold or italics are stripped off. In this case, the standard extension is TXT.

The master index file contains the unique identifier and related indexes for all entities in the database. An example is the identification file for all patient records in a health care system. In most cases, a master file will contain additional information that can be used to ensure the identity of the entity. In a master index for patient files, the additional information usually includes the patient's birth date and social security number.

Database Models

The successful use of a database is dependent on the careful structuring of the files and records within the database. A database provides access to both the data in the database and to the interrelationship within and between the various data elements. Building a database begins by identifying the data elements and the relationships that exist between the data elements. The first step in building the database is to understand the data and the data relationships from the users' perspective. This is referred to as the conceptual model. The conceptual model is then used as a guide for structuring the physical database within the computer.

Conceptual Models

A formal conceptual model includes a diagram and narrative description of the data elements, their attributes, and the relationships between the data. For example, there may be a database system to manage patient medication orders. With each individual order, there will be several data elements. The data elements include the specific medication, the dose, the time and frequency of administration, the route of administration, and any specific directions for administering the medication. Each medication order is an individual order written for one patient. This is referred to as a one-to-one relationship. A one-to-one relationship is diagrammed in Fig. 5.3.

While there is only one order, each order can result in several administrations of the medication. For example, an order for amoxicillin 500 mg q 8 hrs. times 10 days would result in the medication being administered 30 times. This is a one-to-many relationship. A one-to-many relationship is diagrammed in Fig. 5.4.

While Figure 5.4 demonstrated a one-to-many relationship, a simpler form of this type of diagram is demonstrated in Fig. 5.5. Note that in Fig. 5.5 the first box, Medication Order, includes the word "Frequency" while the second box, Medication Administration, includes the word "Time." It is the relationship between frequency and time that creates the one-to-many relationship.

Data in a database may also have many-to-many relationships. For example, a patient may have several caregivers and each caregiver may have several patients or clients.

When completed, the conceptual data model will include all data elements, the definition and attributes of each datum, and all relationships between data. The definitions and the description of each data attribute are used to create the data dictionary. For nursing, this has been a major challenge. Many of the data elements including nursing diagnosis, interventions, and outcomes have not been included in the data dictionaries of DBMSs used in health care. Nursing has had difficulty identifying and defining data elements in a format that can be used in an automated system. In the last few years, there have been several major accomplishments in the development of nursing languages. It is now imperative that nursing leaders share these developments with database system developers in health care.

Conceptual data models for health care systems are usually very large and include several pages. Even when planning a small database for personal use developing the conceptual model is an important first step. There are several questions that can be helpful in thinking through this process.

1. How will the database be used? What kind of information or output will be expected from the system? This includes both on-line queries and written reports.

2. What data elements need to be in the database to produce the desired output? What are the attributes of each data element? What type of data are the data elements, and how much space does each data element require? For example, a first name is an alphanumeric data type. The largest name in the database may require 25 character spaces.

3. What are easy to remember logical names for each of the data fields?

4. What approach will be used to create a unique identifier for each record in the database? Is each table designed so that there is a unique identifier for each record?

5. Is each of the tables designed so that there are no unnecessary overlapping data, and yet there are

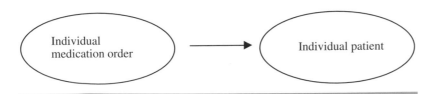

Figure 5.3
One-to-one relationship.

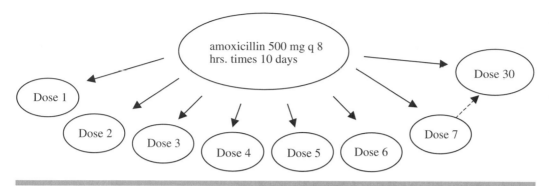

Figure 5.4
One-to-many relationship.

common data fields so that searches can include several tables?

Once developed, the conceptual data model provides the foundation for the physical data model.

Structural or Physical Data Models

The physical data model includes each of the data elements and the relationship between the data elements. There are four primary approaches to the development of a physical data model. These are hierarchical, network, relational, and object-oriented.

Hierarchical   Hierarchical databases have been compared to inverted trees. All access to data starts at the top of the hierarchy, or at the root. The table at the root will have pointers called branches that will point to

tables with data that relate hierarchically to the root. Each table is referred to as a node. For example, a master index might include pointers to each patient's record node. Each of the patient record nodes could include pointers to lab data, radiology data, and medication data for that patient. The patient record nodes are called parent nodes, while the lab, medication, and radiology nodes are called child nodes. In a hierarchical model, a parent node may have several children nodes, but each child node can only have one parent node. Fig. 5.6 demonstrates a hierarchical model and the related terminology.

Hierarchical models are very effective at representing one-to-many relationships. However, they have some disadvantages. Many data relationships do not fit the one-to-many model. Remember the class notes that were put in two folders. In addition, if the data relation-

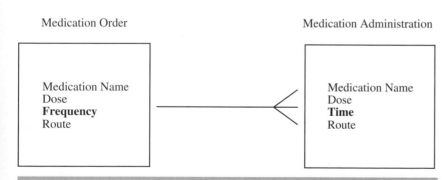

Figure 5.5
Simpler form diagramming the one-to-many relationship.

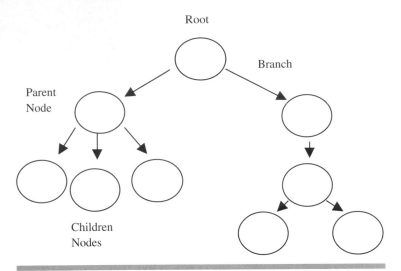

Figure 5.6
Hierarchical database model.

ships change, this can require significant redesign of the database.

Network Model   Network models developed from hierarchical models. In a network model, the child node is not limited to one parent. This makes it possible for a network model to represent many-to-many relationships. However, the presence of multiple links between data does make it more difficult if data relationships change and redesign is needed.

Relational Database Models   Relational database models consist of a series of files set up as tables. Each column represents an attribute, and each row is a record. Another name for a row is "tuple." The intersection of the row and the column is a cell. The datum in the cell is the manifestation of the attribute for that record. Each cell may contain only one attribute. Because of this limitation, the relationships represented are linear and only relate one data element to another.

A relational database joins any two or more files and generates a new file from the records that meet the matching search criteria. Figure 5.7 includes two related tables, Table A and Table B. Both tables include the patient's ID number. This is the common field by which the tables can be joined. By joining these two tables, it is possible to create a new table that identifies all patients who have a diagnosis of CVA. For example, Table C is

created by the DBMC in response to the query, "List all patients with a diagnosis of CVA."

Object-Oriented Model   An object-oriented database consists of objects that essentially represent an entity. In addition, attributes of the entity are stored with the object. An object can store other objects as well. In the object-oriented model the data definition includes both the object and its attributes. For example, amoxicillin is an antibiotic. All antibiotics have certain attributes or actions. Because amoxicillin is an antibiotic, it can be stored in the object antibiotic and inherit the attributes that are true of all antibiotics. In addition to containing numbers and text, an object-oriented approach can contain complex data types such as pictures and sounds. This is a major advantage in health care computing.

Database Life Cycle

The development and use of a DBMS follow a systematic process called the life cycle of a database system. The number of steps used to describe this process can vary from one author to another. In this chapter, the life cycle process will be described in five steps. While the process of developing a database management system moves forward through these steps, there is a recursive pattern to the development. Each step in the process provides the developer(s) with new insights. As these new insights

Table A

ID	L-NAME	F-NAME	SEX	B-DATE
12	Smith	Tom	M	01-23-73
14	Brown	Robert	M	02-01-77
13	Jones	Mary Lou	F	12-12-54
15	Yurick	Edward	M	04-04-38

Table B

ID	DX-1	DX-2	DX-3	DX-4
12	MI	CVA	GLAUCOMA	PVD
14	CVA	HEPATITIS C	COLITIS	UTI
13	DIABETES M	ANGINA	CVA	GOUT
15	CERF	ANEMIA	GLAUCOMA	PEPTIC ULCER

Table C

ID	L-NAME	F-NAME	DX-1	DX-2	DX-3
12	Smith	Tom		CVA	
14	Brown	Robert	CVA		
13	Jones	Mary Lou			CVA

Figure 5.7
Relational database.

occur, it is sometimes necessary to make modifications in previously completed steps of the process.

Initiation

Initiation occurs when a need or problem is identified and the development of a DBMS is seen as a potential solution. This initial assessment looks at what is the need, what are the current approaches, and what are the potential options for dealing with the need. For example, the Staff Development Department in a home health agency may want to automate their staff education records. The current approach is to maintain an index card for each staff member. The index card lists all the programs attended by the individual staff member. When the card gets full, a second card is stapled to the first card. When the department needed to know how many total hours of staff development education had been provided monthly by branch office for the last year, it required paying staff several hours of overtime to review the cards and collect these data. The department had a computer with a DBMS software program; however, no one in the depart-

ment knew how to use the program or structure the data for a database program. A decision was made to request assistance in designing a database from the Information Services Department. The nurse who organized most of the reports for the department would attend in-service classes and work with the database administrator from the Informational Services Department. The Staff Development Department is ready to start planning for their automated DBMS.

Planning and Analysis

This step begins with the development of the conceptual model. What are all the information needs of the department and how is the information used? This includes the internal and external uses of information. External needs for information come from outside the department. What are all the reports that the department produces? What are the requests for information that the department has been unable to fill? What information would the department like to report but has not reported because it is too difficult or time-consuming to collect the data? Internally what information does the department use in planning and/or developing educational programs? How does the department evaluate the quality of individual programs or its overall performance? How does the department evaluate the performance of individual faculty? By understanding the informational needs of the department, it is possible to identify data and the data relationships that will need to be captured in the DBMS. Diagrams and narrative reports will be used to describe the data elements, their attributes, and the overall ideal information flow. With this information, the database administrator will begin to develop the physical model of the database.

Detailed Systems Design

The detailed systems design begins with the selection of the physical model: hierarchical, network, relational, or object-oriented. Using the physical model, each table and the relationships between the tables are developed. At this point, the data entry screens and the format for all output reports will be carefully designed. The users in the department must validate the data entry screens and output formats. It is often helpful to use prototypes and screen shoots to get user input during this stage. Revisions are to be expected.

Implementation

Implementation includes training the users, testing the system, developing a procedure manual for use of the system, piloting the DBMS, and finally "going live." The procedure manual outlines the "rules" for how the system is used in day-to-day operations. For example, what

is the procedure for recording attendance at individual classes, and when is the attendance data to be provided to the data entry clerk? In going live with a database system, one of the difficult decisions is how much previous data must be loaded into the DBMS. The initial request that stimulated the development of the DBMS would have required at least one year of previous data.

Evaluation and Maintenance

When a new database system has been installed, the developers and the users can be very anxious to immediately evaluate the system. Initial or early evaluations may have limited value. It will take a few weeks or even months for users to adjust their work routines to this new approach to information management. The first evaluations should be informal and focus more on troubleshooting specific problems. Once the system is up and running and users have adjusted to the new information processing procedure, they will have a whole new appreciation of the value of a DBMS. At this point, a number of requests for new options can be expected.

Common Database Operations

DBMSs vary from small programs running on a personal computer to massive programs that manage the data for large international enterprises. No matter what size or how a DBMS is used, there are common operations that are performed by all DBMSs. There are three basic types of data processing operations. These include data input, data processing, and data output. The relationship between these operations is demonstrated in Fig. 5.8.

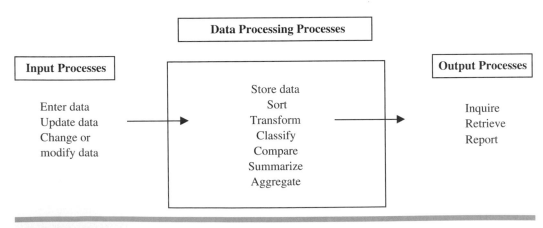

Figure 5.8
Common data processing operations.

Data Input Operations

Data input operations are used to enter new data, update data in the system, or change/modify data in the DBMS. Data are usually entered through a set of screens that have been designed for data entry. A well-designed screen will discourage data entry errors. In addition, the program can be designed to alert the user to potential errors or to prevent obvious data entry errors. It may not accept data that are out of range. For example, if someone tried to enter a blood pressure of 60/180, the system would issue an error message. The error message can be in the form of a sound or a text message on the screen. It is important that text messages are clear and help the user correct the error.

Sometimes data are entered that are unusual but could be correct. For example, a drug dose could be higher than normally recommended for that drug. In these cases, the system may be designed to offer an alert and request that the user re-enter the data to confirm its accuracy. It is important to evaluate how the alert should function. For example, if this is a clerical office dealing with numerical data, there may be no problem with having the clerk re-enter the data. However, if this is an intensive care unit, where drug doses are often higher than the recommended dose in textbooks, requiring busy caregivers to re-enter data may not be a good idea.

One of the most common errors involves inconsistent data entry formats. For example, one user may use all capitals when entering text data. Another user may use a combination of capitals and lowercase letters. If the DBMS is case-sensitive, this inconsistent data entry will have a major impact on query results. When data entry errors are of major importance, programs can be designed for double entry of all data. The first and second entries of the data are compared, and if there is a difference, the system issues an alert. With this approach, the user usually is required to re-enter data.

Database systems also let the user update, modify, or change data that has been previously entered into the system. Depending on the design of the DBMS, the original data may be overwritten and lost, or the original data may be saved in a separate file. With patient data, it is important to be able to track all data modifications. This should include who changed the data, what were the original data, and what modification was made to the data.

Data Processing Processes

Data processing processes are DBMS-directed actions that the computer performs on the data once it is entered into the system. It is these processes that are used to convert raw data into meaningful information. These include common database functions discussed previously in this chapter as well as a number of the processes used with data warehouses.

Data Output Operations

This section will include on-line and written reports. The approach to designing the reports will have a major impact on what information the reader actually gains from the report. Reports that are clear and concise help the reader see the information in the data. On the other hand, poorly designed reports can mislead and confuse the reader.

The development of a database system within a department serves two important purposes. First, both the developers and the users develop a new level of knowledge and skill. Second, as individual departments develop databases, institutional data are being created. However, if each department develops its individual database system, in isolation, islands of automation are then developed.

 ## The Development of Data Warehouses

Health care institutions have been automating their processes and developing databases since the mid 1960s. In most institutions, this process began in two areas, in the financial department and in departmental systems. Some of the oldest and most developed departmental systems are in the labs and the radiology, medical records, and cardiac departments. Initially, the systems developed as islands of automation that were focused on the operational needs of the departments. The development of these systems and the interfaces between these systems were strongly influenced by the fee-for-service approach to financing health care. Room charges are a primary concern in a financial system for a hospital information system (HIS). For financial systems to function, they needed to track patients. When admission, discharge, and transfer modules were added to the financial systems, this automated the process of room charges. However, in a hospital there are a number of other services that involve charges. Most of these services originate with a physician order. This stimulated the development of order entry systems. For most institutions, the financial system with charges and billing was closely tied to the admission, discharge, and transfer (ADT) and order entry systems. In many cases, they were offered by the same vendor, and interface problems were minimal. However, the order entry systems needed to interface with department systems. One of the first approaches was to simply have the computer generate a printed copy of the order requisition in the department. This was then manually entered into the department system. Developing a computer interface with the department where the order entry system on the clinical units could "talk to" the department systems was a problem. Because the department systems had been developed independently, they used different naming and coding structures. The databases reflected different architectures. This was true for systems developed by the same vendors and was even more of a problem for systems that had been developed by different vendors.

Think back to the example of organizing class notes. What if several students agreed to share their class notes, but each student maintained her notes in her own room and had her own filing system? Some of the students may have organized the content by courses, while other students may have organized it by years, and still other students set up their total filing systems by topic. Because the notes were stored in individual rooms, each student who wanted to use another student's notes would need to send a request to the other student(s).

Attempts to share data by building interfaces across automated systems in health care institutions shared many of the same problems as the student example. In health care institutions where interfaces needed to go from the order entry system to **all** departments, the problem was compounded. Of course, any change or update to any of the department computer programs required that changes be made to the interface. This could impact any of the other departmental systems.

While order entry systems automated the manual process for charging, which was a major advantage for the financial department, the results-reporting module of these systems proved to be very valuable to care givers. The results-reporting module sent information back to the clinical units with the results of various tests and exams. This was especially useful for lab results. Without automation, stat lab results had to be phoned back to the clinical units and manually dictated. On-line lab results made it possible for nurses and doctors to make clinical decisions based on the latest information. However, each department system that could send results back to the clinical units functioned independently. Users had to learn how to use each system, and there was no way that the results from different departments could be viewed in an integrated fashion. The departmental systems were used to meet the day-to-day operational needs of the institution. Data were not stored on a long-term basis. Due to systems' storage requirements, the data in the systems were usually purged within a set number of days after the patient left the hospital.

In the late 1980s and early 1990s, a number of changes ushered in a new approach. Computer systems had become much more powerful. Database theory and products were much more sophisticated. Users were becoming computer-literate and developing more requirements. A core of health care informatics leaders had developed. The Institute of Medicine issued its report on the computer-based patient record (Dick and Steen, 1991). The move away from fee-for-service to managed care created a new set of information needs. The data within the computer systems took on a new value. The new approach involved collecting the data from each of the systems and storing it in a warehouse.

A data warehouse is a large collection of data imported from several different systems within one database. Smaller collections of data are referred to as data marts. A data mart might be developed for a department or a small group of departments. A data mart can also be developed by exporting a subset of the data from the data warehouse. Bill Immon, the father of the data warehouse concept, defined a data warehouse as a subject-oriented, integrated, time variant, nonvolatile collection of data used to support the management decision-making process (Lambert). In health care, management includes management of the client/patient as well as the health care institution.

Functions of a Data Warehouse

The management of a data warehouse requires three types of programs. First the data warehouse must be able to extract data from the various computer systems and import that data into the data warehouse. This is a key point for nursing. If nursing data are not in the various computer systems or do not exist in any standardized format, they cannot be extracted and imported into the data warehouse. Nursing data are not limited to the data that nurses generate but include all the data that nurses utilize for client care, administration, research, and education.

Furthermore, the data definitions that were established in the original computer systems must now be revised so that the data from the different systems can be integrated. For example, does the data definition for patient problem(s) include all problems identified by all professional care givers, or is it limited to the medical diagnosis?

Second, the data warehouse must function as a database able to store and process all of the data in the database. This includes the ability to aggregate the data and process the aggregated data. For example, the operational database systems used to manage the institution on a day-to-day basis do not usually offer the opportunity to look at data over time, yet a data warehouse frequently supports integration of data and the analysis of trends over time. The individual data elements that are imported into the warehouse are referred to as primary data. The aggregate data produced by the warehouse database system are referred to as secondary data or derived data.

Third, the data warehouse must be able to deliver the data in the warehouse back to the users in the form of information. Information from a data warehouse is used for decision support systems and executive information systems. These systems show the "big picture" as well as trends over time. For example, the data in a data warehouse may demonstrate that patients with diabetes who attend a diabetic education class increase their number of clinic or office visits. The data may also demonstrate that these same patients show a decrease in their number of hospitalizations and an overall decrease in cost of care. In reviewing these data, the patient manager may need to "drill down" into the data. Does this summary apply to all patients, or are there select groups of patients who are gaining this benefit? It may be that adolescents do not demonstrate this benefit and that a different approach is needed for this group of patients.

Data from a data warehouse can be used to support a number of activities including (AHIMA, 1998):

1. Decision support for caregivers at the point of care

2. Outcome measurements and quality improvement

3. Clinical research and professional education

4. Reporting to external agencies, e.g., Joint Commission on Accreditation of Health Care Organizations

5. Market trend analysis and strategic planning

6. Health services management and process reengineering

7. Targeted outreach to patients, professionals, and other community groups

Quality of the Data

In a data warehouse, data are entered once but used by many users for a number of different purposes. As a result, the quality of the data takes on a whole new level of importance. In addition, the concept of data ownership changes. When dealing with a department information system, the department is usually seen as owning the data and being responsible for the quality of that data. For example, one might expect nurses to be responsible for the quality of data in a nursing information system.

However, when one is responsible for the data in a data warehouse, the concept of a data steward is more appropriate. A data steward does not own the data but ensures its quality. He or she is the "keeper of the data," not the "owner of the data." The data steward must work with the departments that generate the data to ensure the quality of the data coming into the warehouse. In addition, the data steward is responsible for working with care givers and administrative personnel to develop naming standards, entity and attribute standards, rule specifications, data security specifications, and retention specifications (Imhoff, 1998).

Data Mining

As data warehouses have developed, a wide range of tools for extracting the information within that data have also developed. Some of these tools have themselves become automated, and the process is now referred to as data mining. Data mining uses powerful new approaches for the extraction of hidden predictive information from large databases. Data mining makes it possible to automate the prediction of trends and patterns as well as the discovery of previously unknown trends (Thearling). Data mining begins by carefully assessing the questions that users need answered. The second step is to build a model that would answer those questions using known data. For example, there are a number of variables that influence the number and type of medication errors within an institution. Some variables include staffing ratios, number of medications to be given, presence of new or novice staff, and number of new medications. This information is used to build a model that predicts when medication errors can be expected to increase or decrease. The model is then applied to real data where the number and type of errors are known. Adjustments are made to the formulas and assumptions in the model until the model is able to predict the correct results. The model is then installed and issues an alert if a situation is developing where medication errors can be expected to increase. Data mining uses a number of complex techniques to answer these questions. Some of the more commonly used techniques include artificial neural networks, decision trees, genetic algorithms, and if-then rules.

 Summary

This chapter described data processing, which is the primary use for computers in health care. The focus of the chapter was on understanding concepts and issues

necessary to effectively use database systems in health care. The chapter began by discussing the difference between data and information. The process of using an information system to produce information from data was described. The chapter explained data structures and models. The purpose(s), structures, and functions of automated database systems are reviewed. The life cycle of an automated database system is outlined. The chapter concludes with a discussion of concepts and issues related to data warehouses in health care.

References

AHIMA. (1998). Data resource administration: The road ahead. *Journal of AHIMA-Practice Briefs.* 69–10. *http://www.ahima.org/publications/2a/pract.brief.1198.html*

Burch, J., Strater, F. R., Grudnitski, G. (1983). *Information Systems: Theory and Practice.* 3d edition. New York: John Wiley.

Dick, R. S. and Steen, E. B. (1991). *The Computer-Based Patient Record: An Essential Technology for Health Care.* Washington, DC: National Academy Press.

English, L. 1999. Plain English on data quality. *DM Review. http://www.dmreview.com/issues/1999/jan/jan99_index .htm*

Imhoff, C. (1998). Ensuring data quality through data stewardship. *DM Review. http://www.dmreview.com/ issues/1998/apr/apr98_index.htm*

John, M. (1997). *Information Management for Health Professionals.* New York: Delmar Publishers.

Joos, I., Whitman, N. I., Smith, M. J., and Nelson, R. (2000). *Computers in Small Bytes.* New York: Jones and Bartlett Publishers.

Lambert, B. Data warehousing fundamentals: What you need to know to succeed. *DM Review. http://www. datawarehouse.com/resources/articles/*

Stajano, F. (1998). A general introduction to relational and object oriented databases: (ORL technical report TR-98-2.). *http://www.uk.research.att.com/~fms/*

Thearling, K. An introduction to data mining: Discovering the hidden value in your data warehouse. *http://www3. shore.net/~kht/text/dmwhite/dmwhite.htm*

Zielstorff, R., Hudgings, C. Grobe, S. and NCNIP. (1993). *Next-Generation Nursing Information Systems: Essential Characteristics for Professional Practice.* Washington, D.C.: American Nursing Publishing.

Recommended Readings

Andersen, C. M. and Emery, L. J. (1998). Interdisciplinary team teaching of database management. *Occupational Therapy in Health Care, 11*(2), 45.

Arthur, P. (1997). Demonstrating value through information management: Database decision support for physical therapy practice. *Resource, 27*(1), 12.

Beck, C. T. (1996). The practical computer: Use of a meta-analytic database management system. *Nursing Research, 45*(3), 181.

Bersky, A. K. and Krawczak, J. (1995). Building a nursing activity database for processing free-text entry during computerized clinical simulation testing. *Computers in Nursing, 13*(5), 236.

Bertocci, G., Karg, P., and Hobson, D. (1997). Wheeled mobility device database for transportation safety research and standards. *Assistive Technology, 9*(2), 102.

Brazier, H. and Begley, C. M. (1996). Selecting a database for literature searches in nursing: MEDLINE or CINAHL? *Journal of Advanced Nursing, 24*(4), 868.

Burnard, P. (1996). Issues in designing a student database. *Nurse Education Today, 16*(1), 56.

Burnard, P. (1996). Using a database for managing interview data. *Professional Nurse, 11*(9), 578.

Burnard, P. (1994). Using a database program to handle qualitative data. *Nurse Education Today, 14*(3), 228.

Button, P. S. (1997). Computers in practice: Challenges and uses—using standardized nursing nomenclature in an automated careplanning and documentation system. In M. J. Rantz et al. (Eds.) *Classification of Nursing Diagnoses: Proceedings of the Twelfth Conference, North America Nursing Diagnosis Association* (p. 327). Glendale, CA: CINAHL Information Systems.

Carpenter, I. (1997). Addressing the problems of care services for the elderly with a database of primary clinical data. *British Journal of Healthcare Computing & Information Management, 14*(10), 16.

Catrambone, C. (1995). Creating database links between nursing diagnoses and nursing activities. *Issues, 16*(1), 8.

Chang, B. L. (1993). CARIN system—database for Bayes' Theorem applications... computer-aided research in nursing. *Western Journal of Nursing Research, 15*(5), 644.

Cheek, J., Gillham, D., and Mills, P. (1997). Using a computerised clinical database to enhance problem-based learning strategies for second year and undergraduate nursing students. *Australian Electronic Journal of Nursing Education, 2*(2), *http://www.scu.edu. au/schools/nhcp/aejne/aejnehp.htm*

Cheek, J., Gillham, D., and Mills, P. (1998). Using clinical databases in tertiary nurse education: An innovative approach to computer technology. *Nurse Education Today, 18*(2), 153.

Chu, S. C. and Thom, J. B. (1997). Database issues in object-oriented clinical information systems design. In U. Gerdin et al. (Eds.) *Nursing Informatics: The Impact of Nursing Knowledge on Health Care Informatics . . . Proceedings of NI'97, Sixth Triennial International Congress of IMIA-NI, Nursing Informatics of Inter- national Medical Informatics Association* (p. 376). Amsterdam, Netherlands, IOS Press.

Clougherty, J., McCloskey, J. C., Johnson, M., et al. (1991). Creating a relational database for nursing service administration. *Computers in Nursing, 9*(2), 69.

Coenen, A. and Wake, M. (1996). Developing a database for an international classification for nursing practice. *International Nursing Review, 43*(6), 183.

Courtney, R. and Rice, C. A. (1995). Using an encounter form to develop a clinical database for documenting nurse practitioner primary care. *Journal of the American Academy of Nurse Practitioners, 7*(11), 537.

Crothers, D., Ramachandran, S., and Giles, P. (1997). Measuring clinical performance: Database effectiveness in a coronary heart disease prevention programme. *British Journal of Healthcare Computing & Information Management, 14*(8), 19.

Delaney, C. and Moorhead, S. (1995). The Nursing Minimum Data Set, standardized language, and health care quality. *Journal of Nursing Care Quality, 10*(1), 16.

Denwood, R. (1996). Data capture for quality management nursing opportunity. *Computers in Nursing, 14*(1), 39.

Dobrzykowski, E. A. and Nance, T. (1997). The Focus On Therapeutic Outcomes (FOTO) Outpatient Orthopedic Rehabilitation Database: Results of 1994–1996. *Journal of Rehabilitation Outcomes Measurement, 1*(1), 56.

Enkin, M. W. (1995). Effective care in pregnancy and childbirth: The Cochrane Pregnancy and Childbirth Database. *Journal of Perinatal Education, 4*(4), 23.

Gooch, P. M. (1996). Databases: Hom-Inform bibliographic database and information service for homoeopathic literature. *Complementary Therapies in Medicine, 4*(1), 63.

Goodwin, L. (1997). Data mining for improved patient care outcomes. *Tar Heel Nurse, 59*(4), 21.

Horton, B. J., Revak, G. R., and Jordan, L. M. (1994). The computer database for nurse anesthesia education programs. *AANA Journal, 62*(3), 234.

Hudson, R. and Bowen, C., Clinical audit database. *Health Visitor.* 70(6).223, (1997).

Jacobson, T. (1996). Standardized ET nursing database: imagine the possibilities. *Journal of Wocn, 23*(1), 5.

Jacox, A. (1995). Practice and policy implications of clinical and administrative databases. In *An Emerging Framework: Data System Advances for Clinical Nursing Practice* (p. 161). Washington, D.C.: American Nurses Association Publications.

Kilchenstein, J. M. (1995). Working smart. A professional practice forum. Future foundations: Database query languages. *Journal American Health Information Management Association, 66*(5), 35.

Kuehn, A. F. (1998). Establishing an advanced practice nurse database: A four-phase comprehensive study. *Missouri Nurse, 67*(3), 12.

Lang, N. M., Hudgings, C., Jacox, A., et al. (1995). Toward a national database for nursing practice. In *An Emerging Framework: Data System Advances for Clinical Nursing Practice*. Washington, D.C.: American Nurses Association Publications.

Lange, L. L and Jacox, A. (1993). Using large data bases in nursing and health policy research. *Journal of Professional Nursing, 9*(4), 204.

Lee, F. W. (1996). Technology—how to use entity-relationship diagrams in developing personal database systems. *Journal Americal Health Information Management Association, 67*(2), 42.

Loebl, D., Willems, B., and Nordin, M. (1995). Database analysis of injury patterns in an institution for developmental disabilities. *Journal of Occupational Rehabilitation, 5*(3), 169.

Marlett, J. D. and Cheung, T. (1997). Perspectives in practice. Database and quick methods of assessing typical dietary fiber intakes using data for 228 commonly consumed foods. *Journal of the American Dietetic Association, 97*(10), 1139.

McDaniel, A. M. (1997). Developing and testing a prototype patient care database. *Computers in Nursing, 15*(3), 129.

Melillo, K. D. and Futrell, M. (1995). A guide for assessing caregiver needs: Determining a health history database for family caregivers. *The Nurse Practitioner, 20*(5), 40.

Moseley, L. G. and Mead, D. M. (1993). Good relations: The use of a relational database for large-scale data analysis. *Journal of Advanced Nursing, 18*(11), 1795.

Oyri, K (1997). Workload measurement in the ICU. In U. Gerdin, et al. (Eds.), *Nursing Informatics: The Impact of Nursing Knowledge on Health Care Informatics . . . Proceedings of NI'97, Sixth Triennial International Congress of IMIA-NI, Nursing Informatics of International Medical Informatics Association* (p. 512). Amsterdam, Netherlands: IOS Press.

Ozbolt, J. G., Fruchtnicht, J. N., and Hayden, J. R. (1994). Toward data standards for clinical nursing information. *Journal of the American Medical Informatics Association, 1*(2), 175.

Ozbolt, J. G. (1995). From minimum data to maximum impact: Using clinical data to strengthen patient care. *Advanced Practice Nursing Quarterly, 1*(4), 62.

Pheby, D. F. H. and Thorne, P. (1994). The Medical Data Index (MDI) dependency module: A shared database to assist discharge planning and audit. *Journal of Advanced Nursing, 20*(2), 361.

Picella, D. V. (1996). Use of relational database program for quantification of the CNS role. *Clinical Nurse Specialist, 10*(6), 301.

Pohlmann, B. (1995). The Department of Veterans Affairs experience: Development of a database for the patient problem list. In *An Emerging Framework: Data System Advances for Clinical Nursing Practice* (p. 185). Washington, D.C.: American Nurses Association Publications.

Reynolds, J. P. (1996). Are you ready to join an outcomes database? *PT—Magazine of Physical Therapy, 4*(10), 36, 67.

Ribbons, R. M. and McKenna, L. G. (1997). Facilitating Higher Order Thinking Skills in Nurse Education: A

Prototype Database for Teaching Wound Assessment
and Management Skills. In U. Gerdin, et al. (Eds.),
*Nursing Informatics: The Impact of Nursing Knowledge
on Health Care Informatics... Proceedings of NI'97,
Sixth Triennial International Congress of IMIA-NI,
Nursing Informatics of International Medical Informatics
Association* (p. 389). Amsterdam, Netherlands: IOS Press.

Roberts, D. J. (1995). Databases. AMED: A bibliographic
database for complementary medicine and allied health.
Complementary Therapies in Medicine, 3(4), 255.

Rock, B. D., Beckerman, A., Auerback, C., et al. (1995).
Management of alternate level of care patients using a
computerized database. *Health & Social Work, 20*
(2), 133.

Ross, B. A. (1994). Use of a database for managing
qualitative research data. *Computers in Nursing,
12*(3), 154.

Schermer, J., Geisler, E., and Vang, P. (1995). Nursing
Thesis Database Project: A cooperative venture for
nursing faculty and computer science professionals.
Computers in Nursing, 13(2), 50.

Sieler, P. and Adams, J. (1998). Using a database to
integrate technology into the curriculum. *Nursing
Standard. http://www.nursing-standard.co.uk/*

Urden, L. D. (1996). Development of a nurse executive
decision support database: A model for outcomes
evaluation. *Journal of Nursing Administration, 26*
(10), 15.

Warren, J. J. and Hoskins, L. M. (1995). NANDA's
nursing diagnosis taxonomy: A nursing database. In
*An Emerging Framework: Data System Advances for
Clinical Nursing Practice* (p. 49). Washington, D.C.:
American Nurses Association Publications.

Welton, J. M. (1997). Development of a computerized
database for a nursing quality management team. In
U. Gerdin, et al. (Eds.), *Nursing Informatics: The
Impact of Nursing Knowledge on Health Care
Informatics . . . Proceedings of NI'97, Sixth Triennial
International Congress of IMIA-NI, Nursing
Informatics of International Medical Informatics
Association* (p. 82). Amsterdam, Netherlands: IOS.

Wiggers, T. B. (1996) Educators' corner: Use of a computer
database to facilitate management of hematology
teaching slides. *Clinical Laboratory Science, 9*(1), 10.

Zisselman, M. H., Allen, D., Cutillo-Schmitter, T. C, et al.
(1998). The minimum data set and psychotropic drug
use in nursing home residents. *Annals of Long Term
Care, 6*(7), 199.

Computer Systems

Mary L. McHugh

OBJECTIVES

1. Define the term "system," and describe how the term applies to the field of computers.
2. Identify the five defining attributes of a system and define the meaning of each.
3. Discuss computer information systems and their subsets: management information systems and hospital information systems.
4. List the most common administrative and clinical modules in a hospital information system.
5. Define the term "network," and describe the two essential components of network technology.
6. Discuss the history of the Internet, define the key terms used in this modality, and provide an overview of its use.

KEY WORDS

information systems
computer science

This chapter provides an overview of concepts critical to understanding computer systems. Every functioning computer is a system; that is, it is a complex entity, consisting of an organized set of interconnected components or factors that function together as a unit to accomplish results that one part alone could not. At a minimum, a computer must have at least four components to function. These minimum components are a power source, a central processing unit, a peripheral to allow input, and a peripheral to permit output. Of course, computers typically have many more than four components. "Computer system" may refer to a single machine (and its peripherals) that is unconnected to any other computer. However, most health professionals use computer systems consisting of multiple, interconnected computers that function to facilitate the work of groups of providers and their support people in a system called a **network**. The greatest range of functionality is realized when computers are connected to other computers in a network or, as with the Internet, a system of networks.

The use of systems in computer technology is based on systems theory. Previous chapters described computer hardware and computer software and the fundamentals of computer functioning. Systems theory and its subset, network theory, provide the basis for understanding how the power of individual computers has been greatly enhanced through the process of linking multiple computers into a single system and multiple computer systems into networks.

Systems Theory

Systems theory provides the conceptual basis for understanding complex entities that consist of multiple interrelated parts working together to achieve a desired result. Such entities are called **systems**. A system, by its nature, is not random; it is orderly and predictable in its functioning. If a system begins to exhibit unpredictable behavior, one of two conditions pertain. Either the system is malfunctioning for some reason internal or external to the system itself, or the observer does not fully understand the system and thus a proper result is misinterpreted as incorrect (unpredicted). The key concepts of systems theory are parts, interaction (among the parts), interdependency (among the parts), input, output, processing, feedback, and control. The primary propositions of the theory are the following:

1. A system takes in input upon which to perform processes.

2. The processes performed by a system upon input result in system output.

3. The processes in a system are subject to control forces.

4. Feedback is the key mechanism of control in a system.

5. A system's parts interact in such a way that the parts are interdependent with respect to the system's processes.

6. Impingement upon one part in a system will produce effects on the system's processes and may produce distortions upon other parts of the system. A corollary to this proposition is the following.

7. Distortion in one part of a system may be a symptom of a problem in another component. (This is called a secondary malfunction.)

8. Thus, correction of a malfunctioning part will correct the system functioning only if the malfunction was a primary malfunction and not a secondary malfunction.

9. Effects on the system's processing function will affect the system's output.

10. A system is more than the sum of its parts. Thus, while a system can be broken down into its component parts, if the system is broken down into its component parts, the system no longer exists. Corollaries to this proposition are:
    (a) The functioning of a system is different than the functioning of its separate parts.
    (b) The output of each separate part, even if combined, does not equal the output of the system.
    (c) When combined into a system, the component parts form an entirely new entity.

History of Systems Theory

The earliest roots of systems theory must be attributed to Aristotle (384-322 B.C.) when he said, "The whole is more than the sum of its parts." Unfortunately, Aristotle's observations were not vigorously pursued by Western science until the middle of the 20th century. Prior to the general acceptance of general systems theory, mechanistic reductionism was used to explain the workings of nature.

Sir Isaac Newton (1643-1727) articulated the foundations of mechanistic thought with his focus on real-world explanations rather than biblically derived explanations for natural phenomena. An example of a mechanistic explanation is consideration of the heart as a pump. Understood in that light, the heart obeys the laws of a hydraulic/mechanical system. Mechanistic thought viewed nature and the behavior of natural phenomena as additive—which can be summarized as, "A thing is the sum of its parts." As the late 1700s passed into the early 1800s, mechanistic theory formed the foundation of the Industrial Revolution. The key belief engendered by mechanism was that ultimately, nature could be controlled, if only all the mechanics of its workings could be discovered.

Reductionism was a theory added to mechanism during the 1800s to help further "understand" the working of the physical world. Reductionism was a cornerstone of the scientific method. It required that an entity, machine, or other object of interest be **analyzed**; that is, the item of interest must be broken down to its component parts and each part studied so that the item could be better understood. A key theorem of reductionism is that if a phenomenon could be analyzed and understood at its lower levels, then the functioning of its higher levels could be derived logically. The field of modern medicine emerged during that time. Even today, this theory underlies medicine, with all its specialization and emphasis on the malfunctioning body part rather than on the whole person.

Unfortunately, mechanistic reductionism could not explain phenomena that functioned as a gestalt. That is, phenomena whose parts working together produced something quite beyond the capacity of each part separately. A new theory was needed to explain the workings of such phenomena. The beginnings of modern knowledge of complex systems are seen in Niels Bohr's (Petrucciolo, 1993) theory of quantum mechanics. As a physicist working with atoms, Bohr observed that different combinations of the same particles—electrons, protons, and neutrons—produced very different elements. Clearly, he realized that an atom is more than its particles. One proposition of system theory is that experimentation on one part of a system destroys the functioning of complementary parts of the system. Thus, the possibility of learning about the complementary component is lost—the normal state of the component has been destroyed. That principle is usually articulated as follows: "any factor that impinges on one part of a system affects other parts of the system, and ultimately, the system as a whole" (Petrucciolo, 1993).

General systems theory arose from these foundations during the 1950s, when mechanistic reductionism failed as a way of explaining social behavior and biological functions. The most prominent theorist in system theory was the biologist Ludwig Von Bertalanffy (1976). In 1950, he formulated general systems theory as a framework for integrating and interpreting diverse scientific knowledge sets (Von Bertalanffy, 1972). This theory is a framework for: (1) organizing ideas about how multiple parts could work together to produce work that none alone could accomplish and (2) for simplifying the complexity of machine workings. General systems theory has been found useful in many areas of science, including computer science, social sciences, medicine, and nursing.

During the 1960s, general systems theory (GST) greatly influenced the development of nursing theory (Donnelly et al., 1980). Nurse theorists began to develop a holistic nursing model of practice that was distinct from the mechanistic medical model. This did have the somewhat unfortunate effect of dividing nursing and medicine. Nonetheless, leaders in the nursing profession quickly realized that nursing the whole person in the context of his or her social system produced nursing care that was more effective and more satisfying for both patient and nurse. The leaders of the profession expanded their use of system theory concepts through study of the way that the theory was applied in other disciplines. As a result, nursing practice was reformulated in terms of a holistic approach, and new nursing theory was generated. During the 1990s, as the field of nursing informatics became recognized as a new nursing specialty, general systems theory served as a conceptual foundation for much of the work in this field.

System Elements

A system consists of the following six elements: The system's set of interdependent parts, input to the system, system processes, output of the system, system control, and feedback.

Interdependent Parts   The most defining attribute of a system is that its parts interact to conduct some process. Without the interaction, the system process could not occur. Therefore, in the production of the system's process, the parts are interdependent. Each acting alone could not perform the system's process. In computer systems, the process involves mathematical, logical, or data transfer operations requiring interaction among the CPU, RAM, and ROM chips and the motherboard's power source.

Input   Input is any factor from the external environment that is taken into the system. Input in a computer system may serve to initiate system functioning, as when the machine is turned on and the operating system is loaded into RAM. It may consist of data that the system is to process. In living systems, input may consist of energy from the sun, nourishment, or stimulation, or it might be information needed to survive, function, or enjoy life. However, by itself, input is just inert substance or data. The system must act upon input if it is to get use from it.

Process   Process is the activity of the system. A system performs process upon its inputs to produce outputs, or create some sort of result. (Survival is the result of the processes of a living system.) Process in a computer system can be seen in the example of a presentation graphics system. The hardware, software, and peripherals constitute the interdependent parts. The commands entered by the user, the numerical data for a graphic, and the alphanumeric characters used for title, labels, and notations on the graph constitute the input. The system sends the translated data and commands to the CPU, which performs the ordered operations (processes) upon the input to create a graphic image (e.g. pie graph, bar graph, etc.). Then the graphic package further processes the instructions to produce whatever output is ordered by the user of the system.

Output   Output is any product or waste produced as a result of system process. Not all process produces a visible, external product. (The result of life processes may be homeostasis, energy, movement, or feedback within the living system.) However, in many of the systems people work with—such as manufacturing systems—the purpose of the system is to produce output. For example, the output of the manufacturing process at Ford Motor Company is composed of automobiles, trucks, and specialty vehicles. For computer systems, output is the reason the system was created or purchased. Typical computer system output includes electronic data transmission from the main memory to a hard or floppy disk, paper reports, or data transmissions (such as information exchange through the Internet).

For example, many users today have word processors and presentation graphics program packages. The output from the presentation graphics system might be an electronic file stored on the hard drive or on a portable floppy disk. It might be an image printed in either black and white or color on a piece of paper or a transparency; or it might be that same image printed onto color 35-mm film for processing into a color slide. Output from a word processor is usually a professionally formatted and printed text document.

Control   "Control" refers to any component or activity that serves to prevent or correct problems or errors in the system's input, process, or output. A system must function within rules and procedures that keep it functioning smoothly. These rules and procedures constitute a system's **control** operations. Process means activity. Activity must have some beginning and end point, or else the system goes out of control. Cancers are an example of an out-of-control function in a person's body. Cells that need to regrow as part of healing from injury must stop growing once repair is accomplished. When cells continue to grow without control, the result is eventually fatal. Control is an essential function of any system.

In computer systems, a variety of control facilities exist within the operating system. Most application programs also incorporate control functions to help the user avoid erroneous results. Control in computers functions by checking, validating, and verifying input and output data and by checking for and flagging certain conditions during processing. An example of a processing error is division by zero. Such an operation is impossible, and whenever such a problem is detected, processing is terminated and an appropriate error message is displayed on the screen or printout.

A good application program will have special programming that creates "error traps" to detect certain kinds of errors. For example, most word processor programs automatically detect words that are misspelled. In such a program, the concept, "misspelled" means that the word has no match in the word processor's dictionary and therefore is not recognized by the program. The user is notified that the system doesn't recognize the word (by a change in color of the word on the screen, by underlining, or in some other way). Data entry programs for some statistical analysis programs may detect impossible values. The way they do this is that during creation of the data entry screen, the developer identifies upper and lower numerical limits or acceptable/unacceptable characters for the type of data to be stored in that variable. Any value that doesn't fit the defined acceptable codes is considered an "out-of-range" value. Then any time a data entry person enters an out-of-range value, processing stops, and a warning message is issued.

Feedback   Feedback is output from one part of a system process that serves as input to another part of a system process. Feedback is a special case of control.

Feedback within a system is typically used as part of a system's self-regulation function. For example, in human beings, body temperature is regulated by a feedback system. A falling core temperature stimulates temperature-sensitive neurons in the hypothalamus. In response, the hypothalamus (in conjunction with certain higher brain centers) activates a number of temperature response mechanisms, most obviously the shivering response. Shivering consists of rapid muscle movements—and muscle movement produces heat. The heat is disseminated and raises the body temperature; that, in turn, changes the sensations to the hypothalamus temperature-sensing neurons. (This is a much-simplified picture and only a small part of the temperature-regulatory feedback system in a human being.)

In a computer system, feedback components are important functions of the operating system and utility programs. The user will experience the results of feedback if a "save" command orders the system to store a file on a diskette that is already full. The operating system checks the diskette, and the discovery of a "full" condition initiates a subroutine (small program module used repeatedly). The subroutine stops the processing and issues a message to the user that the command has failed because the disk is full.

A clinical computing example of feedback is the ventilation rate in a mechanical ventilator set at "demand." The processor in the ventilator detects its own activity, and based on the timing of the last activity, it initiates or does not initiate another breath. That is, it has a timer that keeps track of the most recent breath taken by (or delivered to) a patient. The ventilator is set to deliver a breath if a certain amount of time has elapsed since the last breath. If the patient's breathing rate is such that each breath is taken prior to the "deadline," the system does not initiate forced inspiration. Otherwise, the machine initiates a breath. In this way, the ventilator controls the rate at which it delivers breaths to the patient—neither too fast nor too slow for optimal oxygenation.

Classification of Systems

There are two types or classes of system, closed systems and open systems.

Closed Systems   A closed system is defined as a system with the following characteristics: differentiation, isolation, independence, and self-sufficiency (sometimes called self-containment or self-regulation). A closed system is clearly differentiated from all other systems and factors in its environment. Its boundaries are clearly defined and rigid. Therefore, it is easy to tell just where the system begins and ends and what is part of the system and what is not part of the system.

By definition, a closed system has sealed boundaries that separate the closed system from the rest of the environment. Access to the system is highly restricted, because the only inputs acceptable to the system are inputs from another part of itself. System outputs are actually forms of internal communication; that is, the output of one part of the system serves as input to another part of the system in a feedback loop. In this sense, a closed system is self-contained.

Closed systems must be independent (i.e., self-regulating) to endure any length of time, because a closed system cannot tolerate significant external interference. Since external influences are destructive to a closed system, it must be able to function fully with only its own resources. It cannot rely on the external environment, so it must be able to control itself fully. No part of the system can grow to excess or fail to grow when needed. It cannot be allowed to consume its own energy sources without renewing them, because without energy, processes cannot take place, and a system is not a system unless it exhibits some process.

A closed system has to be self-sufficient, because any input from the external environment is a threat to the integrity of a closed system. It must therefore be able to provide for all its own energy and processing requirements without going outside its own boundaries. Furthermore, it cannot need an external source to help rid it of its output or waste products. Due to the need for an energy source, it may be that no system is ever truly closed. However, some systems are sufficiently isolated that it makes conceptual sense to consider them closed. More typically, a closed system has a closed feedback loop as its major process. Outside energy is still required to power the system.

For example, animal habitats often function as closed systems. When the boundaries of the environment are breached, and animals from other systems intrude on the formerly closed system, animals originating in the closed system often cannot compete and become extinct. A closed system such as an animal habitat must isolate itself from rather than accommodate to outside influences.

A nursing example of a closed system could be an intravenous hypertension control system (Fig. 6.1). The components of the system include the patient's intravenous line and fluid with the antihypertensive

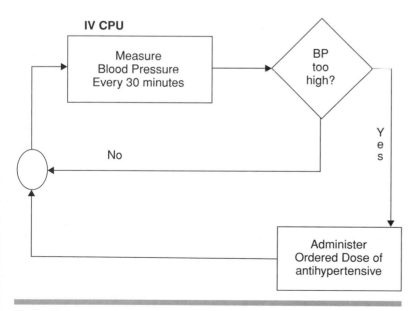

Figure 6.1
Closed system with feedback loop.

medication, the electronic sphygmomanometer, the volumetric pump, and the programmed computer processor (the CPU) that controls the system. In such a system, the computer is programmed to initiate a blood pressure (BP) reading at determined time intervals. At the proper time, the CPU sends a command to the sphygmomanometer to take a reading through the arterial line. The value is returned to the CPU, where it is compared to a preset critical value. The processor determines whether or not the reading is above the critical value. If not, it does nothing until its clock indicates that it is time for another measurement. If the BP is above the critical value, it sends an instruction to the volumetric pump to deliver the correct dose of antihypertensive medication. In reality, a system such as described would never be completely closed. There would always be an alarm system to warn the nurse if the medication was ineffective or if the BP fell too low or rose too high or of other problems requiring system maintenance.

Closed systems are often described as fixed or static. This description is fundamentally flawed, because closed systems do have processes. Therefore, they exhibit some degree of internal fluidity. However, the change must be with internal processing, not through interaction with the external world. From that perspective, to an outsider, the closed system appears to be static and unchanging.

Open Systems   Open systems are systems that exhibit integration, fluid or fuzzy boundaries, and interaction with their environments (Farace et al., 1977). They need not be self-regulating, although they might exhibit that facility. They are fundamentally different from closed systems. An open system overlaps other systems and may be a subsystem within a larger system. Consequently, it is often difficult to determine whether a particular process belongs to a specific system or to a related system. In fact, it can be quite easy to iteratively redefine a system's borders whenever an interaction with another system occurs. The interaction is viewed as a new system function. Taken to extremes, the redefinition continues until the entire universe is included in the system.

For this reason, it is sometimes very difficult to identify the borders or boundaries of an open system. The boundaries are permeable to external influences rather than sealed against them. Open systems fundamentally require the energy of input from the external environment. All living creatures are examples of open systems. They must acquire nourishment from their external environment or die. Unlike closed systems, open systems

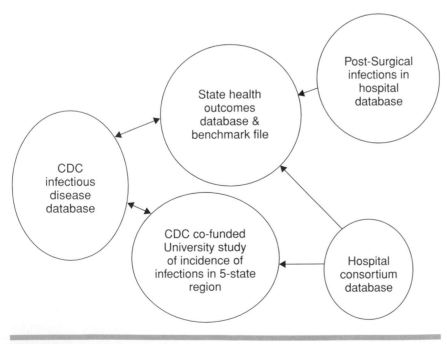

Figure 6.2
Open system interactions.

exhibit change with respect to both internal and external processes. Since they interact with their environment, open systems may not appear to have any clearly identifiable boundaries. However, it is important to define boundaries because any system is defined as much by its boundaries as it is by its processes (Fig. 6.2).

An open system may exhibit self-regulation. More commonly, however, an open system expands until it bumps up against another system's boundary, and the second system takes action to protect itself against the encroachment of the first system.

 ## Computer Systems

The term "computer system" is used to describe the set of peripherals, computer "box," and software that together perform computing functions for one or more users. The actual devices that comprise a computer system depend on the needs of the user. Typically, most users need a keyboard and mouse or trackball for input. Many also use a joystick for games or drawing programs. Peripheral devices that have grown in popularity as use of the Internet has increased include a modem, scanner, microphone, and video camera. Application software usually includes an "office" package that includes word processor, spread sheet, presentation graphics and database programs, an Internet browser, and a Web authoring program such as Front Page or Lotus Notes.

The term "computer system" is vague and could refer to anything from a hand-held personal computer to an organization's entire network of computers. In most nursing settings, nurses work with what is known as an information system and, in hospitals, a hospital information system.

Information Systems

An information system is the collection and integration of various pieces of hardware and software and the human resources that meet the data collection, storage, processing, and report generation needs of an organization. For most large health care organizations, the software requirements are varied and complex. The hardware must always be purchased to fit the software requirements. As a result, most large organizations must retain a sophisticated information systems department to construct, maintain, and interface the various—and sometimes incompatible—hardware and software necessary to support the work of the organization. When an organization is so large and its computing requirements so diverse that the organization simply cannot obtain a single sys-

tem to meet all its needs, the result is usually a hodgepodge of incompatible software and hardware platforms. The IS department must program and maintain the software interfaces that let the systems work together. The key pieces of an information system are the hardware, software, and the database or databases in which the organization's data are stored.

Information Systems Types

Information systems are found almost everywhere in health care, including in hospitals, clinics, community health agencies, research facilities, and educational institutions. Their configuration, power, and functions vary widely depending on how they are used and the type of work performed in the organization. There is a wide range of information systems in health care facilities that provide different functions. They have different titles/names, which overlap depending on the context in which they are used. The major ones to be described include management information systems, bibliographic retrieval systems, stand-alone systems, transaction systems, physiologic monitoring systems, decision support systems, and expert systems.

Management Information Systems

A management information system (MIS) provides managers information about their business operations. An MIS is defined as an organized system for managing the flow of information in an organization in a timely manner. Its primary use is assisting in the decision-making processes. The MIS in a health care facility may be integrated with a large, hospital information system, or it might be a stand-alone system. Most MIS systems have programs that support strategic planning, management control, and operations support.

"Strategic planning" refers to the policy decisions made by the top-level team of administrators. Strategic planning is the work that seeks to position the organization with respect to its customers and competitors. The management control function refers to the program and personnel decisions made by middle-level managers, supervisors, and head nurses. They need information to measure performance standards and to control, plan, and allocate resources. The operations control support functions provide data and information to the first line managers. For example, unit managers need information on the state of the unit budget, on occupancy and workload, and on overtime hours spent. They need information on incident reports, infection rates, and other clinical indicators of care quality. They need the type of information that helps them manage the unit in such a way that patient care is effectively and efficiently carried out.

A health care MIS typically provides information that can be used to generate the balance sheet and cash flow reports, help the finance department gather information for other financial reports, and track inpatient occupancy rates by unit or department, clinic visits, procedures, etc. It also usually has programs that will allow management to analyze trends in the data and project future business given current trends and other assumptions. However, most MIS databases supplement internal data with data from external local, regional, and national databases. Many organizations join private organizations that share buying power and information useful to management.

Increasingly, health care organizations are joining with each other into private consortia whose purpose is the collection of information from all members so that averages and ranges of performance data can be used for benchmarking purposes. The University Hospital Consortium in Oakbrook, Illinois, is one such organization (University Hospital Consortium, 1999). Hospital consortia provide their members with a variety of reports that supplement, and sometimes help managers interpret, their own internal organizational data.

Bibliographic Retrieval Systems

A bibliographic retrieval system is a retrieval system that generally refers to bibliographic data, document information, or literature. Such a system is primarily used to store and retrieve data and not to conduct any computations per se. The textual data are input and stored and are available for retrieval in a user-friendly format that is easy to read and understand. The system is designed to provide bibliographic data on journal articles, books, monographs, and textual reports. It generally contains the full citations, keywords, abstracts, and other pertinent facts on the documents in the database. An example of a bibliographic retrieval system is CINAHL MEDLINE, developed and published by the National Library of Medicine (NLM). In the late 1990s, NLM made MEDLINE, along with a friendly user interface, Grateful Med, available free on-line to anyone who wishes to use it. MEDLINE may be accessed at the NLM URL: *http://igm.nlm.nih.gov/*. The user simply clicks on the word MEDLINE, which is the first choice on the left-hand side of the screen in the "Select Database to Search" menu.

Stand-Alone, Dedicated, or Turnkey Systems

A stand-alone system is a special purpose system. It is developed for a single application or set of functions. A patient classification system is an example of a stand-alone system. Most stand-alone systems are described by their purpose, such as a pharmacy or laboratory system or an imaging system in the radiology department. Until recently, most turnkey systems ran on a microcomputer or PC. However, during the 1990s, most vendors of large hospital information systems changed their design strategy. Formerly, most vendors deliberately designed their systems to be unique rather than easily integrated with other systems. Due to customer demand and the realization that a hospital's needs were simply too large for any one vendor to support completely, most HIS vendors made real efforts to make their products more "friendly" to other products. Advances in networking science have also changed the technology available for transporting information across different products and platforms. Eventually, most organizations should be able to freely move their data from one system to another electronically.

Transaction Systems

A transaction system is used to process predefined transactions and produce predefined reports. It is designed for repeated operations using a fixed list. From this list, displayed on a computer terminal, a user selects the names of transactions to be processed. A computer program is written so that it can be used repeatedly to process the same type of transactions and generate the same type of reports or products. The computer programs and the list of transactions are retained in storage and retrieved as needed.

An inventory system is an example of a transaction system. It is used to monitor the distribution of items as well as to update and reorder supplies. These kinds of operations are repetitive and always processed in the same manner. A standard list of items is initially developed. Inventory systems usually have information about vendors and prices, track inventory, and can generate automatic reorders when stock on hand drops below a certain level. Typically, inventory control systems produce a set of management reports that helps management keep track of which items are increasing in demand so they can take advantage of volume discounts. The transactions can also be summarized and reports developed to produce monthly bills, prepare order vouchers, and summarize the inventory status for any given time period. In this type of system, the computer program is specifically written to process the transactions (raw data). Grocery store scanners are linked to a transaction-based inventory control system.

Pharmacy, laboratory, and admission/discharge/transfer systems are also forms of transaction systems. Transaction systems can also be designed to process routine medical or nursing orders and permit clinicians to update the orders in real time. This activity is done to ensure that the orders once entered are current in the system. The updating of medical and nursing orders can also be summarized for documenting care plans, change of shift reports, discharge summary, quality review, research studies, etc.

Physiologic Monitoring Systems

Physiologic monitoring systems are widely used in hospital patient care units, in surgery, and more and more commonly, in private homes. The heart monitor was one of the first physiologic monitors used by nurses. Primarily due to the heart monitor, survival rates for hospitalized myocardial infarction patients increased by about 30% in the early 1970s. Today, all sorts of physiologic processes are monitored in order that problems can be detected and treated early. In the labor and delivery unit, mothers' uterine contractions and fetal heart rate are routinely monitored so that complications can be recognized and addressed without delay. Brain waves are monitored in seizure and sleep disorders units. Intraventricular pressure is monitored in neurological intensive care units for patients at great risk of cerebral aneurysm rupture.

All of these devices are a form of oscilloscope. An oscilloscope is an electronic device that senses electric impulses and converts them into waveforms on a monitor screen. On the screen, the impulses are represented by a light cursor (a point on the screen that is bright as compared with the darker background). The cursor moves from left to right across the screen at a timed rate (i.e., moves a defined number of centimeters across the screen per second). When the monitor is not connected, the cursor travels at the bottom edge of the usable screen in a straight line, and this line is called the **baseline**. The strength of the impulse deflects the cursor vertically. Thus, when a positive or negative impulse occurs in the human body being monitored, the cursor is deflected up or down from the baseline. As the impulse ebbs, the cursor returns to the baseline (Fig. 6.3).

Physiological monitoring systems are being used more frequently to measure and monitor continuous auto-

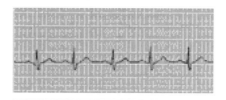

Figure 6.3
An EKG.

matic physiological findings such as heart rate, blood pressure, and other vital signs. Monitoring systems provide alarms to detect significant abnormal findings when personnel are needed to provide patient care and save lives.

Decision Support Systems

A decision support system is a computer system that supports some aspect of the human decision-making process. Decision support systems work with the user to support, but not replace, human judgement in a decision-making situation (Brennan and McHugh, 1988). Decision-making systems also exist, and these tend to be closed systems that function on internal feedback loops. Decision support systems may model the decision process. This type of system guides the user in a highly structured approach that helps identify the salient components of the problem (Brennan and McHugh, 1988).

Certain types of analytic modeling systems may also be considered as decision support systems. Business and engineering applications for decision support include linear programming, computer simulation modeling, trend analysis, and forecasting. Although some merely consider these tools to be analysis tools, others consider them to be decision support systems, since they are used to analyze the outcomes of a variety of possible decisions. Still another form of decision support system is an **optimization** program. Optimization programs take all the information about a problem situation and generate a variety of possible solutions. Then each solution is **implemented** (usually simulated in a computer), and the results of the implementation for each solution are compared. Then the optimization program selects the best solutions based on the outcomes. In an optimization problem, several variables exist such that as one improves, another deteriorates. The difficulty is in producing a solution that jointly maximizes the benefits while minimizing the negative consequences. Nurse staffing is a good example of an optimization problem. If high levels of nursing hours are provided, costs of idle time rise. As staffing levels are lowered, more and more patient care needs are neglected. However, since both nurse supply and patient acuity vary, a perfect staffing level does not exist. So the real challenge is to determine the optimal staffing level for an organization (McHugh, 1997). Other decision support systems provide expert advice to the user.

Expert Systems

An expert system is a computer system containing the information and decision-making strategies of an expert to assist nonexperts in decision-making. An expert system is designed for users to simulate the cause and effect reasoning that an expert would use if confronted with the same situation in a real live environment.

The heart of an expert system has two parts: (1) a knowledge base containing facts and data pertinent to the problem area and (2) an inference engine programmed to replicate the reasoning and decision-making strategies of expert clinicians. The format for decision making allows the rule, "What if?—then . . ." rule of logic. This approach is used to draw inferences about the problem posed by the user so that a solution or possible solutions to the problem can be provided. The inference system is based on a method of reasoning that can be either inductive or deductive. Expert systems can be used for assisting practitioners to implement clinical practice guidelines.

Artificial Intelligence Systems

An artificial intelligence (AI) system is a system that attempts to model human reasoning processes. The field is concerned with symbolic inference and knowledge representation. Symbolic inference is concerned with deriving new knowledge from known facts and the use of logical inference rules. An example of an inference rule is: "if A > B and B > C, then A must be greater than C." Knowledge representation is the field concerned with devising ways to represent and use abstract knowledge and then store those representations and use rules in a computer system. Once abstract phenomena can be represented, and the rules about how to combine facts about phenomena can be determined and programmed into the computer, then new facts can be added as they are discovered. Then the computer can replicate the human process of developing new knowledge by combining new facts with existing knowledge patterns to generate new facts and understandings.

A true artificial intelligence system can also track the accuracy of its predictions and judgements and alter its own decision-making rules, based on new knowledge it generates for itself. This capacity replicates the human power to reason under conditions of uncertainty. AI is a subject that sheds light on the nature of thinking by simulating the process of reasoning. Programs have been devised to solve typical mental problems in an effort to demonstrate that the reasoning process follows a systematic series of rules.

Pattern recognition and problem solving are important aspects of AI. People have longed for computers that they could talk with rather than having to rely on slow and inconvenient methods of data entry such as typing. Unfortunately, understanding natural human language has proven to be a most difficult task, requiring a much higher degree of intelligence than simple serial processing.

Natural Language Systems

A natural language system is a system that can understand and process commands given in the user's own natural, spoken language. It does not require the user to learn a special vocabulary, syntax, and set of programming rules and instructions. Natural language requires the computer to understand a wide range of words, speech styles (accents), syntax, and sentence structures. Some computer programs are marketed to accept and process natural language input. They consist of relatively crude matching technique methods to process the input. The newer natural language systems are used to recognize and process human speech (voice) and/or handwriting.

Hospital Information Systems

A hospital information system (HIS), sometimes called a medical information system (MIS) or patient care system (PCS), provides support for a wide variety of both administrative and clinical functions. The purpose of a HIS is to manage information needed to facilitate daily hospital operations by all health care personnel. Administrators manage financial budgets and establish charges for services; physicians diagnose, treat, and evaluate patient conditions; nurses assess, plan, and provide patient care; other personnel provide ancillary services; and a variety of other personnel support the delivery of patient care services. Blum (1986) asserts that a HIS performs two major functions: (1) communication support and (2) organization of data to facilitate decision-making in a hospital. He indicated that the HIS provides the tools for each operational unit in a hospital to communicate with other units as well as support for internal operations.

A HIS is usually a large package of programs, and it is often purchased from a single vendor. While the hospital may own programs that were not supplied by the HIS vendor, the difficulties of integrating programs from multiple vendors can greatly raise the cost of operating the HIS department. Therefore, most hospitals try to keep the number of different products to a minimum.

Hospital Information System Configurations

A HIS can use several different computer system configurations. The most common configuration uses a mainframe computer with hardwired terminals or workstations. Users are able to work directly with the mainframe through an interactive interface and real-time processing. Another, and increasingly popular, configuration employs a local area network (LAN). The HIS software is either on the mainframe or on a network server. Users access the HIS through their office PC and the network connections.

Many HIS configurations consist of multiple separate systems that are either linked through a network or, in some cases, may not be electronically linked at all. Many hospitals' configuration includes dedicated information systems for special purposes, such as nurse staffing, pharmacy, or laboratory systems (Blum, 1984; Collen, 1983; Shortliffe and Perreault, 1990; Wiederhold and Perreault, 1990).

Program Modules Available in a HIS

Programs typically offered in a HIS include a wide variety of administrative applications (modules) such as admission and discharge, patient tracking, finance, payroll, billing, budgeting support, inventory, and management reporting programs. Clinical support programs are increasingly being viewed as critically important modules in a HIS. As a result, vendors have increased the number and quality of the clinical support tools available in commercial HIS packages.

Administrative Applications

Administrative applications refer to the support of the administrative functions of patient care. They generally include budgeting and payroll, cost accounting, patient billing, inventory control, bed census, and medical records. These are the same systems that are available in almost any management information system. For nursing administration, a variety of administrative support systems are available commercially as part of a HIS, as partially integrated systems, or as completely stand alone systems. Patient classification systems are one of the most popular modules for nursing administration. These systems support the process of assigning nursing staff to units and patients. They function by evaluating the acuity of patients in a particular unit and determining the number of nurses needed to care for that group of patients. Many of these modules can produce a variety of specialized operations reports. Other supports for upper and middle management include staff scheduling and budget support modules.

Semi-Clinical Modules

Two modules in a HIS support both administrative and clinical operations. These are the admission, discharge, and transfer (ADT) and order entry systems. The ADT module monitors and sometimes controls the flow of patients in a hospital from admission to discharge. The ADT module may automatically prepare the midnight census and activity reports. Admissions and discharges constitute the hospital's patient census, which is a key factor in billing and future planning for how to best deploy hospital resources.

Another "semi-clinical" module is the order-entry-results-reporting (OE) module. OE is almost always available in a HIS. Order entry means that staff can enter laboratory, pharmacy, and radiology orders on-line. Results reporting means that the lab, pharmacy, and radiology can enter the results into the computer system and have those results available to the nursing unit. Some are "paperless systems" in which all results are reported and posted to the chart electronically. Others may post the results on-line, but paper reports are still generated and manually posted to the patient chart.

Clinical Support Modules

Charting Systems   Support for nurse charting is highly variable. However, during the 1990s, most vendors greatly upgraded their clinical record products. Many vendors now offer some form of on-line charting. Usually included are the medication administration reports, admission assessment, shift assessments, special assessments (e.g., neurological assessments, labor records, etc.), at least some elements of the nursing care plan (such as nursing diagnosis and interventions), vital signs records, wound care, and hygienic care records. Some provision is usually made for on-line progress notes.

Unfortunately, there is still a major stumbling block to computerizing the record of nursing care. The lack of a universally implemented standard nursing language continues to impede both the development effort and the market success of the systems that are available. Worse, for the profession of nursing, it impedes efforts of nurses to document the outcomes—and therefore the value of nursing care. This problem is not a function of lack of nursing nomenclatures. The American Nurses Association has recognized such nomenclatures as the Home Health Care Classification (HHCC), the Nursing Intervention Classification/Nursing Outcomes Classification (NIC/NOC), North America Nursing Diagnosis Association (NANDA), the Omaha and Grobe systems (Carroll-Johnson and Paquette, 1994; McCloskey and Bulechek, 1996; Grobe, 1996; Martin, 1996; Saba, 1992). For further discussion of nursing nomenclatures, see Chap. 10, "Data Standards."

Point of Service Systems   A point-of-service (POS) or point-of-care system is a special type of clinical system. A POS system uses a hand-held or bedside PC to ensure that data are entered at the point at which they are collected. In other types of clinical systems, the placement of workstations may create a problem for nurses. Typically, workstations have been located at the nurses' station, or in a separate physician's charting room. However, patient data are not collected at those locations. That situation forces the nurse to record information on a "scrap" sheet and later transcribe it to the computer record. This approach produces several suboptimal conditions. First, it is costly to record the same data twice. Second, there is a certain amount of error whenever data are transcribed from one place to another. Third, there is a greater potential that the scrap sheet and the data it contains could be lost or misplaced. Fourth, if the scrap sheet is lost, there is a potential for compromise of patient confidentiality. Fifth, there is always a delay between the time data are collected and the time those data show up on the chart. Finally, the remote workstation approach virtually guarantees idle nursing time because only one person can use the workstation at a time, and there is always competition for access to the workstations. POS systems eliminate all of these problems.

A point-of-service system is designed to save time by recording critical clinical data such as patient assessment, drug administration, vital signs, etc. as they are administered by the provider of the service. It also provides immediate access to key patient information to all care providers involved with the patient. It can retrieve the patient's care plan, latest vital signs, or medication administered. A point of service system is generally installed in a direct patient care unit, such as the inten-

sive or critical care units, but can be also found in patient care units in a facility where an HIS is installed (Massengill; 1993; Wiederhold and Perreault, 1990).

Laboratory, Pharmacy, and Radiology Modules

Laboratory, pharmacy, and radiology support programs are needed by all hospitals. A typical laboratory system, for example, includes a laboratory test request, generates the specimen labels, tracks the specimen through the various laboratory stages, generates the results, and communicates the findings to patient's medical record. Pharmacy systems track medication orders and changes in orders. They often have drug interaction warning programs, dosage calculators, and other supports for the pharmacy function. They generally include a computer-stored database of the Physician Drug Reference (PDR) Manual, which provides a knowledge base for the pharmacists. Radiology systems are usually separate products developed by companies that specialize in diagnostic computer imaging systems. Ideally, they can be linked with the HIS in such a way that the pictures (digitized versions of the radiographic studies) and radiologist report can be viewed at the bedside or unit workstation.

Network Systems

A network is a set of interconnected computers that, through hardware and software technology, work cooperatively for the purpose of information and application program interchange. This definition identifies two essential factors for any network: (1) **hardware** (see Chap. 3), including a physical (electronic) connection (card in the computer) and a physical linkage that permits data and information to be transferred back and forth between the computers in the network (typically co-axial or twisted wire cables) and (2) network communication **software** that allows different computers to make sense of the electronic signals and data streams sent back and forth across the wires (see Chap. 4). The purpose of the hardware and software configuration is to facilitate the transmission of information across different types of computers and computer platforms throughout the system.

Network systems are key to the effective functioning of most hospital computer systems and of many home health, visiting nurse, and clinic computer systems. Increasingly, private and public networks are being used to support the operations of large corporations, educational institutions, governmental operations, and virtually all areas of the economy. Given their importance, it is important that students of informatics science gain an understanding of the fundamental concepts of network science.

The central concept of network science is **cooperation**. All computers in a network must function in an interdependent way. Merely connecting two computers with a wire does not produce a network. In fact, it might not produce any communication. Communication implies mutually understandable interactivity. Simply sending electronic signals from one computer to another does not necessarily mean that the receiving computer can make any sense of the signal. A network, therefore, must have software that can **interpret** the signals it receives. At a minimum, a network must have a set of communication rules. The rules are written into system software programs called **protocols** or networking software.

Advantages of Computer Networks

Networks offer enormous advantages to companies and to individual users. For companies, networking computers often saves money in storage, software purchase prices, reduction of costs attributable to errors in the data, and human time and efficiency.

Efficiencies Related to Storage and Data Integrity

In a HIS, many departments often must use the same data items. Storing the same information in multiple computers increases the cost of storage and may increase the organization's costs of maintaining accurate records. Consider a major hospital that has many inpatient departments and outpatient clinics. Every department in which care or services are provided needs a patient's identifying information. Storing that patient's identifying information in only one record that can be accessed by all of the departments means that storage space is conserved. Even more important, patients may visit multiple departments and clinics over time. Since people's identifying information sometimes changes, the information should be changed *in every instance in which it has been stored*. This might include hospital admissions, pharmacy, laboratory, several clinics, the billing department, medical records, and so on. But patients may move from one residence to another. When information is stored in multiple computers, updates almost never reach all of the various storage sites. Thus, the integrity (accuracy and currency) of data in at least some of the departmental computers is compromised. In a network system in which data are stored in a central location and shared with remote workstations, the networks not only save storage space dollars, they can improve the accuracy of the data in the institution's database.

Software Savings   Many health care organizations have a local area network (LAN) in which most of the workstations use "desktop office" software (e.g., Microsoft Office, Corel Office, etc.). If the organization had to individually purchase the "desktop office" software for each workstation, the purchase cost might be prohibitive. Even worse, each user might select a different brand, and workers could not share work efficiently. As a result, the major software vendors offer what is called a "site network license." When a site license is purchased, the cost per workstation is considerably less than the cost of purchasing the same number of software packages individually.

As an added advantage, the cost of maintaining the software is significantly reduced. This is because only one copy of the software is actually stored on the server. The network version of the software allows each user to access and use the same program. Then, if a problem arises, the HIS department can determine quickly if the problem is encountered everywhere in the network (a program problem) if only one user is experiencing problems (local problem). Problem diagnosis is facilitated. If a program bug is found and must be corrected, it is corrected in only one place.

Savings in Human Time and Efficiency   In many cases, multiple departments in an organization need the same information. When networks allow all of the departments to use the same information, only one has to collect and enter the data. Networks also facilitate the work of groups within an organization. One can initiate a document, and others can add to the document, edit it, and print it. Electronic mail (E-mail) on networks greatly reduces human dependence on real-time communication devices such as telephones. With E-mail, the worker can stop to review messages at a convenient time rather than stopping work in progress to answer a phone. This also reduces stress and anxiety. Stress and anxiety do not constitute states of mind compatible with efficient performance.

Network Functions

Some of the functions performed by networks include (1) file transfer (from one computer to another), (2) information availability (e.g., data and text files can be simultaneously received by more than one recipient at the same time), (3) resource sharing (e.g., programs and data are available to all users simultaneously), (4) on-line transactions (e.g., grocery stores use computer networks for their charging and inventory control programs attached to the laser scanners at the checkout stand), (5) provision of a powerful communication medium among widely separated employees who may use different computer platforms, (6) interactive environment, (7) education and entertainment (sharing privately or publicly developed educational offerings, games, movies, recordings, etc.), and (8) E-mail.

Network Security

The data or information on a network is valuable property to its owner. Loss or damage to health care data can be costly and can create serious legal liability for a facility that loses critical patient care data or other business data and communications. For example, if a baby is later diagnosed with brain damage, and the labor and delivery record is damaged or destroyed, how shall the facility defend itself against a malpractice suit?

Modern security practices weave layers of physical, administrative, electronic, and encrypted security around valuable data. In the early days of computing, data security wasn't a major concern. However, physical safety of the computer itself was quite important. The vacuum tubes were vulnerable to heat and dirt. Therefore, mainframe computer systems required a closed, air-conditioned environment. However, they generally weren't connected to the outside world. They certainly were not connected in any way to other computers, and computer expertise was extremely rare. To steal data from a mainframe computer, one would need physical access to the computer itself. One would also need an in-depth knowledge of machine language. Today, neither physical access nor obscure programming knowledge is necessary to break into another's computer.

Networks have simultaneously opened up enormous opportunities to share knowledge . . . and to engage in a variety of malicious and sometimes criminal activities. Physical security remains an important factor, but electronic security is even more important. It is difficult to produce the requisite security with a group of networked personal computers and a large cohort of highly sophisticated computer users throughout the world.

In many large organizations, the central computer room, or server room, is making a comeback. Server rooms provide cooling, stable electrical power, and physical security. They must also provide highly sophisticated security programs, protocols, and encoding for use in modern network installations.

During the 1980s, several trends combined to make data security a major concern. First, computers became the hub of most modern businesses. They became the storehouse for inventory payroll, employee information,

design, and manufacturing documents. Due to the sensitivity and value of the information, computer installations have become very attractive targets for thieves, disgruntled employees, vandals, and industrial espionage agents. Second, the trend toward networking and open communications led computer makers to adopt common standards for data communication and storage. It became easy to view a file created on an IBM mainframe on a PC. Finally, most large computers became connected to some kind of networking system, either by LAN or modem. Sensitive corporate data came within the reach of anyone clever enough to get it.

In the 1990s, a new criminal, the hacker, emerged. Originally used to describe anyone who was a "clever programmer," the term is now almost exclusively applied to people who illegally break into computers belonging to someone else. Some hackers do it for profit or for hire as a form of corporate or international espionage. But many others break into computer systems purely for the challenge. Many older mainframe computers were designed with few security measures beyond password protection. In some cases, all computers with the same operating system were shipped with the same maintenance password. If an administrator didn't change the maintenance password, a savvy hacker had an unobstructed ride into the system. (This happened to the Mayo Clinic in the 1980s, because nobody bothered to change that system password. Unfortunately, the system password was widely published on hacker bulletin boards.)

Password protection can be enough security for most systems, provided that people give their passwords the proper handling and respect. In nursing, it is absolutely essential that all personnel know there is a policy of severe punishment for disclosing one's password to anyone else and that the policy is rigidly followed. There must be no second chances! Failure to enforce the rules in one case makes it legally difficult to enforce the rules when others break them. Lax security actually leads people to believe security violations are "naughty" or even acceptable rather than helping them understand that these are criminal acts.

An administrative security program focuses on passwords, access rights, and personnel issues. System administrators have to work with managers to ensure that only people with a current need to access information are on authorization lists. The HIS department needs to be sure people know that writing their computer passwords down on a desk calendar on a note taped to their monitors is a serious security violation! The fact is that most intrusions into computer systems involve a compromised password. Passwords should be more than five characters long, random, frequently changed, and protected in order to provide effective security. The most sophisticated electronic security systems are useless without good administrative security practices. Unfortunately, few people can remember such passwords and must have a mnemonic password—which is more easily compromised.

Electronic security techniques are designed to keep hackers away from important data. These techniques operate at different levels, but generally they recognize and accredit the source of the data. Starting with connections from outside the LAN, many modems can receive a call and, on command, dial back the caller at a prestored number to foil a would be intruder. Modems can also use incoming caller ID, an optional telephone company feature, to identify calls as coming from an authorized telephone number. Similarly, network operating systems can recognize the embedded addresses of network adapters and associate certain maximum privileges with specific adapters.

Physical security devices also exist, and they are much more reliable than software methods. They include fingerprint and handprint readers, retinal scanners, and the like. They are the best security available but are very much more expensive and so are hard to sell to cost-conscious managers.

In wide area networks (WANs), particularly those with Internet connections, specialized routers, called firewalls, carefully inspect each incoming packet of information, looking for authorized source addresses and rejecting any unknown addresses or even suspicious packets. A skillful and determined hacker can generate packets with some correct authorized source information, so sometimes illegal packets are only detected by their process and intent. The U.S. National Institute of Standards and Technology has quite a complete discussion of firewalls at the following URL: *http://csrc.ncsl. nist.gov/nistpubs/800-10/main.html.*

Encryption is another layer of protection. Encryption means that the data are converted into a cipher, or a code of some kind. Even if it is intercepted, the hacker probably can't break the code and read the material. Sometimes data are compressed into smaller packets for more economical storage. Interestingly, compression techniques, often used during data transmission and file storage, act as a primitive form of encryption. It takes a lot more effort to hijack compressed data. Beyond compression, serious encryption systems obscure even the volume of information being transmitted and stored. Some operating systems and electronic mail systems encrypt files during storage, and all commercial-quality network operating systems offer encryption of passwords. Several

companies offer encryption modules for routers so that all of the data passing between networked sites is, in practical terms, totally private.

The threat to data exists even in small companies. The larger the monetary stakes, the higher the threat. Good administrative security practices are a must for every organization. We can and should scale electronic protection schemes to match the value of the information and the threat.

Types of Networks

Local Area Network   A LAN is a data network intended to serve a single building or a group of buildings in close proximity to each other. Due to the restricted physical area served by the LAN, the connections among the machines on the network are by means of physical wiring. That is, the communications do not have to go through telephone lines or satellite transmission technology. This direct wiring between the machines is called **hard wiring**, and machines on the network are said to be "hard wired" into the system. Due to hard wiring, very fast data transmission rates are made possible by LAN technology.

Wide Area Network   A wide area network is a system of connected computers spanning a large geographical area, often a continent or country. This network is usually constructed with serial lines, telephone lines, satellites, and FDDI (fiber-optic distributed data interface) cables for WANs. It can also be constructed by connecting local area networks.

Metropolitan Area Network   A metropolitan area network (MAN) is a data network intended to serve an area approximating the size of a large city. Such networks are being implemented by innovative techniques, such as running fiber cables through subway tunnels. A popular example of a MAN is SMDS (switched multimegabit data service).

The Internet

The Internet is a network of networks. It might be visualized as widest of WANs. The Internet is a collection of thousands of networks linked by a common set of technical protocols that make it possible for users of any one of the networks to communicate with or use the services located on any of the other networks. These protocols are referred to as Transmission Control Protocol over Internet Protocol, or TCP/IP. The package of TCP/IP protocols is sometimes called the TCP/IP protocol suite. The Internet began in 1968 with the Advanced Research Projects Agency Network (ARPANET). ARPANET began as a network designed to link certain U.S. Defense Department computers with university computers on campuses performing defense-related research. Today, ARPANET has been subsumed by the National Science Foundation Network (NSFNET), which also includes such networks as the Australian Academic and Research Network (AARNet), the NASA Science Internet (NSI), the Swiss Academic and Research Network (SWITCH), and about 10,000 other large and small, commercial and research, networks. To be part of the Internet, a network must be based on the TCP/IP protocol.

There are other major WANs that are not based on the TCP/IP protocols and are thus often not considered part of the Internet. However, it is possible to communicate between them and the Internet via electronic mail because of mail gateways that act as "translators" between the different network protocols involved.

How to Navigate on the Internet   In order to enter the Internet, the user must have an Internet service provider (ISP) and a Web browser. Most large hospital, corporate, and university computer departments have their own Internet address (node), and serve as an ISP to their faculty and staff. Private home users typically purchase ISP services from public companies like America Online (AOL), Sprint, etc. During the late 1990s, cable companies developed the technology to let users access the Internet directly from their cable provider. Increasingly, users are seeking services from a cable television provider both because cable modem transmissions are often faster than transmissions through private telephone lines and because this produces one less bill to pay at the end of the month. Recently, telephone companies have begun to offer bundled services that include home telephone, cell phone, cable, and Internet access all for one monthly fee.

To search the Internet efficiently, a search engine is essential. Today, most of the popular search engines are supported not by user fees, but by advertising. Some popular search engines and their addresses are:

1. Altavista. Created by Digital Computer Corporation, this is a highly effective and efficient engine. URL: *http://altavista.com*

2. Yahoo!. Originally developed by graduate students Jerry Yang and David Filo at Stanford University, Yahoo is now a privately owned and operated commercial company. URL: *http://www.yahoo.com/*

3. Magellan. Owned and operated by The McKinley Group, a subsidiary of Excite Corporation. URL: *http://magellan.excite.com*

4. 37.com. This is a **metacrawler**. A metacrawler is a search engine that searches for the requested term or phrase on more than one other search engine. URL: *http://37.com*

5. Go2net is another Webcrawler. URL: *http://www.go2net.com/search.html*

Web Browser   A Web browser is a program that is used to visit Web pages. The two most well-known web browsers are Netscape Navigator (part of the Netscape Communicator package) and Microsoft Internet Explorer. Other browsers are available as well but are not as popular. A Web browser has features that allow the user to download and print documents on the Internet; to view the source document, which includes the program codes that format the document; to save images found on the Internet; and to perform a variety of other useful functions. It is the user's window into the Internet. Prior to the development of Web browsers, about the only people who could use the Internet were programmers and other sophisticated users. They had to understand disk operating system commands, because the user's interface with the Internet was not graphical.

A Short History of Web Browsers   The very first Web browser was written by Tim Berners-Lee (creator of the World Wide Web) while at CERN (a European center for physics research). However, Dr. Berners-Lee's browser was not generally available to the public. The first Web browser to capture the public's imagination was Mosaic. Mosaic was written by Marc Andreessen while he was a graduate student at the National Center for Supercomputing Applications at the University of Illinois. Mosaic was highly popular and in fact, was the key that opened the Internet to the general public. The success of Mosaic led eventually to the formation of the company Netscape Communications and the popular Netscape Communicater browser. During the late 1990s, the Microsoft Corporation was also working on a Web browser that would interface smoothly with its desktop office software. With the introduction of Windows '98 and later versions of the Microsoft PC operating system, Microsoft's browser, Explorer, was integrated as a utility attached to the operating system.

How Does a Web Browser Work?   A Web browser is a software program or set of programs that allows users of the Internet to communicate and send/receive files, sound, and graphics. It works by using a special protocol called HTTP (Hypertext Transfer Protocol). Documents on the Internet contain special instructions (written in Hyper-

Text Markup Language (HTML)) that tell the browser how to display the document on the user's screen. The instructions may include references (hyperlinks) to other Web pages, text color and position, locations for various images contained in the document, and where to position them. Some Web pages may use layout instructions contained in separate documents called style sheets.

World Wide Web   The World Wide Web (WWW) is a hypertext-based, distributed information system created by a team of researchers led by Dr. Tim Berners-Lee at CERN in Switzerland. Users may create, edit, or browse hypertext documents. The clients and servers are freely available. This is a subset of the Internet that uses a combination of text, graphics, audio, and video (multimedia) to provide information on most every subject imaginable.

Hypertext and Hyperlinks   Hypertext is a document, written in HTML, which contains automated links (hyperlinks) to other documents, which may or may not also be hypertext documents. Hypertext documents are usually retrieved using the WWW. A hyperlink pointer within a hypertext document points (links) to another document, which may or may not be a hyper-

text document. Hyperlinks are usually a bright blue color (although the person who designs the Web page may change the color). Hyperlinks are also often underlined as well, and often, when the reader places the cursor on the hyperlink, it changes color to be sure the user knows the text is a hyperlink. Hyperlinks are usually documents placed on other sites on the Internet. Clicking on these links activates the necessary protocols and pulls up the chosen site.

Hypertext Markup Language   HTML is the language used to create hypertext documents. It is a subset of the Standardized General Markup Language (SGML) and includes mechanisms to establish hyperlinks in one document that take the user to the address of other documents. With HTML you can build Web pages. It is basically a formatting language. Table 6.1 presents a sample of HTML codes designed to format text on a Web page.

While the codes appear to be complex and obscure, the HTML programmer primarily has to master mnemonic characters such as <B>, which means format the following text in a bold font, and </B>, which means turn off the bold and return the text to a regular font for the next text lines. Note that documents on the World Wide Web must begin with the notation <html> (which

Table 6.1   HTML Formatting Codes Generated in Microsoft Front Page

```
<html>
<head>
<meta http-equiv="Content-Type" content="text/html; charset=iso-8859-1">
<title>Module 2</title>
<meta name="GENERATOR" content="Microsoft FrontPage 3.0">
<meta name="Microsoft Theme" content="none">
</head>
<body>
<h1 align="center"><font color="#FF0000">Module 2</font></h1>
<h1 align="center"><font color="#FF0000">Structured Systems Analysis</font></h1>
<p ALIGN="CENTER"> 
Structured Systems Analysis</p>
<p align="left">    Structured systems analysis (SSA) incorporates
a set of strategies and techniques designed to improve the probability that the
final system designed or purchased actually meets the users; needs for system
support. The process is useful not only in the computer system design and
selection process. The philosophy that underlies SSA has proven so durable and
so effective that many managers find that using it improves the success rate of
their decisions in a variety of managerial as well as computer systems situations.
SSA is so important that failure to use an SSA model in computer system selection
virtually guarantees some degree of failure of the whole project.</p>
</font>
</body>
</html>
```

tells the system that an HTML document will follow) and end with the </html> notation, which signals that the document is complete (see Table 6.1).

Additional Concepts Involved in Interconnecting Computers into Networked Systems

Attenuation As the length of the cable increases, the strength of the signal decreases, which is called attenuation. It may fall below a certain level and may not be possible for the other computers to clearly receive the signal. Hence, there is a maximum limit on the length of a cable that can be used.

Repeater If the computers are placed at a distance more than the allowed cable length, then there must be a way to connect those computers without attenuation. This is done by using repeaters. A repeater is a device that receives a signal, amplifies it, and then sends it along the next leg of its journey. For very long distances, a signal may pass through a series of repeaters before it reaches its final destination.

Bridge If multiple LANs are to be connected, then bridge technology may be employed. Bridges will extract the information from the physical line rather than taking the electrical signal. They will reproduce the information on the other side but will not amplify the signals. In this way they reduce the noise.

Router When two computers in different networks need to exchange information, they must be connected through a common computer. This is called a router. A router is a device (or it may be software installed in a server computer) that determines the next network point to which a packet should be forwarded toward its destination. The router is connected to at least two networks that need to exchange information (same protocol). It is the job of the router to determine which way to send each information packet. To accomplish its mission, a router must develop and maintain a table of available routes, cost, and distance. The router applies an algorithm to these data to determine the fastest and lowest-cost path for each information packet. A router must be located at any juncture of networks (gateway).

Point of Presence In the Internet, the location of a device that serves as an access point or gateway into the Internet is called a point of presence, or POP. When users need to get a new E-mail address working, they have to identify their computer's POP server to the E-mail pro-

gram so it knows where to send the mail. Every POP server has a unique Internet address.

Gateway A gateway is a network's point of access into other computer or networks. A gateway allows users to interconnect computers in different networks of different types. These gateways will extract information at a higher level, reformat it, and then pass it to the other network.

Glossary of Internet Terms

Address: The location of an Internet resource. The address identifies the type of agency. The most commonly encountered are nonprofit organizations (.org), companies (.com), governmental bodies (.gov), and educational institutions (.edu). An E-mail address may take the form of jones@someclinic.com. A Web address looks something like *http://www.charityhospital.org.*

Applet: An applet is a little application program that can be downloaded over a network and launched on the user's computer. Java applets can perform interactive animations, immediate calculations, or other simple tasks without having to send a user request back to the server. Applets make it possible for a Web page user to interact with the page.

Bandwidth: A measurement of the volume of information that can be transmitted over a network at a given time. Think of a network as a water pipe—the higher the bandwidth (the larger the diameter of the pipe), the more data (water) that can pass over the network (through the pipe).

Browser: A program run on a client computer for viewing World Wide Web pages. Examples include Netscape, Microsoft's Internet Explorer, and Mosaic.

Cache: A region of memory where frequently accessed data can be stored for rapid access. A cache (pronounced CASH) is a place to store something more or less temporarily.

CGI: Common Gateway Interface—the specification for how an HTTP server should communicate with server gateway applications.

Chat: A system that allows for on-line real-time communication between Internet users. Since it is a real-time activity, chat discussions disappear as they scroll off your screen. Also, everybody has to be on-line at the same time.

Client: A program (like a Web browser) that connects to and requests information from a server.

Cookies: The collective name for files stored on your hard drive by your Web browser that hold information about your browsing habits, like what sites you have visited, which newsgroups you have read, etc. Many view cookies as an invasion of privacy.

Dial-up Connection: A connection to the Internet via phone and modem. Connection types include Point-to-Point Protocol (PPP) and Symmetric List Processsor (SLIP).

Direct Connection: A connection made directly to the Internet—much faster than a dial-up connection.

Discussion Group: A particular section within the USENET system typically, though not always, dedicated to a particular subject of interest. Also known as a newsgroup. A class discussion board is an example of a discussion group.

Domain: The Internet is divided into smaller sets known as domains, including .com (business), .gov (government), .edu (educational), and others. The WSU domain is an educational domain; thus the .edu at the end of all its server names.

Domain Name: A domain name is the Internet name or identifier of a company, university, or other entity on the Internet.

Download: The process of copying data file(s) from a remote computer to a local computer. The opposite action is upload, where a local file is copied to a server.

FTP: File Transfer Protocol—a set of rules for exchanging files between computers via the Internet.

Gateway: Computer hardware and software that allow users to connect from one network to another.

Home Page: The first or entry level page in an individual's or institution's Web site. Typically, the home page is the default page that is located at the user's URL address.

HTML: HyperText Markup Language—a collection of tags typically used in the development of Web pages. This is actually a formatter rather than a programming language.

HTTP: HyperText Transfer Protocol—a set of instructions for communication between a server and a World Wide Web client.

Hyperlink: A connection between two anchors. Clicking on one anchor will take you to the linked anchor. Can be within the same document/page or two totally different documents.

Hypertext: A document that contains links to other documents, commonly seen in Web pages and help files.

ISDN Line: A category of leased telephone line service, allowing transfer rates of 128 kilobytes per second over the Internet. No longer too expensive for home users (around $50 per month plus one cent a minute), but still more commonly found in business environments. (See T1 line.)

ISP: Internet Service Provider— the company that provides you with a connection to the Internet via either a dial-up connection or a direct connection.

IP Address: Internet Protocol address—every computer on the Internet has a unique identifying number, like 191.1.24.2.

Internet: The worldwide network of computers communicating via an agreed upon set of Internet protocols.

LAN: Local area network—a network of computers confined within a small area, such as an office building.

Link: Another name for a hyperlink.

Mailing List: A list of E-mail addresses to which messages are sent. Users can subscribe to a mailing list typically by sending an E-mail to the contact address with the following in the body of the message: the word subscribe, the name of the list, and their E-mail address.

Mirror Site: An Internet site set up as an alternate to a busy site; it contains copies of all the files stored at the primary location.

Mosaic: One of the first graphical World Wide Web browsers, developed at NCSA.

Netscape: One of the two most widely used Internet browsers. At this time, Netscape dominates the market for World Wide Web browsers and servers; however, Microsoft Explorer is gaining ground.

Network: A system of connected computers exchanging information with each other. A LAN is a relatively small form of a network in comparison with the Internet, a worldwide network of computers.

On-line: When you are on a computer, especially when connected to the Internet, you are on-line.

On-line Service: Another name for an Internet service provider (ISP). Companies such as America Online, CompuServe, Prodigy, and the Microsoft Network provide content to subscribers and usually connections to the Internet.

Page: An HTML document, or Web site.

Protocol: An agreed upon set of rules by which computers exchange information.

Provider: An Internet service provider, or ISP. Specifically, it is a company that sells access to the Internet and often also offers the customer an E-mail address and space on the server on which the user can place his or her own home page and other materials.

Search Engine: A tool for searching information on the Internet by topic.

Server: One half of the client-server protocol, it runs on a networked computer and responds to requests submitted by the client. Your World Wide Web browser is a client of a World Wide Web server.

Site: A single Web page or collection of related Web pages. A site has a URL.

SMTP: Simple Mail Transfer Protocol—a protocol dictating how E-mail messages are exchanged over the Internet.

T1: A category of leased telephone line service, allowing transfer rates of 1.5 megabytes per second over the Internet. Too expensive for home users (around $2,000 per month) but commonly found in business environments. (See ISDN line.)

Telnet: A protocol for logging onto remote computers from anywhere on the Internet.

Upload: To copy a file from a local computer connected to the Internet to a remote computer. Opposite is download.

URL: Uniform Resource Locator—the method by which Internet sites are addressed.

WAN: Wide area network—a system of connected computers spanning a large geographical area.

WWW: World Wide Web, or simply Web. Invented by Tim Berners-Lee, it consists of a set of standards and communication protocols that allow information to be shared, regardless of the owner's platform. HTML, the language of the Web, uses a combination of text, graphics, audio, and video (multimedia) to provide information on most every subject imaginable.

Yahoo!: Yahoo! began as the bookmark lists of two Stanford University graduate students, David Filo and Jerry Yang. Putting their combined bookmark lists organized by categories on a college site, the list began to grow into another Internet phenomenon. Filo and Yang postponed their graduate work, and their search engine became part of a public offering for a multimillion-dollar corporation. Their site (*www. yahoo.com*) is constantly updated and provides an easy way of finding almost any Web page.

Summary

This chapter discussed systems and systems theory. It addressed the history of computer systems, computer networks, and the network of networks, the Internet. The concept of systems, including types, elements, and major characteristics, were discussed. Computer systems and information systems were also defined, followed by a discussion of major types of information systems. Hospital systems and their major program modules, including both administrative and clinical applications, were discussed.

The phenomenon of computer networks was introduced. The types of networks and key terms in network theory and practice were presented. The chapter concluded with a discussion of the Internet. A history of the development of the Internet was presented, followed by an introduction to the functioning and utility programs of the Internet. A dictionary of important terms related to the Internet was included.

References

Blum, B. I. (1986). *Clinical Information Systems*. New York: Springer Verlag.

Blum, B. I. (Ed.). (1984). *Information Systems for Patient Care*. New York: Springer-Verlag.

Brennan, P,. and McHugh, M. (1988). Clinical decision-making and computer support. *Applied Nursing Research, 1*(2), 89–93.

Bulechek, G., and McCloskey, J. (1996). *Nursing Interventions Classification (NIC)* (2nd ed.). St. Louis: Mosby.

Carroll-Johnson, R., and Paquette, M. (Eds). (1994). *Classification of Nursing Diagnoses: Proceedings of The Tenth Conference*. Philadelphia: Lippincott.

Collen, M. F. (1983). The function of a HIS: An overview. In O. Fokkens et al. (Eds.), *MEDINFO 83 Seminars* (pp. 61–64). Amsterdam: North-Holland.

Farace, R., Monge, P., and Hamish, R. (1977). *Communicating and Organizing*. Reading, MA: Addison-Wesley Publishing Company.

Grobe, S. (1996). The nursing intervention lexicon and taxonomy: Implications for representing nursing care data in automated patient records. *Holistic Nursing Practice, 11*(1), 48–63.

Martin, K. (1996). The Omaha System: A model for describing practice. *Holistic Nursing Practice, 11*(1), 75–83.

Massengill, S. (1993). The Four Technologies of the Electronic Patient Record. In *Conference Proceedings: Toward an Electronic Patient Record '93* (pp. 92–94). Newton, MA: Medical Record Institute.

McHugh, M. (1997). Cost effectiveness of clustered versus unclustered unit transfers of nursing staff. *Nursing Economics, 15*(6), 294–300.

Optner, S. L. (1975). *Systems Analysis for Business Management* (2nd ed.). Englewood Cliffs, NJ: Prentice-Hall.

Petruccioli, S. (1993). *Atoms, Metaphors and Paradoxes : Niels Bohr and the Construction of a New Physics*. Massachusetts: Cambridge University Press.

Saba, V. K. (1974). Basic consideration in management information systems for public health/community health agencies. In National League for Nursing (Ed.), *Management Information for Public Health/Community Health Agencies: Report of the Conference* (pp. 3–13). New York: National League for Nursing.

Saba, V. (1992). The classification of home health care nursing diagnoses and interventions. *Caring, 11*(3), 50–57.

Shortliffe, E. H., and Perreault, L. E. (Eds.). (1990). *Medical informatics: Computer Applications in Health Care*. Reading, MA: Addison-Wesley Publishing.

University Hospital Consortium (UHC). (1999). *The University Hospital Consortium: An Overview. http://www.radsci.ucla.edu:8000/uhc/description.html*

Von Bertalanffy, L. (1976). *General System Theory: Foundations, Development, Applications*. New York: George Braziller.

Wiederhold, G., and Perreault, L. E. (1990). Hospital information systems. In E. H. Shortliffe and L. E. Perreault (Eds.), *Medical Informatics: Computer Applications in Health Care* (pp. 219–243). Reading, MA: Addison-Wesley Publishing.

7

The Internet: A Nursing Resource

Linda Q. Thede

OBJECTIVES

1. Discuss the history of the Internet.
2. Define protocols that make up the Internet.
3. Identify the functions for which one can use the Internet.
4. Explore the customs used with Internet communication.
5. Describe evaluation steps that one should use with information obtained on the Internet.
6. Discuss the steps for using the Internet.

KEY WORDS:

Internet
World Wide Web
communication
evaluation of Web resources
creation of Web pages

Although relatively new, the Internet is creating many changes in world society, changes that will affect nursing. From its beginning as a technology for the Cold War to the World Wide Web, it has changed how we communicate. Starting with E-mail, communication tools have grown to include such things as mailing lists, news groups, on-line journals, movies, and real-time exchanges. With the freedom of communication has come access to information that heretofore was unavailable to all but a few, necessitating that nurses as well as everyone learn the skills of finding, evaluating, and managing information.

The Internet and Communication

Internet users in the Americas can often truthfully say, "Yesterday I received a message from tomorrow." Time zones and a date line are becoming arbitrary divisions in the world made possible by the Internet in which messages sent from the Far East, where it is tomorrow, are received by computers in the Americas while it is still today. The changes in communication that the Internet is creating are affecting, and will affect, all of us professionally and personally.

The Internet itself is a worldwide system for linking smaller private and public computer networks together to form a global medium for citizens to use for the communication of everything from the written word to movies. In the next decade, it is predicted that over one half of the world will be connected to the Internet (Fulton, 1999; Grush, 1998), giving it the power to democratize communication and make knowledge available to anyone who can use a computer at work, in a library, or at home. The result is that information, which once was a rare commodity owned by a few, will be available to all.

The changes in how knowledge is acquired will affect nurses as well as all other health care disciplines. More and more laypeople are using the Internet as a source of health care information. Patients are starting to come to health care professionals and institutions with a basic knowledge of their condition. This is creating situations different from those of traditional health care in which the health care professional was the source of most of the knowledge about medical conditions. She or he had the power to distribute this knowledge when and if the health care professional felt it would be helpful to a patient. As Internet usage becomes more common, health care professionals will find that instead of deciding who to tell what and giving the appropriate information, they will be helping patients to understand what they have read on the Internet and correcting misinformation they may have found.

Nurses will find the Internet to be a constant source of up-to-date information. All health care institutions will have access to the information that previously was available only in large medical and nursing libraries. Nurses are already using the Internet to network with colleagues all over the world, sharing their knowledge and learning from colleagues in their own and other lands, thus broadening their nursing knowledge. They are also searching the Internet for information about approaches to specific nursing situations. The sheer scope of the Internet and speed of the spread of information will cause care standards to evolve from community to regional to national to international.

These changes are creating new issues and challenges for nursing as well as providing many benefits. In these next few pages, we will explore the multitude of ways that one can use and benefit from the Internet both professionally and personally.

The Origins of the Internet

The Internet might never have come about, or at least would have been much longer in appearing, if in 1957 the Russians had not jolted the United States out of its complacency by launching Sputnik (Hudson, 1996). The result was the creation of the Advanced Research Project Agency (ARPA) by the Pentagon Department of Defense (DOD) and the involvement of the RAND Corporation's think tank to solve the problem of how U.S. authorities could communicate after a nuclear war (Sterling, 1993). These individuals realized that no matter how thoroughly a conventional network such as the telephone network was protected, the switching and wiring would be vulnerable to attack. The result was to devise a network that had no central authority and would be assumed at all times to be unreliable. To facilitate this they devised a system known as "packet switching." The packets would be the result of dividing messages into smaller pieces, each individually addressed. The route that each packet took to its destination would be dependent on the availability of routing at the nanosecond it was being transmitted. Thus, packets from the same message could be switched to different routes. When all of the packets arrived at their destination, the receiving computer would reassemble the packets, and do a little arithmetic to arrive at a checksum. This would be compared with the checksum originated by the sending computer. If they did not agree, a resend would be requested from the originating computer. If part of the network were gone it would not make any difference; the packets would bounce from node to node until they found a route to their destination. It was not a very efficient delivery system, but one that was and still is rugged, a fact that was evident in the earthquake in Los Angles in 1994, when communication was quickly reestablished via the Internet.

The Beginning

This brainchild was first put into operation in the fall of 1969 and named ARPANET, after its DOD Pentagon sponsor the Advanced Research Projects Agency (Sterling, 1993). The first node was installed at the University of California Los Angeles. Within a few months, other nodes were established at Stanford Research Institute, University of California Santa Barbara, and the University of Utah. Not only did this system provide protection against an interruption in communication, but it provided a convenient service to scientists and researchers, allowing them to share what were then scarce computer resources.

Others also felt a need to share computer resources, resulting in the development of many other networks. Each network, however, used a different method for sending and receiving transmissions with the result that it was impossible for the various networks to communicate with each other. To solve this problem, it was necessary to develop communication standards, or protocols, and to gain agreement from other networks to use these standards. The creation of the Transmission Control Protocol and the Internet Protocol (TCP/IP) accomplished the first step. Any computer or network who would agree to use these protocols could join ARPANET. The brand name of the computer, its content, and even its ownership were irrelevant. This decentralized structure together with standard communication methods made expansion easy. By the mid-1980s, many networks had adopted the standards, and a world Internet became a reality. However, it was not until the mid 1990s that the commercial networks such as CompuServe and Prodigy became a part of the Internet. Prior to this, users of these networks could only communicate with those using the same service.

Today, the connection of all major networks to the Internet represents the pinnacle of computer communication. The Internet itself has no owners, censors, bosses, board of directors, or stockholders. In principle, any computer or network that obeys the protocols, which are technical, not social or political, can be an equal player (Sterling, 1993). It is an example of a true, modern, functional anarchy. It does, however, have voluntary groups that develop and coordinate standards, resources, and day-to-day issues of operation (MacPherson, 1997). The overall organizing force is the Internet Society, which sponsors the Internet Architecture Board (IAB), the Internet Research Task Force (IRTF), and the Internet Engineering Steering Group (IESG) (Carpenter, 1996).

Future Plans

Two projects are currently under way to improve the Internet: Internet2 and the Next Generation Internet (NGI). The Internet2 is a project to develop advanced Internet technologies in research and education to support higher education (Internet2, 1999). It is a collaborative effort by more than 120 U.S. universities that are working with partners in industry and government under the umbrella of the University Corporation for Advanced Internet Development (UCAID). The NGI is a government research and development project involving many agencies. Their aim is to increase the speed of transmission on the Internet. Besides working independently, there is a large amount of cooperation between these two groups.

 ## The Technology Behind the Internet

We have mentioned earlier that it was standardized communication protocols that enabled the Internet to function. A protocol, in plain English, is just an agreed upon format for doing something. On the Internet, protocols determine how data will be transmitted between two devices, the type of error checking that will be performed, how data compression, if any, is accomplished, how the sending computer will signal that it has finished sending a message, and how the receiving computer will signal that it has received a message (PC Webopaedia, 1996). As a user, the only issue that need concern you is to be sure that either your software or hardware supports the protocols of the computer or device with which you wish to have your computer communicate. To make it easy for all computer users to use the Internet, most computers sold in the last few years were sold with software that supports these protocols already installed.

The main protocols of the Internet are the TCP/IP. Each of these protocols performs a different job. The TCP protocol carries out the task of breaking a message into the small packets, which was described earlier, and generating the checksum at the beginning and end of a transmission as well as requesting a resend if there is an error. The Internet protocol is responsible for routing the message; it allows Internet computers to find one another

(Quiggle, 1999). All of the functions of the Internet are dependent on these and other protocols. E-mail, or electronic messages sent via the Internet, is supported by several protocols. Some other Internet protocols are HTTP (HyperText Transmission Protocol), which supports the World Wide Web (WWW); FTP (File Transmission Protocol), which permits users to send all types of electronic files over the Internet; and Telnet, which is a protocol allowing users to access a distant computer as though they were sitting in front of it.

 ## What Can One Do on the Internet?

The Past

Even though the original networks were supposed to be for computer sharing, it did not take long for users to realize that they could also send messages to one another. Indeed, they became far more enthusiastic about this function than computer sharing (Sterling, 1993). The first E-mail software appeared in 1972. Like today's E-mail software, it allowed users to list, selectively read, file, forward, and respond to messages (Leiner et al, 1998). For the next decade, E-mail was the largest network application.

The E-mail software was made freely available to anyone who wanted it, which was typical of the atmosphere of the Internet in its first 2 decades. The people involved developed applications that they freely shared with others. These applications could be software for any purpose, files of information, or pictures. To share these items, host computers became "anonymous FTP" sites. Anyone connected to the Internet could use the FTP protocols to connect to the host computer and download any of the available files. This involved learning some commands, which by itself was not difficult. Finding what one wanted, however, was. Most information about available files was spread by word of mouth, particularly E-mail, although there was file locator software called Archie that allowed searching of these sites. Several sites around the world served as Archie sites; they pooled the information from their searches and made it available to users at other sites. The Archie sites were extremely busy, which made it difficult to use them. Further difficulties with FTP were that users could only see the name of the file, which often was not indicative of the contents. It was also impossible to look at the file before downloading it. Still, many useful things were shared by FTP, and it kept the spirit of sharing on the Internet alive.

The next improvement in finding resources on the Internet was the Gopher program developed at the University of Minnesota. Like most networks, it was a client server program. Under this system, a client computer is one that has software that allows it to retrieve files from a distant computer, while a server is a computer that has software that allows it to respond to a client by sending a requested file (Thede, 1999). A computer can be both a client and a server, although most computers have only client software.

The Gopher program provided users a menu of items that the server had available. Users entered the number of their selection, and the file contents were sent to the user's computer, where the user could then read the contents. Like on the WWW, it was possible to bookmark the file, a process in which one sets a pointer to that file so it can be easily accessed again, or download the file to one's own computer, where it could be accessed without using the Internet. A search program called Veronica allowed users to search the Internet for subjects of interest. Gopher, however, only supported text files. Although it supported a form of hypertext, it did not support point and click hypertext, which is the ability to click on an item and retrieve information about that item. The WWW with its graphical files and hypertext interface has made Gophers fairly extinct. The WWW, however, can access Gopher pages and every now and then while using the WWW one accesses a document that looks like a typewritten page and has no links, an indication that it is probably an old Gopher document.

E-mail

E-mail, or electronic mail, is mail that is sent and received by computer. It was, and continues to be, a very important use of the Internet. As more and more people become connected to the Internet, having an Internet E-mail address is becoming more and more expected of people. Most educational institutions and many organizations provide an E-mail account for their people. Some even allow use of the account from a home computer. Commercial Internet service providers (ISPs) are available for those who do not have this privilege or wish to have a private E-mail address.

E-mail Address Anatomy   Given the wide use of E-mail addresses in society, even if you do not yet have one, it is probable that you have seen a few, perhaps on a business card, or in an advertisement. At first glance, they may look confusing, but they all follow the same scheme. They have two parts, separated by the "@." The first part is what may be called the user name, user ID, or login name. Some organizations let the user select their user name, while others assign them based on a

system such as first initial and last name or first name dot (a period) last name. You may find such symbols as an underline (_), a hyphen (-), or even the percent sign (%) or pound sign (#) in the user name. What you will not find are spaces.

In the E-mail address in Fig. 7.1, the user name is "Clara.Barton." The characters after the user name are the name of the computer that assigned the user name. In Fig. 7.1, this name is "RedCross.org." Notice the last three letters of the computer name. They are assigned to the computer under the domain name system. This system was developed to assign responsibility for naming computers to various groups yet still keep all computer names unique. Table 7.1 lists the original top six U.S. domains, although with the growth of the Internet, expect to see this list increase.

The domain name of the computer in Fig. 7.1 is "org," indicating that this address is for a computer in a nonprofit organization. Some computer names have more than one dot in them. This too is part of the domain name system. Each of the top level domains (see Table 7.1) delegated responsibility to groups within their domain who may have further delegated naming responsibility. If you see a computer name of "peds.nursing.xyz.edu," you would know that the educational institution "xyz" named the computer for the nursing area "nursing," while the nursing group named the computer for the pediatric area, "peds." This is another example of the distributed responsibility characteristic of the Internet.

You may also see a country code in a computer address. Outside of the U.S., and even for some addresses inside the U.S., the last two letters of the E-mail address

Table 7.1   Top Level Domain Names

Domain	Usage
edu	Educational institution
gov	Government organization
net	A network resource
org	A nonprofit organization
com	A business
mil	Military
Some possible new domain names	
firm	A business
store	A business offering merchandise for sale
web	Web-related activities

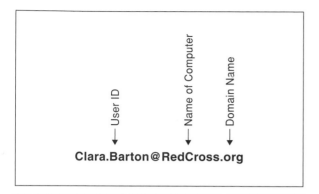

Figure 7.1
An E-mail Address.

indicate the country of origin. CA is Canada, UK is Great Britain, and DE is Germany. A full list of country codes can be found at *ftp://rs.internic.net/netinfo/iso 3166-countrycodes*.

Like user names, computer names do not have any spaces. Currently, most E-mail addresses are not case-sensitive; that is, whether you use a capital letter or a lowercase letter will not affect the address. Omitting any characters, or typing just one incorrectly, however, will.

Using E-mail   To participate with E-mail, besides having an account on the Internet that provides an E-mail address and having a computer, you need communication software. Computers purchased in the last few years have communication software included as part of the operating system. Additionally, all of the World Wide Web browsers (software programs that allow you to use the WWW) have built-in E-mail programs. There are also other E-mail packages available; some are available free, and most can be downloaded from the Internet.

The functions that E-mail software provides vary with the package, but all permit a user to receive and read a message, send a reply, initiate a new message, forward a received message to someone else, and organize received messages in folders. The steps for accomplishing each task vary from program to program, but help in using an E-mail package is available for all of the major packages, often by first getting "on-line" or connecting to the Internet and then using the help option.

Cautions in Using E-mail   E-mail communication is different from either telephone or face to face communication. On the telephone, you can hear voice inflections,

and in face-to-face communication, you can see and hear the other individual. E-mail is also different from a written letter in that it is often done "on the fly" and is usually posted immediately after finishing. For these reasons, some customs and E-mail common sense apply.

Many people have learned the hard way that E-mail is not considered private as is mail delivered by the post office. Nor is any E-mail sent from an account on a business or educational computer protected from oversight by an administrator. This may hold true even if the user has been told that their E-mail is private (Atkins, 1998). Records of what you send can exist in many places besides your hard drive. Additionally, it is very easy for a recipient to forward a message you send to someone else either accidentally or on purpose. To avoid embarrassing moments, or worse, think carefully before you send any E-mail message. If something makes you angry, do not post an immediate reply. If you must write one, save it, let time pass, and then edit it before sending it.

Use of Emoticons and Abbreviations   To make up for the inability of message recipients to accurately judge the mood of the sender, small icons called emoticons or smileys, that can be created on the keyboard, are often used to denote a mood. For example, saying something jokingly is often denoted with the icon :-). If you tilt your head to the left you can see a sideways smiling face. Some other emoticons can be seen in Table 7.2.

Given that voice has not yet displaced the keyboard as the most common method of text entry, abbreviations are often used in E-mail. Table 7.3 has some examples. Both emoticons and abbreviations should be used cautiously; if the recipient of the message does not understand the symbol, communication is lost.

E-mail Etiquette   E-mail etiquette consists of the same consideration that you would show when writing to anyone. Given the nature of E-mail, there are a few

Table 7.2   Some Emoticons

Icon	Meaning
:-*	Blowing a kiss
;-(	Crying
:-)	Happy
;-)	I think I am being funny
:-D	Laughing
:-(	Sad

Table 7.3   Abbreviations

Abbreviation	Meaning
BTW	By the way
FTF	Face to face
<G>	Grin
IMHO	In my humble opinion
LOL	Laughing out loud
OTOH	On the other hand

additional things that one should consider. Using all capital letters is considered "shouting;" additionally it is about 50 percent harder to read than the traditional upper- and lowercase text. It is also good form to always use a subject for your E-mail, even if it is as simple as "Hi!" This helps the recipient, who may have 50 or more messages to read, to decide if your message needs to be read "stat" or if it can wait until she or he has more time. Additionally, there are people who just delete any message that does not have a subject.

Another custom is that all messages should be signed; assuming that the recipient will know who you are leads to problems. If you have received E-mail you may have noticed that some of the messages have rather lengthy signatures, perhaps a full identification of the sender, plus even an icon created on the keyboard or a saying. These are not typed in for every message or even pasted in. These users have learned how to use a signature file. A signature file contains the information that you want added to every message that you send. Once created, the preferences section of your mailing program is directed to add it to every message. At a minimum, a signature file should include your name and E-mail address; at a maximum, it should not be longer than six lines.

Organizing Received Files   Once you start using E-mail, you will find that you want to keep some of the messages that you receive. E-mail packages provide a way to create folders and transfer a received message to them. This allows you to keep your "inbox" or mailbox area clear for messages that you still have to attend to and allows you to keep messages you may want in the future in an organized manner.

File Attachments   E-mail is a plain text file. A plain text file, often referred to as an ASCII file or a DOS file, can be read by all E-mail software and all word processors. Text files, however, have no formatting; that is,

text placement cannot be determined by the individual who created the file, nor can this individual add any attributes such as boldface or italics. For most E-mail communication, this is not a problem.

Sometimes, however, you may wish to send someone a file that will preserve the formatting. To do this, you will want to send a file created by a word processor or other application program. These programs create what are called proprietary files, or a file format that can only be read by the program that created it.

In these cases, you can send the file itself instead of the text the file contains. This is known as attaching a file. Use the E-mail software help to discover how your E-mail package fulfills this function. When you attach a file, the recipient must have the same software package to read the file that you used to create the file. If you send a Word Perfect file to a Word user, the Word user will not be able to read it. Before sending a file attachment, check to be sure your recipient will be able to read it.

Mailing Lists

E-mail communication between individuals led to a desire to be able to send one message to many people to enable group discussions. To enable this, mailing list software was developed in the early 1980s. It was Eric Thomas, however, in 1986, who created the first software that automated many of the functions necessary to maintain a list. Reflecting the ambiance of the Internet at the time, the software was free to anyone who wanted to use it. It was called Listserv™ after the earlier manual product, a name that is often used to denote any mailing list, even though today there are several other software products that manage mailing lists.

Mailing lists are set up to provide an arena for discussion of a specific topic (Bowers, 1997). They are "owned" by an individual who manages the day-to-day affairs of the list. Although the term "owner" is used, the owner pays no money to manage the list and in most cases receives no remuneration for this chore. The owner is responsible for taking care of error messages or messages that cannot be delivered, handling requests from members who have not learned how to use the automated functions of the list or who for other reasons are unable to carry them out, and for handling any disputes that degenerate into "flame wars." A flame war is a series of flames, or ill-considered, knee-jerk expressions of anger that are insulting.

When one subscribes to a list, one receives all messages that other members send to the list. A reply to a list message is automatically sent to the list, not the individual who sent the message to the list. Subscriptions are free, but thoughtful list members assume responsibilities that make the life of the owner easier.

Mailing lists have found many uses. They enable nurses from the entire world to communicate. On lists, students as well as graduate nurses can and do get into discussions with faculty, deans, and other nursing leaders. Ideas are explored, and individuals find solutions to situations and new ideas for approaching a situation. Many teachers open a mailing list for their class to enable students to ask and answer questions of the teacher and their classmates. They are also being used as support groups for people with chronic illnesses, such as asthma or cancer. Some organizations now use them to keep their members informed.

List Fundamentals   Mailing lists have two addresses. One is the address of the software that manages the list. This address is used to subscribe to the list, unsubscribe, or use some of the functions that the software makes available such as getting a list of other subscribers. The functions that are available vary with the software that manages the list. Once one is subscribed, a message is sent by the software that contains information about the functions that are available and how to use them. It is necessary to keep this message so that it can be referred to when needed. It can be filed along with other messages that one wants to keep.

The second address for a mailing list is the one that subscribers use to post a message to the mailing list. That is the only purpose that this address has, although it is the address that subscribers use the most frequently. Sending a message to be posted on the list is done the same way as sending a message to an individual. Most users "lurk," or just read list messages for a few days or weeks, to gain a feel for the list, before posting a message.

Finding a List   Several WWW sites maintain lists of mailing lists. Mailing lists increase so rapidly that it is a constant job to keep such a list updated. Rod Ward in the UK maintains a list of health-related mailing lists at *http://www.shef.ac.uk/~nhcon/nulist.htm* along with simple instructions for subscribing to each.

List Etiquette   List etiquette follows that for E-mail, with some added features that are a reflection of the nature of lists. Any messages that are posted to a list will be read by all members of the list. This number can run from ten to thousands. Thus, one will not want to use the reply function to send a personal message to a message received via the list. Instead, initiate a new mes-

sage using the private E-mail address of the poster, which is found on the "From line."

When sending a message, use descriptive subjects; not all list members are interested in everything on the list, and on a busy list members often choose what to read based on the subject. If you are initiating a new subject, do not use the reply function, because it will pick up the original subject and be misinterpreted; instead use a new message.

Avoid sending file attachments; not only cannot everyone read them, but they are a source of viruses, and many people discard them. Because members subscribe using a great variety of computers, messages should only be sent in text format. The default in some E-mail programs is to send hypertext messages; turn this off in the mail section of preferences.

If you will be unable to read your E-mail messages for a while, either unsubscribe from a list or, if the mailing list software permits this, set your mail to "nomail." If your E-mail supports the ability to generate an automatic reply stating when you will be gone and when you will return, do not use it when you have a subscription to a list. The message that it generates will create a loop in which messages bounce back and forth, creating hundreds of messages that fill subscribers' mailboxes and causing problems for other subscribers as well as the list owner.

These items are common sense when one considers how mailing lists and E-mail work. The most important item is a "Do." Do share your information and knowledge, and do ask questions. A good list has member participation. A mailing list is one venue where you can speak out and everyone will listen.

Usenet News and On-line Forums

There are two other types of discussion groups on the Internet: newsgroups and on-line forums. Newsgroups are sort of a worldwide bulletin board system that is accessed using software called a newsreader. Most WWW browsers contain a newsreader that tracks the messages that you have read and can be set up to allow you to easily access new messages. It also allows you to post a message to the group. There are newsgroups on almost every topic. They were originally organized hierarchically under seven main headings, but with the explosion of the Internet there are now more upper level headings.

On-line forums are often organized by organizations to allow members, or anyone, depending on how the forum is organized, to share ideas. They often require that a user register and either create or be given a password, which is used to access the site. Forums were originally accessed by Telnet, but today they are usually accessed through a Web site.

Messages on both forums and newsgroups as well as the archives for mailing lists are organized by the subject entered by the poster. This same subject is also automatically assigned from the subject line when a reply to a subject is made. This type of organization is called threading, and it allows users to select the topics for which they will read messages and to read all of the messages on a given topic in the order they were received or from latest to earliest. Etiquette for both these groups is similar to that for a mailing list except that one does not need to be concerned with items that pertain to E-mail.

Telnet

Telnet was mentioned earlier as one of the protocols used on the Internet. It is a terminal emulation protocol that is part of the TCP/IP protocols. Telnet allows a connecting computer to behave like a terminal for a distant computer regardless of the type of computer that is either the target or originator of the Telnet session. Once connected using Telnet, the user is able to perform any functions that he or she would be able to if she or he were sitting in front of a terminal directly connected to the target computer no matter how separated in distance the two computers may be. Although not as common as it was a few years ago, some ISPs use Telnet behind the scenes to connect their subscribers to proprietary forums or the Internet (Sparks, 1996). There are, however, still some Internet features that can only be accessed using telnet such as MOOs and MUDs. These are programs that let users interact in a text-based virtual environment. They started as Dungeons and Dragons-type gaming programs and have found a use in education (Thede, 1999).

File Transfer Protocol

The File Transfer Protocol (FTP) was mentioned above as the method used by early Intranauts (those who people the Internet) to upload to and download files from distant computers. Uploading a file refers to the process of moving a file from the user's computer to a distant computer, generally one that is larger. Downloading a file means to transfer the file from the distant computer to the user's computer. FTP is still in use today, but most use is transparent to the user. When you use the WWW to download software to your computer, the browser is giving commands to an FTP program behind the scenes.

FTP is also used by individuals when they upload or post files to a WWW site. There are many programs available that make this task easy, unlike in the early 1990s when individuals had to perform these tasks by entering commands and setting the scene for the transfer of the type of file.

World Wide Web

Today it is impossible to discuss the Internet without mentioning the WWW. To many the WWW has come to symbolize the Internet, despite the fact that it is only one part of the Internet. However, except for E-mail, today most people interact on the Internet using a WWW browser. A browser is a client program that translates WWW files to the image you see on the screen. Before the browser interprets it, a WWW file is text that contains what are called tags that tell the browser how to display the file. Figure 7.2 shows the text that a browser receives, and Fig. 7.3 shows how the browser uses the tags to display the information. In Fig. 7.2, the text enclosed between the less than sign ($<$) and greater than sign ($>$) are the tags. These tags and many others comprise hypertext markup language (HTML), which is used to format documents for the Web. There are several choices in browsers, but the most common today are Netscape and Internet Explorer.

Where Did the World Wide Web Come from?   To many it may seem as if the WWW suddenly appeared in the last half of the 1990s. Like most things on the Internet, its history is very short. It was first proposed in 1989 by Tim Berners-Lee at CERN (Conseil Européene pour la Recherche Nucléaire, or the European Particle Physics Laboratory) in Geneva, Switzerland as a means to make it easier to share resources over distances. The first prototype appeared in 1990 with a subsequent release in 1991. It was, however, 1992 before the first browser was released to the public as freeware (Cailliau, 1995). By the end of 1995, there had been improvements in browsers, and there were 73,500 Web servers all over the world. Today, Web servers number in the millions. The speed with which the WWW has gone from a proposal to full acceptance is indicative of the speed of change that the Internet is creating in society.

What Makes the World Wide Web Function? Like Gopher, the Web is built on the client/server model common to most networks. The client software is the browser making any computer with this software a client.

```
<HTML>
<HEAD>
<TITLE>Mailing Lists</TITLE>
</HEAD>
<BODY TEXT="#000000" BGCOLOR="#FFFFC0" LINK="#0000FF" VLINK="#800080"
ALINK="#FF00FF">
<P>After confirming your subscription you will receive information about the list. KEEP
THIS INFORMATION. It gives useful items such as the address to use to post to the list,
how to unsubscribe from the list and other functions that the software provides such as setting
your mail to nomail when you will temporarily be unable to read your mail, and where the
archives for the list are located.</P>
<CENTER><A  HREF="INFO.htm">Return to the main INFO page</A></CENTER>
</BODY>
</HTML>
```

Figure 7.2
A WWW file before interpretation.

A computer that functions as a server has special software that allows it to receive, interpret, and send to the client computer the requested file. The Web uses the HTTP (HyperText Transmission Protocol) protocol that enables the transmitting and interpretation of all types of files, not just text.

What Is a URL?   The address for a specific document on the Web is called a universal resource locator (URL). URLs are very similar to E-mail addresses except there is no @ in them and they contain names of directories (division of a storage disk that is called a folder in PC graphical operating systems) where the specific document is located and often the file name. They all start with "http." Following that, you will see a colon (:) and two forward slashes (//). Sometimes the next entry is "www," and sometimes the name of the computer follows. Fig. 7.4 shows an imaginary URL with the parts labeled.

What Makes the World Wide Web Valuable?   Having access to the WWW is like having a library in your computer. This library, however, is worldwide. It is as

After confirming your subscription you will receive information about the list. KEEP THIS INFORMATION. It gives useful items such as the address to use to post to the list, how to unsubscribe from the list and other functions that the software provides such as setting your mail to nomail when you will temporarily be unable to read your mail, and where the archives for the list are located.

Return to the main INFO page

Figure 7.3
The WWW file from Figure 7.2 as interpreted by a browser.

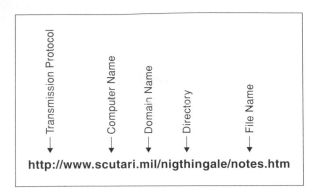

Figure 7.4
Anatomy of a URL.

easy to access information on a computer in Hong Kong as on one across the street. One can also access a library catalog from a library anywhere in the world as well as do a bibliographic search. Another Web feature is on-line journals, including several for nursing, most of which are free. Additionally, many print journals have an on-line presence that varies from just the table of contents to abstracts to the full text of some articles.

Continuing education (CE) is also available on the Web. On-line CE offers many benefits including no travel, lodging, or meal costs as well as the ability to complete the offering on your own timetable (Plank, 1998). Many CE sites provide the ability to print the course certificate as soon as you successfully complete the course and pay the fee.

There are excellent tutorials available on-line, not only for using the various features of the Internet, but also for nursing. Easy access is also provided to information about National Institute of Health (NIH) grants. One can find information about specific hospitals, products that one wishes to buy, the weather for any place in the world, and generally any topic that one wishes to know more about.

Searching the Web   Finding this information, however, is not always easy. The Web is still vastly unorganized. Unlike a print-based library, where one can locate information in the card catalog, the Web is not catalogued. Given the wide breadth of types of available information, this is not surprising. There are browser programs that will search the Web to help you find information. They do not all search the same way. Basically, there are three different types: directories, search engines, and metasearchers.

Directories, or catalogs as they may be called, only search those sites that they have approved. Yahoo and Magellan are directories. Programs that are basic search engines, such as Alta Vista, Excite, or Infoseek, create a data set of sites by searching the Web and bringing back information. How they search and what they bring back varies from engine to engine. Some look at titles and the first few lines of text, while others look at metastatements. A metastatement is text inserted into the source document by the author that is not placed on the screen by the browser and contains some key words about the document. The third category, metasearchers, search more than one site, eliminate most of the duplicates, and return the results to you. MetaCrawler and Inference Find are metasearchers.

Deciding which type of search service to use should depend on the topic. If you are searching for a topic on which there is a lot of information, a directory searcher will find relevant information and avoid much of the clutter that sometimes shows up with other search services. On the other hand, if you are searching for something that is relatively uncommon, a metasearcher will be the place to start. Sometimes you need to use all three. A site, maintained by the Nueva Library that can help you select an appropriate search engine is located at *http:// nuevaschool.org/~debbie/library/research/adviceengine.html*. There are also specialized search services that will assist you in locating such things as E-mail addresses, regular and Web addresses for businesses, and even a map and driving directions from one location to another. The search engines also differ in how they request input to narrow or expand searches. For the best results, tailor your search request using the help that each search service provides.

A site worth mentioning is the Study Web (*http:// www.studyweb.com/*). This site is in the directory category. The listings, while of a very high quality, are fairly limited. It would be a good place to start looking for a topic that is fairly common, such as obesity. Its limited offerings and lack of ability to search the entire site are made up for by the quality of the links as well as the information provided about each link.

Evaluating Information from the Web   The fact that anyone can and does publish on the Web and that many search engines are not discriminatory in the selections in their databases gives rise to a need to carefully evaluate information that one finds on the Internet. Of particular concern to nurses is health care information. Attempts are being made to rate various sites, but this presents many other questions, such as who is doing the rating and what changes, if any, occurred after the rating was done.

There are several excellent sites on the Web that discuss evaluation of Web information including one with checklists for many different types of sites. Efforts are currently under way by three organizations—Mitretek Systems and the Health Information Technology Institute (HITI) (both nonprofit organizations) and the Agency for Healthcare Research and Quality (AHRQ), formerly Agency for Health Care Policy and Research (AHCPR)— to assess the quality of health information on the WWW. Mitreteck's white paper, which they hope will promote discussion of the topic, puts forth seven areas that they feel are important. (1) The first item, credibility, asks the user to consider the source of the document, its context, currency, relevance, and the editorial review process (Ambre et al. 1997). (2) Regarding content, the next item, they believe one needs to consider the accuracy, hierarchy of evidence, whether original sources are stated, any disclaimers on the information, and if there are any omissions. (3) Disclosure, the third item, would have the user consider the purpose of the site, who is sponsoring it, and what the site owners will do with any information that they collect. (4) These groups next consider links and suggest that the user consider the quality of the links provided. (5) They are also concerned with how easy the site is to navigate and what types of interactivity such as feedback or chat rooms are provided. (6) These groups would also have a user be very careful about sharing personal information with a Web site and to carefully evaluate the sponsoring organization instead of relying on a name, which can be crafted to appear very prestigious. (7) They also suggest that the user be skeptical of the use of expressions such as of "amazing results," "earthshaking breakthroughs," or "miracles."

Real-Time Communication

In addition to access to information, the Internet can be used for real-time communication, or two-way communications that are occurring at the same time. This is known as synchronous communication. One of the more interesting of these technologies is CU-SeeMe, which allows users to participate in visual communication across the net. Due to the large amount of data that must be transmitted and the current state of Internet connections, this technology is still in its infancy. Instead of the usual 30 frames per minute, most transmissions only allow for 4 to 10 and occasionally 15 frames a minute, producing movement that appears very spastic. Additionally, there is often a lag between any audio and the visual. Expect, however, to see improvements in this technology.

 ## How Does One Use the Internet? (Getting Aboard)

Using the Internet requires a computer, a modem, communications software, and an Internet service provider (ISP).

Hardware and Software

Any computer into which a modem can be installed can be used to communicate with the Internet. If, however, one wishes to use a graphical browser on the WWW, a computer capable of graphics such as a Windows or Macintosh computer is necessary. A modem is a device that translates computer output, which is digital, to an output that can be transmitted using the telephone lines' analog signal and then back to a digital signal for the receiving computer. The price varies with the speed; a 56 kilobits per second (Kbps) modem, which translates data much faster than a 28.8 Kbps modem, is also more expensive. Some people now use cable modems, modems that use the television cable into a house. These modems transmit information that is downloaded very rapidly, but they upload information at the same speed as regular modems.

Most institutions connect to the Internet with high speed lines such as ISDN (integrated services digital network) that can transmit knowledge at speeds from 64 to 128 Kbps or T1 lines, which are capable of simultaneously carrying 24 channels of information at 64 Kbps (Thede, 1999). The ultimate connection is fiber-optic cable, which today transmits information at about 2 gigabytes per second, although technically it is capable of speeds up to 250 gigabytes per second.

Internet Service Provider

ISPs are companies that provide access to the Internet for a monthly fee. They provide users with a software package, a user name, password, and access phone number. Many also make available from one to five megabytes of space on their server for users to post Web pages. ISPs can also be called Internet access providers (IAPs).

Finding an ISP   Most people today are aware of the large ISPs such as America Online and Microsoft Network, but there are many others. These large ISPs provide Internet access and many proprietary features such as chat rooms and games. Some, however, will not give direct access to a site in a URL without first connecting you to their version of the type of feature that URL represents. Also, they have many subscribers, and many find it difficult to get on-line in the evenings and weekends.

They do, however, provide access from much of the world and may be the ISP of choice for those who access the Web from multiple points.

Evaluating an ISP   There are also many lesser known ISPs that often provide more flexibility in use as well as protection from "spam," or unsolicited E-mail that is sent from a phony address. Additionally, technical help is usually easily available via phone. Smaller ISPs often do not present the access problems that one can run into with the more well-known ISPs.

The yellow pages now have a separate listing for ISPs, but an excellent place to start is often the Web, if you can gain access. The List, at *http://thelist.internet. com/*, offers a chance to search for an ISP by area code, while Dawn McGatney's site at *http://dogwolf.seagull. net* offers user reviews of many ISPs.

There are several questions that you should ask of a potential ISP. Find out how many subscribers they have per modem; the more in excess of 20 the more busy signals you will get. Also ask what type of connection they have to the Internet. These can vary from a simple 56 Kbps to fiber-optic cable, all of which will affect the speed at which you can use the Internet. Getting a recommendation from someone who has used an ISP for over 6 months and is very satisfied is probably the best way to determine if the ISP is good.

How Does One Contribute to the Internet? (Creating Web Pages)

Creating a Web page is not difficult. All of the major office suites (Corel's Office Perfect, Microsoft's Office, and Lotus's Smart Suite) provide the ability to publish documents and graphics to the Web, although the result is generally not polished. They do, however, make the information readable on the Web. Most of these products even provide the ability to insert links in the document.

Although using a word processor may be a good way to start a page, most people will want to modify the resulting HTML tags a little to get a desired effect. When one first looks at a document with the HTML tags such as the one in Fig. 7.2, she or he may think that this is very difficult. It is not. Basic HTML can be learned in about 3 hours. A search with any search engine for "HTML tutor" will yield a multitude of very good sites that will help one learn HTML. There are also excellent HTML editors available, some of which are WYSIWIG; that is, you make your changes on the actual page just as you would to a word processing document, and the program automatically creates the code. These programs often provide some site management tools also. Examples are

Adobe's Page Mill, Macromedia's Dreamweaver, and Microsoft's Front Page. Several of these allow a free 15- to 30-day trial period.

Home Page

A home page is the main page of a Web site. Generally, it serves as an index or table of contents to either other documents at that site or other sites. Some individuals have home pages for biographical information, or they may provide a list of links for a topic about which they are very interested. Whenever you see a URL with a tilde (~) in it, you are usually looking at the URL for an individual's home page.

Home Page Design

Like all computer projects, the amount of time that one spends in planning a home page and any connected documents greatly reduces the amount of time that the construction takes. Saba (1996) mentions seven things that should be considered when building a home page: purpose, scope, structure, enhancements, links, forms, and maintenance.

Purpose and Scope   A Web site needs to have a focus. Decide what your purpose for creating the site is. If it's personal, is it to provide information about yourself, or about your interests? If for an organization, is the purpose to provide information for the group members or to showcase the organization? These decisions will determine what is on your page and how you organize it. One of the most difficult things about designing a web page, especially if it is a site for a group, can be obtaining the necessary information. Some printed material that organizations want posted are copyrighted; be sure to clear up any copyright issues before posting information on a page.

Structure and Enhancements   How you place items on a page and the types of enhancements you use determine the usability of your page. Planning for the structure should start with your audience. Organize information in a logical way for them, not you. Look at other home pages and analyze how the ones that you find easiest to use are set up. Talk with some members of your potential audience to get their opinions. Be consistent in design throughout the entire site. If you place a link to return to the home page at the bottom on one linked document, be sure that this placement is followed for all of the pages (Saba, 1996). Using paper to sketch the pages first will make this phase easier.

Be consistent in how you use color and fonts. The objective is to give the user a feel for the page so that she or he can pay attention to the content, not try to determine how to proceed. Remember that using too many colors or fonts can be distracting. Use colors for the text that contrast with the background color. If you use "wallpaper," or a design for the background, be sure that it does not detract from the readability of the information.

Many sites choose to use graphics, or images, to enhance the site. Although they can add immeasurably to the looks of a site, they also increase download time. If the majority of your audience will be accessing your site from a home computer, give careful consideration to the size of the graphics; a long download time will decrease use. Also include alternative text for a graphic picture. This permits those who are accessing the site with a text browser or who have turned off their graphics display to decrease download time to know what the graphic is that they are not seeing. Copyright is also a consideration when using graphics. Before you use art on a site, be sure you know the copyright status. This holds true whether the clip art is from a software package or from the Web.

Some sites now use frames, or two or more files that appear in different places on the screen. If you use these, you may need to provide an alternate site for users who are using browsers that do not have frame capability. When using frames, if you include links to a site outside your site, be sure to include code to open this site in another window.

Links, Forms, and Maintenance   Links either within a site or to other sites are a hallmark of the Web. If you link to outside sites, they should relate to the purpose of the site. Providing a brief description of what a user can expect to find at a site prevents unpleasant surprises. Whether the links are internal or external they should be checked before posting and periodically after posting. Most of the HTML editors provide a way to check the links.

If the site is for an organization, you may wish to include a form to request more information which users can download and mail, fax, or E-mail to the organization (Saba, 1996). It is also possible to design a form that users can use to enter information on-line, but this will require additional programming and the appropriate programs on the server. The use of the "mailto:" tag, which turns into a preaddressed E-mail message when the user clicks it, is another way to request information.

Many sites are started with a great deal of excitement and then left to fend for themselves, a result readily apparent to users. Plans for a site also need to include plans for who will update the site and when. If provisions are made for a user to request information, it is imperative that requests are answered promptly.

Summary

Changing the mode of communication has always produced social change (Fulton, 1999). The Internet has, and is, a huge change in communication, rivaling that of the printing press, but happening on a much faster and broader scale. What changes the Internet will produce in today's society can at this point only be predictions, but some changes are already appearing. From the preceding you can see that the Internet has made it easy for anyone to communicate with anyone, regardless of social standing, class, or culture. This has resulted in the leveling of many organizations. The Internet has also been shown to make knowledge formerly available to only those in a profession freely available to all, a fact that we see with many patients. It also makes it possible for citizens of the world to be able to bypass traditional broadcast and print media and obtain information they want from other sources, a factor that makes geographical boundaries seem contrived.

The sheer amount of available information creates a situation in which it is practically physically impossible to absorb it (VanCuilenburg, 1987). Not many years ago, we talked about computer literacy; now the theme has shifted to information literacy. Nurses, like all citizens, need to learn how to select, evaluate, and use the information they find (VanCuilenburg, 1987). The computer and the Internet are merely tools that allow us to find this information; what we use and how we use it are functions that we as thinking beings will need to consider.

References

Ambre, J., Guard, R., Perveiler, F. M., et al. (1997). White paper: Criteria for assessing the quality of health information on the Internet. *http://hitiweb.mitretek.org/docs/criteria.html*

Atkins, L. (1998). Big brother is watching—and reading your email. *Cleveland Plain Dealer*, January 21, 11B.

Bowers, L. (1997). Constructing international professional identity: What psychiatric nurses talk about on the Internet. *International Journal of Nursing Studies*, 34(3), 208–212.

Cailliau, R. and VanCuilenburg, J. J. (1995). *A Short History of the Web*. Paper presented at the European branch of the W3 Consortium on Nov 2, 1995. *http://www.inria.fr/Actualites/Cailliau-fra.html*

Carpenter, B. (1996). What does the IAB do, anyway? *http://www.iab.org/iab/connexions.html*

Fulton, B. (1999). The information age: New dimensions for U.S. foreign policy. In *Great Decisions*, 1999 Edition. Hanover, NH: Dartmouth Printing Company.

Grush, M. (1998). Raising the bar for Networking in Education: The next generation Internet. *Syllabus*

Magazine, 12(4). *http://www.syllabus.com/nov98_magfea2.html*

Hudson, D. (1996) Rewired. *Journal of a Strained Net.* *http://www.internetvalley.com/intvalold.html*

Leiner, B. M., Cerf, V. G., Clark, D. D., et al. (1998). A brief history of the Internet. *http://www.isoc.org/brief.htm*

MacPherson, K. I. (1997). Menopause on the Internet: Building knowledge and community on-line. *Advanced Nursing Science, 20*(1), 66–78.

PC Webopaedia. (1996). *http://www.pcwebopaedia.com/*

Internet2 and the NGI: Complementary and Interdependent. (1999). *http://www.internet2.edu/html/internet2-ngi.html*

Plank, R. K. (1998). Nursing on-line for continuing education credit. *The Journal of Continuing Education in Nursing, 29*(4), 165–172.

Quiggle, A. (1999). Personal communication.

Saba, V. (1996). Developing a home page for the World Wide Web. *American Journal of Infection Control, 24*(6), 468–470.

Sparks, S. (1996).Use of the Internet for infection control and epidemiology. *American Journal of Infection Control, 24*(6), 435–439.

Sterling, B.(1993). History of the Internet. *The Magazine of Fantasy and Science Fiction.* *http://www.eff.org/pub/Net_culture/Cyberpunk/Bruce_Sterling/FSF_columns/fsf.05*

Thede, L. Q. (1999). *Computers in Nursing: Bridges to the Future.* Philadelphia: Lippincott-Williams & Wilkins.

VanCuilenburg, J. J. (1987). The Information Society: Some trends and implications. *European Journal of Communication, 2*, 105–121.

■ Selected Readings

Anthony, D. (1998). Web worries . . . a major concern is over security and provision of relevant high quality information. *Nursing Standard, 12*(43), 28.

Anthony, D. (1996). *Health on the Internet.* Cambridge, MA: Blackwell Science.

Bachman, J. A., and Panzarine, S. (1998). Enabling student nurses to use the information superhighway. *Journal of Nursing Education, 37*(4), 155–161.

Bowers, L. (1997). Constructing international professional identity: What psychiatric nurses talk about on the Internet. *International Journal of Nursing Studies, 34*(3), 208–212.

Brown, L. P., Bair, A. H., Meier, P. P., et al. (1998). Connecting points. Accessing on-line information at the National Institutes of Health: Highlights and practical tips. *Computers in Nursing, 16*(4), 198–201.

Clark, D. J. (1998). Course redesign: Incorporating an Internet web site into an existing nursing class. *Computers in Nursing, 16*(4), 219–22.

Coiera, E. (1997). *Guide to Medical Informatics, the Internet and Telemedicine.* New York: Chapman & Hall.

Conrad, S. A., and Rensink, Y. (1997). Using intranet technology in the ICU. *Nursing Management, 28*(7), 34–36.

Davis, J. (Ed.) et al. (1998). *Health & Medicine on the Internet* (Professional Edition). New York: Chapman & Hall.

Davison, D., and Rhodes, D. (1996). The virtual university. *Nursing Standard, 10*(27), 21–22.

DuBois, K., and Rizzolo, M. A. (1994). Cruising the "information superhighway." *American Journal of Nursing, 94*(12), 58–60.

Edwards, M. J. A. (1995). *The Internet for Nurses and Allied Health Professionals.* New York: Springer.

Fawcett, J., and Buhle, E. L., Jr. (1995). Using the Internet for data collection. An innovative electronic strategy. *Computers in Nursing, 13*(6), 273–279.

Fleitas, J. (1998). Computer monitor. Spinning tales from the World Wide Web: Qualitative research in an electronic environment. *Qualitative Health Research, 8*(2), 283–292.

Frandsen, J. L. (1997). The use of computers in cancer pain management. *Seminars in Oncology Nursing, 13*(1), 49–56.

Gee, P. M. (1997). The Internet—a home care nursing clinical resource: Part 1. *Home Healthcare Nurse, 15*(2), 115–21.

Gibbs, M. A. (Ed.). (1997). *Mosby's Medical Surfari: A Guide to Exploring the Internet and Discovering Top Health Care Resources.* St. Louis, MO: Mosby.

Guard, J. R., Morris, T. A., Schick, L., et al. (1997). A community approach to serving health information needs: NetWellness. *Health Care on the Internet, 1*(1), 73–82.

Hamff, C. L., and Glaser, J. P. (1997). Internet policy and procedures for health care organizations: The approach of Partners Healthcare System, Inc. *Topics in Health Information Management, 17*(4), 40–61.

Henry, N. I. (1997). Getting acquainted with support and self-help groups on the Internet. *Health Care on the Internet, 1*(2), 27–32.

Jenkins, J., and Erdman K. (1998). Web-based documentation systems. *Home Health Care Management & Practice, 10*(2), 52–61.

Kirkpatrick, M. K., Brown, S., and Atkins, T. (1998). Electronic education. Using the Internet to integrate cultural diversity and global awareness. *Nurse Educator, 23*(2), 15–17.

Klemm, P., and Nolan, M. T. (1998). Internet cancer support groups: Legal and ethical issues for nurse researchers. *Oncology Nursing Forum, 25*(4), 673–676.

Klemm, P., Reppert, K., and Visich, L. (1998). A nontraditional cancer support group: The Internet. *Computers in Nursing, 16*(1), 31–6.

Kolesar, M. S. (1997). Realizing the competitive advantage of the Internet. *Caring, 16*(12), 56, 58, 60.

Lakeman, R. (1997). Using the Internet for data collection in nursing research. Presented as a paper at a qualitative research conference for health researchers held at the Eastern Institute of Technology, Taradale, New Zealand, January 1997. *Computers in Nursing, 15*(5), 269–75.

Laws, J. (1998). Computer applications: Safety & health on the Internet. *Occupational Health & Safety, 67*(4), 25.

Lewis, A. (1998). Information technology in the next millennium: Five trends reshape home care's future. *Remington Report, 6*(2), 4–6.

Lybecker, C. J. (1998). Professionally speaking. Surfing the Net. *American Journal of Maternal Child Nursing, 23*(1), 17–21.

MacPherson, K. I. (1997). Menopause on the Internet: Building knowledge and community on-line. *Advances in Nursing Science, 20*(1), 66–78.

Mangan, P. (1998). Site perfect. *Nursing Standard, 12*(39), 22–25.

McKenzie, B. C. (1997). *Medicine and the Internet: Introducing Online Resources and Terminology.* New York: Oxford University Press.

Morris, D. A., Guard, J. R., Marine, S. A., et al. (1997). Approaching equity in consumer health information delivery: NetWellness. *Journal of the American Medical Informatics Association, 4*(1), 6–13.

Murray, P. J. (1996). Nurses' computer-mediated communications on NURSENET: A case study. *Computers in Nursing, 14*(4), 227–234.

Neray, P. (1997). End paper. Security on the Internet: Is your system vulnerable? *Nursing Management, 28*(7), 64.

Nicoll, L. H. (1994). An introduction to the Internet: History, structure, and access. Part 2. *Journal of Nursing Administration, 24*(5), 11–13.

Nicoll, L. H. (1994). An introduction to the Internet: History, structure, and access. Part 1. *Journal of Nursing Administration, 24*(3), 9–11.

Nicoll, L. H. (1998). *Computers in Nursing's Nurses Guide to the Internet.* Philadelphia: Lippincott-Williams & Wilkins.

O'Carroll, D., and McMahon, A. S. (1998). Research & development co-ordinating centre. *Nursing Standard, 12*(38), 32–33.

Payne, W. (1996). Medical consultation on the Internet. *British Journal of Healthcare Computing & Information Management , 13*(10), 30–32.

Plank, R. K. (1998). Nursing on-line for continuing education credit. *Journal of Continuing Education in Nursing, 29*(4), 165–172.

Pomeroy, B. (Ed.). (1997). *A Beginner's Guide to the Internet and the World Wide Web.* San Diego: Harcourt Brace Professional Publishing.

Puetz, B. E. (1997). Resume writing in a wired age. *RN, 60*(2), 28–31.

Ryan, J. M., and Southern, J. (1998). Soapbox. A&E nursing and the Internet. *Accident & Emergency Nursing, 6*(2), 106–109.

Schell, C. L., and Rathe, R. (1996). Geri Ann: Designing educational programs for the Internet. *Gerontology & Geriatrics Education, 16*(4), 15–25.

Simpson, R. L. (1996). Technology: Nursing the system. Will the Internet supplant community health networks?. *Nursing Management, 27*(2), 20; 23.

Simpson, R. L. (1997). Technology: Nursing the system. Internet security concerns. *Nursing Management, 28*(12), 24–25, 27.

Sinclair, M. (1997). Education: Midwives, midwifery and the Internet. *Modern Midwife, 7*(9), 11–14.

Skiba, D. J. (1997). Intellectual property issues in the digital health care world. *Nursing Administration Quarterly, 21*(3), 11–20.

Sparks, S. M. (1996). Using the Internet for urology nursing. *Urologic Nursing, 16*(4), 131–134.

Sparks, S. M. (1997). Using the Internet for nursing administration. *Journal of Nursing Administration, 27*(3), 15–20.

Taira, F. (1993). Driving down the electronic highway . . . the Internet. *Computers in Nursing, 11*(5), 219–221.

Thorwaldson, J. (1997). "PAN Islands" experiment may be an answer to problem of Internet-access "have-nots." *Health Care on the Internet, 1*(1), 35–41.

Thede, L. Q. The Internet unraveled. *Orthopaedic Nursing.*

Tomaiuolo, N. G. (1995). Accessing nursing resources on the Internet. *Computers in Nursing, 13*(4), 159–64.

Walker, G. D., and Burnham, L. D. (1997). Putting the Web to work. *Caring, 16*(12), 52–54.

Ward, R., and Haines, M. (1998). Don't get left behind—get on-line. *Practice Nurse, 16*(3), 164–166.

Ward, R. (1997). Network. Implications of computer networking and the Internet for nurse education. *Nurse Education Today, 17*(3), 178–183.

Wink, D. M. (1996). Electronic education. An introduction to nursing on the Internet: Part two. *Nurse Educator, 21*(1), 8–12.

Wink, D. M. (1995). Electronic education. An introduction to nursing on the Internet. Part one. *Nurse Educator, 20*(6), 9–13.

Wootton, J. C. (1997). The quality of information on women's health on the Internet. *Journal of Women's Health, 6*(5), 575–581.

PART 3

Issues in Informatics

8

Nursing Informatics and Health Care Policy

Carole A. Gassert

OBJECTIVES

1. Consider the policy implications of nursing informatics as a specialty within the health care environment.
2. Identify the impact of national initiatives that focus on information and information technologies on nursing informatics practice.
3. Discuss the national nursing informatics agenda.

KEY WORDS

information systems
social sciences
public policy
health policy

The professional workforce of the new millennium continues to experience significant changes in health care. To practice effectively in this environment, informatics professionals need to be aware of existing and proposed health care policy. Policy is defined as a course of action that guides present and future decisions. It is based on given conditions and selected from among identified alternatives (Webster, 1985). Health care policy is established on local, state, and national levels to guide the implementation of solutions for the population's health needs. Both existing conditions and emerging trends in the health care industry influence policy decisions. Because these decisions have a significant impact on health care, policy makers need data to guide their thinking.

If decisions are to be data-driven, policy makers must be able to access appropriate, complete, and accurate data about the status of health care. Interestingly, most existing information systems (IS) are not able to collect data adequately from multiple sources, track patient outcomes across a continuum of care, and aggregate data as needed to guide policy decisions (Amatayakul, 1998). The need for continued improvement of IS is echoed by most health policy-setting organizations. For example, the President's Advisory Commission on Consumer Protection and Quality in the Health Care Industry states that to build the capacity to improve the quality of health care, there must

be significant investment in health information systems (President's Advisory Commission on Consumer Protection and Quality in the Health Care Industry, 1998).

Not only is there a need for more adequate IS, there is a need to prepare health care providers, including nurses, to use information technology to collect and manage data needed for providing care and making policy decisions (National Advisory Council on Nurse Education and Practice, 1997; Pew Health Professions Commission, 1998; American Nurses Association, 1994). Preparing nurses to be computer-literate, i.e., to use computers, is not enough. Nurses need to understand the thought processes, language, and decision-making that goes into the data being collected and manipulated by the computer (Thompson, 1997). A cadre of informatics nurses with an even higher level of understanding of information, information management, and computers is needed to ensure appropriate data are available as needed for health policy decisions.

Nursing informatics professionals need to become more cognizant of health care policies that will affect their practice. In this chapter, nursing informatics and its role as a specialty within a changing health care system will be examined. Second, pertinent national health policy and its impact on the role of informatics will be discussed. And finally, the national nursing informatics agenda will be presented.

Nursing Informatics and Health Care

Nurses have contributed to the purchase, design, and implementation of information systems since the 1970s. It has only been since 1992 that informatics roles have been recognized as a specialty practice for nurses by the American Nurses Association (Milholland, 1992). To be acknowledged as a specialty within nursing, informatics has had to demonstrate a differentiated practice base, identify the existence of educational programs in the field, show support from nationally recognized organizations, and develop a research agenda (Panniers and Gassert, 1995). The term nursing informatics (NI) first appeared in the literature in 1984 and has evolved as the field of nursing informatics has matured (Ball and Hannah, 1984; Hannah, 1985; Grobe, 1988). In a classic article that describes its domain, NI is defined as the combination of nursing, information, and computer sciences to manage and process nursing data into information and knowledge for use in nursing practice (Graves and Corcoran, 1989).

The domain of NI is focused on data and its structures, information management, and the technology, including databases, needed to manage information effectively. Yet it also includes significant use of theory from linguistics, human-machine interface, decision science, cognitive science, communication, engineering, library science, and organizational dynamics. Because the knowledge base is so extensive, informatics nurses tend to develop expertise in one aspect of the domain. For example, informatics nurses working in acute care settings might focus on system selection and implementation, while informatics nurses employed in the research arm of vendor corporations develop expertise in data structures and databases.

What is common among informatics nurses is that they have strong clinical backgrounds but cease to deliver care directly to patients. They refocus their career on the informatics domain of interest to provide indirect health care services. As technology becomes ubiquitous in health care, this differentiation of practice is extremely important. Nurses will increasingly use information technologies as tools to deliver clinical services. And they will need to be trained to use the tools effectively with patients. But the profession has to be careful that it does not declare a unique clinical specialty has emerged just because providers are using a particular type of information technology to deliver clinical services. An example is the current effort of some nurses to declare telehealth nursing as a specialty. In this example, nurses are using telecommunication tools to deliver clinical services from a location that is distant from the patient. The nurses focus on the clinical care they are providing; the technology is simply a tool they use to provide clinical services. Informatics nurses should accept responsibility for developing and implementing technology tools and for evaluating the effectiveness of the technological tools being used by the clinical nurses.

Differentiated and Interdisciplinary Practice

A description of NI as a differentiated practice has been established through the activities of defining the scope of practice (American Nurses Association, 1994), writing standards (American Nurses Association, 1995), and developing a testing mechanism for certification as a generalist in informatics (American Nurses Credentialing Center, 1999). As the scope of practice document emphasizes, NI brings an added dimension to nursing practice that focuses on knowledge and skill in information and information management techniques. Although all nurses must process information, informatics nurses demonstrate specialized knowledge of "identifying, naming, organizing, grouping, collecting processing, analyzing, storing, retrieving, or managing data and information" (American Nurses Association, 1994, p. 3). Added to the knowledge of information management is a sophisticated level of understanding of information technology. This knowledge exceeds the ability to use technology that is expected of all nurses.

The need to differentiate NI practice from other specialties within nursing has often led health informatics disciplines to misinterpret that action and accuse nursing of trying to practice informatics in isolation. NI practice differentiates itself from other areas of nursing practice but emphasizes its interaction with informatics disciplines such as mathematics, statistics, linguistics, engineering, computer science, and health informatics (American Nurses Association, 1994). In fact, NI has been described as one example of a specific domain of informatics that falls under a broader umbrella of health informatics (National Advisory Council on Nurse Education and Practice, 1997). Other examples of domain-specific informatics practices are medical informatics, dental informatics, and consumer informatics.

In its 1998 report, the Pew Commission discusses a need to prepare all health professionals, including nurses, to work in interdisciplinary teams (Pew Health Professions Commission, 1998). The NI community also believes it is essential to practice within an interdisciplinary team. It supports the interdisciplinary philosophy because patient care is increasingly delivered by a team of providers from different professions rather than by individual providers (Bruegel, 1998) and because vocabulary systems need to be linked across health care disciplines to enable meaningful data to be shared for making health policy decisions. The interdisciplinary focus of NI practice was emphasized by two conferences held in 1999. The Spring American Medical Informatics Association (AMIA) conference brought interdisciplinary representatives together to identify core competencies shared by all health informatics professionals. A vocabulary summit brought nursing and medical informatics vocabulary experts together to explore how further language development can facilitate the integration of computerized languages among health care disciplines (Ozbolt, 1998).

Specialty Practice

To become a specialty, it was necessary for NI to show that educational programs are available to prepare nurses to practice in the field. Between 1988 and 1992 the Division of Nursing (DN), Bureau of Health Professions, Health and Human Services Administration (HRSA), funded two Master's programs (Heller et al., 1989; Graves et al., 1995) and one doctoral program in NI (Gassert et al., 1992). The program at the University of Maryland has demonstrated an interdisciplinary approach to education by requiring that students take their information management courses through an information systems department outside of nursing. The University of Utah program also has demonstrated an interdisciplinary approach but has developed courses taught in the school of nursing by faculty from both nursing and medical informatics.

Authorizing legislation passed in 1992 prevented the DN from funding other programs in NI. This action halted the implementation of additional NI specialty programs for several years. Finally, in 1997 a NI specialty program opened at New York University, and in 1998 a fourth specialty program was implemented at Duquesne University in Pittsburgh. The Duquesne program offers NI courses on the Internet. Both of these programs offer a post-Master's certificate in NI and informatics specialty preparation at the graduate level. Additional schools of nursing have developed certificate programs in NI or NI courses as part of graduate preparation in related graduate specialties such as administration (AMIA, 1998). Due to increased interest in informatics in health care and changes in authorizing legislation for the DN, it is anticipated that more schools of nursing will develop NI programs in the next few years. This will help to increase the number of nurses who have advanced skills in informatics.

As the number of graduate programs in NI increases, there will be a larger cadre of informatics nurses eligible for certification. The certification examination currently available through the American Nurses Credentialing Center is for a generalist in NI. Perhaps it is time for the profession to develop a specialist level of certification for nursing informatics.

In her discussion of specialization, Styles included the identification of a research focus as one of the criteria for a specialty (Styles, 1989). NI researchers described seven areas needing scientific study in 1993 (National Center for Nursing Research, 1993). Those needs still exist. Even though the research agenda was defined, except for studies that focus on the development of nursing vocabulary, researchers have found it difficult to obtain funding for informatics projects within nursing. To be successful in obtaining funding, researchers need to tie informatics projects to clinical problems within nursing. NI researchers also need to consider projects that can be examined from a multidisciplinary focus and submit them outside of traditional nursing funding sources for financial support.

A final requirement for a specialty is representation by at least one organization. NI has the support of both nursing and multidisciplinary organizations. Within nursing, there is organizational support within the National League for Nursing, the American Organization of Nurse Executives, and the American Nurses Association. Increasingly, organizations outside of nursing encourage informatics nurses to become actively involved in their organizations to help solve informatics practice issues. Informatics nurses have responded and become active within multidisciplinary organizations. Two examples are the American Medical Informatics Association and the Health Information Management Systems Society; informatics nurses have served as president of both of these organizations. Multidisciplinary organizations work to bring together system designers, developers, managers, users, consultants, and educators from various health informatics disciplines to solve issues of information management. It is helpful for informatics nurses to be involved in multidisciplinary organizations, because their structure mirrors the nature of health care.

Health Care Trends and Nursing Informatics

Six health care trends have been identified that will impact information management and technology (Lorence, 1998) and consequently the roles of informatics nurses. One trend is the move from alphanumeric to multimedia information within IS. Generally, health care information system vendors have been slow to incorporate innovations into their systems. For example, graphical user interfaces have been available for years but have been included only recently in health care information systems. To keep pace with the format of data being produced, IS will need to be more responsive to innovative technologies. IS will soon be expected to include graphics and sound, especially with increased use of telehealth technologies. As systems are designed, built, or purchased in the future, informatics nurses must consider the need to capture multimedia information from distant sites and the need for larger storage capacities, and they must have skills to store or retrieve information from dissimilar storage media.

A second trend is the move to providing health care services in international markets. Regulations for patient documentation and requirements for licensing differ from country to country. To avoid potential legal issues, informatics nurses must become familiar with the rules and regulations governing documentation and licensing in all countries included in health care networks managed in their practice. Issues associated with equipment incompatibilities and transmitting data over long distances will also command informatics nurses' attention.

A third trend of great importance to informatics nurses is the increasing effort to solve the issue of confidentiality of patient and provider information. As information systems are connected over wider geographic areas, it is even more important to ensure that existing data are secured adequately to protect confidentiality. Security policies will be challenged as organizations outside of health care, such as law enforcement agencies or corporations, demand access to sensitive information. In addition, the Health Insurance Portability and Accountability Act of 1996 (HIPAA) requires that legislation or federal regulations concerning security be passed in 2000. Since legislation was not passed, federal standards are being finalized. Organizations must be compliant with these regulations or experience financial consequences. Informatics nurses, therefore, will need to be prepared to implement the regulations. Informatics nurses also can expect more complex encryption systems to be implemented and more detailed security policies to be written.

A fourth trend that is impacting NI is health care consumerism. Breugel refers to this trend as patient empowerment (Bruegel, 1998). Information technologies are considered to be key enablers in patient empowerment. For example, a 1997 report analyzing American consumers' demand for health and medical information on the Internet identified them as a new market segment for using Internet services. At that time health information retrievers accounted for about 37 percent of the Internet traffic. In less than 2 years the Harris Poll reports the

number of Americans seeking health information from the Internet has risen to 68 percent.

As patients have easier access to medical information, through sources such as the Web, TV, and other media, they have a greater ability to participate in their treatment decisions and influence their health status. And as patients become more knowledgeable and refocus their concern on customer service, they will expect providers to know their preferences in health care. Information systems, therefore, will need to be designed to capture data about patient preferences. IS may also be expected to generate reports that will be given to patients as a routine part of their health care encounters. In keeping with patients' expectations for greater access to information, providers will need to establish policies for using E-mail with patients as part of their individual clinical practices. With the increase in consumerism, informatics nurses in collaboration with other health informaticists will need to design IS that place greater emphasis on providing information for patients.

A fifth health care trend that impacts informatics nurses is the need for comparative outcome databases in health care. These databases will provide organizations with tools that are essential for analyzing their performance across time and comparing their achievement against external benchmarks. Agencies such as the Joint Commission for Accrediting Healthcare Organizations (JCAHO) and the National Committee for Quality Assurance are requiring organizations to use performance standards to report clinical outcomes. JCAHO is integrating outcomes and other performance measurement data into the accreditation process through an initiative called ORYX. Criteria are written for assessing candidates' measurement systems in terms of their ability to be integrated into accreditation. The evaluation attributes relate to the following: characteristics of performance measures; system technical capabilities; data quality and measurement accuracy; risk adjustment; performance measure-related feedback; and relevance to the accreditation process. JCAHO does not expect immediate integration of candidates' existing measurement systems into the accreditation process, but over time it will require compliance (Joint Commission for Accreditation of Healthcare Organizations). Informatics nurses will need to follow data requirements of accreditation bodies to assist in the development of appropriate IS. Informatics nurses increasingly will need to use advanced data analysis and database management skills to maintain the larger and more complex comparative databases.

The sixth and final health care trend to be presented is that increasingly health care providers include nonphysician providers. This trend is in direct response to regulations that have increased reimbursement for non-physician providers. As computerized credentialing systems are developed, informatics nurses should be certain that data elements are appropriate for the credentialing of both physician and nonphysician providers.

National Health Policy and Nursing Informatics

The practice of NI is impacted not only by health care trends but also by national health policy that has been adopted. Within this section, seven health care policy initiatives will be discussed that have a significant potential to influence the roles of informatics nurses.

National Information Infrastructure

The National Information Infrastructure (NII) is an initiative to enhance the basic infrastructure for telecommunications and computer technology throughout the United States (Public Health Data Policy Coordinating Committee, 1995). The NII is described as a web that links computers, telephones, and televisions to each other and to other technologies connected within the web. Included in the infrastructure are technologies, standards, applications, and persons needed to integrate these components.

The NII initiative has assumed that a health information infrastructure (HII) is one component of its structure. The health component, however, has not applied information and telecommunication technologies as vigorously as other sectors, is underrepresented in the NII, and is not viewed by the American public as important in the NII as other components such as education or defense. The National Committee on Vital and Health Statistics (NCVHS) has suggested that Department of Health and Human Services (DHHS) develop a detailed vision for the HII and a plan for reaching the vision as a partner with other public and private entities (National Committee on Vital and Health Statistics, 1998). With the health care trends identified earlier in this chapter, it is essential that greater attention be paid to the HII. As representatives of the largest health care provider group, nurses who are experts in informatics need to be among the stakeholders included in further delineation of the HII.

The NCVHS has identified the four major work areas needing development within the HII as population-based data, computer-based health records, knowledge management/decision support, and telemedicine. IS need to aggregate data from computer-based health records and individual patient encounters to produce population-based data that can be used to make decisions about health care in America. NCVHS has further identified

six processes needing work that cut across the HII and all other components of the NII. They are as follows:

- Protection of privacy
- Protection from discrimination
- Development of standards and measures
- Research, education, and development
- Universal access to information resource
- International collaboration.

Areas needing further work within the NII are certainly within the domain of interest for informatics nurses.

In 1995, the Vice President underscored the importance of the NII initiative in health care by designating the Secretary of DHHS to lead an interagency effort to resolve issues that slow or block development of the HII. The issues of health data standards, privacy, enhanced information for consumers, and telemedicine were assigned priority. To address these areas of concern, the Secretary formed the Data Council. To assist the Data Council in meeting its goals, six working groups were formed as follows: Survey Integration Work Group, Joint Working Group on Telemedicine, Interagency Health Privacy Working Group, Committee on Health Data Standards, Working Group on Racial and Ethnic Data, and Working Group on International Health Data Collaboration. The Data Council remains the focal point for data policy issues and advises the Secretary on data standards and privacy issues. With the passage of HIPAA, the DHHS Data Council assumed responsibility for the administrative simplification provisions (Department of Health and Human Services, 1999). In addition, HIPAA has mandated that the NCVHS serve as an external advisory group on national health data standards to the Data Council.

Simplifying Administration of Health Care

Within HIPAA, known as the Kassebaum-Kennedy insurance reform legislation, Subtitle F mandates simplification of the administration of the health system. Administrative simplification is intended to improve public and private health programs by establishing standards to facilitate the efficient transmission of electronic health information (Joint Healthcare Information Technology Alliance; Health Care Financing Administration, 1998). HIPAA preempts state law and payer-specific variations of data standards; mandates input from private, standard-setting organizations; and gives DHHS authority to move ahead with standard setting. The law also designates financial penalties for noncompliance with standards related to specific transactions. Given the reluctance of the informatics community to adopt uniform standards, the provisions of HIPAA are essential to move this aspect of the HII forward. Hopefully, the quip that the nice thing about standards is that there are so many of them to choose from will cease to be relevant in health care.

HIPAA mandates the adoption of standards for financial and administrative transactions and associated data elements. The Standards for Electronic Transactions and Code Sets will effect ten different transactions. To avoid further duplication of effort, the law requires DHHS to adopt standards from those already approved by private standards-setting organizations. The Notice of Proposed Rule Making (NPRM) for Standards for Electronic Transactions and Code Sets was published in the Federal Register on May 7, 1998 for public comment (Health Care Financing Administration, 1998; Coffey et al., 1997; Department of Health and Human Services, 1998). The comment period ended on July 6, 1998, but no final regulations have been posted by DHHS as of publication.

In addition to data standards, HIPAA mandates the adoption of standards for unique identifiers for individuals, employers, health plans, and health care providers. Currently no universally accepted national identification system exists for health care providers. Often providers must use multiple numbers to submit claims from different practice sites. Because data are not easily transmitted between systems, redundant data are collected, leading to higher costs to complete needed transactions. The NPRM for the National Provider Identifier was published in the Federal Register on May 7, 1998 for public comment (Health Care Financing Administration). The comment period ended July 6, 1998, but final regulations have not been posted by DHHS as of publication.

One of the most important problems to block progress of the HII is lack of a data security standard. Without this, providers and organizations are reluctant to share information electronically or submit data that can be aggregated and used to address population needs (Amatayakul, 1998). Security is such an important issue that the NCVHS supports a policy of not implementing a Unique Health Identifier for Individuals (UHII) until a law is passed that protects health information. Even though DHHS had issued a Notice of Intent to publish a white paper on the UHII, it has put this issue on hold until the security issue is resolved (Joint Healthcare Information Technology Alliance, 1998).

HIPAA mandates that a security standard be adopted to protect the integrity and confidentiality of information transmitted and to prevent unauthorized uses of that information. The standard will apply to health plans, health care clearinghouses, and health care providers and to all health care data electronically maintained or used in an electronic transmission. This includes magnetic tape, disk, CD media, and transmissions over the Internet, Extranet, leased lines, dial-up lines, and private networks (Public Law 104-191, 1996). The NPRM for security and electronic signatures was published in the Federal Register on August 12, 1998 for public comment (Health Care Financing Administration, 1998). The comment period ended October 13, 1998. There was such a large number of comments received that to allow adequate time to analyze and respond to the inquiries, HCFA had again delayed release of the final rules on security (Waldo, 1998).

According to HIPAA, Congress needed to enact security legislation by August 20, 1999 that includes provision for privacy and confidentiality. Since that did not occur, the DHHS Secretary issued regulations on security and public comment ended in February 2000. To achieve more comprehensive provisions than DHHS-issued regulations would cover, health care organizations and policy makers hoped that Congress would create protection for privacy and confidentiality through legislation (Carrington, 1999). Informatics nurses will need to follow development of the security standard closely to be able to plan for being compliant with the requirements.

HIPAA regulations will have a tremendous impact on health informatics, including NI. There have been opportunities to comment on proposed regulations as they have been developed, but data indicate that even though advanced nurse providers are directly impacted by proposed NPI standards, only two of 152 responses received were from nursing organizations—one state organization and one national organization (Department of Health and Human Services, 1998). Nursing organizations may feel inadequate to comment about informatics issues. So it is important that informatics nurses either individually or through their professional organizations offer consultation to allow nursing issues to be represented in decisions that impact nursing practice.

Outcomes Measurement

One of the changes in the private health care sector has been a paradigm shift from documenting process to documenting outcomes. The Government Performance and Results Act (GPRA) of 1993 has mandated that federal programs also document outcomes. GPRA was passed to improve the confidence of the American people in program outcomes and to improve the performance of programs by setting goals and measuring outcomes against those goals. GPRA's provisions require a series of steps designed to improve performance. By fiscal year 1998, all federal organizations were required to have strategic plans developed for their programs. During fiscal year 1999, organizations must develop performance plans that are based on their strategic plans. Beginning in March 2000, all organizations must write annual performance reports that will be made public. The reports must compare actual outcomes to stated goals (Whittaker, 1997).

GPRA will have a meaningful impact on recipients of federal funding. Because federal agencies will be measuring their own performance, all grantees will be required to submit requested data on outcomes of their programs. The Bureau of Health Professions, HRSA, has developed a Comprehensive Performance Management System (CPMS) that identifies indicators that cut across all programs within the Bureau. Initially, data will be collected for seven indicators within CPMS. For example, schools of nursing receiving moneys from the Division of Nursing to support advanced education nursing programs would be required to collect and transmit data for the CPMS on the number of graduates, minority/disadvantaged graduates, underrepresented minorities serving as faculty, and graduates who enter practice in underserved areas. Additional programmatic indicators will be needed to measure the performance of DN programs. Agencies within HRSA are developing Web-based technologies for grantees to submit data directly to their funding agencies. Because the Web is a telecommunications medium that is platform-neutral, there is less concern about hardware and software incompatibilities. Informatics nurses within schools of nursing need to facilitate the development of data collection and transmission techniques in their environments. They also may need to help nursing faculty update their informatics skills to smooth the process of grantee compliance with data submission requirements.

With increased attention to the identification and measurement of clinical outcomes during the past decade, data have emerged that allow the formulation of clinical guidelines for evidence-based practice or "best practices." The Agency for Health Policy and Research (AHCPR), now the Agency for Healthcare Research and Quality (AHRQ) has developed and distributed several clinical guidelines. In December 1998, AHCPR in partnership with the American Medical Association and the American Association of Health Plans activated the National Guidelines Clearinghouse (NGC) Web site to make evidence-based clinical practice guidelines widely available.

Within NGC, data on each guideline include a structured abstract of information about the guideline and how it

was developed, a comparison of similarities and differences in guidelines that cover the same topic, and either full text or a link to full text of the guideline. AHRQ reviews guidelines submitted to them for inclusion in NGC and judges whether they meet minimal criteria for inclusion. Criteria were published in the Federal Register on April 13, 1998 (Agency for Health Care Policy and Research, 1998). Efforts to compare guidelines highlight the language problems that face the informatics community. Informatics professionals believe the development of an integrated language is the most pressing need within informatics. Informatics nurses need to work with other informatics professionals to link terminology through a unified language to ease efforts to compare outcomes through mechanisms such as guidelines.

Statistical data are produced for public use by more than 70 federal organizations. The Federal Interagency Council on Statistical Policy maintains a web site called FEDSTATS that links users to appropriate agencies for statistical data (Federal Interagency Council on Statistical Policy, 1999). Data on minorities can be accessed from the Directory of Minority DHHS Data Resources (Department of Health and Human Services, 1999).

Consumer Bill of Rights

The trend of patient consumerism or empowerment discussed earlier will likely see patients accessing, reviewing, and inserting information into their medical records. Even though patients insist on greater access to their medical records, they will continue to have legal concerns about violations of privacy and confidentiality. The issues of patient access to information and confidentiality of patient records are two areas addressed in a proposed Consumer Bill of Rights.

With its appointment on March 26, 1997, the 34-member Advisory Commission on Consumer Protection and Quality in the Health Care Industry was directed to recommend the best way to promote and ensure consumer protection and health care quality (Joint Healthcare Information Technology Alliance; Advisory Commission on Consumer Protection and Quality in the Health Care Industry, 1998). The Commission's recommendations have framed a proposed Consumer Bill of Rights and Responsibilities that Congress has been asked to pass. There are eight areas of rights and responsibilities identified in the bill. Three of the areas having significance for informatics nurses are information disclosure, participation in treatment decisions, and confidentiality of health records. The bill of rights document states that consumers have a right to receive accurate and easily understood information about their health plans, professionals, and facilities. Patients also have a right to information about their treatments that is easily understood. The goal is to enable patients or their representatives to have enough information to choose from available treatment options. As consumers and providers communicate in confidence about health care, they have a right to have any information that can be linked to them individually protected from unauthorized disclosure. The role of informatics nurses in assuring the confidentiality of patient records has been discussed previously.

To ensure that adequate information is available, informatics nurses will need to use technology to facilitate the collection and presentation of health care information in a format that is easily understood by patients. Whenever possible, multimedia approaches should be used to explain more complex treatment options to patients. Informatics nurses will need to partner with content experts to ensure the accuracy of information presented to patients. Information resources, including Web sites, that target patients will need to reflect a reading level appropriate for general audiences. An example of an excellent patient-focused Web site is Healthfinder, a site developed by the Department of Health and Human Services in collaboration with other federal agencies. The goal of this web site is to "improve consumer access to selected health information from government agencies, their many partner organizations, and other reliable resources that serve the public interest" (Department of Health and Human Services, 1999). Healthfinder does not provide health information directly, but links consumers to information sharing sites that have met specified criteria. It has received awards for its concept, design, and focus on patients and serves as an outstanding model for providing information to consumers.

Federal Credentialing Project

Credentialing is a process to assure that providers have the necessary knowledge, education, and skill to practice in a given health care environment. It involves a systematic procedure of screening, evaluating, and authenticating the qualifications of providers by each facility in which they practice. Credentialing information includes professional education, postgraduate training, professional experience, professional affiliations, and licensure data. The National Provider Data Bank (NPDB) is queried for reported adverse actions. Generally, each employing entity conducts an independent credentialing review of the provider, resulting in tremendous duplication of effort for both initial and subsequent reviews.

The Federal Credentialing Program (FCP) proposes to link existing credentialing databases to facilitate the sharing of primary source credentialing information across federal systems. The FCP was initiated jointly by the Departments of Defense, DHHS, and Veterans Affairs to standardize and streamline the credentialing process. A computerized credentialing system, known as VetPro, is being developed through an interagency agreement between the Veterans Health Administration and Bureau of Health Profession, HRSA. VetPro will use regular and Web-based data entry and imaging techniques to capture credentialing information and eliminate the need for paper files, to share verified credentials, to facilitate the identification of qualified health care providers at times of national or international disaster, and to support telehealth. The prototype system has been developed and will be beta tested in eight sites during 1999 before deployment throughout VA medical centers (Division of Quality Assurance, 1999).

With the increased use of nonphysician providers to deliver primary care, issues surrounding credentialing will become even more important in health care. Through the Quality Interagency Coordination (QuIC) Task Force, established by an Executive Order, efforts are under way to expand the FCP to three nonphysician provider groups, including nursing. A meeting of professional and licensing representatives will be convened during 1999 to identify discipline-specific and common core data elements needed for credentialing providers from all of the disciplines. To eliminate redundant efforts associated with credentialing and to expedite the process, informatics nurses will need to ensure core data elements for credentialing are included in information systems as they are designed or implemented.

Next Generation Internet

In October 1996, the Next Generation Internet (NGI) initiative was announced (The White House Office of the Press Secretary, 1996). This multiagency federal research and development initiative has three goals: developing advanced networking technologies to connect universities and national laboratories, encouraging development of applications that require advanced networking, and demonstrating new applications on networks 100 to 1000 times faster than the present Internet. The initiative uses public-private partnerships to accomplish its objectives.

Evidence of successful implementation of the NGI has been reported in the literature (Young, 1998). The InternetII Project, a collaborative group of about 135 universities, unveiled a high-speed backbone called Abilene in April 1998. Many of the InternetII projects have been funded by the NGI. In December 1998, Gemini2000 was announced as the first coast-to-coast, NGI backbone network to carry traffic from both commercial and research communities. Gemini2000 uses a logical, hierarchical architecture that includes zones, regions, and core sites to ensure high-speed performance (IXC Communications, Inc., 1998).

What will be the impact of NGI on informatics nurses? One anticipated outcome of the NGI is to produce the capacity for using real-time, multimedia applications such as video-conferencing and video streaming and for transferring huge volumes of data. Both of these outcomes will benefit telemedicine and distance education efforts in health care and increase the demand for such technologies. Informatics nurses will likely become involved in implementing telehealth technologies. As electronic commerce increases over high-speed networks, some predict that for the economically disadvantaged, electronic inequalities will intensify (Guernsey, 1999). Informatics nurses need to study the social impact of the Internet, monitor the ability of all individuals to access information as needed, and propose initiatives to reduce electronic inequities.

Telehealth

Telehealth is a new frontier for nursing informatics. It is a broader concept than its predecessor telemedicine, a term that is used by the Health Care Financing Association (HCFA) to mean a consultation delivered interactively through telecommunications equipment that includes a video display. Telehealth has been defined as the use of communication and information technologies to provide or support a diverse group of health-related activities such as health professionals' education, community health education, public health research, the administration of health services, or the delivery of health services. The World Health Organization has used the word "telematics" to depict this same notion. The broader concept describes more accurately how the technology can be used to complete many different activities without creating artificial distinctions between them (Conrad, 1997). Such distinctions could be detrimental to the development of integrated, multiuse systems.

Three major issues—reimbursement, licensure, and security—have prevented widespread adoption and use of telehealth. Policy makers have begun to address these issues legislatively. As discussed earlier, HIPAA has mandated security legislation by August 2000, so that aspect of telehealth will be addressed. Limited reimbursement for telehealth has been available through private insurance, and only 11 states currently reimburse physicians who use interactive video telecommunications equipment for consultation services to Medicaid patients. The Balanced Budget Act passed in 1997 should increase reimbursement, because it has mandated the first national reimbursement policy for Medicare. Since January 1, 1999, physician and nonphysician providers, including nurse practitioners, nurse midwives, and clinical nurse specialists, must be reimbursed for Medicare teleconsultation in rural health professional shortage areas. The consultation must be interactive, and an eligible provider must present the patient to an eligible consulting provider. At present, if store and forward technologies are used for the consultation, it cannot be reimbursed. HCFA is aware of concerns among providers that the regulations as implemented are not inclusive enough to meet health needs in rural areas and have indicated that future changes may be considered.

Licensure is becoming a big issue in telehealth practice. Although policy makers have suggested that state licensure regulations should not become barriers for practicing telehealth, delivering telehealth services across state lines remains an issue. More than 19 states have recently passed laws requiring physicians to obtain full and unrestricted licenses to deliver interstate telehealth services. The model suggested by the Federation of State Medical Boards to allow limited practice across state lines has been largely ignored.

The National Council of State Boards of Nursing has proposed a model of mutual recognition in which nurses obtain a state-based license that is nationally recognized and locally enforced (National Council of State Boards of Nursing, 1998). In other words, the nurse obtains one license in the state of residence and can practice in other states that agree to participate in the compact without obtaining additional licenses. Nurses remain accountable for their practice in states in which they are delivering services. States agree to recognize the nursing licenses of other states through a compact, a legal document that regulates business between two or more states. As of May 2000, 10 states have passed the Nursing Compact and several states are introducing it for consideration.

Informatics nurses must keep up to date on both licensure and reimbursement issues in telehealth. They will need to implement health policy as it is made and be certain that their systems comply with any regulations that pertain to interstate use of information technologies. Informatics nurses, while largely focused on IS, generally have failed to recognize the need to integrate telehealth technologies with existing IS. Telehealth and informatics professional groups have developed in isolation from each other. Informatics nurses need to help to integrate telehealth technologies and IS so that patient encounters became part of the computerized patient record and informatics issues such as standards and language are systematically addressed.

National Nursing Informatics Agenda

The Division of Nursing is responsible for setting national policy to guide the preparation of the nursing workforce, including preparation in the area of nursing informatics. The DN recognized the importance of information management and technology long before the title "nursing informatics" was used to describe the field of practice and has funded projects focused in this area since 1972. During the 1970s, funding efforts focused on increasing awareness of the need for IS that could be used to support nursing practice and developing a nursing language that could be applied to public health settings. Funding during the 1980s and early 1990s enabled four different educational models to be developed for NI; two models focused on specialty practice in NI, and two models incorporated NI skills into administration and community health programs, respectively. In 1987 and since 1994, the DN has funded projects that either focus on distance learning methodologies or use them to deliver advanced nursing education. Faculty development in NI was the focus of funding for three regional compacts in 1996.

Although the DN has supported NI projects, the nursing workforce has continued to be deficient in informatics skills. As a result, in 1997 the Division convened the National Nursing Informatics Work Group (NNIWG) to make recommendations to the National Advisory Council for Nurse Education and Practice (NACNEP) for setting the nation's Nursing Informatics Agenda (NIA) for nursing education and practice. There were 19 experts on NNIWG who identified nursing informatics needs from the perspectives of patient care settings, commercial business, government service, and nursing education. NNIWG members are experts in decision support, distance education, informatics education, information systems, language and taxonomies, and telecommunications.

Identifying Needs and Initiatives

A nominal group technique was used to help NNIWG members identify NI needs and initiatives. Within two subgroups, NNIWG members in turn each stated a need. Needs were recorded without discussion until the end of the specified time period. Each of the identified needs was then discussed and either maintained as written,

expanded, combined with other needs, rephrased, or eliminated with the consent of the originator of that idea. Using a weighting scheme, NNIWG members prioritized items within their respective subgroups.

The lists of prioritized needs were returned to the experts, and they were asked to suggest initiatives that would offer solutions for the informatics needs that were identified. Nine initiatives were developed and ranked from highest to lowest priority by NNIWG. The ranking process resulted in a score for each initiative; results were circulated electronically to NNIWG members for comment. The experts suggested that two sets of initiatives should be combined, leaving five initiatives to be forwarded to NACNEP for consideration as a nursing informatics agenda.

NACNEP reviewed the recommended initiatives at their Spring 1997 meeting and approved them with minor changes. The Advisory Council's recommendations were sent to the Secretary of DHHS as a National Nursing Informatics Agenda. The Council's report is titled *A National Informatics Agenda for Nursing Education and Practice, December 1997* and can be obtained from the Division of Nursing (National Advisory Council on Nurse Education and Practice, 1997).

Strategic Directions for Nursing Informatics

There are five assumptions considered by NACNEP to be a basis for all further discussion of nursing informatics initiatives:

- Learners are students, faculty, and clinicians.
- Nursing informatics must be considered within an interdisciplinary context of partnerships and collaboration.
- Efforts should target disadvantaged and underserved populations.
- Initiatives should be responsive to other government funding priorities.
- Collaboration among federal agencies and between federal and private entities is necessary.

Five key directions for informatics in nursing education and practice were recommended to the Secretary in the NACNEP report. The recommendations are as follows:

- Educate nursing students and practicing nurses in core informatics content.
- Prepare nurses with specialized skills in informatics.
- Enhance nursing practice and education through informatics projects.

- Prepare nursing faculty in informatics.
- Increase collaborative efforts in nursing informatics.

The existence of a national strategic direction for nursing informatics combined with new authorizing legislation for the DN should enhance the field of nursing informatics and the roles of informatics nurses. In November 1998, the President signed Public Law 105-392, The Health Professions Education Partnership Act of 1998, Title VIII, Subtitle B, The Nursing Education and Practice Improvement Act of 1998. This legislation gives authority to the DN to fund nursing education and practice programs needed to prepare a nursing workforce to meet the nation's health needs. It amends the previous Title VIII legislation passed in 1992. Part D of the new legislation addresses the need for strengthening capacity for basic nurse education and practice. Informatics is specifically named as one of the seven priority areas for strengthening capacity. The priority is to provide education in informatics, including distance learning methodologies (Public Law 150-392, 1998).

The new legislation is consistent with the NIA's first strategic direction to include core informatics knowledge and skill in all undergraduate, graduate, and continuing education programs. Interestingly, NI experts have published lists of informatics skills and knowledge but have not distinguished informatics skills needed for different levels of nursing practice or validated them using research methodologies. Such activity is needed to accurately identify core informatics skills and knowledge to be included in all educational programs. This author is collaborating with faculty and informatics experts at the University of Utah, New York University, Slippery Rock University, and the Hershey-Geisinger Medical Center to validate NI competencies and recommend core content for nursing education programs.

Generally, the NI community believes that core informatics skills include computer literacy, i.e. being able to use word processing, spreadsheets, databases, E-mail, the Internet, presentation graphics, and literature-searching techniques. Core informatics knowledge includes the ability to use information systems to collect and record data and retrieve information needed to provide care. It also includes the ability to implement policies that address the privacy, confidentiality, and security of information (American Nurses Association, 1994). Many informatics nurses also suggest adding knowledge about information management, standard nomenclatures for nursing language, and decision-making to nursing programs.

If core content is included in educational programs, the nursing workforce increasingly will be prepared to use the information technologies that have been installed in their health care delivery environments. This will decrease the length of time informatics nurses need to teach new graduates about information systems in their work environments or eliminate the need for training altogether. Of concern, however, is how to improve core informatics skills and knowledge of practicing nurses who graduated more than 2 or 3 years ago. Innovative projects are needed to help this large population of nurses become more competent in informatics.

The second strategic direction for nursing informatics is to increase the number of nurses who have specialized skills in informatics. As stated before, amendments to the Public Health Service Act in 1992 prohibited the DN from funding more than the two initial graduate programs in nursing informatics. The 1998 legislation has reinstated administration as an eligible focus to receive funds for advanced education nursing. Since informatics curricula usually have been aligned with nursing administration programs, this change might produce applications for delivering informatics specialty skills in advanced education nurse programs. Having more opportunity to complete advanced informatics preparation should help to increase the number of NI specialists in practice. This, in return, should increase nursing involvement in IS and information technology design, purchase, and implementation. Because of their advocacy roles for patients, nurses should be able to address the information needs of patients.

The Pew Commission has strongly recommended that health providers receive educational experiences as members of interdisciplinary teams. Given the interdisciplinary nature and technological focus of informatics practice, it would be interesting to see unique models of nursing informatics programs emerge. One interesting model would be to develop collaborative educational programs that cut across traditional disciplinary lines. Schools of medicine, nursing, dentistry, and information systems management could be full partners in these programs, collaborating to share financial burdens, decision-making, curriculum planning, teaching, and evaluation. Collaborative programs could provide core informatics content to students from multiple disciplines and then allow the students to apply knowledge within their individual professional domains. To make certain graduates have the necessary credentials to advance within their licensed professions, degrees should be awarded so that students retain their professional identify.

A third strategic direction for NI is to enhance nursing practice and education through informatics projects. There is a critical need to improve the skills of the public health workforce to meet the needs of at risk and underserved populations. Fewer than 50 percent of nurses working in public health have a baccalaureate degree in nursing; most have an associate degree. It is the baccalaureate program that includes coursework in public health. Because almost twice as many nurses graduated from associate degree programs as from baccalaureate programs in 1996, nursing leaders are concerned that the problem will continue (Moses, 1996). As stated earlier, there is also a need to improve the informatics skills of the nursing workforce, particularly with nurses who have been out of school for a few years. Telehealth projects could be used to address both of these workforce issues. Informatics nurses are encouraged to work with academic, public health, and other health care delivery entities to develop programs that use telehealth technologies to improve nursing workforce skills.

The fourth strategic direction for NI is to improve faculty skills in NI so that they in turn can promote the development of informatics competence in students. Unless faculty members are prepared to use all of the basic software packages—that is, unless they are computer literate—they are unlikely to require students to use information technology as part of their assignments. Faculties are under tremendous pressures from issues brought about by a rapidly changing health care environment. They are older, have larger classes, are required to bring in money to supplement their salaries, and are constantly asked to increase their scope of practice. To add the need for increasing informatics skills so that they can teach these classes might be overwhelming to some faculty members. And can faculty reasonably be expected to have expertise in all areas of health care? Existing technology could facilitate innovative ways to meet the informatics needs of both faculty and students.

The teaching of computer literacy skills could be contracted to companies who specialize in such education. Faculty and students could pay a nominal laboratory fee to cover expenses; both groups would gain expertise in basic computer skills. Faculty could learn more advanced informatics skills through collaborative arrangements between schools of nursing or between a school of nursing and a department of information systems management. Teleconferencing could be used for faculty to "attend" informatics courses offered on other campuses to improve their skills. Collaborative arrangements might also allow informatics nurse experts on one campus to educate students on another campus, thereby decreasing the unmet demand for faculty prepared to teach NI. This model would also decrease stresses placed on faculty members to increase their skills in so many important areas of health care all at once. Collaborative

models need exploration to identify the best practices for faculty preparation in NI.

The fifth and final strategic direction is to increase collaborative efforts in nursing informatics. What is obvious in higher education is that the limited resources available will need to be used efficiently and economically. Many health care policy makers advocate that collaborative efforts are key to using resources wisely. Competitive educational models may need to be replaced by collaborative models, particularly in informatics.

The NIA also advocates collaborative efforts between federal agencies and among public and private organizations to identify and fund needed informatics research and projects. In 1998, the National Library of Medicine, National Heart, Blood and Lung Institute, and the health informatics community collaborated to identify ways that information technologies could be used to accomplish the goals of the National Heart Attack Alert Program. Informatics nurses served on the planning committee for a 2-day conference that successfully identified projects for funding. A second example of collaboration between private and public organizations to advance NI is a Vocabulary Summit that was hosted by Vanderbilt University during 1999. Both the Division of Nursing and the American Medical Informatics Association's Nursing Informatics Working Group were among the financial supporters of this important meeting designed to advance work being done on nursing data structures. These are but two of the collaborative efforts that have occurred in nursing informatics.

Summary

In summary, nursing informatics is well established as a specialty within nursing. Current and proposed health care policy will impact NI in several ways. Given the emphasis on interdisciplinary practice, NI needs to broaden its educational and practice perspectives to include a more interdisciplinary focus. More graduate programs in NI have been established. Certification as a generalist in nursing informatics is currently available, but a specialist level of certification is needed to acknowledge more advanced informatics skills. Even though opportunities for specialty preparation in informatics are increasing, there is a tremendous need to improve the general informatics skills of nursing faculty, students, and clinicians. Collaborative efforts are needed to link schools so that informatics resources can be shared.

When reimbursement, licensure, and security issues in telehealth are solved, the use of these technologies will increase dramatically. NI needs to embrace telehealth as part of informatics practice. As a result of the patient con-sumerism movement, NI will also need to focus more on patients' demands for access to information that is easier to understand.

And finally, the nursing informatics community needs to become more aware of health policies that have been established or are under consideration. Issues need to be addressed through position papers, proposed regula-tions need to be reviewed and comments submitted if necessary, and funding agencies need to be encouraged to include nursing in informatics initiatives.

References:

Advisory Commission on Consumer Protection and Quality in the Health Care Industry. (1998). Consumer Bill of Rights and Responsibilities. *http://www.hc qualitycommission.gov/cborr/exsumm.html*

Agency for Health Care Policy and Research. (1998). Invi-tation to submit guidelines to the National Guideline Clearinghouse. *Federal Register, 63*(70), 18027.

Amatayakul, M. (1998). The state of the computer-based patient record. *Journal of AHIMA, 1. http://www. ahima.org/publications/2f/focus.1.1098.html*

American Medical Informatics Association Nursing Informatics Working Group. (1998). *Education in Nursing Informatics. http://www.parsons.umaryland. edu/amia/Niprogram.htm*

American Nurses Association. (1994). *Scope of Practice for Nursing Informatics*. Washington, D.C.: American Nurses Publishing.

American Nurses Association. (1995). *Nursing Informatics Standards of Practice*. Washington, D.C.: American Nurses Publishing.

American Nurses Credentialing Center. (1999). ANCC Informatics Nurse Certification Catalog. *http://www. ana.org/ancc/inform98/informat.htm*

Ball, M. J., and Hannah, K. J. (1984). *Using Computers in Nursing*. Reston, VA: Reston Publishers.

Bruegel, R. B. (1998). Patient empowerment: A trend that matters. *Journal of AHIMA, 1*, September. *http://www. ahima.org/publications/2f/focus.1.998.html*

Carrington, C. (1999). Congress unlikely to meet privacy legislation deadline. *Telehealth Magazine, 5*(1), 19.

Coffey, R. M., Ball, J. K., Johangen M., et al. (1997). The case for national health data standards. *Health Affairs, 16*(5), 58–72.

Conrad, K. (1997). Introduction. *North Dakota Law Review, 73*(1), 1–6.

Department of Health and Human Services. (1998). Milestones in Health Information Standards. *http:// aspe.os.dhhs.gov/admsimp/asmiles.htm*

Department of Health and Human Services. (1998). Who Submitted Comments on the National Provider

Identifier Notice of Proposed Rule Making. *http://aspe.os.dhhs.gov/admnsimp/npicom.htm*

Department of Health and Human Services. (1999). Current Selection Policies and Procedures. *Healthfinder. http://www.healthfinder.gov/aboutus/ selectionpolicy.htm*

Department of Health and Human Services. (1999). Directory of Minority Health and Human Services Data Resources. *http://www.os.dhhs.gov/progorg/ aspe/minority/mintoc.htm*

Department of Health and Human Services. (1999). The DHHS Data Council. *http://aspe.os.dhhs.gov/datacncl/ index.htm*

Division of Quality Assurance. (1999). Federal Credentialing Project. *http://www.credentialing.org*

Federal Interagency Council on Statistical Policy. (1999). *FEDSTATS. http://www.fedstats.gov*

Gassert, C. A., Mills, M. E., and Heller, B. R. (1992). Doctoral specialization in nursing informatics. In P. D. Clayton, (Ed.), *Proceedings of the Fifteenth Annual Symposium on Computer Applications in Medical Care* (pp. 263–267). New York: McGraw-Hill.

Graves, J. R., Amos, L. K., Heuther, S., et al. (1995). Description of a graduate program in clinical nursing informatics. *Computers in Nursing, 13*(2), 60–70.

Graves, J. R., and Corcoran, S. (1989). The study of nursing informatics. *Image: Journal of Nursing Scholarship, 21* (4), 227–231.

Grobe, S. J. (1988). Nursing informatics competencies for nurse educators and researchers. In H. E. Peterson and U. Gerdin Jelger (Eds.), *Preparing Nurses for Using Information Systems: Recommended Informatics Competencies* (pp. 25–33). New York: National League for Nursing.

Guernsey, L. (1999). Scholars call for research on how computers may be widening the global economic gap. *The Chronicle of Higher Education. http://chronicle. com/daily/99/02/99021701t.htm*

Hannah, K. J. (1985). Current trends in nursing informatics: Implications for curriculum planning. In K. J. Hannah, E. J. Guillemin, and D. N. Conklin (Eds.), *Nursing Uses of Computers and Information Science* (pp. 181–187). Amsterdam: Elsevier.

Health Care Financing Administration. (1998). Data standards. *Federal Register Notice, 63* (88), 25271–25320.

Health Care Financing Administration. (1998). Security and electronic signature standards. *Federal Register Notice, 63*(155), 43241–43280.

Health Care Financing Administration. The National Provider Identifier. *http://www.hcfa.gov/stats/npi/ overview.htm*

Heller, B. R., Romano, C. A., Moray, L. R, and Gassert, C. A. (1989). Special follow-up report: The implementation of the first graduate program in nursing informatics. *Computers in Nursing, 7*(5), 209–213.

IXC Communications, Inc. (1998). Gemini2000. *http://www.ixc-comm.com*

Joint Commission for Accreditation of Healthcare Organizations. *Mission. http://www.jcaho.org/about_jc/govt.htm*

Joint Healthcare Information Technology Alliance. (1998). Advocacy Paper. *http://www.jhita.org/admsimp.htm*

Joint Healthcare Information Technology Alliance. Advocacy Paper: Patient's Bill of Rights. *http://www.jhita.org/pbr.htm*

Joint Healthcare Information Technology Alliance. Factsheet. *http://www.jhita.org/secstd.htm*

Lorence, D. P. (1998). Planning for the future of HIM Practice: Healthcare trends to watch. *Journal of AHIMA, 1*, July/August. *http:www.ahima.org/publications/2f/focus.2.798.html*

Milholland, D. K (1992). Congress says nursing informatics is a specialty. *American Nurse* July/August: 1.

Moses, E. B. (1996). *The Registered Nurse Population.* Rockville, MD: Department of Health and Human Services, Health Resources and Services Administration.

National Advisory Council on Nurse Education and Practice. (1997). *A National Informatics Agenda for Nursing Education and Practice: A Report to the Secretary of the Department of Health and Human Services.* Rockville, MD: Department of Health and Human Services, Health Resources and Services Administration, Bureau of Health Professions, Division of Nursing.

National Center for Nursing Research. (1993). *Nursing Informatics: Enhancing Patient Care.* Bethesda, MD: Department of Health and Human Services, National Institutes of Health, National Center for Nursing Research.

National Committee on Vital and Health Statistics. (1998). *Assuring a Health Dimension for the National Information Infrastructure. http://aspe.os.dhhs.gov/ncvhs/hii-nii.htm*

National Council of State Boards of Nursing. (1998). *Mutual Recognition of Nursing Licenses Benefits Both Nurses and Health Care Consumers. http://www.ncsbn.org/files/newsreleases/nr981125mr.html*

Panniers, T. L., and Gassert, C. A. (1995). Standards of practice and preparation for certification. In B. R. Heller, M. E. Mills, and C. A. Romano (Eds.),

Information Management in Nursing and Health Care. Springhouse, PA: Springhouse Corporation.

Pew Health Professions Commission. (1998). Executive summary. In *Recreating Health Professional Practice for a New Century.* San Francisco, CA: University of California, San Francisco.

President's Advisory Commission on Consumer Protection and Quality in the Health Care Industry. (1998). *Quality First: Better Health Care for All Americans.* Columbia, MD: Consumer Bill of Rights.

Public Health Data Policy Coordinating Committee. (1995). *Making a Powerful Connection: The Health of the Public and the National Information Infrastructure.* Bethesda: National Library of Medicine.

Public Law 104-191. (1996). *Health Insurance Portability and Accountability Act of 1996.*

Public Law 150-392. (1998). *Health Professions Education Partnership Act of 1998, Title VIII, Subtitle B, The Nursing Education and Practice Improvement Act of 1998.*

Styles, M. M. (1989). *On Specialization in Nursing: Toward a New Empowerment.* Kansas City, MO: American Nurses Foundation, Inc.

The White House Office of the Press Secretary. (1996). Background on Clinton-Gore Administration's Next-Generation Internet Initiative. *http://www.npr.gov/library/news/101096-2.html*

Thompson, C. B. (1997). Informatics and computer literacy. In American Association of Colleges of Nursing, *Master's Education via Interdisciplinary Links, Case Management, and Nursing Informatics: Proceedings of the American Association of Colleges of Nursing's Master's Education Conference* (pp. 41–50). Washington, D.C.: AACN.

Waldo, B. H. (1998) Managing data security: Developing a plan to protect patient data. *Nursing Economics, 17*(1), 49–52.

Webster. (1985). *Webster's Ninth New Collegiate Dictionary.* Springfield MA: Merriam-Webster, Inc.

Whittaker, J. B. (1997). *The Government Performance and Results Act: A Mandate for Strategic Planning and Performance Measurement.* Arlington, VA: ESI International.

Young, J. R. (1998). High-speed research connections advance on public and private fronts. *The Chronicle of Higher Education. http://chronicle.com/daily/98/12/98121602t.htm*

CHAPTER **9**

Privacy, Confidentiality, and Security

Suzy Ann Buckovich

OBJECTIVES:

1. Understand the privacy, confidentiality, and security of health information.
2. Discuss relevant privacy, confidentiality, and security laws.
3. Describe technical mechanisms available to protect health care data.
4. Discuss the importance of an organizational policy for protecting the privacy, confidentiality, and security of health data.
5. Outline the key issues involved in the federal privacy and confidentiality law debate.

KEY WORDS

information systems
computer science
security measures
confidentiality
privacy

s the health care marketplace changes with the growth in managed care, integrated delivery systems, and computer use, protecting the privacy, confidentiality, and security of health information has never been more critical for ethical/legal reasons. This change involves an increase in the collection and storage of data as well as an increase in the entities requesting access to health information across the continuum of care and organizational boundaries. This opens the door for easier access and the potential misuse of personal information, especially in light of inadequate federal and state legal protections. Technical applications do exist to aid in protecting health information, but they should be combined with organizational policies to fully protect the personal information "near and dear" to a patient. This chapter discusses the privacy, confidentiality, and security of health information; the technical applications available to protect health data; the importance of organizational policies; the current legislative environment; and accreditation requirements.

 Privacy

Privacy is defined as "The right of individuals to be left alone and to be protected against physical or psycholog-

ical invasion or the misuse of their property. It includes freedom from intrusion or observation into one's private affairs, the right to maintain control over certain personal information, and the freedom to act without outside interference" (ASTM Committee E-31 on Healthcare Informatics, 1997). In the medical information context, privacy involves the rights of individuals to control the disclosure and use of their health information.

■ **Patients' Concerns**

Individuals consider their health information to be private as they willingly share information with health care professionals. They expect this information to be safeguarded and not disclosed or used for unauthorized purposes without their knowledge. Based upon these sound expectations, the public has reacted to the dissemination of personal health information with real concern. A recent poll by Louis Harris & Associates reported that 75 percent of respondents said they feared their health care information would be used for purposes other than health care services. Twenty-seven percent of respondents reported that their medical information had been improperly disclosed at some time, and almost 35 percent of that group said the disclosure had resulted in embarrassment or personal harm (Kibbe and Bard, 1997).

The media has heightened the public's privacy awareness with news reports on the misuse of information. In 1998, a pharmacy and supermarket sold consumers' prescription information to a marketing company without consumers' authorization (Senate Panel to Study Health Privacy Issue, 1998). The New York Post published details on a past suicide attempt by Rep. Nydia Velazquez (D-New York) during her 1992 election. She later won her congressional race but sued a hospital for failing to maintain the confidentiality of her medical records (Siwicki, 1997a). In 1995, state employees (who were later prosecuted) illegally sold health maintenance organization (HMO) recruiters the names and Social Security numbers of Maryland Medicaid recipients (Siwicki, 1997a). Out west, a Nevada computer consultant bought a used computer from a California company and found information on 2,000 customers from a Smitty's Supermarkets Pharmacy in Arizona. The information contained patients' names, Social Security numbers, and medication lists (Siwicki, 1997a). More recently, in February 1999, several thousand patient records at the University of Michigan Medical Center inadvertently remained on public Internet sites for 2 months. The records contained identifying information such as names, addresses, Social Security numbers, employment status, and treatments (George, 1999). From these real examples, it is clear why the public has concerns regarding the "whereabouts" of their personal health information.

Federal Laws

Federal laws intend to appropriately balance the public's right to access and control information gathered by the government against the individual's right to protect personal information from misuse or other unauthorized disclosures (Fig. 9.1). Table 9.1 details the federal case and statutory laws that exist in the attempt to protect people's privacy; however, they each have limits in their scope of protection.

Implications of Federal Laws

The existing federal laws have limits in the scope of their protection. For example, the Privacy Act only applies to information collected by government agencies, thus not reaching the health information typically collected and maintained by the private sector (*For the Record*, 1997). Federal protection is also limited to specialized classes of information, such as information pertaining to sub-

stance abuse patients, and to information gathered in federally funded programs (federal alcohol and drug abuse statutes) (Recommendations of the Secretary of Health and Human Services, retrieved February 12, 1999). This lack of comprehensive protection has been a driving factor towards the push for enactment of the Health Insurance Portability and Accountability Act (HIPAA)-mandated federal privacy and confidentiality law.

Confidentiality

Confidential is defined as the "status accorded to data or information indicating that it is sensitive for some reason, and therefore it needs to be protected against theft, disclosure, or improper use, or both, and must be disseminated only to authorized individuals or organizations with a need to know" (ASTM Committee on Healthcare Informatics, 1997).

Health Care Providers' Obligation

Health care providers have an ethical, legal, and professional duty to protect the confidentiality of patient information. This fiduciary duty has been a long-standing doctrine in medical ethics. The American Medical Association states that patient information is "confidential to the greatest degree possible" (American Medical Association, 1999, p. 187). The Hippocratic Oath states: "Whatever, in connection with my profession, or not in connection with it, I may see or hear in the lives of men which ought not be spoken abroad I will not divulge as reckoning that all should be kept secret" (American Medical Association, 1999, p. 188). Additionally, *The Code*

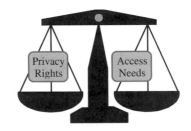

Figure 9.1
There is a balance to be struck between protecting privacy and assessing data for legitimate needs by authorized persons. The goal is to balance sometimes competing interests.

Table 9.1 Legal Federal Protections of Health Information

Legal Protection	Purpose
Whalen v. Roe, 429 U.S. 589 (1977)	The Supreme Court recognizes a limited constitutional right in privacy of personal medical information. Despite the Court upholding a New York statute allowing the state to keep a list of prescription records for dangerous drugs and requiring physicians to disclose the names of patients for whom they prescribed those drugs, it acknowledged an "individual interest in avoiding disclosure of personal matters" (*For the Record*, 1997, p. 43).
Freedom of Information Act of 1966	Allows individuals access to their personal data collected by federal agencies, except for those records that fall under exceptions (*For the Record*, 1997, p. 38).
Fair Credit Act of 1970	Allows individuals access to their credit records (Saba and McCormick, 1996).
Privacy Act of 1974	A very significant act that allows individuals the right to access their information collected by federal agencies; grants individuals the right to copy, correct, or amend their records kept by the government; mandates that federal agencies cannot keep secret record systems; and requires that personal information should be used only for its intended purposes (*For the Record*, 1997, p. 38).
United States Code, Sections 290dd-3 and 290ee-30	Creates specific federal regulations to protect the records of patients who seek drug or alcohol abuse treatment at federally funded facilities; provides for limited exceptions for release of patient information without the patient's written consent (*For the Record*, 1997, p. 41).
Medicare Conditions of Participation for Hospitals	Requires hospitals to have procedures for ensuring the confidentiality of patient records; requires hospitals to only release information to authorized individuals (*For the Record*, 1997, p. 41).
Health Insurance Portability and Accountability Act of 1996 (HIPAA)	A monumental act that mandates Congress to enact medical privacy legislation by August 1999. Since Congress failed to act, the Department of Health and Human Services is responsible for promulgating privacy regulations. HIPAA also provides penalties ranging from $50,000 to $250,000 and 1 to 10 years in jail for wrongful disclosure of individually identifiable health information (*For the Record*, 1997, p. 53).

for Nurses clearly expresses, "The nurse safeguards the client's right to privacy by judiciously protecting information of a confidential nature" (American Nurses Association, 1975; Saba and McCormick, 1996, p. 167). This is an important doctrine to uphold in order to maintain patients' trust to fully disclose information to their providers. This open communication leads to the optimal diagnosis and course of treatment.

Breaches of Confidentiality

There are many types of breaches that threaten confidentiality concerns. They include the following examples:

- Accidental disclosures—inadvertent actions, unintentional mistakes.
- Insider curiosity—curious employees accessing celebrities' or friends' information.
- Insider subornation—disgruntled employees wanting revenge.

- Uncontrolled secondary usage—use of information for unintended purposes such as for marketing (use without patient's authorization).
- Unauthorized access—unauthorized users accessing the system either through hacking or the use of another's password (Rindfleisch, 1997).

Interestingly enough, most known confidentiality violations involved fired workers or other insiders motivated by revenge, humiliation, blackmail, or curiosity (Siegel, 1997).

Impact of Breaches

While patient disclosure of all personal health information is beneficial for patient care, breaches of confidential information can have devastating consequences, leading to loss of employment and housing, health and life insurance problems, and social stigma (Computer-based Patient Record Institute, retrieved February 10, 1999). There is real concern for potential employment discrimination cause the Employee Retirement Income Security Act allows, in certain situations, self-funded employers to request and review employee medical records (Siegel, 1997; Roach, 1998). There is also public concern regarding potential insurance discrimination in light of genetic testing that is becoming available.

Key Steps to Protect Confidentiality in a Computer Environment

Health care organizations are responsible for taking appropriate measures to protect the confidentiality of health information in the computer age. These measures may include the following:

- Adopt appropriate security measures (see "security" below).

- Educate all (employees, third parties, etc. who handle health information) about computer technology and the contents of health records.

- Institute technical and administration controls (see "technology" below). These include tools to identify users, verify authorization, determine legitimacy of use, restrict retrieval to "need-to-know" information, and track all access (Computer-based Patient Record Institute, undated).

Confidentiality Legislation

Federal Law

On the federal level there is a lack of comprehensive protection for the confidentiality of health information. However, the Health Insurance Portability and Accountability Act (HIPAA) may foster a change in this protection. HIPAA mandated Congress to enact a medical information confidentiality law by August 1999. Even though many bills were introduced and there was much debate, Congress failed to enact legislation. Therefore, the Department of Health and Human Services (DHHS) is responsible for promulgating confidentiality regulations. As of the writing of this chapter, DHHS has published a Notice of Proposed Rulemaking but has not yet issued final regulations. A critical limitation in DHHS's proposed confidentiality regulation is that the protection only applies to *electronic* health information and not to all formats of health information (i.e., paper) (*Comprehensive Guide to Electronic Health Records*, 1999).

State Law

The obligation of health care providers and health care organizations to keep medical information confidential (in paper and computer format) is generally governed by state statutes that vary widely from state to state. Statutory provisions concerning health information often are scattered throughout a state's code (hospital licensing act, medical records act, HMO act, etc.) and differ in the scope of their coverage (Roach, 1998, p. 93). Many states' statutes apply only to specific categories of persons and/or categories of information (Roach, 1998, p. 297) and not all health information is protected at the same level. Typically, states impose stricter confidentiality requirements for HIV, drug and alcohol abuse information, and psychiatric records (Roach, 1998, p. 103). Virtually all states specifically prohibit the disclosure of AIDS or HIV infection except in limited circumstances (Comprehensive Guide to Electronic Records, 1999, p. 189).

Examples of Specific State Laws

Some states do not impose similar confidentiality requirements on all entities that hold patient information. For example, in New York, licensed health professionals must maintain patient privacy, but there are no laws governing nonlicensed workers in health care institutions and no laws or regulations obligating insurance companies to maintain privacy (Riley, 1996). A few states have begun to target insurers and managed care organizations with statutory provisions requiring them to keep patient information confidential (Roach, 1998, p. 93). Most states require patients' authorization before disclosing their information except under limited circumstances such as for emergency situations and peer review purposes. State statutes, hospitals, and health care organizations generally allow certain staff members to access medical records without patient consent for authorized purposes such as for patient care and some administrative functions (e.g. billing) (Roach, 1998, pp. 111–112). A few state patient rights statutes, such as New Jersey's Patient Bill of Rights Act cover confidentiality protections. That statute states that all patients admitted to a hospital licensed in that state are entitled to privacy and confidentiality of their records (Roach, 1998. p. 94). Some states, such as Montana and Washington, have enacted comprehensive health information statutes. Both have adopted the Uniform Healthcare Information Act (UHCIA), which, among other things, prohibits a health care provider from disclosing health care information without the patient's written authorization. The statute also provides for exceptions such as disclosure for the peer review process (Roach, 1998, p. 95).

Liability for Health Care Providers

Statutory requirements should be taken very seriously. Health care providers and institutions may face civil and criminal liability and/or professional disciplinary sanctions for releasing medical record information that has not been either authorized by the patient or made pursuant to other regulatory or legal authority (Roach, 1998, p. 259). Additionally, under HIPAA, there are penalties for wrongful disclosure of information that carry fines up to $250,000 and prison terms as long as 10 years (*For the Record*, 1997). You should become aware of your state's, health care institution's, and profession's confidentiality requirements to avoid liability. Additionally, until federal confidentiality legislation is passed, if you practice across state lines, you should be familiar with each state's confidentiality requirements.

 ## Security

Health care organizations have an enormous responsibility for securing information that they collect, record, transmit, store, and make available internally and to external entities. This entails being responsible for the security of computer systems, organizational data including patient data, data transport mechanisms (e.g. cables and switches), network layers, information layers (database and file servers), and software applications (Computer-based Patient Record Institute, retrieved February 11, 1999). The majority of security leaks, breaches, and attacks occur when insiders with authorization to access medical records simply misuse or abuse their access rights. Unauthorized users gaining access to confidential information is the next most frequent cause of data security breaches (Kibbe and Bard, 1997). The following definitions are for two types of security.

Data Security

Data security is "the result of effective data protection measures; the sum of measures that safeguard data and computer programs from undesired occurrences and exposure to: (1) accidental or intentional access or disclosure to unauthorized persons, or a combination thereof, (2) accidental or malicious alteration, (3) unauthorized copying, (4) loss by theft or destruction by hardware

failures, software deficiencies, operating mistakes; physical damage by fire, water, smoke, excessive temperature, electrical failure or sabotage; or combination thereof." (ASTM Committee E-31 on Healthcare Informatics, 1997, p. 3).

System Security

System Security is the "totality of safeguards including hardware, software, personnel policies, information practice policies, disaster preparedness, and oversight of these components. Security protects both the system and the information contained within from unauthorized access from without and from misuse from within" (ASTM Committee E-31 on Healthcare Informatics, 1997, p. 3).

Security Legislation

Maintaining the security of computer systems is critical for protecting the privacy of personal information. As more computers are used today and as they become more sophisticated in their scope and capability of functions, protecting the vast amount of data now available and easily shared is imperative. Table 9.2 details the laws that affect data on individuals that can be stored in computer systems.

Key Features of a Secure System and Network

The key tools to incorporate in a security policy for securing a system and network include the following:

- Authentication
- Authorization and access control
- Data integrity
- Accountability
- Availability
- Data storage
- Data transmission

Authentication   Authentication is the means of verifying the correct identity and/or group membership of users or other entities (e.g. external entities) prior to granting access to a requested system or application. For example, a health care provider must be authenticated to the laboratory system, or the user of an E-mailbox must be accurately identified (Quinn et al., 1997). Authentication uses mechanisms such as user names, passwords,

Table 9.2   Security Legislation

Legal Protection	Purpose
Privacy Protection Act of 1980 (Title 11)	Enables the attorney general to access documents that are confidential, such as medical records (Saba and McCormick, 1996, p. 167).
Electronic Communications Privacy Act of 1986	Makes it a crime to own an electronic, mechanical, or other device primarily for the purpose of the surreptitious interception of wire, oral, or electronic communication (Saba and McCormick, 1996, p. 167).
Computer Fraud and Abuse Act of 1984 (amended in 1986)	Specifies that it is a crime to access a federal computer without authorization in order to alter, destroy, or damage information (Saba and McCormick, 1996, p. 167).
Copyright Act	Protects the textual, pictorial, or musical expression embodied in a work; makes it a federal offense to reproduce computer software without authorization (Saba and McCormick, 1996, p. 167).
Health Insurance Portability and Accountability Act of 1996	Monumental legislation that mandates the federal government to propose health data security rules. The 1998 Proposed Security Rules require organizations to implement "specific administrative, physical safeguards, and technical procedures to ensure the security and confidentiality of health care data." The use of encryption software is also required for the transmission of health information over the Internet or other "open" networks, such as dial-in lines (Siwicki, 1998).

and biometric identification (such as fingerprint or retinal scan). Typically, a user identifies himself or herself to the system and then authenticates his/her identity by providing a second piece of information that is known only by the user (e.g. a password), held only by the user (e.g. digital signature), or attributable only to the user (e.g. fingerprint).

Authorization and Access Control   Authorization determines who has the privilege of access to a system or application (both within and outside of the organization). Access is the privilege to approach, inspect, review, and make use of data or information (Quinn et al., 1998). Access control limits the resources of a system to only those users, programs, processes, and other systems that are properly authorized. Therefore, organizations should establish and update an information use policy to prevent unauthorized access. Further mechanisms should also be employed to control subsequent reading, writing, modification, and deletion of applications and data (Quinn et al., 1998). The traditional mechanism for implementing access control is an access control list (ACL), which is typically associated with a particular resource (e.g. files and databases) and specifies permissions that predefined users may perform on these resources.

Integrity   Integrity is used to support information accuracy to ensure that data have not been altered or destroyed in an unauthorized manner. It is imperative to

have program integrity (protecting software design), system integrity (protecting the system's capabilities to perform its functions), and network integrity (protecting local and wide area networks) for tight computer and system security. Without integrity, there could be inaccessible data, garbled data, the insertion of viruses, or the misidentification of a patient by a destination system. Undetected integrity problems could have detrimental results such as the wrong demographic information being associated with a piece of clinical data or claims made for services that were not rendered (Quinn et al., 1998). Mechanisms for protection of data integrity include error detection/error correction protocols.

Accountability   Accountability ensures that the actions of any entity can be traced during the movement of data from the source to the recipient. It holds users responsible for actions tracked, such as breaching confidentiality or not complying with operational procedures (Quinn et al., 1998). Auditing is typically accomplished through audit trails that are chronological records of activities occurring in the system during use. These records typically contain the identification of the user, data source, person about whom the health information is recorded, provider facility, time and date, and nature of the activity (e.g. modify, copy, append) (Computer-based Patient Record Institute, retrieved February 10, 1999). Audit trails involve a reactive process, since they capture system activity as it happens; thus, they do not prevent the activities from occurring. However, if users are aware of the auditing process, they may be deterred from misuse.

Availability   Availability ensures that information is immediately accessible and usable for an authorized entity. This is imperative as health care providers use information systems to make decisions that affect patient care outcomes, treatment choices, and diagnosis (Quinn et al., 1998). To ensure system availability, one should consider using system, data, and communications backups; protecting and restricting system access; and protecting against computer viruses. Typically, physical and/ or procedural control mechanisms provide the primary support for system availability.

Data Storage   Data storage requires protecting and maintaining the physical location of the data as well as the data itself. An organization must establish security policies that include procedures for physically protecting processors, storage media, cables, terminals, and workstations. The policies should also include system maintenance responsibilities and procedures for protection against sabotage. Additionally, there are legal and regulatory mandates regarding the retention of data such as preservation of format and storage period of time requirements (Quinn et al., 1998).

Data Transmission   Data transmission involves "the exchange of data between person and program, or program and program, when the sender and receiver are remote from each other" (Quinn et al., 1998). Transmitting and accessing health data in a secure manner that ensures integrity and confidentiality is critical as systems are used to share information with many requestors (e.g. payers, other providers). Security features must be employed that both protect the data as well as the network itself. Encryption and firewalls are typically utilized to protect health information. Encryption is a method that scrambles readable information into a mess of characters as it travels between computer users (Siwicki, 1997c). Only the original senders and receivers (with the appropriate "keys") are then able to unscramble and "read" the information. This ensures both the integrity of the information and that unauthorized persons can't "understand" the information. Firewalls can provide a strong defense against outsider attacks. They reduce the attacks on a private network from other networks, including the Internet and other corporate networks (both internal and external) and restrict the set of external services available to insiders. A firewall serves as a "filtering" mechanism in that only authorized "traffic" going in

and out of the network will be allowed to pass through (Computer-based Patient Record Institute, retrieved February 11, 1999).

Data Security Technologies

There are a number of security technologies available to protect data storage, maintenance, and transmission in the electronic age. Technological tools can help ensure the granting and restriction of access to users with legitimate needs. This is accomplished through the use of passwords, access codes, other identifying mechanisms such as biometrics (e.g. iris scans and fingerprints), and lockout of communications, computers, and display systems (*For the Record*, 1997, p. 93–94; Morrissey, 1996). Encryption, firewalls, and system back-up technologies can be utilized to maintain and transmit health data in a secure manner as well as to keep others from entering into a network. Technology provides an electronic mechanism to track users including details about information access, identity of the requester, the date and time of the request, the source and destination of the request, a descriptor of the information retrieved, and the reason for access (*For the Record*, 1997, p. 97). This helps to identify unauthorized users and to hold them accountable for their illegal actions. Technical mechanisms also offer means for authentication such as by using digital signatures and digital certification to verify users. Tools can also be employed to de-identify personal health data for research purposes to protect privacy interests in personally identifiable information (*For the Record*, 1997, p. 192). Technological improvements will continue to enhance the capability to protect health care information as the health care marketplace continues to change.

Organizational Privacy, Confidentiality, and Security Policies

It is important to recognize that technological applications alone are not successful in protecting health information. Just as important is the need for an organization to establish a clear information security policy that covers privacy and confidentiality, information security, and personnel policies. This policy defines and documents a health care organization's philosophy on security, their protection of health care data, and establishes guidelines for personnel. It should include new staff and ongoing privacy and security awareness and training programs as well as enforcement mechanisms for violations (Olson et al., 1998). In addition to security and personnel procedures, the policy should address the following important confidentiality issues:

- Access rights—who should have access to what type of information and for which purposes (should provide written policies for staff to understand)
- Release of information—procedures for release to the patient, other health care providers, and third parties (should have written confidentiality agreements in place for employees and external entities to sign)
- Specific information—determine if there should be different levels of protection or any special handling for certain information (such as HIV results or psychiatric notes)
- Integrity of medical information—procedures for positively identifying users, handling of information revisions or addenda
- Methods for communication of medical information—determine the approved methods for communicating such as Internet, fax, E-mail (Olson et al., 1998).

Summary of the Current Legislative Environment

Inadequate Legal Protections

From the previous sections, it is clear that there is an inadequate legal environment for protecting the privacy, confidentiality, and security of health information. Currently, there exists no comprehensive federal law and only a patchwork of inconsistent state laws that protect health information. This inadequate legal environment continues to serve as a barrier when data are transmitted electronically across state borders. It also proves difficult for patients, health care providers, health care organizations, integrated delivery organizations, research institutions, and information system vendors to determine their appropriate rights, responsibilities, and duties.

Does HIPAA Provide Hope?

There may be some legislative hope for protecting the privacy, confidentiality, and security of health information with the passage of the 1996 Health Insurance Portability and Accountability Act. As previously mentioned, HIPAA is a monumental act that attempts to address and incorporate all three issues within one law.

As briefly mentioned, HIPAA mandates the development of a national health information privacy law, data security standards, and specific electronic transactions standards. It provides penalties for standards violations

and wrongful disclosures of health information. It calls for the Secretary of DHHS to adopt standards for a universal health identifier (UHI) for each individual, employer, and health care provider within the health care system (Lander and Daniel, 1997). To date, UHI standards for employers and health care providers have been proposed, but the Clinton Administration has put off creating a UHI for each individual, at least until privacy protections have been put in place (Health Care Financing Administration, 1998). The idea of assigning every person a number has caused deep concern, especially from privacy advocates and the public (Charles and Edwards, 1998). HIPAA's impact will be felt by almost all involved in health care, since most must comply with its somewhat daunting mandates or face severe penalties. It is at least a first step in the right direction, but time will tell how well the law's intent and expectations will be met. DHHS's proposed security rules and privacy recommendations have already resulted in the emergence of controversial issues and tension in many organizations.

HIPAA's Data Security Standards

In August 1998, in accordance with HIPAA's mandate, DHHS proposed security standards to protect all electronic health data from improper access or alteration and to protect against loss of records. The proposed regulations included technical guidance and administrative requirements for those using electronic health information. Specifically, DHHS proposed that "All health plans, healthcare providers, and healthcare clearinghouses that maintain or transmit health information electronically will be required to establish and maintain responsible and appropriate safeguards to ensure the integrity and confidentiality of the information" (Health Care Financing Administration, 1998). The regulations allow for flexibility by recognizing that not all security needs are the same for all entities; thus, security plans may vary in sophistication level depending on the entity. DHHS recommended training for employees, administrative procedures (internal audits, maintaining an emergency plan), physical safeguards, and technical security mechanisms to protect data during transmission and storage (Health Care Financing Administration, 1998). The proposed rules also state that digital signatures must be used when an electronic signature is required for one of the standard transactions specified in the law (Health Care Financing Administration, 1998).

Many provider and health plan associations have openly opposed the proposed rules due to concerns that the regulations would increase administrative burdens and costs. The American Medical Association (AMA) likens the rules to "micromanagement of physicians' offices." The AMA Executive Vice President and CEO E. Ratcliffe Anderson Jr., MD, stated in his letter to HCFA, "The depth and volume of regulatory detail proposed are totally incompatible with, and even hostile to, the administrative simplification envisioned by the law's drafters. We anticipate that the cumulative effect of the mandatory implementation measures, practices and procedures would overwhelm many physicians' practices" (Aston, 1998). Bruce Bagley, MD, American Academy of Family Physicians president-elect reported that the set of regulations, "smells like the CLIA—They're [HCFA] asking you to do the right thing but in a way that is onerous" (Aston, 1998). The American Association of Health Plans states that the rules require security technologies "that are immature, lack standardization and are not sufficiently robust to adopt within the given time line" (Aston, 1998). HCFA must take into consideration the provider-oriented concerns as well as other regulatory comments from the industry before promulgating the final rules expected in 2000. Compliance is mandated 24 months after the date of the final regulations. Small health plans have 36 months to comply (Health Care Financing Administration, 1998).

The Privacy Law Debate

HIPAA required DHHS to deliver recommendations to Congress to enact federal legislation to protect the privacy of healthcare information. In September 1997, the Secretary of DHHS, presented recommendations to Congress that detailed five principles healthcare officials should consider as they set up information systems.

- Boundaries—restrict data to healthcare uses
- Security—require protections against misuse and unauthorized disclosure
- Consumer Control—patients have the right to see and correct (or amend) data
- Accountability—penalties for violations
- Public Responsibility—limited access for the public good.

Congress failed to enact legislation by its mandated deadline of August 1999; therefore, DHHS must promulgate privacy regulations. As of the writing of this chapter, DHHS has published a Notice of Proposed Rulemaking but has not yet issued final regulations.

Once final regulations are promulgated, Congress may still enact medical privacy legislation.

Issues to Consider in Federal Law

Many controversial issues must be resolved in the medical information privacy debate before DHHS promulgates the final regulations or Congress passes national privacy legislation. The following lists the key issues in the debate and the major users and their interests. Where do you stand on these issues? Do you think all of these issues can be resolved in a manner to serve all interest groups?

- How to appropriately balance privacy rights with those who need access to information.
- What categories of information should be protected ("identifiable" versus all health information).
- What entities or persons should have access to what type of information (employers, insurance companies, individuals, research institutions, etc.).
- Should law enforcement require a warrant or a less stringent legal proceeding to access medical information.
- Should there be a "ceiling" or "floor" preemption (determines how this federal law interacts with state laws—"ceiling" preemption means federal law supercedes all state laws, and "floor" preemption means that states may pass more stringent laws).
- When is patient authorization required for disclosure of information for primary (medical care) and secondary (research, marketing, etc.) uses of information.
- What patients' rights should be granted (access, amend, copy medical information/medical records).
- How to enforce these provisions.

Users of Health Data

As listed below, there are many users with legitimate needs in the medical information law debate. Again, the goal is to adequately balance the sometimes competing needs— privacy rights of individuals and the needs of those who require access to health information for the public good.

- Health care providers (need access to accurate information; safeguard privacy in order to maintain trust in the health care provider/ patient relationship for best medical care)

- Patients (understand legal rights; access to records; authorize information disclosure; amend records; copy records)
- Privacy right advocates (make sure patients' rights are safeguarded and understood; ensure accountability for violations)
- Health care organizations (need for ready access to accurate data; ease of access to data; delivering high quality care)
- Research institutions and associations (ease of access to needed data for research)
- Public health departments, government agencies (need data for research; public health reporting)
- Insurance companies (need data for processing claims; determining fraud)
- Law enforcement (need for evidence of criminal activity in such cases as sexual abuse or shootings; need to detect fraud and abuse)
- Accrediting bodies (ensuring information is kept confidential and secure; obtaining accurate data on such elements as outcomes measures).

Accreditation Requirements

Hospitals, HMOs, and health care organizations seeking accreditation from private authorities are required to meet standards regarding privacy, confidentiality, and security of health information.

The Joint Commission on Accreditation of Healthcare Organizations (JCAHO) requires accredited hospitals to maintain the "confidentiality, security, and integrity of data and information" (Joint Commission of Accreditation of Healthcare Organizations, 1997a). JCAHO also requires hospitals to identify and establish what type of information is considered "secure and confidential" (Joint Commission of Accreditation of Healthcare Organizations, 1997b) and extends the security and confidentiality standards to situations "where external data bases are contributed to or used" (Joint Commission of Accreditation of Healthcare Organizations, 1997c). JCAHO also created information management standards for "networks," which covers the following:

- Information management processes protecting the confidentiality, security, and integrity of information (Joint Commission of Accreditation of Healthcare Organizations, 1996a).

- The network and its components determining appropriate levels of security and confidentiality of data and information and safeguarding records against tampering, loss, destruction, and unauthorized access or use (Joint Commission of Accreditation of Healthcare Organizations, 1996b).
- Timely, easy data retrieval without compromising security and confidentiality (Joint Commission of Accreditation of Healthcare Organizations, 1996c).

The National Committee for Quality Assurance (NCQA), the body that accredits managed care entities, requires physician organizations seeking accreditation to have established policies and procedures to protect the confidentiality of medical records (National Committee for Quality Assurance, 1997).

In November 1998, JCAHO and NCQA jointly issued a report, "Protecting Personal Health Information: A Framework for Meeting the Challenges in a Managed Care Environment," that provided recommendations to address the demands for personal health information by managed care organizations, health care providers, employers, quality oversight organizations, regulators, and researchers. The report focused on the following issues:

- Dealing with consent in an evolving health care delivery and financing system
- Ensuring accountability
- Educating about policies, practices, rights, and responsibilities
- Using technology as a solution
- Providing legislative support
- Guiding research (Mitka, 1998).

These recommendations may surface in future accreditation requirements.

Summary

The National Research Council reported in 1997 that the greatest concerns regarding the privacy of health information come from (1) widespread sharing of patient information throughout the health care industry and (2) the inadequate federal and state laws for systemic protection of health information (Siwicki, 1997b). This chapter addressed these two major concerns and others. It provided an overview of the privacy, confidentiality, and security of health information. It emphasized the importance of protecting data in the electronic age. It recognized the balance to be struck between protecting privacy and accessing data for legitimate needs by authorized persons. It described the technological mechanisms available to help ensure data security and briefly defined key security terms. It emphasized that adequate protection of health care information depends on both technological and organizational policies. It reviewed the current state and federal legislative environment for protecting the privacy, confidentiality, and security of health information. The importance of federal privacy legislation, the issues in the current debate, and the key players were also discussed. The chapter concluded with accreditation requirements.

References

American Medical Association. (1999). *Comprehensive Guide to Electronic Health Records.* New York: Faulkner & Gray.

American Society for Testing and Materials Committee E-31 on Healthcare Informatics, Subcommittee E31.17 on Privacy, Confidentiality, and Access. (1997). *Standard Guide for Confidentiality, Privacy, Access, and Data Security Principles for Health Information Including Computer Based Patient Records,* Philadelphia: ASTM Designation: E 1869-97.

Aston, G. (1998). Doctors, health plans reject data security proposal. *American Medical News,* 5(1) November 2.

Charles, D., and Edwards, B. (1998). Privacy concerns kill medical database. NPR Morning Edition, November 26.

Computer-based Patient Record Institute. Confidentiality of CPRs. *http://www.cpri.org/conf.html* (retrieved February 10, 1999).

Computer-based Patient Record Institute. *Security Features for Computer-Based Patient Record Systems. http://www.cpri.org/docs/features.html/* (retrieved February 11, 1999).

For the Record: Protecting Electronic Health Information. (1997). Washington, DC: National Academy Press.

George, M. (1999). U-M fixes error, takes medical files off web. *Detroit Free Press,* State Edition, Section: NWS, Page 3B, February 12.

Health Care Financing Administration. (1998). HHS *Proposes Security Standards For Electronic Health Data.* Press Release, Tuesday, August 11. *http://aspe.os.dhhs.gov/admnsimp/nprm/press3.htm*

Joint Commission for the Accreditation of Healthcare Organizations. (1996a). *Comprehensive Accreditation Manual for Hospitals,* IM.2.

Joint Commission for the Accreditation of Healthcare Organizations. (1996b). *Comprehensive Accreditation Manual for Hospitals,* IM.2.1, IM.2.3.

Joint Commission for the Accreditation of Healthcare Organizations. (1996c). *Comprehensive Accreditation Manual for Hospitals,* IM.2.2.

Joint Commission for Accreditation of Healthcare Organizations. (1997a). *Comprehensive Accreditation Manual for Hospitals,* IM.2.

Joint Commission for the Accreditation of Healthcare Organizations. (1997b). *Comprehensive Accreditation Manual for Hospitals,* IM.2.1.

Joint Commission for the Accreditation of Healthcare Organizations. (1997c). *Comprehensive Accreditation Manual for Hospitals,* IM.10.3.

Kibbe, D., and Bard, M. R. (1997). How safe are computerized patient records? *Family Practice Management. http://www.aarp.org/family/fpm/9/ 0500fm/lead.html*

Lander, M. L., and Daniel, A. (1997). The journey to the electronic health record. *Healthcare Informatics,* October 1997, Industry Report Supplement, page IR 8.

Mitka, M. (1998). Do-it-yourself report on patient privacy. *Journal of the American Medical Association,* December 9.

Morrissey, J. (1996). Data security: As healthcare invests heavily in computer technology, confidentiality issues may be shortchanged. *Modern Healthcare,* September 30, 35–36.

National Committee for Quality Assurance. (1997). *Standards for the Certification of Physician Organizations.* Standard MR 1.

Olson, L. A., Peters, S. G., and Stewart, J. B. (1998). Security and confidentiality in an electronic medical record. *The Journal of the Healthcare Information and Management Systems Society,* 12, 29.

Quinn, J., Jaworski, S., and Toole, J. Security and the Internet: Healthcare's concerns and approaches to think, build, and operate solutions today. *The Journal of the Healthcare Information and Management Systems Society,* Volume 12, 85.

Recommendations of the Secretary of Health and Human Services. *Confidentiality of Individually-Identifiable Health Information. http://aspe.os.hhs.gov/admnsimp/*

Riley, J. (1996). Open secrets/Your medical records/Will Bill cure ills?/Legislation on access to medical data sparks debate. *Newsday,* April 3, Section: News, page A08.

Rindfleisch, T. (1997). Privacy, information technology, and health care. *Communications of the ACM,* 40(8), 95–96.

Roach, W. H. (1998). The Aspen Health Law and Compliance Center. *Medical Records and The Law,* (3rd ed.) Maryland: Aspen Publishers.

Saba, V. K., and McCormick, K. A. (1996). Data processing: *Essentials of Computers For Nurses* (2nd ed.) New York: McGraw-Hill.

Senate Panel to Study Health-Privacy Issue. (1998). *Boston Globe,* February 26, p. D2. Pledger, M. (1998). Patients worry about privacy customers complain about telemarketing. *The Plain Dealer,* February 21, p. 1C.

Siegel, L. (1997). Privacy in the computer age; medical records: It's easy for others to make your business their business; records can fall into wrong hands. *The Salt*

Lake Tribune, April 25, Section: Nation-World; page A1.

Siwicki, B. (1997a). Health data security: A new priority. *Health Data Management, 5,* 47, September.

Siwicki, B. (1997b). Health data security: A new priority. *Health Data Management, 5,* 48, September.

Siwicki, B. (1997c). Health data security: A new priority. *Health Data Management, 5,* 56, September.

Siwicki, B. (1998). Can chief security officers protect data from prying eyes? *Health Data Management,* October, 6, 55–67.

10 Data Standards

Robert Mayes

OBJECTIVES

1. Discuss the need for data standards.
2. Describe the standards development process.
3. Identify standards development organizations.
4. Describe health care data standards initiatives.

KEY WORDS

organization and administration
standards
legislation and jurisprudence
HIPAA

There is a need to be able to share health care information across organizational boundaries, whether those are different departments within a single institution, or, as is increasingly the case, among a varied cast of providers, payers, regulators, and others. In order to enable this communication, it is necessary that there be a common set of rules and definitions, both at the level of data meaning as well as at the technical level of data exchange. In addition, there must be a socio-political framework that recognizes the benefits of shared information and supports the adoptions of such standards.

This chapter examines health care data standards in terms of the following:

■ System level communications
■ Shared meaning at the data content level.

These various standards are then placed within an organizational context through an overview of the various standards development organizations and their current efforts. A discussion of current national and international initiatives shows the interlocking nature of standards activities and the potential impact on the future of health care delivery. Specific topics described in this chapter include the following:

■ Need for data standards
■ Health care data communication standards
■ Health care data content standards
■ Data standards development

■ Health care data standards development organizations
■ Health care data standards initiatives.

Need for Health Data Standards

The National Standards Policy Advisory Committee defines standards broadly as follows: "A prescribed set of rules, conditions, or requirements concerning definition of terms; classification of components; specification of materials, performance or operations; delineation of procedures; or measurement of quantity and quality in describing materials, products, systems, services or practices" (National Standards Policy Advisory Committee, 1978, p. 6). In the domain of information management, standards can be further categorized as those that support the generic infrastructure and are not domain-specific, those that support the exchange of information and are domain-specific, and those that support activities and practices within a specific domain. Examples of the first type of standard would include equipment specifications such as processor type or network transmission protocols such as Ethernet or token ring. The second type of standard typically involves the specification of data structures and content and would include such standards as messaging formats and core data sets. The third type of standard addresses how information should be interpreted and acted upon within a particular context. An example of this type of standard would be practice guidelines. It is the second class of standards, which are commonly described as data standards, that will be the focus of the following discussion.

Health care is fundamentally a process of communication. For much of history, direct person-to-person dialog between a patient and a health care provider characterized this communication. The temporal and physical proximity of the communicators provided ample opportunity to clarify any ambiguity that might have arisen as to the meaning of what was being communicated.

Today the care process is far more complex, and even a single episode may take place across multiple settings and involve numerous parties including the patient and his social support system, providers working directly and indirectly with the patient, administrators, and payers. In addition, the information about a patient and his care is now used not only for the direct care process but also for many other purposes including reimbursement, research, public health, education, policy development, and litigation.

It is this tremendous increase in the distribution and amount of information, both physically and temporally, that has driven the need for modern information management systems in the health care domain. However, while current information technology is able to move and manipulate large amounts of data, it is not as proficient in dealing with ambiguity in the structure and semantic content of that data. Data standards are an attempt to reduce the level of ambiguity in the communication of data so that actions taken based on the data are consistent with the actual meaning of the data.

While the term "data standards" is generally used to describe those standards having to do with the structure and content of health information, it may be useful to differentiate data, information, and knowledge. Data are the fundamental building blocks upon which health care decisions are based. Data are collections of unstructured, discrete entities (facts) that exist outside of any particular context. When data are interpreted within a given context and given meaningful structure within that context, they become information. When information from various contexts is aggregated following a defined set of rules, it becomes knowledge and provides the basis for informed action (Saba and McCormick, 1996, p. 231). Data standards cover both data and their transformation into information. Analysis generates knowledge, which is the foundation of practice standards.

Data Communication Standards

Data communication standards address, primarily, the format of messages that are exchanged between computer systems and the coding and classification schemes used within the messages. In order to achieve data compatibility between systems, it is necessary to have prior agreement on the syntax of the messages to be exchanged. The receiving system must be able to parse the incoming message into discrete data elements that reflect what the sending system wishes to communicate. In addition to a common message format, it is also necessary that the individual data elements be structured in a common way as well. Although there is a great deal of activity around the development of natural language processing capabilities, most health data exchange still involves coded, or structured, information. The following section describes some of the major organizations involved in the development of message format and coding and classification standards.

Message Format Standards

Four broad classes of message format standards have emerged in the health care sector: medical device communications, digital imaging communications, administrative data exchange, and clinical data exchange. It should be noted that there is considerable overlap among standards development activities, and there may be more than one standard available for each of these classes.

Institute of Electrical and Electronic Engineers   The Institute of Electrical and Electronic Engineers (IEEE) has developed a series of standards known collectively as P1073 Medical Information Bus (MIB), which support real-time, continuous, and comprehensive capture and communication of data from bedside medical devices such as those found in intensive care units, operating rooms, and emergency departments. These data include physiological parameter measurements and device settings. These standards are used internationally.

National Electrical Manufacturers Association   The National Electrical Manufacturers Association (NEMA), in collaboration with the American College of Radiologists (ACR) and others, formed the Digital Imaging Communication in Medicine Standards Committee (DICOM) to develop a generic digital format and a transfer protocol for biomedical images and image-related information. The specification is usable on any type of computer system and supports transfer over the Internet. The DICOM standard is the dominant international data interchange message format in biomedical imaging.

Accredited Standards Committee X12N/Insurance   Accredited Standards Committee (ASC) X12N has developed a broad range of electronic data interchange (EDI) standards to facilitate electronic business transactions. In the health care arena, X12N standards have been proposed for adoption as national standards for such administrative transactions as claims, enrollment and eligibility in health plans, and first report of injury under the requirements of the Health Insurance Portability and Accountability Act of 1996 (HIPAA). Due to the uniqueness of health insurance practices from country to country, these standards are primarily used in the United States.

National Council for Prescription Drug Programs

The National Council for Prescription Drug Programs (NCPDP) develops standards for information processing for the pharmacy services sector of the health care industry. This has been a very successful example of how standards can enable significant improvements in service delivery. Since the introduction of this standard in 1992, the retail pharmacy industry has moved to almost 100% electronic claims processing in real time. As with the X12N standards, the NCPDP standards are primarily used in the United States.

Health Level 7   Health Level 7 (HL7) standards focus on facilitating the interchange of data to support clinical practice both within and across institutions. The major areas covered by the standard include medical orders; clinical observations; test results; admission, transfer, and discharge; and charge and billing information. Since 1997, HL7 and ASC X12N have been collaborating on the development of a joint standard for claims attachments, with X12N supplying the transmission envelope and HL7 the internal message structure. HL7 is widely supported by health information systems vendors worldwide, and there are over a dozen foreign affiliates, which have adapted the basic standard for use in their particular settings.

Coding and Classification Standards

A fundamental requirement for effective communication is the ability to represent concepts in an unambiguous fashion between both the sender and receiver of the message. Natural human languages are incredibly rich in their ability to communicate subtle differences in the semantic content, or meaning, of messages. While there have been great advances in the ability of computers to process natural language, most communication between health information systems relies on the use of structured vocabularies, code sets, and classification systems to represent health care concepts. The following examples describe a few of the major systems.

International Statistical Classification of Diseases and Related Health Problems: Ninth Revision and Clinical Modifications (World Health Organization, 1980)   The International Statistical Classification of Diseases and Related Health Problems: Ninth Revision and Clinical Modifications (ICD-9-CM) is the latest version of a mortality and morbidity classification that originated in 1893. The ICD-9-CM has been the sole classification used for morbidity reporting in the United States since 1979. It is widely accepted and used in the health care industry and has been adopted for a number of purposes including data collection, quality-of-care analysis, resource utilization, and statistical reporting. It is the basis for the diagnostic related groups (DRGs), which are used extensively for hospital reimbursement. ICD-9-CM is used primarily in the United States. Internationally, ICD-9 is used for death tabulation.

International Statistical Classification of Diseases and Related Health Problems: Tenth Revision (World Health Organization, 1992)   The International Statistical Classification of Diseases and Related Health Problems: Tenth Revision (ICD-10) is the most recent revision of the ICD classification system for mortality and morbidity, which is used worldwide. In addition to diagnostic labels, the ICD-10 also encompasses nomenclature structures. The U.S. version, ICD-10-CM, is currently planned for implementation in October 2000.

Current Procedural Terminology, Fourth Revision (American Medical Association, 1992)   The Current Procedural Terminology, Fourth Revision (CPT-4) is a listing of descriptive terms and codes for reporting medical services and procedures. In addition to descriptive terms and codes, it contains modifiers, notes, and guidelines to facilitate correct usage. While primarily used in the United States for reimbursement purposes, it has, like ICD-9-CM, been adopted for other data purposes. Its use internationally has slowly increased.

Systemized Nomenclature of Human and Veterinary Medicine International (College of American Pathologists, 1993)   SNOMED International is a comprehensive, multi-axial nomenclature and classification system created for indexing human and veterinary medical vocabulary, including signs and symptoms, diagnoses, and procedures. It has gained increasing international acceptance as a standard for recording medical record information since its introduction in 1993. It is being used by a number of health professional specialty groups, and a subset of SNOMED is used in the DICOM imaging standard.

There are many more vocabularies, code sets, and classification systems in addition to those described above. These include the Logical Observation Identifier Names and Codes (LOINC), Nursing Interventions Classification (NIC), Current Dental Terminology (CDT), International Medical Terminology (IMT), and Diagnostic and Statistical Manual of Mental Disorders (DSM-III-R) to name just a few. There have been a number of efforts to develop mapping and linkages among various code sets, classification systems, and vocabularies. One of the most successful is the Unified Medical Language System (UMLS) project undertaken by the U.S. National Library of Medicine.

Unified Medical Language System   There are specialized vocabularies, code sets, and classification systems for almost every practice domain in health care. Most of these are not compatible with one another, and much work needs to be done to achieve usable mapping and linkages between them. In 1986, the U.S. National Library of Medicine began an ambitious long-term project to map and link a large number of vocabularies from a number of knowledge sources to allow retrieval and integration of relevant machine-readable information. Currently, the UMLS consists of a metathesaurus of terms and concepts from dozens of vocabularies; a semantic network of relationships among the concepts recognized in the metathesaurus; and an information sources map of the various biomedical databases referenced.

Data Content Standards

In addition to standardizing the format of health data messages and the lexicons and value domains used in those messages, there has been a great deal of interest in defining common sets of data for specific message types. The concept of a minimum data set is that of "a minimum set of items with uniform definitions and categories concerning a specific aspect or dimension of the health care system which meets the essential needs of multiple users" (Health Information Policy Council, 1983). A related concept is that of a core data element. It has been defined as "a standard data element with a uniform definition and coding convention to collect data on persons and on events or encounters" (National Committee on Vital and Health Statistics, 1996). Core data elements are seen as serving as the building blocks for well-formed minimum data sets and may appear in several minimum data sets.

As with vocabularies and code sets, there are many minimum data sets in place or under development. A

recent survey of public and private sector efforts in the development of minimum data sets and core data elements reported on 17 such sets in use nationally (McCormick et al., 1997). The following are some brief examples of minimum, or core, data sets currently in use. As with code sets, professional specialty groups are the best source for current information on minimum data set development efforts. A number of the standards development organizations (SDOs) who develop messaging format standards, such as HL7 and ASC X12N, have been increasingly interested in incorporating domain-specific data sets into their message standards.

National Uniform Claim Committee Recommended Data Set for a Noninstitutional Claim (American Medical Association, 1997)

The National Uniform Claim Committee (NUCC) was organized in 1995 to develop, promote, and maintain a standard data set for use in noninstitutional claims and encounter information. The Committee is chaired by the American Medical Association, and its member organizations represent a number of the major public and private sector payers. The current NUCC data set forms the basis for the proposed noninstitutional claim and encounter standard proposed for national adoption under HIPAA.

Standard Guide for Content and Structure of the Computer-Based Patient Record (ASTM E1384-96) (American Society for Testing and Materials, 1996)

The American Society for Testing and Materials (ASTM) is one of the largest SDOs in the world and publishes over 9,000 standards covering all sectors in the economy. Committee E31 on Healthcare Informatics has developed a wide range of standards supporting the electronic management of health information. E1384-96 provides a framework vocabulary for the computer-based patient record content. It proposes a minimum essential content drawn from a developing annex of dictionary elements. It is used in conjunction with ASTM E1633-95, Standard Specification for Coded Values for the Computer-Based Patient Record (American Society for Testing and Materials, 1995).

Data Elements for Emergency Department Systems (Centers for Disease Control and Prevention, 1996)

The Data Elements for Emergency Department Systems (DEEDS) data set was developed by the Division of Acute

Care, Rehabilitation Research and Disability Prevention, National Center for Injury Prevention and Control, Centers for Disease Control and Prevention (CDC). It is intended for use in hospital-based emergency departments and to provide the basis for sharing of data among local, state, and national organizations involved in tracking injury statistics. The data elements have been designed to be incorporated into computer-based patient records, and each element is also linked to a HL7 message segment.

The Standards Development Process

The development and adoption of data standards is not only a technical process; it takes place within a socio-political context. Initially, there must be recognition that potential ambiguity exists at a level that would significantly impair communication and that this impairment is unacceptable within the social context. In health care, there is an increasing recognition that there exist significant opportunities to improve the quality of care provided and the outcomes associated with that care. It has also been recognized that any potential improvement in quality of care depends greatly on the ability to communicate health care information efficiently and effectively. In its final report, the President's Advisory Commission on Consumer Protection and Quality in the Health Care Industry identified improving information systems as one of the key elements for building the capacity to improve the quality of health care on a national level. Among its specific recommendations, the Commission stated that, "National standards for the structure, content, definition, and coding of health information should be established to support improvements in information systems" (President's Advisory Commission on Consumer Protection and Quality in the Health Care Industry, 1998, p. 17).

Identification of a need for standardization, while necessary for development and implementation of standards, is not, in itself, sufficient. As with all things in life, there is never only one way to accomplish consistent communication of health information. Indeed, an old joke among standards developers is that the nice thing about standards is that there are so many to choose from. Standards are resource-intensive to develop and to implement, particularly if an organization is already using a different way to do things. For this reason, widespread adoption of particular standards always involves "winners and losers" and so becomes a political process.

While standards, when adopted, drive a consensus approach to data and information exchange and management, it does not follow that the development and adoption processes themselves are the result of a consensus-based methodology. There are primarily three ways in which standards are commonly developed and adopted: proprietary standards developed by vendors who hold a dominant position in the market; legislated standards developed by government organizations; and consensus-based standards developed by SDOs and adopted by virtue of their utility. An example of the first is CPT-4, developed by the American Medical Association and used for reimbursement of medical services and procedures. There are numerous examples of government-developed and -mandated standards, such as the Long-term Care Minimum Data Set required by the U.S. Health Care Financing Administration (HCFA) to be reported for all long-term care residents in Medicare-certified long-term care facilities. An example of the third group is the messaging standards developed by the HL7 standards development organization and supported by a majority of health information systems vendors. Each of these approaches has its advantages and disadvantages.

Proprietary standards can often be developed quickly and are supported by available implementations and tools. If the developer can maintain a dominant market position, the standards can gain widespread acceptance quickly. While proprietary standards can respond quickly to technological changes, they can, paradoxically, also result in a delay in the adoption of new technologies as the creator of the standard wishes to gain a maximum return on the investment required to develop the standard in its current form. It may also not be responsive to changes in the environment, since it will reflect primarily the view of the creating organization and its market interests. Finally, in a sector as fragmented as health care, it is difficult for any organization to gain and retain the requisite dominant market position.

Legislated, government-developed standards are able to gain widespread acceptance by virtue of their being required by either regulation or in order to participate in large, government-funded programs, such as Medicare. Because government-developed standards are in the public domain, they are available at little or no costs and can be incorporated into any information system. However, they are often developed to support particular government initiatives and not be as suitable for general, private sector use. Also, given the amount of bureaucratic overhead attached to the legislative and regulatory process, it is likely that they will lag behind changes in technology and the general business environment.

Standards developed by SDOs are consensus based and reflect the perspectives of a wide variety of interested stakeholders. They are generally not tied to specific systems. For this reason, they tend to be robust and adaptable across a range of implementations. However, most SDOs are voluntary organizations that rely on the commitment of dedicated individuals and organizations to develop and maintain standards. This often limits the amount of work that can be undertaken. In addition, the consensus process can be time consuming and result in a slow development process, which does not always keep pace with technological change. Perhaps the most problematic aspect of consensus-based standards is that there is no mechanism to ensure that they are adopted by the industry, since there is usually little infrastructure in place to actively and aggressively market them. This has resulted in the development of many technically competent standards that are never implemented.

It is increasingly recognized that combining the strength of these approaches tends to minimize their weaknesses and can lead to significant gains for the health care sector as a whole. This melding of approaches is being achieved both at the organizational level by the development of coordinating bodies and consortia, and through the development of several national, government-directed initiatives.

Standards Coordination Efforts

It has become clear to both public and private sector standards development efforts that no one entity has the resources to create an exhaustive set of health data standards that will meet all needs. In addition to the various SDOs described above, the following organizations have been developed at the international, regional, and national levels to try and create a synergistic relationship between their member organizations. These larger organizations are involved in standards development across all sectors of the economy. Since many of the data standards issues in health care, such as security, are not unique to the health care sector, this breadth of scope offers the potential for technology transfer across sectors. The following is a brief description of some of the major international, regional, and national organizations involved in broad-based standards development and coordination.

International Standards Organization

The International Standards Organization (ISO) is an organization that develops and publishes standards internationally. ISO standards are developed, in large part, from standards brought forth by member countries. Often, these national standards are further broadened to reflect the greater diversity of the international community. In 1998, ISO Technical Committee 215 on

Health Informatics was formed to coordinate the development of international health care information standards, including data standards.

European Technical Committee for Standardization

In 1990, Technical Committee 251 on Medical Informatics was established by the European Committee for Standardization (CEN). CEN TC251 works to develop a wide variety of standards in the area of health care data management and interchange. CEN standards are adopted by its member countries in Europe and are also submitted for development into ISO standards.

American National Standards Institute

The American National Standards Institute (ANSI) serves as the coordinator for voluntary standards activity in the United States. Standards are submitted to ANSI by member SDOs and are approved as American National Standards through a consensus methodology developed by ANSI. ANSI is also the U.S. representative to ISO and is responsible for bringing forward U.S. standards to that organization. In 1991, the ANSI Healthcare Informatics Standards Planning Panel was convened to act as a coordinating forum for both SDOs and other stakeholders in the area of health information standards. Rechartered as the ANSI Healthcare Informatics Standards Board (HISB) in 1996, ANSI HISB does not write standards but serves as a forum to identify needs and coordinate activities related to health care information standardization. All of the major health care SDOs are HISB members, as well as a number of government agencies involved in health data standards and several major vendors of health information systems.

Object Management Group

While the organizations described so far are made up of voluntary SDOs, the Object Management Group (OMG) is representative of a different approach to standards development. OMG is an international consortium of over 800 organizations, primarily for-profit vendors of information systems technology, who are interested in the development of standards based on object-oriented technologies. While its standards are developed by private organizations, it has developed a process to lessen the potential problems noted above with proprietary standards. Standards developed in OMG are required to be implemented in a commercially available product by their developers within one year of the standard being accepted. However, the specifications for the standard are made publicly available. The OMG CORBAMed working group is responsible for development of object-based standards in the health information arena.

National Health Data Standards Initiatives

In its revised edition of its seminal 1991 report, *The Computer-Based Patient Record*, the Institute of Medicine (IOM) wrote in the preface: "Leadership at the Federal level is required to ensure that standards necessary to preserve and enhance health care in the United States are developed. Until standards exist for uniquely identifying individuals and coding and exchanging health data, the value from capturing and aggregating data will go unrealized and each organization will be its own pioneer" (Dick and Steen, 1991).

This sentiment reflects a growing recognition in the United States (and indeed has corollaries in other countries) that the adoption of health data standards on a national level is unlikely to occur in a timely fashion without the involvement of the federal government. However, it is also recognized that merely creating another layer of regulatory oversight is not effective and that a new approach that partners the federal government with a wide range of public and private stakeholders, including SDOs, is more likely to achieve success. There are several current initiatives that reflect this new approach.

Health Insurance Portability and Accountability Act

Perhaps the single most important advance in the adoption of national health data standards was the passage in 1996 of HIPAA. It has been estimated that, on average, 26 cents of every dollar intended for health care is spent on administrative overhead. Administrative overhead includes such tasks as enrolling an individual in a health plan, paying health insurance premiums, checking insurance eligibility, getting authorization to refer a patient to a specialist, filing a claim for insurance reimbursement for delivered health care, requesting additional information to support a claim, coordinating the processing of a claim across different insurance companies, and notifying the provider about the payment of a claim. These processes involve numerous paper forms and telephone calls and many delays in communicating information between different locations, creating problems and costs for health care providers, plans, and insurers

alike. To address these problems, the health care industry has been attempting to develop standards to allow these transactions to be accomplished electronically, but it has been very difficult to get voluntary agreement from all of the competing parties involved to adopt a uniform set of such standards. Consequently, at the request of the industry, and with bipartisan support, Congress included the Administrative Simplification provisions (Title II, Subtitle F) in the HIPAA (Public Law 104-191, 1996), which was signed into law August 21, 1996. The industry estimates that full implementation of these provisions could save up to $9 billion per year from administrative overhead without reducing the amount or quality of health care services (Workgroup for Electronic Data Interchange (WEDI), 1993).

To make these savings in cost and administrative efficiency a reality, the law charges the U.S. Secretary of Health and Human Services with establishing standards for a broad range of health information, including health insurance claims and encounters; health claims attachments; health insurance enrollment and eligibility; health identifiers for providers, health plans, employers, and individuals; code sets; and classification systems. To address concerns about the potential for abuse of electronic access to this type of information, the law also requires standards for the security and confidentiality of health information that might be associated with an individual. In addition to general security and confidentiality standards, the HIPAA requires the adoption of a standard for electronic signatures. Civil and criminal penalties are prescribed for failure to use standards or for wrongful disclosure of confidential information. The schedule for adoption and implementation of these standards is an aggressive one. Within 24-36 months after adoption of the standards by regulation, all health plans, providers, and insurers engaged in electronic health care commerce are required to implement these standards. In addition, the HIPAA also requires privacy protections to be enacted by Congress or, as a back-up, issued by HHS to accompany the implementation of the new standards.

The law envisions that the standards adopted would, in general, be standards that have been developed, adopted, or modified by an ANSI-accredited SDO. In addition, the law requires the Secretary to rely upon the recommendations of the National Committee on Vital and Health Statistics (NCVHS), a federal advisory committee on issues in health data, standards, privacy, and health information policy. The law also requires consultation with the NUCC, the National Uniform Billing Committee (NUBC), the Workgroup on Electronic Data Interchange (WEDI), and the American Dental Association (ADA).

The Administrative Simplification subtitle of the HIPAA represents the first time that the federal government has mandated health data standards on a national level. As can be seen from this very brief overview, this standards activity is likely to have a major impact on the development of electronic health care records beyond the administrative and financial realms. In today's world of quality-focused health care delivery, the line between administrative and clinical data is very blurred indeed. While the transaction sets specified in this legislation are, perhaps, narrowly focused, the same cannot be said of the wide variety of supporting standards that must be adopted. Standards for such things as patient identifier, vocabularies, and electronic signatures have impact directly on anyone designing or implementing an electronic clinical system. In addition, the privacy legislation/regulation will cover health information in the broad sense and will apply to any system handling personally identifiable information. Another important aspect of this legislation is that it preempts state law in most cases, thus establishing a consistent legal framework for electronic exchange of certain health care data.

National Committee for Vital and Health Statistics Computer-Based Patient Record Workgroup

In addition to its focus on administrative and financial transactions, the Administrative Simplification provisions also begin the process of addressing the broader standards issues of electronic health care records in general. The subject of these recommendations and legislative proposals are set forth in Section 263 of the Administrative Simplification provisions of HIPAA. These provisions state that NCVHS:

"(B) shall study the issues related to the adoption of uniform data standards for patient medical record information and the electronic exchange of such information;
(C) shall report to the Secretary not later than 4 years after the date of the enactment of the Health Insurance Portability and Accountability Act of 1996 [August 2000] recommendations and legislative proposals for such standards and electronic exchange." (Public Law 104-191, 1996)

In order to meet this charge, the NCVHS formed the Computer-based Patient Record Workgroup. This workgroup develops recommendations based on public hearings and input from informed stakeholders and domain experts. The workgroup has identified six major areas of interest:

1. Message format standards that contain patient medical record information. This area of focus includes message format syntaxes, document format standards, the role of information models to enable the development of message format standards, and the need to coordinate standards.

2. Medical terminology related to patient medical record information including data element definitions, data models, and code sets. This area of focus includes issues related to convergent medical terminologies, coordination and maintenance of vocabularies, coordination of drug knowledge bases, and other issues related to medical terminologies.

3. Business case issues related to the development and implementation of uniform data standards for patient medical record information. This area of focus includes return-on-investment issues and the cost burden of vendors, SDOs, code set developers, and users to participate in the standards development processes.

4. National Healthcare Information Infrastructure (NHII). The vision of NHII and identification of issues related to it are being defined within the NHII workgroup of the NCVHS. The CPR workgroup will identify the standards issues necessary to support this vision.

5. Data quality, accountability, and integrity related to patient medical record information. This area of focus includes data quality issues beginning with the initial capture or recording of data, the communication of data, the translation and encoding of data, and the decoding or presentation of data. It also includes the guidelines or standards for accountability and data integrity (e.g. accuracy, consistency, continuity, completeness, context, and comparability).

6. Inconsistencies and contradictions among state laws that discourage or prevent the creation, storage, or communication of patient medical record information in a consistent manner nationwide. Inconsistencies include laws for record retention, document authentication, access to records, etc.

While it is unlikely that these recommendations will result in a complete set of legislated requirements for health data standards, the process of developing the recommendations offers a tremendous opportunity to bring together a broad coalition of stakeholders to better define specific areas where further standardization is needed.

Government Computer-Based Patient Record Project

Another federal project that has great potential for furthering health data standards is the Government Computer-Based Patient Record (GCPR) project, a collaboration between the U.S. Department of Defense, the U.S. Department of Veterans Affairs, and the U.S. Department of Health and Human Services, Indian Health Service. The goal of this ambitious project is to develop and implement a standard means of exchanging and managing health information across federal health providers. It is not attempting to develop a single federal electronic health record, but rather, it is focusing on standardizing the interface between health information systems in terms of how data are defined, structured, and exchanged.

While this project is focused solely on federal health care providers, three factors increase its general interest and impact. First is the size of the population these organizations serve. Combined, these three organizations are the largest providers of health care in the United States by a considerable margin, both in terms of persons served and organizationally in terms of number of facilities and hospital beds. They are also geographically distributed throughout the United States and, in the case of the Department of Defense, in many parts of the world. This size makes them the largest purchaser of health information system technology in the United States, and any specifications developed for the GCPR project will have a significant impact in the vendor community. A second characteristic of the project extends this potential influence further. It was decided from the outset that the project would rely on standards-based solutions and that where standards did not exist, an effort would be made to foster their development through recognized SDOs. In addition, any technologies developed for this project are to be held in the public domain and will be available freely for use by other health care organizations, both public and private sector. Finally, an explicit effort is being made to coordinate the GCPR activities with those of the NCVHS CPR Workgroup. Key individuals participate in both initiatives, and it is hoped that the GCPR experience can provide "real world" testing of some of the potential recommendations that the NCVHS will be making to the Secretary and Congress.

Summary

This chapter discussed health data standards, organizations that develop them, the process by which they are developed, and examples of current standards initiatives. Data standards that deal with data communications include those describing common message formats and those that specify standardized code sets, classification systems, and vocabularies. Data standards that focus on the content of messages specify minimum data sets for specific purposes and commonly defined core data elements. A number of standards development organizations involved in the development of these types of standards were profiled.

A discussion of the standards development process highlighted the socio-political context in which standards are developed and the potential impact it has on the availability and currency of standards. The increasingly significant role of the federal government in influencing the development and adoption of health data standards is discussed. Several key initiatives, including HIPAA and GCPR were described, and their potential impact was highlighted.

References

American Medical Association. (1992). *Current Procedural Terminology* (fourth revision). Chicago, IL.

American Medical Association. (1997). *The National Uniform Claim Committee Data Set.* Chicago, IL.

American Society for Testing and Materials. (1995). *Standard Specification for Coded Values for the Computer-Based Patient Record E1633-95.* West Conshohocken, PA.

American Society for Testing and Materials. (1996). *Standard Guide for Content and Structure of the Computer-Based Patient Record E1384-96.* West Conshohocken, PA.

College of American Pathologists. (1993). *SNOMED International: The Systemized Nomenclature of Human and Veterinary Medicine.* Northfield, IL.

Centers for Disease Control and Prevention. (1996). *Data Elements for Emergency Department System (DEEDS).* Atlanta, GA.

Dick, R. S., and Steen, E. B. (Eds.). (1991). *The Computer-Based Patient Record: An Essential Technology for Health Care* (2nd ed.). Washington, D.C.: National Academy Press.

Health Information Policy Council. (1983). *Background Paper: Uniform Minimum Health Data Sets.* Washington, D.C.: U.S. Department of Health and Human Services; [Unpublished].

McCormick, K. A., Renner, A. L., Mayes, R. W., et al. (1997). The Federal and private sector roles in the development of minimum data sets and core health data elements. *Computers in Nursing, 15*(2) Supplement, S23–S32.

National Committee on Vital and Health Statistics. (1996). *Report of the National Committee on Vital and*

Health Statistics: Core Health Data Elements. Washington, D.C.: Government Printing Office.

National Standards Policy Advisory Committee. (1978). Washington, D.C.: Government Printing Office.

President's Advisory Commission on Consumer Protection and Quality in the Health Care Industry. (1998). *Quality First: Better Health Care for All Americans.* Washington, D.C.: Government Printing Office.

Public Law 104-191. (1996). *Health Insurance Portability and Accountability Act of 1996.* Washington, D.C.: Government Printing Office.

Saba, V. K., and McCormick, K. A. (1996). *Essentials of Computers for Nurses* (2nd ed.).New York: McGraw-Hill.

Workgroup for Electronic Data Interchange. (1993). *WEDI Report.* Washington, D.C.

World Health Organization. (1980). *International Classification of Diseases: 9th Revision: Clinical Modifications (ICD-9-CM).* Geneva, Switzerland.

World Health Organization. (1992). *International Statistical Classification of Diseases and Related Health Problems (ICD-10).* Geneva, Switzerland.

Recommended Readings

The field of data standards is a very dynamic one with existing standards undergoing revision and new standards being developed. The best way to learn about specific standards activities is to get involved in the process of actually developing standards. All of the organizations discussed in this chapter provide opportunities to be involved directly in the process. Listed below are the World Wide Web addresses for each organization. Most sites describe current activities and publications available and many have links to other related sites.

Accredited Standards Committee (ASC) X12. *http://www.disa.org* or *http://www.wpc.edi.com*

American National Standards Institute (ANSI). *http://www.ansi.org*

American Society for Testing and Materials (ASTM). *http://www.astm.org*

Digital Imaging Communication in Medicine Standards Committee (DICOM). *http://www.nema.org*

European Technical Committee for Standardization Technical Committee 251 on Medical Informatics (CEN TC251). *http://www.centc251.org*

Government Computer-Based Patient Record Project (GCPR). *http://www.cba.ha.mil/projects/gcpr*

Health Insurance Portability and Accountability Act (HIPAA). *http://aspe.os.dhhs.gov/admnsimp*

Health Level 7 (HL7). *http://www.hl7.org*

Institute of Electrical and Electronic Engineers (IEEE). *http://www.ieee.org*

International Standards Organization (ISO). *http://www.iso.org*

International Statistical Classification of Diseases and Related Health Problems (ICD-9, ICD-9CM, ICD-10). *http://www.cdc.gov/nchswww/*

National Committee for Vital and Health Statistics (NCVHS). *http://aspe.os.dhhs.gov/ncvhs*

National Council for Prescription Drug Programs (NCPDP). *http://www.ncpdp.org*

Object Management Group (OMG). *http://www.omg.org*

Systemized Nomenclature of Human and Veterinary Medicine (SNOMED®) International. *http://www.snomed.org*

Unified Medical Language System (UMLS). *http://www.nlm.nih.gov/research/umls/*

PART **4**

Informatics Theory

11

Nursing Informatics Theory

Kathleen Milholland Hunter

OBJECTIVES

1. Discuss the relationship between health care informatics and nursing informatics.
2. Discuss different definitions and models of nursing and health care informatics.
3. Discuss core concepts of nursing informatics.
4. Describe nursing informatics as a distinct specialty.
5. Discuss key aspects of the electronic health record (EHR).
6. Identify national and international informatics organizations.
7. Describe opportunities for nursing informatics education and research.

KEY WORDS

informatics
electronic health record
nomenclatures

Nursing informatics is an established and growing area of specialization in nursing. All nurses employ information technologies in their practice. Informatics nurses are key persons in the design, development, implementation, and evaluation of those technologies and in the development of the knowledge underlying them.

This chapter addresses the concepts of nursing and health care informatics, their interrelationships, and their definitions. The core concepts of nursing informatics are described and related to one another. The recognition of nursing informatics as a distinct nursing specialty, its scope of practice, and certification are discussed. Nursing informatics concepts and practices are described within the context of the electronic health record (also known as the CPR and EMR). Opportunities for academic preparation of informatics nurses are presented. The role of nursing informatics in nursing research and the priorities for research in nursing informatics are described.

Background

"Information is power." Information is critical to making decisions. In the course of daily work, this link between information and decision-making may not be obvious; nonetheless, it is there. Nursing is a cognitive profession; the core of nursing takes place in our heads. It is the thinking that occurs before physical action. Assessment (data collection), diagnosis (or interpretation of assessment data), and planning are cognitive components of nursing. Implementation of a plan is the visible operationalization of this thinking. (Evaluation of a plan's implementation is another form of assessment and decision-making.) The collection of data about a situation (client, management, education, and research) is guided by a nurse's knowledge: knowledge built from formal education and from experience. The decisions a nurse makes are guided by his or her knowledge, as well. In health care, as in most areas of our lives, information and knowledge are increasing at astronomical rates. In clinical nursing practice, alone, the amount of data that *must* be collected (for legal, regulatory, quality, and other reasons), the data and knowledge related to specific client health conditions, and the information and knowledge about the health care environment are growing steadily. Collecting data in a systematic, thoughtful way, organizing data for efficient and accurate transformation into information, and documenting thinking and actions are critical to successful nursing practice. Nursing informatics is a nursing specialty that endeavors to make the collection and management of data, information, and knowledge easier for the practitioner, regardless of the domain and setting.

Informatics Definitions

Informatics and Health Care Informatics

What, then, is informatics? At its simplest, imagine the words "information" and "automatic." Combining "inform" and "atic" gives "informatics"; that is, informatics deals with information through the use of automated technologies.

More formally, informatics is a science that combines a domain science, computer science, information science, and cognitive science. Thus, it is a multidisciplinary science drawing from varied theories and knowledge applications. Thus, health care informatics may be defined as the integration of health care sciences, computer science, information science, and cognitive science to assist in the management of health care information. Health care informatics is a subdiscipline of informatics. Imagine a large umbrella (informatics) and imagine many persons under this umbrella. Each person represents a different domain science, one of which is health care informatics.

Because health care informatics is a relatively young addition to the informatics umbrella, you may see other terms that seem to address this same area: e.g. health informatics or medical informatics. Medical informatics historically has been used simultaneously with health care informatics. However, as health care informatics matures, there is more clarity in terms and scopes. Medical informatics is more clearly a subdomain of health care informatics. Health informatics is commonly noted to mean informatics used in educating health care clients and/or the general public.

Health care informatics addresses the study and management of health care information. Consider Fig. 11.1. Here, health care informatics is depicted as a large circle encompassing multiple health care-related disciplines. Note that the circles inside the larger circle overlap. This indicates that there are areas of common knowledge and use among the disciplines. But each discipline also has areas that are unique to that discipline.

Figure 11.2 represents multiple aspects of health care informatics. Health care informatics is the largest oval and encompasses all of the aspects. The vertical and horizontal ovals are the different aspects that intersect with each other. These aspects include information retrieval, ethics, security, decision support, patient care, evaluation, human-computer interaction, standards, telehealth, health care information systems, imaging, knowledge representation,

electronic health records, education, and information retrieval. The intersections illustrate the interdependencies of these aspects. This same model applies to the subdomains of health care informatics; that is, each subdomain, such as nursing informatics, must address these aspects as they apply to that health care discipline.

Nursing informatics is a subdomain of health care informatics (as shown in Fig. 11.1). It shares common areas of science with other subdomains and therefore supports multidisciplinary education, practice, and research in health care informatics. As shown in Fig. 11.1, nursing informatics also has unique areas that address the special information needs of the discipline of nursing.

A discipline, or a body of knowledge, illuminates the values and beliefs that are fundamental to services provided by the practitioners of the discipline. It is the foundation for how practitioners approach and treat clients. The body of knowledge making up a discipline includes knowledge that is unique to the discipline. This unique knowledge is evident in the language of the discipline. Discipline is what distinguishes nursing from medicine or medicine from dentistry (Brennan, 1994).

This is an important distinction to remember. Nurses work collaboratively with other health care disciplines and independently when engaged in nursing practice. Nursing informatics reflects this duality as well, moving in and out of integration and separation as situations and needs demand.

Nursing Informatics

Kathryn Hannah proposed a definition of nursing informatics in 1986. For Hannah, it is using information technologies in relation to any of nursing's functions and any actions of nurses (Hannah, 1985).

Health care Informatics

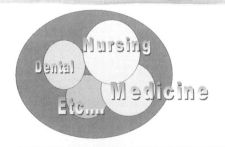

Figure 11.1
Health care informatics and subdomains of health care informatics.

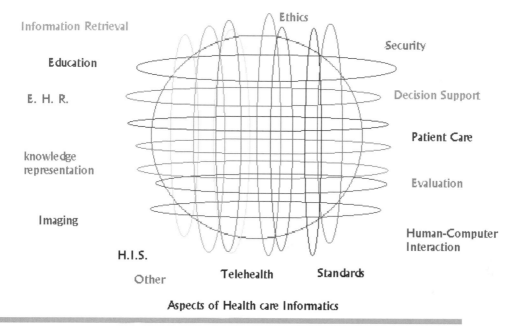

Aspects of Health care Informatics

Figure 11.2
Aspects of health care informatics. E.H.R., electronic health record; H.I.S., health
information system.

In their classic article on the science of nursing informatics, Graves and Corcoran presented a more complex
definition of nursing informatics. Nursing informatics is
a combination of computer science, information science,
and nursing science designed to assist in the management
and processing of nursing data, information, and knowledge to support the practice of nursing and the delivery of
nursing care (Graves and Corcoran, 1989). Suzanne Henry
uses this definition in her 1995 update on the state of the
science in nursing informatics (Henry, 1995).

The American Nurses Association (ANA) modified
the Graves and Corcoran definition when it developed
the scope of practice for nursing informatics. The ANA
defines nursing informatics as the specialty that integrates
nursing science, computer science, and information science in identifying, collecting, processing, and managing
data and information to support nursing practice, administration, education, research, and the expansion of nursing knowledge (American Nurses Association, 1994).

As health care informatics matures, scholars and practitioners are expanding the vantage points from which one
approaches this discipline. Patel and Kaufman (1998) advocate a place of prominence for cognitive science in the
informatics framework. There is growing belief that medical informatics and nursing informatics (and other subdomains of health care informatics) are more than the

intersection of computing and practice. More emphasis
is needed on communication and collaboration than on
computing (Patel and Kaufman, 1998).

An exhaustive presentation of all nursing informatics
definitions proposed during the last few decades is outside
the scope of this chapter. What is important to remember is that nursing informatics is a dynamic discipline,
comprised of many aspects (see Fig. 11.2) and defined in
many ways. Definitions reflect the definer's perspectives
and the emergence of new knowledge in nursing informatics and the sciences with which it is integrated. Turley
(1996) presents and analyzes historic and current definitions of nursing informatics.

Computer science encompasses the engineering and
technology of hardware, software, and communications
(Collen, 1994). Rapid technological advances in these
areas have radically changed how most of us live and
work today. These advances have made possible the advance of nursing informatics as well. Computer scientists
also are becoming more engaged in studying aspects of
information science and cognitive science (just as those
disciplines are incorporating more computer science into
their studies and knowledge bases).

Information science, like nursing informatics, is an
evolving discipline. Modern information science began
in the 1950s, following the publication of Shannon's

information theory (Meadows, 1990). Information science can imply the exploitation of scientific and technical information of all kinds and by all means. It may also imply the application of science and technology to general information handling (Hanson, 1971). Branches of modern information science include information retrieval, information handling as part of a system, and human-computer interaction (Meadows, 1990).

In cognitive science, theories and methods from psychology, linguistics, philosophy, anthropology, and computer science are incorporated to study the processes of perception, comprehension, reasoning, decision-making, and problem-solving (Patel and Kaufman, 1998). In nursing informatics, the focus of cognitive science is on these processes as they apply to nursing practice.

Nursing science is the representation of nursing's understanding of human behavior (psychological, biological, social) in health and illness (Gortner, 1980). It is distinguished from nursing practice and nursing knowledge. Nursing science provides empirical substantiation for nursing practice. Nursing knowledge derives from the practice of nursing science (Ryan and Nagle, 1998).

Models of Nursing Informatics

Models are representations of some aspect of the real world. Models show particular perspectives of a selected aspect and may illustrate relationships. Models change as knowledge about the selected aspect changes and are dependent upon the "world view" of the model developer(s). It is important to remember that different models reflect different viewpoints and are not necessarily competitive; that is, there is no one "right" model.

Different scholars in nursing informatics have proposed different models. These models are presented here to provide further perspectives on nursing informatics, to demonstrate how differently scholars and practitioners may view what seems to be the same thing, and to show that nursing informatics is an evolutionary theoretical and practical science. Again, remember that there is no one right model, nor are any of the models presented here exhaustive of the possible perspectives of nursing informatics.

Graves and Corcoran's seminal work included a model of nursing informatics. Their model placed data, information, and knowledge in sequential boxes with one-way arrows pointing from data to information to knowledge. Over these three boxes is management processing, with arrows pointing in one direction to each of the three boxes (Graves and Corcoran, 1989). The model is a direct depiction of their definition of nursing informatics.

In 1986, Patricia Schwirian proposed a model of nursing informatics intended to stimulate and guide systematic research in this discipline (Schwirian, 1986). Her concern at that time was over the sparse volume of research literature in nursing informatics. The model provides a framework for identifying significant information needs, which in turn can foster research. There are four primary elements arranged in a pyramid with a triangular base. The four elements are the raw material (nursing-related information), the technology (a computing system), the users (nurses and students), and the goal or objective toward which the preceding elements are directed. The goal element is placed at the apex of the pyramid to show its importance. The raw material, user, and computer interact to form the pyramid's base. All interaction among the elements is bi-directional (Schwirian, 1986).

Turley, writing in 1996, proposed another model in which the core components of informatics (cognitive science, information science, and computer science) are depicted as intersecting circles. Nursing science is a larger circle that completely encompasses the intersecting circles. Nursing informatics is the intersection between the discipline-specific science (nursing) and the area of informatics (Turley, 1996).

Core Concepts

Data, Information, and Knowledge

The data, information, and knowledge involved in nursing are the core phenomena of nursing informatics (American Nurses Association, 1994, p. 15). These core phenomena may come from any of the four domains of nursing: education, clinical practice, research, and administration.

A datum is a fact; a value assigned to a variable. For example, a systolic blood pressure is a datum. Another datum may be a nursing intervention, a patient problem, skin integrity, etc.

Information is the result of processing data. Data processing occurs when raw facts are transformed through the application of context to give those facts meaning or via the organization of data into a structure that connotes meaning (Graves and Corcoran, 1989).

Knowledge emerges from the transformation of information. Knowledge may be conceived as new or different information, as shown in Fig. 11.3. (Note, however, that processing of information does not always result in knowledge. Further, knowledge is necessary to the processing of data and information.) Knowledge itself may be processed to generate decisions and new knowledge (Graves and Corcoran, 1989).

Knowledge Work Model

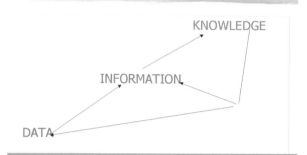

Figure 11.3
Relationship of data, information, and knowledge.

Registered Nurses as Knowledge Workers

Knowledge work is the exercise of specialist knowledge and competencies (Blackleaf, 1995). The United States is becoming a nation of knowledge workers. Futurists predict that in the second millennium, the primary domestic product of the United States will be knowledge and related knowledge services. Knowledge workers will be valued contributors to these products.

Registered nurses are consummate knowledge workers for the 21st century. Their skills in assessment, planning, critical thinking, and evaluation are transferable to many different settings but are most exquisitely employed in nursing practice. Ozbolt and Graves (1993) support the concept of nurses as knowledge workers. They point out that clinical judgement is the application of knowledge to information for deciding what observations to make, evaluating observations, assigning meanings, and determining what actions to take (Ozbolt and Graves, 1993).

Knowledge work, of course, depends on access to data, information, and knowledge. Atomic level data are the foundation for the transforming processes by which knowledge work is accomplished. Atomic level data are raw, uninterpreted facts whose values cannot be further subdivided (i.e. made any smaller). These data are captured at their source in the course of clinical care. Atomic level data are very useful in tracking the effectiveness of nursing decisions and are amenable to inclusion in electronic information systems as well as multiple forms of manipulation (Graves and Corcoran, 1989; Zielstorff et al., 1993). Analysis, combination, aggregation, and summari-

zation are ways in which an information system can transform atomic level data to information and knowledge.

Concept representation involves the set of terms and relationships that describe the phenomena, processes, and practices of a discipline, such as nursing. Data elements and nomenclatures, vocabularies, and languages are some of the ways in which nursing concepts may be represented. Data elements are terms for which data are collected (i.e. for which values are assigned). A specific, purposeful group of data elements, representing a subset of concepts within a discipline, is a data set.

The Nursing Minimum Data Set (NMDS) developed by Harriet Werley is a data set for fostering the comparison of nursing data across time, settings, and populations (Werley and Lang, 1988). This data set contains 16 data elements, divided into patient, service, and nursing care elements. These elements are listed in Table 11.1. Most of these data elements, except for the nursing care elements and the unique identifier for the primary

Table 11.1   Nursing Minimum Data Set

Nursing care elements
1. Nursing diagnosis
2. Nursing intervention
3. Nursing outcome
4. Intensity of nursing care

Patient or client demographic elements
5. Personal identification
6. Date of birth
7. Sex
8. Race and ethnicity
9. Residence

Service elements
10. Unique facility or service agency number
11. Unique health record number of patient or client
12. Unique number of principal registered nurse provider
13. Episode admission or encounter data
14. Discharge or termination date
15. Disposition of patient or client
16. Expected payer

Source: Werley H, Lang N. (1988). The consensually derived nursing minimum data set: Elements and definitions. In: H. Werley and N. Lang, (Eds.), *Identification of the Nursing Minimum Data Set*. New York: Springer Publishing Co.

registered nurse, have long been captured in health care information systems. Werley and her colleagues envisioned collecting these data from everywhere nursing care is delivered, aggregating and storing these data in large databases, and using these data for policy analysis, evaluation of care, strategic planning, and nursing research. As increasing numbers of nursing concepts are integrated into clinical information systems, Werley's vision is an emerging reality.

There are other data sets that contain nursing data elements. These include, but are not limited to, the Minimum Data Set (MDS) developed for long-term care facilities and the Home Health Data Set that is used by home health agencies.

Nursing Nomenclatures, Vocabularies, Classifications, and Taxonomies

Nursing nomenclatures and classification systems offer systematic, standardized ways of describing nursing practice. Nomenclatures are terms or labels for describing concepts in nursing such as diagnoses, interventions, and outcomes. Classifications are the ordering of entities (such as nomenclatures) into groups or classes on the basis of their similarities (Gordon, 1998).

Taxonomy is the study of classification, and simultaneously refers to the end product of a classification. It often is used interchangeably with classification (Gordon, 1998). Similarly, classification is an ordering of entities into groups according to a set of criteria as well as the end result of the ordering (Gordon, 1998). The International Classification of Diseases (ICD) orders medical diagnosis terms into specified groups or classes. A nomenclature or vocabulary is a set of word labels for naming concepts. For example, the set of nursing diagnoses adopted by the North American Nursing Diagnosis Association (NANDA) is a nomenclature. For the sake of simplicity, "nomenclature" will be the term used in further discussions in this chapter of nursing nomenclatures, classifications, and taxonomies to represent all of these permutations of nursing concept representation.

Nursing has many nomenclatures that address the nursing process components of diagnosis, interventions, and outcomes. There are, as well, systems for classifying nursing research. In this chapter, the discussion on nursing nomenclatures focuses on those that have been recognized by the American Nurses Association (ANA). Table 11.2 lists the nomenclatures recognized by ANA as of 1998. A brief description of each of these nomenclatures follows.

Why are informatics nurses and nurse scholars so interested in nomenclatures? Nursing nomenclatures

Table 11.2   American Nurses Association Recognized Nursing Practice Classification Systems, 1998

North American Nursing Diagnosis Association Approved List of Diagnostic Labels (NANDA)

Nursing Interventions Classification (NIC)

Nursing Outcomes Classification (NOC)

The Omaha System

Home Health Care Classification (HHCC)

Ozbolt's Patient Care Data Set (PCDS)

increasingly are important as electronic health records become more and more an integral component of health care delivery. These nomenclatures are used to capture, store, and manipulate data in electronic health records (EHRs). Key functions of nomenclatures within an EHR include the following: provide the legal record of care; support clinical decision-making; facilitate billing, costing, and accounting functions; accumulate a structured database for administrative and clinical queries, quality assurance, and research; and exchange data with internal and external systems (Zielstorff, 1998).

Nursing is both blessed and challenged by the wealth of nomenclatures available for describing nursing practice and nurses' contributions to health care. The multiple nomenclatures offer practitioners choices in how to describe their practice. However, not all nomenclatures are created equal, and not all nomenclatures address all of the functions demanded by modern and future electronic health records. Zielstorff identifies and discusses several key characteristics needed by nursing nomenclatures that will provide data capture, storage, analysis, and reporting for electronic systems. These characteristics are domain completeness, granularity, parsimony, synonymy, nonambiguity, nonredundancy, clinical utility, multiple axes, and combinatorial functionality.

A detailed presentation of these issues is outside the scope of this chapter, and interested readers are referred to the original article. What is important to remember is that none of the ANA-recognized nomenclatures achieves all of these characteristics. In most instances, this is because nomenclatures very often are developed for specific purposes, and many have been built over time, while these ideal characteristics are of recent vintage.

North American Nursing Diagnoses Association Approved List of Diagnostic Labels   The North American Nursing Diagnoses Association (NANDA) is a private membership organization that has developed structures and processes for approving nursing diagnostic labels for testing and research. NANDA defines nursing diagnosis as a clinical judgement about an individual's, a family's, or a community's responses to actual or potential health problems and life processes (Hoskins, 1998). Each diagnosis is classified into one of nine human response patterns: choosing, communicating, exchanging, feeling, knowing, moving, perceiving, relating, and valuing. NANDA is working to improve the consistency in the conceptual and methodological bases of the nursing diagnoses (Hoskins, 1998). The results of these efforts will be evident in future writings.

Home Health Care Classification   The Home Health Care Classification (HHCC) is a system based on the conceptual framework of the nursing process. It is designed to support holistic client assessment and the documentation of home health care via a standard nomenclature (Saba, 1998a). The HHCC has 20 clinical care components for conducting a holistic assessment, 145 nursing diagnoses, 3 expected outcome goals, 160 nursing interventions, 4 nursing intervention actions, and 4 actual outcomes. Used as a system, the HHCC makes it possible to assess clients and document care and track nursing care across time, settings, and distances (Saba, 1998a).

The Omaha System   The Omaha System is a taxonomy of terms for guiding nursing practice, documenting that practice, and managing information in a structured and comprehensive way. It is organized from the general to the specific and includes three major components. These are the Problem Classification Scheme, the Intervention Scheme, and the Problem Rating Scale for Outcomes. Originally developed for use in home health practice, the Omaha System is now being adopted into diverse other clinical practice sites both nationally and internationally (Martin, 1998).

Nursing Interventions Classification   The Nursing Interventions Classification (NIC) is a standardized set of terms and a classification of those terms, focused on treatments (interventions) that nurses may perform. NIC defines an intervention as "any treatment, based upon clinical judgement and knowledge that a nurse performs to enhance patient or client outcomes." These can include direct and indirect care activities. They can be initiated by nurses or requested by other licensed independent health care practitioners. The set of NIC interventions, which continues to grow, is intended to cover all settings and

nursing specialties. The interventions are organized by six domains and 27 classes (McCloskey, 1998).

Nursing Outcomes Classification   The Nursing Outcomes Classification (NOC) is a taxonomy of standardized nursing-sensitive client outcomes. (Nursing-sensitive client outcomes are those that nursing care can affect. This does not mean that other disciplines cannot affect these outcomes.) These outcomes apply to an individual recipient of nursing care or a lay caregiver for the individual. The outcome terms describe states and behaviors including perceptions and subjective states. NOC is developed to encompass the entire continuum of care in order to provide a consistent measure of client and lay caregiver status (Johnson and Maas, 1998).

Patient Care Data Set   The Patient Care Data Set (PCDS) is a structured vocabulary, consisting of a data dictionary with terms and codes for 363 patient problems, 308 therapeutic goals, and 1,357 patient care orders. The PCDS provides a familiar language for recording clinical data and the knowledge work of nursing. The PCDS was developed by Judith Ozbolt, using the paper forms for planning and documenting nursing and some multidisciplinary care from nine acute care hospitals distributed over the United States (Ozbolt, 1998).

Nursing Informatics as a Specialty   In early 1992, the American Nurses Association established nursing informatics as a distinct specialty in nursing. This designation as a specialty, unique among the health care professions, provides official recognition that nursing informatics is a part of nursing and that it has a distinct scope of practice. Following recognition of nursing informatics as a specialty, the American Nurses Credentialing Center (ANCC) established a certification examination. Successful candidates earn the right to place a "C" after their names (e.g. RN, C).

The scope of nursing informatics practice includes developing and evaluating applications, tools, processes, and strategies that assist registered nurses in managing data to support decision-making. This decision-making can encompass any and all of the following areas of nursing practice: client care, research, education, and administration. Information handling—the processes involved in managing data, information, and knowledge—includes naming, organizing, grouping, collecting, processing, analyzing, storing, retrieving, and transforming data and information. The core phenomena of nursing informatics are the data, information, and knowledge of nursing. It is this special focus on the information of nursing that distinguishes nursing informatics from other nursing specialties. As noted earlier in this chapter, nursing informatics is one component of the broader field of health care informatics. Nursing informatics intersects with other domains and disciplines concerned with the management of data, information, and knowledge. The boundaries and intersections are flexible and allow for the inevitable changes that come with time and growth (American Nurses Association, 1994).

Electronic Health Record

Earlier in this chapter, data elements and data sets were defined and described. In essence, data sets are comprised of data elements brought together for a specific reason. When values are assigned to the elements in a data set, the resulting data most often are stored in a database. Modern databases are used for storing data in a way that maintains the logical relationships among data elements, and modern databases are stored in a computer. Note, however, that the logical structure of a database is determined by the conceptual or theoretical views held by the database developers; that is, the same data elements may be organized and related in entirely different ways by different developers.

In health care and nursing, there are different types of databases, including bibliographic, payment claims, research, and the client record. Our focus in this chapter is on the client health record as a database. Any client health record, whether paper-based or computer-based, is a database made up of the myriad data elements for which data are gathered and which are used in health and health care decision-making by health care practitioners, providers, and individuals and families. A simple perspective is that the EHR is a client health record database supported by computer and electronic technologies.

The concept of the EHR emerged, initially, as a computer-based patient record or CPR and was given significant impetus by a 1990 report from the Institute of Medicine that advocated the adoption of the CPR as the primary source of client health care data and information (Dick and Steen, 1990). In this seminal work, the CPR was conceived as a longitudinal medical record receiving data from multiple worldwide sources, not simply an electronic copy of the traditional paper medical record. Naturally, this concept and its definitions have evolved over time. Other terms for the CPR have been used (e.g. electronic medical record (EMR), electronic patient record, computerized patient record, computerized medical record). Gradually, the informatics community has been adopting "electronic health record" as a name more in keeping with modern perspectives on comprehensive

health care, health maintenance, and multidisciplinary practice. The EHR is defined as health status and health care information collected over an individual's lifetime. An EHR encompasses the entire scope of health information in all media forms (Stetson, 1998).

Earlier in this chapter, the primary functions of the electronic health record were identified by Zielstorff (1998). When implemented as part of an information system, the electronic health record is the primary source for information about a client. As a result, it is the place where client information is recorded or documented.

There are many reasons why health care data and information are documented. These include compliance with law and regulations, adherence to the standards of accrediting agencies, communication with others providing health care to the client, providing a basis for costing out services, and creating claims for payment of services. For a clinical nurse, the recording of nursing care and the status of the client usually are very important reasons. It is in the documentation of the nursing process and the delivery of nursing care that nurses accumulate the data that demonstrate their impact on client health outcomes. In the modern health care environment, the availability of empirical evidence that one's discipline and practice positively affect an individual's or a community's health is critical.

Prior to the emergence of the EHR, it was nearly impossible to extract nursing data from the paper health record in an efficient and affordable way. The logical structure of the database, that is, the EHR, along with the development of standardized terms for describing nursing practice, have made data collection a more reasonable and effective exercise. Thus, the NMDS and the standardized nomenclatures described earlier are essential components of an electronic health record. These important developments in nursing informatics foster comprehensive and accurate data collection and documentation of the nursing process. They also support nursing practice research, the development of nursing theory, and health services research. Informatics nurses serve an important role in designing, developing, implementing, monitoring, evaluating, and modifying electronic health records so these records facilitate nurses' work and the growth of the discipline.

Informatics Organizations

There are many diverse organizations associated with nursing informatics and health care informatics. State nurses associations and other state-level nursing organizations frequently have informatics committees. Other organizations are multidisciplinary in their memberships.

Some organizations restrict their membership to other organizations, while others allow only individuals to join. The nature, purposes, and activities of the multiple informatics organizations have sufficient differences that there is bound to be at least one, if not more, organization for everyone interested in nursing informatics. Information about a few of these organizations is provided here. This is in no way an exhaustive presentation. To learn more about these organizations and others, consult the Internet, informatics colleagues, and the literature.

American Medical Informatics Association

The American Medical Informatics Association (AMIA) is an individual membership organization dedicated to the development and application of medical informatics in the support of patient care, teaching, research, and health care administration. (Note: AMIA believes that the term "medical informatics" represents all of the diverse interests, issues, and aspects of informatics in health care.) AMIA serves as an authoritative body in the field of medical informatics and frequently represents the United States in the informational arena of medical informatics in international forums. It is the United States member of the International Medical Informatics Association (IMIA). Members include developers of many of the most significant clinical information systems in the United States, a large number of academically based health care professionals devoted to the applications of computers in clinical care, and a representative number of users of health care information systems. Professionals who are members of AMIA include physicians, nurses, educators, computer and information scientists, biomedical engineers, medical librarians, and academic researchers (American Medical Informatics Association, 1999).

Healthcare Information and Management Systems Society

Healthcare Information and Management Systems Society (HIMSS) is an individual membership organization representing over 12,000 informatics leaders in four professional areas: clinical systems, information systems, management engineering, and telecommunications. HIMSS members are responsible for developing many of today's key innovations in health care delivery and administration, including telehealth, computer-based patient records, community health information networks, and portable/wireless health care computing. HIMSS promotes the organized exchange of experiences, personal and professional growth, the highest standards of professional conduct, and lifelong learning

in the areas of health care information, technology, and change Healthcare Information and Management Systems Society, 1999).

Center for Healthcare Information Management

The Center for Healthcare Information Management (CHIM) is the major trade association for vendors and consultants who provide information technology products and services to the health care industry. Its mission is to positively impact the health care industry through the promotion of health care information technology (HIT), promote the collective business interests of its members, and earn recognition and respect as a HIT industry authority. Informatics nurses who work in the vendor and consulting arenas may become members of CHIM and CHIM's nursing council (Center for Healthcare Information Management, 1999).

The American Nurses Association Council on Nursing Systems and Informatics

The Council on Nursing Systems and Informatics is a membership council of the American Nurses Association. The Council focuses on issues related to managing and practicing in various nursing systems and on issues in nursing informatics. Further, the ANA Congress of Nursing Practice assigns the council specific work to assist the Congress in its mission.

National League for Nursing Council for Nursing Informatics

The Council for Nursing Informatics is one of the membership councils of the National League for Nursing (NLN). The purpose of the Council for Nursing Informatics is to create a multidisciplinary network for assessing needs, providing information, and presenting programs on the impact of the information age and computer technology upon health care and higher education in general, and nursing education and practice specifically.

Nursing Informatics Education

Education about nursing informatics increasingly is a standard component of nursing curricula at both the undergraduate and graduate levels. The content and the ways in which nursing informatics are taught vary tremendously. Some schools provide informatics content throughout every course. Others mandate a minimum number of specific informatics courses. Still others provide informatics courses as an option. There is steadily growing recognition by faculty and students that knowledge and skills in nursing informatics are essential to successful nursing practice.

For registered nurses already in practice, continuing education offerings and participation in informatics meetings, such as the annual AMIA or HIMSS conventions, are two approaches to informatics education. During the process of an information system implementation, nurses may receive informatics content along with information about the technical aspects of the system.

Preparation of nurses in the specialty of nursing informatics begins at the graduate level and may continue through the earning of a doctoral degree. The University of Maryland School of Nursing was the first to offer a Master's of Science in nursing informatics and later followed with the first Doctor of Philosophy degree. The University of Utah in Salt Lake City was next, with a strong focus on clinical practice. Slowly, other graduate programs have been developed, such as the one at New

York University. At this writing, there are still too few programs to meet the demand of interested nurses and employers. As health care and nursing informatics continues to be a strong force in health care, the demand for informatics nurses also will be strong. Table 11.3 lists some of the educational institutions that offer certificate and/or degree programs in nursing informatics (Nursing Informatics Work Group, 1999). More programs are in development, and the AMIA Nursing Work Group provides updated information on its Web site.

 ## Nursing Informatics Research

Nursing informatics contributes to nursing research and is itself an important area for study. Earlier, the challenges to studying nursing practice via the paper health record were discussed. Nursing informatics is critical to overcoming these challenges and other information- or data-based problems in the conduct of research. Hard-

Table 11.3 Academic-Based Certificates and Degrees in Nursing Informatics

Certificates in Nursing Informatics	Graduate Degree with Specialization in Informatics	Graduate Degree with Informatics Courses	Doctoral Degree in Informatics
	University of Maryland at Baltimore, School of Nursing		University of Maryland at Baltimore, School of Nursing
	University of Utah, College of Nursing, Salt Lake City		University of Utah, College of Nursing, Salt Lake City
New York University, New York City	New York University, New York City		New York University, New York City
	St. Louis University		
Duke University, School of Nursing, Durham, NC			
		Northeastern University Graduate School of Nursing, Boston	
University of Arizona, College of Nursing, Phoenix		University of Arizona, College of Nursing, Phoenix	
University of Iowa, College of Nursing, Iowa City			
	University of North Carolina– Chapel Hill, School of Nursing		

Source: NIWG. AMIA Nursing Informatics Work Group. *http://amia-niwg.org*, 1999.

ware and software are used to design research tools, to collect data, and to facilitate data and information analyses in nursing and interdisciplinary research. The nursing data elements in the electronic health record can be used to examine individual client outcomes, document nursing practice, and evaluate quality indicators (Saba, 1998b).

In 1993, the National Institute of Nursing Research (NINR) formed a priority expert panel on nursing informatics. The task of this panel was to identify the nursing informatics research priorities in the United States. The panel focused its work on three questions and recommended priorities for each of them.

- What are nursing data and how can these data be represented in computer-based systems?

- How do nurses manage and process data, information, and knowledge for clinical decision-making?

- How can information technology support the management and processing of nursing data, nursing information, and nursing knowledge (NINR Priority Expert Panel on Nursing Informatics, 1998)?

While a young science, nursing informatics shows great promise in its practice and in its scholarly work. Nursing informatics has great potential to advance nursing's knowledge and its boundaries as a science. To accomplish this potential, it is essential that (1) more informatics nurses be educated (especially at the doctoral level), (2) collaborative nursing informatics research be encouraged, and (3) research funding be available at local, state, national, and international levels (Henry, 1995).

Summary

Through the use of definitions and models, the concepts of informatics, health care informatics, and nursing informatics were explained, and their relationships to each other were discussed. The core concepts of nursing informatics were presented and described in detail. The establishment of the specialty of nursing informatics was explained. The electronic health record was described and related to nursing informatics. Several informatics organizations and opportunities for academic preparation in nursing informatics were presented. Priorities for nursing informatics research were noted.

References

American Medical Informatics Association. (1999). *http://www.amia.org*

American Nurses Association. (1994). *The Scope of Practice for Nursing Informatics*. Washington, D.C.: American Nurses Publishing.

Blackleaf, F. (1995). Knowledge, knowledge work and organizations: An overview and interpretation. *Organization Studies, 16*(6), 1021–1046.

Brennan, P. F. (1994). On the relevance of discipline to informatics. *Journal of the American Medical Informatics Association, 1*(2), 200–201.

Center for Healthcare Information Management. (1999). *http:/www.chim.org*

Collen, M. F. (1994). The origins of informatics. *Journal of the American Medical Informatics Association, 1*(2), 91–107.

Dick, R., and Steen, E. (1990). *The Computer-Based Patient Record: An Essential Technology for Change*. Washington, D.C.: Institute of Medicine.

Gordon, M. (1998). Nursing nomenclature and classification system development. *Online Journal of Issues in Nursing. http://www.nursingworld.org/ojin/Tpc7/tpc7_1.htm*

Gortner, S. (1980). Nursing science in transition. *Nursing Research, 29,* 180–183.

Graves, J.R., and Corcoran, S. (1989). The study of nursing informatics. *IMAGE: Journal of Nursing Scholarship, 21*(4), 227–231.

Hannah, K. (Ed.). (1985). Current trends in nursing informatics: Implications for curriculum planning. In K. Hannah, E. J. Guillemin, and D. N. Conklin (Eds.), *Nursing Uses of Computer and Information Science*. Amsterdam: North-Holland.

Hanson, C. W. (1971). *Introduction to Science-Information Work*. London: Aslib.

Healthcare Information and Management Systems Society. (1999). *http://www.himss.org*

Henry, S. B. (1995). Nursing informatics: State of the science. *Journal of Advanced Nursing, 22,* 1182–1192.

Hoskins, L.M. (1998). NANDA. In J. J. Fitzpatrick (Ed.), *Encyclopedia of Nursing Research* (pp. 320–322). New York: Springer Publishing.

Johnson, M., and Maas, M. (1998). Nursing outcomes classification. In J. J. Fitzpatrick (Ed.), *Encyclopedia of Nursing Research* (pp. 378–379). New York: Springer Publishing Company.

Martin, K. S. (1998). The Omaha system. In J. J. Fitzpatrick (Ed.), *Encyclopedia of Nursing Research* (p. 399). New York: Springer Publishing Company.

McCloskey, J. C. (1998). Nursing interventions classification. In J. J. Fitzpatrick (Ed.), *Encyclopedia of Nursing Research* (pp. 371–374). New York: Springer Publishing.

Meadows, A. J. (1990). Theory in information science. *Journal of Information Science, 16,* 59–63.

NINR Priority Expert Panel. (1993). *Nursing Informatics: Enhancing Patient Care* (vol. 4). Bethesda, MD: US Department of Health and Human Services, U.S. Public Health Service, National Institutes of Health.

Nursing Informatics Work Group. (1999). *http://amia-niwg.org*

Ozbolt, J. (1998). *Introducing Ozbolt's Patient Care Data Set.* Charlottesville, VA: Care Data Corporation.

Ozbolt, J., and Graves, J. (1993). Clinical informatics: Developing tools for knowledge workers. *Nursing Clinics of North America, 28*(2), 407–425.

Patel, V. L., and Kaufman, D. R. (1998). Medical informatics: and the science of cognition. *Journal of the American Medical Informatics Association, 5*(6), 493–502.

Ryan, S. A., and Nagle, L. M. (1998). Nursing informatics: The unfolding of a new science. In V. K. Saba, D. B. Pocklington, and K. P. Miller, (Eds.), *Nursing and Computers. An Anthology, 1987–1996.* New York: Springer.

Saba, V. K. (1998a). Home health care classification. In J. J. Fitzpatrick (Ed.), *Encyclopedia of Nursing Research* (pp. 250–253). New York: Springer Publishing.

Saba, V. K. (1998b). Nursing informatics. In J. J. Fitzpatrick (Ed.), *Encyclopedia of Nursing Research* (pp. 366–368). New York: Springer Publishing Company.

Schwirian, P. M. (1986). The NI Pyramid-A model for research in nursing informatics. *Computers In Nursing, 4*(3), 134–136.

Stetson, N. (1998). The computer-based patient record: Its role in the healthcare enterprise. *Journal of Healthcare Information Management, 12*(4), 1–2.

Turley, J. (1996). Toward a model for nursing informatics. *IMAGE: Journal of Nursing Scholarship, 28*(4), 309–313.

Werley, H., and Lang, N. (1988). The consensually derived nursing minimum data set: Elements and definitions. In H. Werley and N. Lang, (Eds.), *Identification of the Nursing Minimum Data Set.* New York: Springer Publishing Co.

Zielstorff, R., Hudgings, C., and Grobe, S. (1993). *Next-Generation Nursing Information Systems: Essential Characteristics for Professional Practice.* Washington, D.C.: American Nurses Publishing.

Zielstorff, R. D. (1998). Characteristics of a good nursing nomenclature from an informatics perspective. *Online Journal of Issues in Nursing.*

12

Concept-Oriented Terminological Systems

Suzanne Bakken

Nicholas R. Hardiker

Charles N. Mead

OBJECTIVES

1. Describe the need for concept-oriented terminological systems.
2. Identify the components of a concept-oriented terminological system.
3. Compare and contrast two approaches for representing nursing concepts within a concept-oriented terminological system.

KEY WORDS

concept representation
terminology
vocabulary
standardized nursing language

The failure to achieve a single, integrated terminology with broad coverage of the health care domain has been characterized as the "vocabulary problem." Evolving criteria for health care terminologies for implementation in computer-based systems suggest that concept-oriented terminological systems are needed to support the data needs of today's complex, information system-driven health care and health management environment. This chapter focuses on providing the background necessary to understand recent approaches to solving the vocabulary problem. It also includes several illustrative examples of these approaches from the nursing domain.

Background and Definitions

The primary motivation for standardized terms in nursing is the need for valid, comparable data that can be used across information system applications to support clinical decision-making and the evaluation of processes and outcomes of care. Secondary uses of the data for purposes such as clinical research, development of practice-based nursing knowledge, and generation of health care policy are dependent upon the initial collection and representation of the data. Given the importance of standardized terminology, one might ask, "Why, despite the extensive work to date is the 'vocabulary problem' not yet solved?"

The Vocabulary Problem

Several reasons for the vocabulary problem have been posited in the literature. First, the development of multiple specialized terminologies has resulted in areas of overlapping content, areas for which no content exists, and large numbers of codes and terms (Chute et al., 1998). Second, as opposed to being optimized for a specific function, existing terminologies are most often developed to provide sets of terms and definitions of concepts for human interpretation, with computer interpretation as only a secondary goal (Rossi et al., 1998). Unfortunately, knowledge that is eminently understandable to humans is often confusing, ambiguous, or opaque to computers, and, as a result, current efforts have often resulted in terminologies that are inadequate to meet the data needs of today's complex, information system-driven health care and health management environment. This chapter focuses on providing the background necessary to understand recent concept-oriented approaches to solving the vocabulary problem. It also includes several illustrative examples of these approaches from the nursing domain.

Concept Orientation

An appreciation for the approaches discussed in this chapter has as its prerequisite an understanding of what it means for a terminology to be concept oriented. The literature provides an evolving framework that enumerates the criteria (Table 12.1) that render health care vocabularies suitable for implementation in computer-based systems. In particular, it is clear that such vocabularies must be concept oriented (Chute et al., 1998; Cimino et al., 1989; Cimino, 1988). Recent evaluations have reported that existing nursing terminologies do not meet the criteria related to concept orientation (Henry et al., 1998a; Henry et al., 1998b). In order to appreciate the significance of concept-oriented approaches, it is important to first understand the definitions of and relationships among things in the world (objects), our thoughts about things in the world (concepts), and the labels we use to represent our thoughts about things in the world. These relationships are depicted by the figure commonly called the semiotic triangle (Fig. 12.1) (Ogden and Richards, 1923). International Standards Organization (ISO) Standard 1087 provides definitions for each vertex of the triangle:

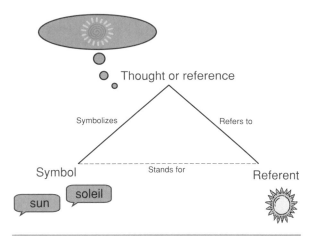

Figure 12.1
The semiotic triangle depicts the relationships among objects in the perceivable or conceivable world (referent), thoughts about things in the world, and the labels (symbols or terms) used to represent thoughts about things in the world.

Table 12.1   Evaluation Criteria Related to Concept-Oriented Approaches

Atomic-based—concepts must be separable into constituent components (Chute et al., 1998)

Compositionality—ability to combine simple concepts into composite concepts, e.g. pain *and* acute = acute pain (Chute et al., 1998)

Concept permanence—once a concept is defined it should not be deleted from a terminology (Cimino, 1998)

Language independence—support for multiple linguistic expressions (Chute et al., 1998)

Multiple hierarchy—accessibility of concepts through all reasonable hierarchical paths with consistency of views (Chute et al., 1998; Cimino et al., 1989; Cimino, 1998)

Nonambiguity—explicit definition for each term, e.g., patient teaching related to medication adherence defined as an activity with *delivery mode* of teaching, *care recipient* of patient, and *focus* of medication adherence (Chute et al., 1998; Cimino et al., 1989; Cimino, 1998)

Nonredundancy—one preferred way of representing a concept or idea (Chute et al., 1998; Cimino et al., 1989; Cimino, 1998)

Synonymy—support for synonyms and consistent mapping of synonyms within and among terminologies (Chute et al., 1998; Cimino et al., 1989; Cimino,1998)

Concept: a unit of thought constituted through abstraction on the basis of properties common to a set of objects.

Object: any part of the perceivable or conceivable world.

Term: designation of a defined concept in a special language by a linguistic expression (International Standards Organization, 1990).

The word "terminology," defined as the set of terms representing a system of concepts, will be used throughout this chapter. As specified by the criteria in Table 12.1 and illustrated in Figure 12.1, a single concept may be associated with multiple terms (synonymy); however, a term should represent only one concept.

Components of a Concept-Oriented Terminological System

Within the high-level information model provided by the Nursing Minimum Data Set (NMDS) (Werley and Lang, 1988), there has been extensive development and refinement of terminologies for describing patient problems, nursing interventions, and nursing-sensitive patient outcomes (Martin and Scheet, 1992; Saba, 1992; McCloskey and Bulechek, 1996; Ozbolt et al., 1994; Mortensen and Nielsen, 1996; North American Nursing Diagnosis Association, 1994; Johnson and Maas, 1997). These terminologies are described in the text. The main component of a concept-oriented terminological system, however, is a terminology model representing a set of concepts and their interrelationships. The model is constructed using a representation language that is implemented by a software system.

Terminology Model

A terminology model is a concept-based representation of a collection of domain-specific terms that is optimized for the management of terminological definitions. It encompasses both schemata and type definitions (Campbell et al., 1998; Sowa, 1984). Schemata incorporate domain-specific knowledge about the typical constellations of entities, attributes, and events in the real world and as such reflect plausible combinations of concepts; e.g. dyspnea may be combined with severe to make severe dyspnea. Schemata may be supported by either formal or informal composition rules (i.e. grammars). Type definitions are obligatory conditions that state only the essential properties of a concept; e.g. a nursing activity must have a recipient, a delivery mode, and a focus (Sowa, 1984). Recently there have been a few published reports related to terminology models for nursing (Hardiker and Rector, 1998; Henry et al., 1999; International Council of Nurses, 1999).

Representation Language

Terminology models are formulated using representation language or description logic (e.g. GALEN Representation and Integration Language (GRAIL) (Rector et al., 1997) or Knowledge Representation Specification Syntax (KRSS)) (Campbell et al., 1998). Description logics represent concepts and relationships between concepts (known as roles or attributes). They support the creation of composite concepts from more elementary concepts and reasoning about those concepts.

Computer-Based Tools

A representation language is implemented by a software system that enables (1) management and internal organization of the model, (2) automatic classification of composite concepts based on their internal structure ("medication teaching" is a kind of "teaching"), and (3) transformation of composite concepts into canonical form ("cardiomegaly of the heart" is transformed to "cardiomegaly," since the location of the pathology is inherent in the term itself). In addition, the software may support a set of sanctions that test for sensibility of a

proposed composite concept (e.g. "decubitus ulcer of the heart" and "impaired, normal cognition" are not coherent terms). Other software support may be provided for knowledge engineering, operations management, and conflict detection and resolution.

The extent to which a terminology is concept-oriented and possesses the categorical structures (i.e. terminology model) that render it suitable for computer processing has been characterized as the "generation" of a language system (Rossi Mori et al., 1998). First generation systems consist of a list of enumerated concepts, possibly arranged as a single hierarchy. They serve a single purpose or a group of closely related purposes. Second generation systems include a "categorial structure" that describes the organization of the main categories used in a particular terminology or set of terminologies. The categorial structure is complemented by a thesaurus of elementary descriptors and templates or rules (i.e. grammar) for defining how categories and descriptors may be combined. For example, "pain" and "severe" can be combined into "severe pain." Second generation systems can be used for a range of purposes, but they allow only limited formal processing by computer; i.e. automatic classification of composite concepts is not possible. Third generation systems support sufficient formalisms to enable computer-based processing (i.e. a grammar that defines the rules for automated generation and classification of new concepts, as well as combination of concepts). Third generation language systems are also referred to as formal concept representation systems (Ingenerf, 1995) or reference terminologies (Spackman et al., 1997).

Because they were designed primarily for classification purposes, the majority of existing nursing terminologies (e.g. Home Health Care Classification, Nursing Interventions Classification) can be characterized as first generation systems. The evolving International Classification of Nursing Practice (ICNP) is an example of a second generation language system (International Council of Nurses, 1999). Third generation, concept-oriented terminological systems are the focus of the remainder of this chapter.

 ## Advantages of Concept-Oriented Terminological Systems

Computer-based systems that support clinical uses such as electronic health records and decision support require more finely granular data (less abstract) than that typically contained in terminologies designed primarily for the purpose of classification (Chute et al., 1996; Campbell et al., 1997). Concept-oriented terminological systems allow much greater granularity through controlled composition, and this factor is a major motivating factor behind their development.

In addition, as described previously in this chapter, concept-oriented terminological systems facilitate two important facets of knowledge representation for computer-based systems that support clinical care: describing concepts and manipulating and reasoning about those concepts using computer-based tools. Information content advantages resulting from the first facet include (1) nonambiguous representation of concepts, (2) facilitation of data abstraction or deabstraction without loss of original data (i.e. lossless data transformation), (3) nonambiguous mapping among terminologies, and (4) data reuse in different contexts. These advantages are particularly important for the clinical uses of the terminology. Advantages gained from the second facet include automated classification of new concepts and ability to support multiple inheritance of defining characteristics. Both advantages are vital to the maintenance of the terminology itself as well as to the ability to subsequently support the clinical utility of the terminology (Campbell et al., 1998; Rector et al., 1997).

 ## Concept-Oriented Terminological Approaches in Nursing

Recently, there have been a number of efforts that support the development of concept-oriented terminological systems for the nursing domain. Following a brief description of two approaches, a set of nursing terms is represented using each system in order to illustrate the similarities and differences between the two terminology models and representations.

GALEN

A concept-oriented approach has been developed within the GALEN Program. GALEN can be used in a range of ways, from directly supporting clinical applications (Kirby and Rector, 1996) to supporting the authoring, maintenance, and quality assurance of other kinds of terminologies (Rogers et al., 1998).

GRAIL is a language for representing concepts and their interrelationships—the source material for the construction of terminology models (Rector et al., 1997). Two integrated sets of tools are used in the development of a GRAIL model: a computer-based modeling environment and a terminology server. The modeling environment facilitates the collaborative formulation of models. It allows authoring of clinical knowledge at differ-

ent levels of abstraction. The terminology server is a software system that implements GRAIL. It performs a range of functions including (1) managing and representing internally the model, (2) testing the validity of combinations of concepts, (3) constructing valid composite concepts, (4) transforming composite concepts into canonical form, and (5) automatically classifying composite concepts into the hierarchy. The terminology server is also used to deliver the model for use by clinical applications and other kinds of authoring environments.

GALEN has been applied successfully in other areas of health care (Kirby and Rector, 1996). A major motivation for applying GALEN to nursing has been the desire to meet the requirements of users of clinical applications (Healthfield et al., 1994). An additional factor has been the need to provide a reusable and extensible model of nursing terminology. It is important to recognize that GALEN does not seek to replace existing nursing terminologies; rather, it seeks to contribute to the development of those terminologies, to supplement them, to allow comparisons among them, and to make them available for describing day-to-day nursing care.

For example, as part of another European project, TELENURSE, GALEN has been applied to the ICNP. ICNP is the first attempt in nursing to provide a formalized vocabulary of elementary concepts (the alpha version of the ICNP classification of nursing interventions consists of over 1,000 elementary concepts distributed among six axes) (Mortensen and Nielsen, 1996). However, the mechanism by which composite concepts are generated is poorly specified. Within the TELENURSE project, GALEN has provided a formalized mechanism for defining the syntax for sensible combinations of elementary ICNP concepts (Hardiker and Rector, 1998). In this experiment, the resulting GRAIL model of nursing terminology was shown to meet evolving evaluation criteria related to health care terminologies (Chute et al., 1998; Cimino, 1998). In so doing, it reinforces the view that concept-oriented approaches can overcome many of the difficulties associated with existing nursing terminologies.

SNOMED RT

An alternative concept-oriented approach has been developed based upon SNOMED International. SNOMED RT is a reference terminology optimized for clinical data retrieval and analysis (Spackman et al., 1997). It includes more than 150,000 terms (e.g. topography, procedures, function, findings). The only nursing-specific terminology currently integrated into SNOMED is the North American Nursing Diagnosis Association (NANDA) Taxonomy 1 (North American Nursing Diagnosis Association, 1992). The primary development partners for SNOMED RT are the College of American Pathologists and Kaiser Permanente. Content is enhanced through collaboration and liaison activities between SNOMED and other groups including clinical specialty organizations (e.g. American Nurses Association) and individual terminology developers.

SNOMED RT includes a high-level structure 12 axes plus a set of models for combining concepts from the axes into nonambiguous concept definitions. SNOMED editorial policy supports provider-neutral representations of observations and interventions. The initial focus of development has been findings (e.g. signs, symptoms, diseases, nursing diagnoses) and procedures.

Concepts and relationships in SNOMED RT are represented using modified KRSS (Campbell et al., 1998). Concept definition and manipulation are supported through a set of tools with functionality such as (1) acronym resolution, word completion, term completion, spelling correction, display of the authoritative form of the term entered by the user, and decomposition of unrecognized input (Metaphrase) (Tuttle et al., 1998), (2) automated classification (Ontylog), and (3) conflict management, detection, and resolution (Galapagos) (Campbell et al., 1998).

Evaluations of SNOMED International have demonstrated broad coverage of the health care domain and of the terms nurses use to describe patient problems (Henry et al., 1994; Humphreys, et al., 1997). However, in order to support the representation of nursing concepts, SNOMED RT requires the development of terminology models appropriate for nursing diagnoses and interventions. Additional concepts are also required to support the nursing domain.

Illustration of Representations Using GALEN and SNOMED RT Approaches

Table 12.2 illustrates the representation of four nursing activities using GRAIL and modified KRSS. Although the two representations use different syntax, similarities between the terminology models include the inclusion and explicit modeling of (1) an attribute focused on the type of action used in the activity (e.g. isEnactmentOf *Teaching* and usesTechnique *Teaching*), (2) the recipient of care (e.g. actsOn *Client* and hasObject *Client*), and (3) the focus of the activity (e.g. hasTopic *SafeSex* and hasObject *SafeSex*). A major difference is the number of attributes available to model concepts in each approach.

The GALEN approach has optimized expressiveness in representation, whereas SNOMED has emphasized parsimony of defining attributes.

 ## Summary and Implications for Nursing

Studies have supported the need for concept-oriented terminological systems that facilitate composition of complex concepts from primitive concepts, provide for nonambiguous concept definitions, and support mapping among terminologies (Chute et al., 1996; Campbell et al., 1997; Henry et al., 1994). Because of the magnitude of resources and collaboration required, development of concept-oriented terminological systems is a fairly recent phenomenon, and there is little documentation of the clinical impact of the approach. However, a number of benefits have been proposed: (1) facilitation of evidence-based practice (e.g. linking of clinical practice guidelines to appropriate patients during the patient-provider encounter), (2) matching of potential research subjects to research protocols for which they are potentially eligible, (3) detection of and prevention of potential adverse drug effects, (4) linking on-line information resources, (5) increased reliability and validity of data for quality indicators, and (6) data mining for purposes such as clinical research, health services research, or knowledge discovery.

The developers of nursing and health care terminologies and informatics scientists have made significant progress towards achievement of a concept-oriented terminological system that supports nursing concepts. From decades of nursing language research, there exists an extensive set of terms describing patient problems, nursing interventions and activities, and nursing-sensitive patient outcomes (Martin and Scheet, 1992; Saba, 1992; McCloskey and Bulechek, 1996; Ozbolt, et al., 1994; Mortensen and Nielsen, 1996; North American Nursing Diagnosis Association, 1994; Johnson and Maas, 1997). Health care terminologies include terms that nursing informatics research has shown to be useful for representing concepts of interest to nursing (Henry et al., 1994; Lange, 1996). Representation languages supported by suites of tools have been developed within the context of terminologies with broad coverage of the health care domain (Campbell et al., 1998). Applicability of these tools to the nursing domain has been demonstrated (Hardiker and Rector, 1998; Zingo, 1997).

A major remaining challenge is the development and dissemination of a terminology model that supports

Table 12.2   Representation of Nursing Activity Concepts Using GRAIL and modified KRSS

Activity/Intervention Phrase	GRAIL Representation	Modified KRSS Representation

Assisting a patient with feeding	*Process[1] which*
	   <playsClinicalRole[3] NursingRole[4]
	   isCharacterizedBy (performance[5] which
	     isEnactmentOf (Assisting which
	      actsOn (Person which
	       <playsSocialRole PatientRole[6]
	       performs Eating>)))>
		(define-concept assisting patient with feeding
		(and procedure)
		(has object patient)
		(has object feeding)
		(uses technique assisting)))

Teaching a client about safe sex	*NursingIntervention which*
	   isCharacterizedBy (performance which
	    isEnactmentOf (Teaching which
	     <actsOn Client
	     hasTopic SafeSex[7]>)).
		(define-concept teaching client safe sex
		(and procedure)
		(has object client)
		(has object safe sex)
		(uses technique teaching)))

Coordinating preoperative care for an individual	*NursingIntervention which*
	   isCharacterizedBy (performance which
	    isEnactmentOf (Coordinating which
	    actsOn (CareProcess which
	     <actsOn Person
	     occursBefore SurgicalIntervention[8]>))).
		(define-concept coordinating preoperative care for an individual
		(and procedure)
		(has object individual)
		(has object preoperative care)
		(uses technique coordinating)))

Assessing the ability of a family to cope	*NursingIntervention which*
	   isCharacterizedBy (performance which
	    isEnactmentOf (Assessing which
	    actsOn (Capability which
	     <isFeatureOf (Multiple[9] which
	      <isMultipleOf Person
	      playsSocialRole FamilyRole>)
	     isWithReferenceTo Coping>))).
		(define-concept assessing ability of family to cope
		(and procedure)
		(has object family)
		(has object coping ability)
		(uses technique assessing)))

[1]*Process* is an example of a concept or "entity."

[2]The operator *which* is used for the creation, normalization, and classification of composite concepts.

[3]*playsClinicalRole* is an example of an attribute. More accurately, it is a directed arc labeled by a special kind of entity called an "attribute." Elementary entities and attributes are asserted into a subsumption taxonomy. Entities can be further described, which causes them to be classified possibly under multiple parents.

[4]The purpose of *playsClinicalRole NursingRole* is merely to flag up that in this particular instance the activity is considered a nursing activity. In another instance the same activity might be regarded as a dietetic activity. This would be reflected in GRAIL by substituting *playsClinicalRole DieteticRole* for *playsClinicalRole NursingRole*. In the following examples, the concept *Process which playsClinicalRole NursingRole* has been given the unique name "NursingIntervention."

[5]A common feature of many terminologies is the inclusion of expressions such as "with" to represent conjunction within a single rubric (e.g. the Nursing Interventions Classification rubric "Airway insertion and stabilization"). In the GRAIL representation, rubrics from other representations are mapped to "Nursing Interventions" rather than to individual actions. More than one action is handled, as is explicit omission of an action (i.e. "without"), by including "performance" and "nonPerformance" as states.

[6]The purpose of *playsSocialRole PatientRole* is to flag up that in this example the person plays the role of a patient. In the second example, the person plays the role of a client. This is reflected in GRAIL by substituting *playsSocialRole ClientRole* for *playsSocialRole PatientRole*. The concept *Person which playsSocialRole ClientRole* has been named "Client."

[7]The concept *SafeSex* is not decomposed, as the essence or meaning behind the concept is embodied in this label.

[8]"SurgicalIntervention" represents the concept *Process which playsClinicalRole SurgicalRole*.

[9]*Multiple which isMultipleOf* allows collections of individuals. In this case, the collection is a group of people playing the role of a family.

nursing concepts. However, there is significant progress in that area as well. The existing standardized nursing terminologies are an excellent source of concepts and relationships. In addition, a number of efforts within nursing and the larger health care arena are aimed towards the achievement of a concept-based termino-logic system that supports semantic interoperability across health care information systems (Chute et al., 1998; Rossi Mori et al., 1998; Spackman et al., 1997; Zingo, 1997). Such interoperability is a prerequisite to meeting the information demands of today's complex health care and health management environment.

References

Campbell, J., Carpenter, P., Sneiderman, C., et al. (1997). Phase II evaluation of clinical coding schemes: Completeness, taxonomy, mapping, definitions, and clarity. *Journal of the American Medical Informatics Association, 4*, 238–251.

Campbell, K. E., Cohn, S. P., Chute, C. G., et al. (1998). Scalable methodologies for distributed development of logic-based convergent medical terminology. *Methods of Information in Medicine, 37*, 426–439.

Chute, C. G., Cohn, S. P., and Campbell, J. R. (1998). A framework for comprehensive terminology systems in the United States: Development guidelines, criteria for selection, and public policy implications. ANSI Healthcare Informatics Standards Board Vocabulary Working Group and the Computer-based Patient Records Institute Working Group on Codes and Structures. *Journal of the American Medical Informatics Association 5*, 503–510.

Chute, C. G., Cohn, S. P., Campbell, K.E., et al. (1996). The content coverage of clinical classifications. *Journal of the American Medical Informatics Association, 3*, 224–233.

Cimino, J. J. (1998). Desiderata for controlled medical vocabularies in the twenty-first century. *Methods of Information in Medicine, 37*, 394–403.

Cimino, J. J., Hripcsak, G., Johnson, S. B., et al. (1989). Designing an introspective, multi-purpose, controlled medical vocabulary. In L. C. Kingsland III (Ed.), *Symposium on Computer Applications in Medical Care* (pp. 513–518). Washington, DC: IEEE Computer Society Press.

Hardiker, N. R., and Rector, A. L. (1998). Modeling nursing terminology using the GRAIL representation language. *Journal of the American Medical Informatics Association, 5*, 120–128.

Healthfield, H. A., Hardiker, N., Kirby, J., et al. (1994). The PEN & PAD medical record model: Development of a nursing record for hospital-based care of the elderly. *Methods of Information in Medicine, 33*, 464–472.

Henry, S. B., Cashen, M. S., and O'Brien, A. (1999). Evaluation of a type definition for representing nursing activities within a concept-oriented terminologic system. In N. Lorenzi (Ed.), *1999 AMIA Annual Symposium, Journal of the American Medical Informatics Association Symposium Supplement.* Philadelphia, PA: Hanley & Belfus, Inc.

Henry, S. B., Elfrink, V., McNeil, B. et al. (1998b). The ICNP's relevance in the US. *International Nursing Review, 45*, 153–158.

Henry, S. B., Holzemer, W. L., Reilly, C. A., et al. (1994). Terms used by nurses to describe patient problems: Can SNOMED III represent nursing concepts in the patient record? *Journal of the American Medical Informatics Association, 1*, 61–74.

Henry, S. B., Warren, J., Lange, L., et al. (1998a). A review of the major nursing vocabularies and the extent to which they meet the characteristics required for implementation in computer-based systems. *Journal of the American Medical Informatics Association, 5*, 321–328.

Humphreys, B. L., McCray, A. T., and Cheh, M. L. (1997). Evaluating the coverage of controlled health data terminologies: Report on the results of the NLM/AHCPR Large Scale Vocabulary Test. *Journal of the American Medical Informatics Association, 4*, 484–500.

Ingenerf, J. (1995). Taxonomic vocabularies in medicine: The intention of usage determines different established structures. In R. A. Greenes, H. E. Peterson, and D. J. Protti (Eds.), *MEDINFO 95* (pp. 136–139), Vancouver, B.C.: HealthCare Computing & Communications, Canada, Inc.

International Council of Nurses. (1999). *ICNP Update.* Geneva, Switzerland: International Council of Nurses.

International Standards Organization. (1990). *International Standard ISO 1087: Terminology—Vocabulary.* Geneva, Switzerland: International Standards Organization.

Johnson, M., and Maas, M. (Eds.). (1997). *Nursing Outcomes Classification (NOC).* St. Louis, MO: Mosby.

Kirby, J., and Rector, A. L. (1996). The PEN & PAD data entry system: From prototype to practical system. In J. J. Cimino, (Ed.), *AMIA Annual Fall Symposium (Formerly SCAMC)* (pp. 707–713). Washington, D.C.: Hanley & Belfus.

Lange, L. (1996). Representation of everyday clinical nursing language in UMLS and SNOMED. In J. J. Cimino (Ed.), *AMIA Annual Fall Symposium (Formerly SCAMC)* (pp. 140–144). Washington, D.C.: Hanley & Belfus.

Martin, K. S., and Scheet, N. J. (1992). *The Omaha System: Applications for Community Health Nursing.* Philadelphia: Saunders.

McCloskey, J. C., and Bulechek, G. M. (1996). *Nursing Interventions Classification* (2nd ed.). St. Louis, MO: Mosby.

Mortensen, R. A., and Nielsen, G. H. (1996). *International Classification of Nursing Practice (version 0.2).* Geneva, Switzerland: International Council of Nursing.

North American Nursing Diagnosis Association. (1992). *NANDA Nursing Diagnoses: Definitions and Classification 1992–1993.* Philadelphia, PA: North American Nursing Diagnosis Association.

North American Nursing Diagnosis Association. (1994). *Nursing Diagnoses: Definitions & Classification 1995–1996.* Philadelphia: North American Nursing Diagnosis Association.

Ogden, C., and Richards, I. (1923). *The Meaning of Meaning.* New York: Harcourt, Brace, and World.

Ozbolt, J., Fruchtnicht, J. N., and Hayden, J.R. (1994). Toward data standards for clinical nursing information. *Journal of the American Medical Informatics Association, 1*, 175–185.

Rector, A. L., Bechhofer, S., Goble, C. A., et al. (1997). The GRAIL concept modelling language for medical terminology. *Artificial Intelligence in Medicine, 9,* 139–171.

Rogers, J. E., Price, C., Rector, A. L., et al. (1998). Validating clinical terminological structures: Integration and cross-validation of read Thesaurus and GALEN. In C. G. Chute (Ed.), *1998 AMIA Annual Fall Symposium, Journal of the American Medical Informatics Association Symposium Supplement* (pp. 845–849). Orlando: Hanley & Belfus.

Rossi Mori, M. A., Consorti, F., and Galeazzi, E. (1998). Standards to support development of terminological systems for healthcare telematics. *Methods of Information in Medicine, 37,* 551–563.

Saba, V. K. (1992). The classification of home health care nursing: Diagnoses and interventions. *Caring Magazine, 11,* 50–56.

Sowa, J. (1984). *Conceptual Structures.* Reading, MA: Addison Wesley.

Spackman, K. A., Campbell, K. E., and Cote, R. A. (1997). SNOMED RT: A reference terminology for health care. In D. Masys (Ed.), *1997 AMIA Annual Fall Symposium, Journal of the American Medical Informatics Association Symposium Supplement* (pp. 640–644). Nashville: Hanley & Belfus.

Tuttle, M. S., Keck, K. D., Cole, W. G. et al. (1998). Metaphrase: An aid to the clinical conceptualization and formalization of patient problems in healthcare enterprises. *Methods of Information in Medicine, 37,* 373–383.

Werley, H. H., and Lang, N. M. (Eds.). (1988). *Identification of the Nursing Minimum Data Set.* New York: Springer.

Zingo, C. A. (1997). Strategies and tools for creating a common nursing terminology within a large health maintenance organization. In U. Gerdin, M. Tallberg, and P. Wainwright (Eds). *Nursing Informatics: The Impact of Nursing Knowledge on Health Care Informatics* (pp. 27–31). Stockholm, Sweden: IOS Press.

13

Implementing and Upgrading Clinical Information Systems

Marina Douglas

OBJECTIVES

1. Describe the eight phases in developing, implementing, or upgrading a clinical information system.
2. Describe the personnel requirements for implementing or upgrading a clinical information system.
3. Describe the roles and responsibilities of nursing for implementing or upgrading a clinical information system.
4. Identify the various tools of the trade used in developing, implementing, and upgrading a clinical information system.
5. Describe the methods of evaluating a clinical information system.
6. Describe new challenges in implementing and upgrading clinical information systems.

KEY WORDS

information systems
information science
integrated advances
information management systems
hospital information systems
clinical information system

 ## What Is a Clinical Information System?

Today's health care delivery system requires clinicians of varying specialties to make clinical decisions based on data from many sources. Articles describe the clinician's demands to view all automated data from a single source. Clinicians evaluate how the computer affects work flow and the ease of use. "If a computer system isn't faster and easier to use than paper and pencil, physicians don't want it" (Cook, 1998). The goal of many organizations is to have not only a complete electronic medical record (EMR), encompassing the demographic, payer, as well as clinical data, but to provide clinical departments with information regarding their management service delivery. Support of the clinical departments must include accessibility to reference materials and current literature (Zielstorff et al., 1988).

The clinical realm of the electronic medical record has been particularly difficult to automate. Technology limited the ability to view analog data (EKG tracings, fetal monitor strips, intercranial pressure monitoring strips) via digital clinical information systems (CISs). New digital technology has all but eliminated these constraints, holding promise for the eventuality of the electronic medical record. A CIS, therefore, strives to provide all clinicians with the automated data required to assess and treat patients. Data collected from the laboratory, radiology, pharmacy, and cardiopulmonary departments, as well as consultative notes, traditional doctors' and nurses' notes, admission history and physical reports, and operative reports are just a few of the sources of data required by clinicians in their evaluation of patients.

Just as multiple clinical disciplines and departments are necessary for the delivery of a health care system, a CIS must incorporate multiple automated sources of clinical data and present the data in a meaningful way to each clinician, discipline, or department. This has been a formidable task for organizations. Incremental technology advances have brought the reality of the CIS from its infancy stages in the 1970s to its current late adolescent status. Web browser technology has provided the first giant step to achieving the goal of a CIS and an EMR. Informatics nurses, with their overall knowledge of the coordination of services required for patient care and their knowledge of automation, have proven to be invaluable in the evolution of the CIS.

Nursing involvement in the design and implementation of clinical systems is required at many levels of the process. Nurses have been instrumental members of departmental teams in addition to their active involvement on nursing-focused projects. The nursing process utilized to deliver direct patient care (i.e. to observe, assess, plan, implement, and evaluate care) provides a strong parallel framework for nurses to succeed in the design and implementation of CIS projects (Douglas, 1995). The skills required to deliver direct patient care necessitate the ability to coordinate patient care involving multiple disciplines and departments. This provides nurses a knowledge of the many aspects of health care delivery orchestrated for effective, efficient health care delivery. Informatics nursing was recognized as a specialty area by the American Nurses Association in 1993.

> Nursing informatics is the specialty that integrates nursing science, computer science, and information science in identifying, collecting, processing, and managing data and information to support nursing practice administration, education, research and the expansion of nursing knowledge. The practice of nursing informatics includes the development and evaluation of applications, tools, processes and structures which assist nurses with the management of data in taking care of patients or in supporting the practice. It involves collaboration with other health-care and informatics professionals in the development of informatics products and standards for nursing and healthcare informatics. (American Nurses Association, 1994)

The roles filled by nurses are at the heart of many development, implementation, and upgrading projects; these roles include being a member of departmental teams and serving as project team leaders, and experienced informatics nurses may be chosen to direct overall projects as project managers.

A CIS assists clinicians with data necessary for decision-making and problem-solving. Clinical disciplines and specialty services share common user requirements as well as having specialized practice requirements. Just as multiple departments work in concert for optimum patient care delivery, the components of a CIS interact in much the same coordinated fashion. Nursing is but one discipline interacting with the patient. Medicine, dietary, laboratory, pharmacy, radiology, and physical therapy departments, etc. are other major disciplines involved. If each discipline acted independently, the care of the patient would be fragmented, causing duplication of efforts and delays in treatment (Selker et al., 1989). A clinical information system must serve the organization and the patient in much the same way a smoothly running health care delivery system involves all appropriate departments in establishing health care delivery processes. The benefit of coordinated efforts to the patient and to the entire organization outweighs the singular advantage to any one discipline's or department's processes.

The nursing requirements of a CIS described in this chapter will focus on the requirements of nursing department of a health care facility providing direct patient care. As described, it is one department in a complex health care delivery system; to be effective, nursing must act in concert with the entire organization. The major CIS requirements for nursing are to (1) administer a nursing department, (2) assist the management of nursing practice, (3) assist nursing education, and (4) support nursing research (Zielstorff, 1988). The nursing component of a CIS can be designed as a stand-alone system, a subsystem of a larger system, or an integral part of the health care organization's overall information system (Simpson, 1993a). It can be programmed for processing by a mainframe, minicomputer, or microcomputer, and it may share the same equipment other departmental systems in the facility use. The advantages of the nursing components (applications) being part of a subsystem or an integrated application are significant. These advantages will be described in detail later in this chapter.

Because of increasingly complex technology and information requirements of health care, few hospitals and/or nursing departments have the resources to develop or create their own CIS or nursing computer applications. Some organizations have implemented CISs and maintained and even completed an evaluation of their nursing components. From the evaluation, new uses of the system have been demonstrated or suggested. To meet new legislation, new regulations, and new professional standards, CISs as young as 5 years old need to be upgraded. The issues related to upgrading already existing computer applications are a feature of this chapter.

Regardless of the size or type of system, any CIS or single application design/implementation or upgrade must complete the eight phases of implementation listed below. The implementation of a clinical information is a process introducing an application or information system to an organization, ensuring the full benefit and potential of the system are realized (Ritter and Glaser, 1994). The phases of implementation utilize a problem-solving, scientific approach. The problem-solving begins with observation of the operations or problem in question. The second step requires an in-depth assessment of the issues. Developing and implementing a plan to resolve the problem are the third and fourth steps. The last step, evaluation, provides feedback on how well the solution resolves the problem. Countless iterations of the problem-solving approach are utilized during software implementation or upgrading. Inherent in the implementation process is the need to recognize and manage change and its impact. "The ability to manage change often marks the difference between the success and failure of implementing a change initiative and moving an organization forward" (Ritter and Glaser, 1994, p. 168). The eight phases of implementation are planning, system analysis, system design/system selection, development, testing, training, implementation, and evaluation (Fig. 13.1). Each of these phases is detailed later in this chapter. The process of upgrading a clinical information system, entailing all eight phases of implementation, will be discussed.

Attempting to implement or upgrade a system without accomplishing the tasks associated with each phase generally results in system failure in one or more of the following areas:

EIGHT PHASES OF DESIGN, IMPLEMENTATION, and UPGRADING

Planning

System Analysis

System Design/System Selection

Development

Testing

Training

Implementation

Evaluation

Figure 13.1
Eight phases of designing, implementing, or upgrading a nursing information system.

- CIS does not meet the stated goal of the project.
- There is failure to gain end user acceptance.
- Expenditures exceed budget.
- Anticipated benefits are unrealized.

The Planning Phase

The planning phase of the project begins once an organization has determined an existing need or problem may be filled or solved by the development or implementation of a clinical information system or application. Establishing the committee framework to research and make recommendations for the project is an important first step.

Clinical Information System Committee Structure and Project Staff

The nursing administrator's involvement in the establishment of a CIS committee structure is paramount to the success of the project. The nursing administrator, in conjunction with the information system's management team, works to develop a committee structure and participation to best guarantee the success of the project. Assigning the appropriate resources, whether financial or personnel, is a critical success factor (Spillane et al., 1990; Protti and Peel, 1998). A three-tiered committee approach is recommended to accomplish the design, implementation, or upgrading of a complete CIS—a steering committee, a project team, and departmental teams.

Clinical Information System Steering Committee
Before a CIS is developed or selected, the organization must appoint a CIS steering committee. The CIS steering committee generally includes representatives from the following areas:

- Hospital administration/hospital finance
- Nursing administration
- Medical staff
- Information systems department at the director or manager level
- Major ancillary departments (lab, radiology, pharmacy, dietary, medical records/patient registration, patient accounting)
- Health information management (medical records)
- Legal affairs
- Outside consultants (as needed)
- Other appointed members (as needed)

The CIS steering committee is charged with providing oversight guidance to the selection and integration of a new CIS into the organization. The collective knowledge of the Steering Committee's members relative to the organization's operations provides global insight and administrative authority to resolve issues. This committee may need to meet frequently during the early planning phase and the implementation phases of the project, with less frequent meetings required during the middle stages (Fig. 13.2).

Project Team   The project team is led by an appointed project manager and includes a designated team leader for each of the major departments affected by the system selection, implementation, or upgrade proposed. The objectives of the project team are to (1) understand the technology and technology restrictions, if any, of a proposed system, (2) understand the impact of intradepartmental decisions, (3) make decisions at the interdepartmental level for the overall good of the CIS within the organization, and (4) become the key resource for their application. A stated goal for the selection, implementation, or upgrading of a CIS is to improve patient care; gains made by one department at the expense of another department rarely work to improve overall patient care delivery. The project team's ability to evaluate multiple departments' information desires in light of the capabilities of the proposed system is important to the overall success of the project.

The project manager must be acutely familiar with the phases of implementation. Larger scale CIS implementations necessitate a project manager with significant implementation experience. The project manager is

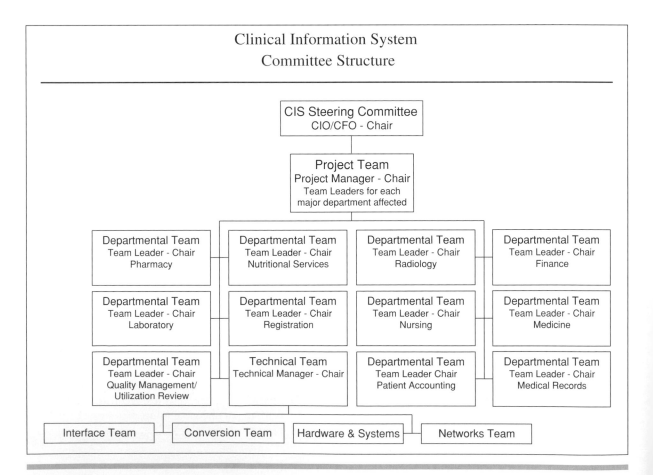

Figure 13.2
Committee structures.

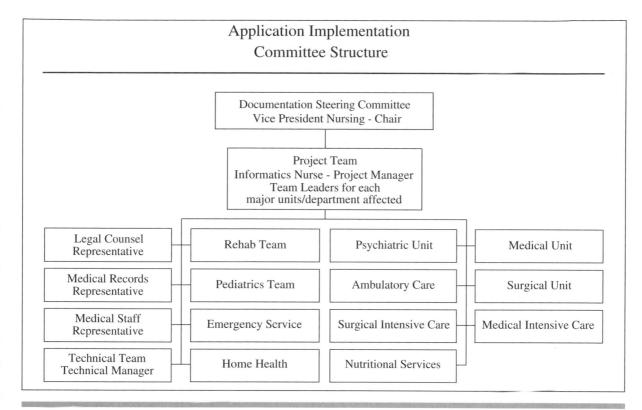

Figure 13.3
Application implementation committee structure.

responsible for managing all aspects of the project. This management includes software application develop ment, hardware, and networks, as well as oversight management of the interfacing and conversion tasks. The project manager must have good communication, facilitation, organizational, and motivational skills to be successful. A sound knowledge of health care delivery, hospital processes, and politics is important. The project manager must have full-time dedication to a large scale design or implementation project (Fig. 13.3).

Departmental Teams   The charge of the departmental teams is (1) to thoroughly understand the department's information needs, (2) to gain a full understanding of the software's features and functions, (3) to merge the new system's capabilities with departments' operations, (4) to assist in the system testing effort, (5) to participate in developing and conducting end user education, and (6) to provide a high level of support during the initial activation period of the new system. The team leaders must

possess a sound knowledge of the hospital and departmental policies and procedures (both formal and informal) good organizational and communication skills, and must be adept at gaining consensus and resolving conflict. Successful implementations have provided decision-making authority at the level of project teams whenever possible.

A smaller scale project requires committee representation of a smaller scope. As an example, representation on the committees to implement an automated documentation project will have an emphasis on nursing members with less involvement from radiology, laboratory, and finance. Each of the major nursing subspecialty areas and ancillary departments scheduled to use the system for patient documentation is represented. A health information management representative and legal counsel assist the committee in planning for regulatory compliance. Physician involvement early in the planning process is recommended to ensure understanding of the information needs of the medical staff relative to patient documentation. The physician committee member assists in easing the medical staff's transition to the new documentation system. If the system will affect nursing interactions or communications with other departments, each of the major areas affected have committee representation and all areas/disciplines have involvement to ensure acceptance of the implementation plan at an early stage. The implementation of software for interdepartmental care planning is an example of a committee structure requiring a wider range of participants. Active involvement by social services, dietary, occupational therapy, and physical therapy departments as well as medicine and nursing ensures greater acceptance of the interdepartmental care planning application.

Planning

During the planning phase, the information requirements necessary to solve the problem or accomplish the goal are assessed. The information needs for selecting, implementing, or upgrading a CIS, including their implications for nursing services, nursing practice, and quality care, must also be identified. In the American Society for Testing and Materials (ASTM) standards, the planning phase is referred to as the project definition. Commercial software developers and consultants rank this phase as the most critical factor in the selection of a system, even more important than the system itself (Zinn, 1989). Excellent planning is time-consuming and seemingly costly. It is estimated the process can take up to 2 years to design and develop or to select and implement a new system (Ginsburg and Browning, 1989). This phase is critical whether a system is actually being developed or existing commercial systems are being evaluated for selection.

The planning phase involves the following steps:

- Definition of the problem and/or stated goal
- Feasibility study
- Documentation and negotiation of project scope agreement
- Allocation of resources

Definition of the Problem

Definition of the problem and/or stated goal precisely is essential and often not readily apparent. Not until the information requirements of the problem and/or stated goal and outcomes are precisely defined will the real characteristics of the problem be revealed (Fitzgerald et al., 1981).

For example:

- Unfair nurse staff assignments may relate to an invalid patient classification tool (inaccurate grouping of patients) rather than to workload measurements and/or acuity score.
- Duplicate health department reports may result in inappropriate statistics being collected instead of the collection of unique atomic-level data elements.

The project definition includes a description of how the system will be evaluated. Establishing the evaluation criteria early in the process supports the successful management philosophy of beginning with the end in mind (Convey, 1992). The results and improvements expected from implementing the system are described by realistic goals for the system. They might include increased processing capabilities, savings in processing time, decreased costs, or increased personnel productivity. When updating or expanding the CIS, the project definition includes the identification of equipment currently available, its age, the degree of amortization, and the need for hardware or operating system software upgrades prior to undertaking an upgrade project.

Feasibility Study

A feasibility study is a preliminary analysis to determine if the proposed problem can be solved by the implementation of a CIS or component application. The feasibility study not only clarifies the problem and/or stated goal but helps to identify the information needs, objectives, and scope of the project. The feasibility study helps the CIS steering committee understand the real problem and/or goal by analyzing multiple parameters and by presenting possible solutions. It highlights whether the proposed solution will produce usable products and whether the proposed system's benefits outweigh the costs. Operational issues are reviewed to determine if the proposed solution will work in the intended environment. Technical issues are reviewed to ensure the proposed system can be built and/or will be compatible with the proposed and/or current technology. Legal and statutory regulations are reviewed to ensure compliance with local and federal law. The feasibility study includes a high level description of the human resources required and how the selected system will be developed, utilized, and implemented. The feasibility study describes the management controls to be established for obtaining administrative, financial, and technical approvals to proceed with each phase of the project.

The feasibility study seeks to answer the following questions:

- What is the real problem to be solved and/or stated goal to be met?
- Where does the project fit into the overall strategic plan of the organization?
- What specific outcomes are expected from the project?
- What are the measurable criteria for determining project success from the above outcomes?
- What research and assumptions support the implementation project?
- What are the known limitations and risks to the project?
- What is the timing of the remaining phases of the project?
- Who will be committed to implementing the project?
- What are the estimated costs in both dollars and personnel time?
- What is the justification for the project, including the relationship between costs and benefits?

A feasibility study includes the following areas?

Statement of Objectives   The first step in conducting a feasibility study is to state the objectives for the proposed system. These objectives constitute the purpose(s) of the system. All objectives are outcomes-oriented and are stated in measurable terms. The objectives identify the "end product" and what the CIS will do for the end users. For example:

- An objective relating to a nursing resource scheduling component to a CIS might be stated as: "Implement a nurse staffing and scheduling application based on a valid and reliable patient classification system."
- An objective relating to statistical reporting in a community health agency might be stated as follows: "Develop a system for reporting the detailed statistical data as required by local, state, and federal authorities."

Environmental Assessment   The project is defined in terms of the support it provides to both the mission and the strategic plans of the organization. The project is evaluated relative to the organization's competition. The impact of legal, regulatory, and ethical considerations is reviewed.

Determination of Information Needs   This step, sometimes called a needs assessment, outlines the high-level information required by the users. Identifying the information needed helps clarify what users will expect from the system. Such knowledge is essential in designing the system's output, input, and processing requirements. For example:

- A nurse staffing system based on patient classification would need the following information:
  - A valid and reliable patient classification tool for determining staffing requirements
  - Number of nursing personnel required by shift to staff each medical and surgical unit
  - Types of nursing personnel required to staff the units
- A statistical reporting system designed to meet local, state, and federal reporting for community/home care nursing might require the following information:
  - Time spent by personnel making visits
  - Cost of visits by type of provider
  - Number of clients per program
  - Number of services provided to clients by nurses

Determination of Scope   The scope of the proposed system establishes system constraints and outlines what the proposed system will and will not produce. For example:

- The scope of a nurse staffing system might be stated as follows: "The system will provide nurse staffing schedules for in-patient care units. Home health and outpatient staffing schedules will not be included."
- The scope of a system relating to community health statistical reporting might be stated as follows: "The system will collect data needed for routine, ongoing reports. Specialty reports will be handled via a separate structured query language reporting system."

Development of a Project Timeline   A project timeline is developed providing an overview of the key milestone events of the project. The projected length of time for each major phase of the project is established. Often called a project workplan, the major steps required for each phase are outlined in sufficient detail to provide the steering committee background on the proposed development or implementation process.

Recommendations   Committees may forget that not all projects are beneficial to the strategic mission of the organization, and a decision can be made not only to proceed, but also not to proceed, with a project. The viability of the project is based on the review of the multiple factors researched in the feasibility study. It is critical to consider whether more personnel or equipment is necessary rather than more computerization. In addition to identifying potential hardware and software improvements, the costs and proposed benefits are factored into the project's viability decision. In upgrading or considering expansion of a system, a concerted effort to maximize use of the current system and to make process improvements in the current management and coordination of existing systems should be undertaken before deciding to procure a new system(s).

If, based on the findings of the feasibility study, the project steering committee determines to continue with the project, a project scope agreement is prepared.

Documentation and Negotiation of a Project Scope Agreement

A project scope agreement is drafted by the project team and submitted to the project's steering committee for acceptance. The project scope agreement includes the scope of the project, the application level management requirements, the proposed activation strategy for implementing the CIS or application, and the technical management and personnel who will maintain the equipment. The agreement is based on the findings of the feasibility study.

The project scope agreement becomes the internal organizational contract for the project. It defines the short- and long-term goals, establishes the criteria for evaluating the success of the project, and expands the workplan to include further detail regarding the steps to be accomplished in the development or implementation of the CIS.

Allocation of Resources

The last step in the planning phase is determining what resources are required to successfully complete the project scope agreement. A firm commitment of resources for development of the entire CIS project scope agreement (including all phases of implementation) is needed before the system can fulfill its stated objectives. The following points should be considered when planning for resources:

- Present staffing workload

- Human resources (i.e. numbers of personnel, experience and abilities, percentage of dedicated time to the project)
- Present cost of operation
- Relationship of implementation events with non-project events (i.e. JCAHO reviews, state certification inspections, peak vacation and census times, union negotiations, house staff turnover)
- Anticipated training costs
- Space availability
- Current and anticipated equipment requirements for the project team

Highly successful projects have spent the requisite amount of time to thoroughly complete the planning phase. Further, the successful organizations have communicated senior management and administration's project expectations through dissemination of the project scope agreement to all departments in the organization.

The Key Role of the Nurse Administrator

Nurse administrators are key to the successful implementation and/or upgrading of a CIS. They play an integral part in the planning phase as they establish a "vision" for nursing and health care delivery where the importance of information is foundational. This vision must encompass: (1) a business vision of the impact on the nursing department's resources, (2) a management vision of the policies and action plans supporting the planning, implementation, and maintenance of these systems, and (3) a nursing vision of enhancing clinical nursing practice (American Association of Nurse Executives, 1993). Nurse administrators need to be engaged in system selection, implementation, evaluation, and upgrading initiatives. In 1991, their involvement and participation in the selection process was mandated by the Joint Commission on Accreditation of Healthcare Organizations (JCAHO). JCAHO guidelines require nurses to be involved in evaluating, selecting, and integrating all systems that affect patient care and that this participation be documented as part of the Commission's accreditation reviews.

Successful implementations of a CIS have been accomplished by many facilities; the active involvement of the nurse executive is considered a critical success factor of any CIS implementation or upgrade. Visionary nursing leaders who have implemented CISs and/or nursing components at their institutions have shared their recommendations and urge that a business plan be developed and incorporated into the process. The following features should be discussed in the business plan:

- An executive summary strongly supporting the power of timely and accurate information.
- An introduction, outlining the purpose and objectives of the proposed CIS and/or nursing application(s).
- An environmental assessment of the CIS and/or nursing components in use by similar hospitals.
- An analysis of the nursing department culture, infrastructure, policies, and information needs.
- An overview of the design and implementation plan describing the objectives, activation strategy to be utilized, a listing of equipment needs, staffing projections, time resources, potential costs, and evaluation methodologies for the CIS as a whole and the nursing component(s) in particular.
- A financial plan projecting staffing, budget, expenses, capital expenditures, and miscellaneous expenditures.

System Analysis Phase

The system analysis phase, the second phase of developing a CIS, is the fact-finding phase. All data requirements related to the problem defined in the project scope agreement are collected and analyzed to gain a sound understanding of the current system, how it is utilized, and what is needed from the new system. Process analysis is foundational to the actual system design, since it examines the objectives and project scope in terms of the end user requirements, the flow of information in daily operation, and the processing of required data elements. Through the analysis effort, the individual data elements, interfaces, and decision points of the project are identified (Yourdon, 1989). Current costs and resources required for processing the data are compared with estimates for the cost of processing with the new system. If a system is being upgraded or expanded, the current equipment and functions are described. Careful evaluation is undertaken to ensure compatibility with the new system's requirements and to maximize the use of available equipment as long as possible. Depreciation costs of available equipment and projected budget expenditures are reviewed.

The importance of this phase should not be underestimated. Design changes made during the analysis stage often add minimal costs to the project; as the project progresses to the development and implementation phases, the cost of programmatic or design changes increases dramatically. According to one source, when a project is in the planning phase, the relative cost to make a design change or fix an error is one; in the analysis phase, the relative cost to fix the error/design change is three to six times that of the planning phase. The relative cost to fix an error or change a system design jumps to 40-1,000 times once the system is operational (Gause and Weinburg, 1989).

The system analysis phase consists of the following five steps:

- Data collection
- Data analysis
- Data review
- Benefits identification
- System proposal development

Data Collection

The collection of data reflecting the existing problem or goal is the first step in the system analysis phase. As a result of thorough data collection, refinements to the project scope agreement may occur. Added benefits to the organization may be realized through the small refinements. Larger project scope refinements should be carefully researched and evaluated (utilizing the steps outlined in the feasibility study methodology above) prior to requesting a major project scope change. Large or small, all changes must continue to support the goal(s) of the project and the strategic plan of the organization.

Two important documents are created as a result of data collection. The first is the creation of a workflow document for each major goal or problem to be resolved by the implementation of the new software or system; the second is a functional design document outlining how the new system will resolve the identified goals/problem.

Work Flow Document The work flow document assimilates the data collected above into logical sequencing of tasks and subtasks performed by the end users for each goal or problem area. Departmental standards of care, ordering patterns, procedures, operating manuals, reports (routine, regulatory, and year-end), and forms used in day-to-day operations are collected. Individual data elements required by clinicians in each department are identified and analyzed for continuity and duplication both inter- and intradepartmentally. The work flow document includes the following:

- A list of assumptions about the process or work effort
- A list of the major tasks performed by the user
- A list of the subtasks and steps the user accomplishes and outlines whether:
  - The determination of optional or required status for each task
  - The frequency of the task being performed
  - The criticality and important factors of the tasks/subtasks
  - The order of the subtasks
- The number and frequency of alternate scenarios available to the end user to accomplish a particular task

There are multiple sources of data for completing a work flow document. These include the following:

- Written documents, forms, and flow sheets
- Policy and procedure manuals
- Questionnaires
- Interviews
- Observations

Written Documents, Forms, and Flow Sheets Many institutions have a forms committee through which all forms used in the institution's legal record are approved. This committee is an excellent first source for forms collection. Individual specialty units may utilize self-developed forms. Reviewing a representative sample of medical records from each of the nursing units or clinics will be helpful in identifying data elements, the presentation of data (from the forms design), and documentation patterns of the institution.

Questionnaires Questionnaires, another method of data collection, provide useful information without consuming large amounts of team members' time. Questionnaires, tailored toward the potential users, can ascertain the needs of the different types of users. Questionnaires can collect the opinions of the potential users regarding multiple topics, such as essential data elements for computerization, the format in which data should be presented, and the products or outputs that should be produced by the system.

Interviews Interviews are one of the best sources of information for clarifying an existing patient care delivery problem or stated goals. Interviews with selected personnel at all organizational levels can elicit specific information on how, when, where, and in what kinds of situations data are processed. Moreover, standard interview tools help to document, in a logical sequence, the kinds of information required by the end user and the sequence in which it is needed.

Observations Observations can reveal how staff members relate to each other, how they manage or view information, and how the information is utilized in patient care. Direct observation provides an understanding of the environment in which the system will be utilized, often revealing duplication of efforts and/or redundant data collection.

Functional Design Document The functional design document is the overview statement of how the new system will work. It utilizes the work flow documents as its base, adding the critical documentation of the integration of each of the work flow documents to create a new system, implement a commercial software application, or upgrade a system. The functional design document, in this phase, outlines the human and machine procedures, the input points, the processing requirements, the output from the data entry, and the major reports to be generated from the new system. The functional design is a concise description of the functions required from the proposed computerized system and describes how the application will accomplish its task. From the functional design document, database structure will be determined.

When new software is being created, the functional design document provides the programmers with a view of screens, linkages, and alternate scenarios to accomplish a task. Initial programming efforts can begin once the functional design is accepted. In the instance where a commercially available system or application is being implemented, the functional design outlines how the end users will utilize the system's programs to accomplish their tasks. In some cases, commercial software provides multiple pathways to accomplish a single task; the functional specification may suggest deploying a limited number of available pathways. For example, a functional specification for creating a new patient care plan application may develop four programmatic pathways to identify a patient problem.

1. Clinicians select a problem from the list of North American Nursing Diagnosis Association (NANDA) approved nursing diagnoses without associated nursing standards of care (interventions). Nurses will be required to add specific interventions to the selected nursing diagnosis.

2. Clinicians select a NANDA-approved nursing problem with nursing standards of care (interventions) defined. The defined interventions may be tailored to the individual patient.

3. Clinicians define a problem utilizing a free text field and build nursing interventions required for the patient.

4. Clinicians select suggested nursing diagnoses derived from rules-based logic applied to an automated patient assessment. (e.g., 4+ pitting edema bilaterally is documented in the patient assessment; the rules-based logic suggests a nursing diagnosis of "alteration in fluid balance, more than required").

In the instance where the above commercial software is available, the functional specification for selection of a nursing diagnosis may limit the end user to the second and fourth options only, since these pathways may more closely support the philosophy of patient care delivery at the institution.

Data Analysis

The analysis of the collected data is the second step in the system analysis phase. The analysis provides the data for development of an overview of the nursing problem and/or stated goal defined in the project scope agreement.

Several tools can be utilized in the development of the work flow and functional design documents. Some of the more common tools are:

- Data flowchart
- Grid chart
- Decision table
- Organizational chart
- Model

Data Flowchart   A data flowchart, one of the most important tools in data analysis, graphically illustrates the sequential steps found in processing the nursing problem or accomplishing the stated goal. It provides a "road map" of the flow of information. A flowchart of the data traces where and when the flow of information begins, where it goes, and where it ends.

Grid Chart   A grid chart, also called a data analysis chart, analyzes the interrelationships of the data used to process the nursing problem and/or stated goal. It generally includes a listing of all the data elements collected as input that are processed and generated as output. A grid chart can also be used to list the kinds of information generated as output, including purpose and recipient.

Decision Table   A decision table, sometimes called a decision-logic table, illustrates the logical decisions and possible alternatives for solving the nursing problem and/or accomplishing the stated goal. It provides a tabular display for all relevant data, lists all possible choices, and highlights the logical rules used for processing the data.

Organizational Chart   An organizational chart depicts the levels of authority and the formal lines of interorganizational communication. It helps clarify who is responsible for what and how current data are processed.

Model   A model provides an abstraction of a real situation, thus helping to analyze circumstances too complex for actual presentation. Moreover, it is more economical to develop a model, graphically displaying the proposed system, than to reconstruct each real-life situation.

The two major types of modeling relevant to data analysis are forecasting and simulation. Forecasting helps with decision-making. For example, it may be used to predict future staffing needs based on certain assumptions. Simulation, on the other hand, presents an abstraction of reality. Simulations can be used to present how different staffing needs will vary based on different ground rules. Both models can be used to determine the best method of predicting staffing.

Computerized planning models can highlight resources, timeframes, materials, and major activities relevant to a given project. Both the program evaluation review technique (PERT) and the critical path method (CPM) are models for planning, scheduling, and controlling a system or project activities. The CPM generally highlights the timeframe and anticipated cost for completing a project. Commercial automated programs are readily available to assist with the management of large-scale, complex models as well as smaller projects.

Data Review

The third step in the analysis phase is to review the data collected in the feasibility study, the work flow documents, and the functional specification and provide recommendations to the project steering committee for the new system. The review focuses on resolving the problems and/or attaining the goals defined in the feasibility study based on the best methods or pathways derived from the work flow documents and the functional design. Recommendations for streamlining work flow are suggested. The success of a CIS implementation project rests on the ability of the departmental and project teams to analyze the data and propose solutions benefiting the total organization without favoring certain departments at the expense of others. The benefits of a thorough structured analysis provide objective data to support these decisions. The careful analysis of end user requirements and potential solutions have been proved to reduce the cost of design and implementation (Gause and Weinburg, 1989).

Benefits Identification

The overall anticipated benefits from the system are documented in the fourth step in the system analysis process. The benefits reflect the resolution of the identified problem, formulated and stated in quantifiable terms. The proposed benefits statements become the criteria for measuring the success of the project. For example:

1. Within 30 days of the system's activation, the new results reporting system will reduce the length of time between the routine collection of a patient's blood sample and the time the result is available to the clinician by X minutes.

2. The new results reporting application will decrease the number of calls by clinicians to the lab for routine lab results by X% within 30 days of the system's activation.

System Proposal Development

The final step in the system analysis stage is to create a system proposal document. The proposal is submitted to the project's steering committee for review and approval. It sets forth the problems and/or goals and the requirements for the new system's overall design. It outlines the standards, documentation, and procedures for management control of the project, and it defines the information required, the necessary resources, anticipated benefits, a detailed workplan, and projected costs for the new system. The system proposal furnishes the project steering committee with recommendations concerning the proposed CIS or application. The system proposal document answers four questions:

1. What are the major problems and/or goals under consideration?

2. How will the proposed CIS solution correct or eliminate the problems and/or accomplish the stated goals?

3. What are the anticipated costs?

4. How long will it take?

The system proposal describes the project in sufficient detail to provide a management level understanding of the system or application without miring in minutiae. Much of the information required in the system proposal is collected in the earlier phases of the analysis. It has been suggested that this proposal is best accepted when presented as a business proposal and championed by a member of the project's steering committee. The format of the final system proposal includes the following information.

1. A concise statement of the problem(s) and/or goal(s)

2. Background information related to the problem

3. Environmental factors related to the problem

   (a) Competition

   (b) Economics

   (c) Politics

   (d) Ethics

4. Anticipated benefits

5. Proposed solutions

6. Budgetary and resource requirements

7. Project timetable

Acceptance of the system proposal by the project steering committee provides the project senior management support. Following acceptance by the project steering committee, it is not unusual for major CIS proposals to be presented to the institution's governing board for their acceptance and approval and to receive funding. Often the requirement for board approval is dependent on the final cost estimates of the system. Acceptance of the proposal by the project steering committee and the governing board assures not only funding for the project but critical top-down management and administrative support for the project. The final system proposal is an internal contract between the CIS committees/teams (steering, project, and departmental) and the institution. When commercially available software is under consideration, the system proposal document assists the institution's legal team in formulating a contract with the software vendor as well as providing the basis for the development of a formal request for proposal (RFP) to potential vendors.

As noted earlier, the active support and involvement of the nursing executive in the development of the feasibility study are essential. The championing of the final system proposal greatly enhances the chances of acceptance of the system proposal.

The System Design Phase

In the system design phase, the design details of the system and the detailed plans for implementing the system are developed for both the functional and the technical components of the system. Acceptance of the system proposal by the steering committee heralds the beginning of the system design phase.

There are three major steps in the system design phase:

- Functional specifications
- Technical specifications
- Implementation planning

Functional Specifications

The functional specifications utilize the functional design document developed in the system analysis phase of a CIS and builds on the design by formulating a detailed description of ALL system inputs, outputs, and processing logic required to complete the scope of the project. It further refines what the proposed system will encompass and provides the framework for its operation. For example, when creating a new application for a nursing documentation application, the functional specifications include all pathways for entering or editing a nurse's note, marking a note entered in error, and the interface functions with the hospital's registration application (allowing automatic updating of the nursing unit census). The functional specification for the "edit note" pathway details the conditions necessary to allow a user to edit a nurse's note (i.e. only the author of the note or an authorized supervisor can edit a note), the method to identify that the note has been edited, the date and time of the original note, the date and time of the edited note(s), how many versions (original and edited) of the note will be available to the end user, and the limit, if any, to the number of edited versions to be saved.

Commercial software vendors generally provide a detailed functional specification document for their system or application in the form of manuals. The manuals, usually application-specific, include an introduction, a section for each pathway, and a technical section. From the provided documentation, the hospital's departmental and project teams produce the organization's functional specification by evaluating the available commercial software's functions with the work flow documents and

making decisions on the pathways and functions to be utilized by the institution.

Data Manipulation and Output There are several considerations for handling data manipulation and output (American Society for Testing and Materials, 1993). The detailed functional specifications are critical to the system's acceptance; each screen, data flow, and report the user can expect to see is analyzed. A significant level of detail with sketches, explanations, and/or examples is necessary (Hewlett-Packard, 1993). With a sketch, the standards incorporated into the design can be shown and will minimize ambiguity in communicating the design intent to the programming staff. From a new system development perspective, these sketches decrease the programming time required for the project. The examples incorporate real data into the explanations and drawings.

During this step, the departmental teams and users determine what the actual data will look like in its output form and gain consensus from the departmental teams for the proposed design. A number of factors are considered. Are slopes or maximum and minimum values required? How will data values outside their normal range be identified? How will panic values be identified for easy recognition by the clinicians? How long should the electronic data remain accessible to clinicians?

When a system or application is being created, there is fluidity between the functional design, functional specification, and initial programming prototype efforts. The design team creating the new application often works closely with the programmers, making adjustments in the design and specification based on new perspectives, programming logic, and/or technologies. As the functional specification matures and major design decisions (e.g. selection of the underlying application technology and database structure) have occurred, a design "freeze point" is established. This indicates that the functional specification is complete and full programming efforts are established.

Once completed, the functional specification provides not only the road map for programming efforts, but the starting point for developing testing plans for verification of the software. It provides developers and the project teams of an implementation with the source for determining testing needs prior to releasing the application into a production, or "live," environment. The advantages of establishing testing plans in concert with the development of the functional specification include a more thorough test plan (pathways are not missed), and "what if" questions often spark the need to develop or allow alternate pathways for a function. For example:

1. The design team reviews the editing function of an automated documentation system under development. The informatics nurse on the design team asks, "What if a student nurse goes home without completing her nurse's note?" Permutations of both the editing and security features of the application must be reviewed. Consideration may be given to development of a specific editing pathway intended for use in the teaching situation. A scenario is developed to test the "what if" possibility of a student nurse leaving before completing her patient documentation.

2. A commercially available clinical documentation application is being implemented at a hospital. The departmental team for nursing reviews the feature for editing a note of a student and determines that this function will not be implemented, since the organization does not have a teaching affiliation for nursing. No testing scenario will be necessary.

The following criteria are considered essential in selecting a clinical information system and can be used as a basis for evaluation. They include the following areas:

- Applications
- Overall system performance
- Evaluation features and pathways
- Ease of system use
- Configuration or programming performance
- Security
- Simplification of reports
- Database access
- Hardware and software reliability
- Connectivity
- System cost

Technical Specifications

In the system design phase, technical personnel work closely with the project and departmental teams to ensure the technical components of the proposed system work in concert with technology and end user needs and to assist in the development of the implementation plan. As stated earlier, a dedicated technical manager is required. He or she is responsible for the coordination of efforts in four major areas. Each area requires that a detailed technical specification be developed. The project's technical manager and the project team leaders ensure that all of the components/applications of the CIS works in concert with all the other components. The four major areas are as follows:

- Hardware
- Software
- Interfaces
- Conversions

Hardware In the case of new software development, the technical project manager ensures that the new software utilizes the best technology platform available. The ability to operate the new application on multiple hardware platforms is often desired. Technical specifications describing the recommended equipment are developed and tested in the development laboratory.

When commercial software is being implemented or upgraded, the technical project manager ensures that the physical environment for the new system conforms with the new system's technical specifications. This may include the need to build a new computer room, establish or upgrade a network, and procure the correct devices for the new system. The types of devices to be utilized (PCs versus hand-held versus bedside devices) require dialog and testing with team leaders and department team members. The testing and deployment of the new equipment (terminals, printers, and/or hand-held devices) are the responsibility of the technical manager. Ongoing maintenance for the new computer's central processing unit (CPU), operating system, and network are coordinated by the project's technical manager.

Application Software The project's technical manager is responsible for establishing the technical specifications outlining the operational requirements for the new system. The specifications detail the procedures required to maintain the application software on a daily, weekly, and monthly basis. The specifications are compiled as the starting point for determining the operations schedule for the system and/or the institution. The operations plan includes detailed information related to when the system will be scheduled for routine maintenance, plans for operations during system failures, and acceptable periods during the week/month for the system to be unavailable to the users. Additional requirements for assuring data reliability and availability following planned and unplanned system downtime, as well as procedures outlining data recovery following a downtime are developed. "Change control" policies and procedures for identifying, tracking, testing, and applying software fixes are established.

Interface Systems An interface system defines those programs and processes required to transmit data between two disparate systems. The project's technical manager coordinates all interfacing activities for the new application. The level of interface complexity for clinical systems continues to grow. While utilization of the industry's Health Level 7 (HL7) interface standards has greatly reduced the effort required to establish clinical interfaces by providing a standard specification for the transmission of data, the number of clinical interfaces in a CIS has increased dramatically. It is not unusual for a CIS to interface with separate registration, patient billing, laboratory, radiology, and pharmacy systems. More complex environments may include interfaces to cardiac and fetal monitors and radio frequency-based portable devices and provide remote access into the hospital's clinical system for physicians and home care nursing staff.

The interface specification details whether the interface will be one way or bi-directional. A bi-directional interface implies that data are flowing both to and from a system. Conversely, a one-way interface may either send data to or receive data from a separate system but not do both. For example, an interface between the existing CIS and a new clinical documentation system is being planned to automatically establish a patient in the documentation system once the patient has been admitted into the existing CIS. The interface will eliminate the need for the clinicians to re-register the patient in the documentation

system. The interface will be a one-way interface—patient registration data from the CIS registration application will go to the clinical documentation system.

The informatics nurse assists in development of the interface specification by assisting with the comparison of data elements in each system and helping to determine which data elements will be included in the interface.

Recent technology has further streamlined interfacing requirements through the availability of interface engines. The interface engine utilizes the concept that similar data element requirements exist among multiple clinical applications. Very similar patient registration data elements, for example, are required by the laboratory, radiology, pharmacy, and clinical documentation systems. The benefits of the interface engine are to decrease the number of transactions being processed by the system and to provide interface management capabilities through a single source. For example, the interface engine receives a message from the registration system indicating the admission of a patient and relays the message to each of the ancillary systems (laboratory, radiology, pharmacy, clinical documentation, etc.) (Figs. 13.4 and 13.5).

It is not uncommon for a separate interface implementation workplan to be created and managed by the project's technical manager. Informatics nurses and/or departmental team members must be intimately involved

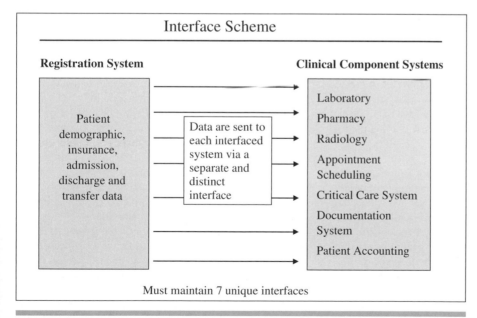

Figure 13.4
Interface scheme.

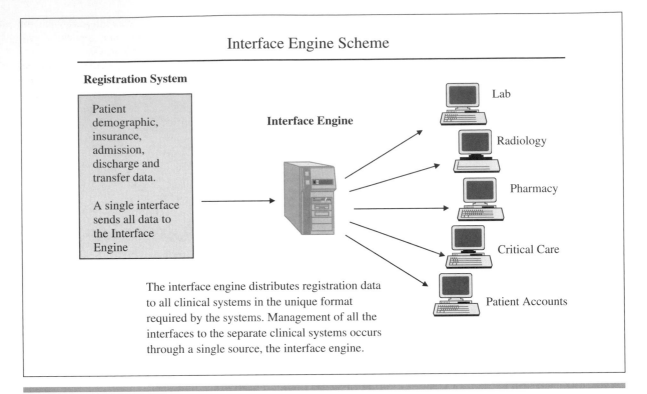

Figure 13.5
Interface engine.

in determining and testing each interface. Their knowledge of the use of clinical data and end user work flow requirements are invaluable to the interface team.

Strenuous testing of the interfaces by the interface team must be completed prior to the full system's integrated test. When pharmacy interfaces are being implemented, a 100% test of all data elements scheduled to cross the interface is recommended.

Conversions   The conversion of data from legacy systems to the new system is the fourth major area of coordination for the project's technical manager. Most hospitals currently utilize automated registration and billing systems; determining the conversion requirements and developing and testing the conversion programs are critical steps in implementing a new system or application.

A series testing pattern is recommended for conversions. An initial test of 10 records will provide the first functional evaluation of the conversion programs. The second level of testing may include 50 records. Departmental teams must carefully review each data element in each record to ensure that appropriate infor-

mation has been converted correctly. It is advisable for the departmental teams to not only review the data, but to simulate their work flow using the converted data. The conversion team may increase the sample size to 500 records before completing a test of 100% of the records to be converted. The 100% test conversion will provide valuable information for the project team regarding the length of time required to actually convert all data into the new system. This is particularly helpful for institutions converting a legacy registration/medical records/patient accounting system to a new system where the CIS will be unavailable to the users for the duration of the final conversion activities.

While all steps are important in the implementation of a new system, the interface and conversion design and testing tasks are frequently areas that cause project delays for the implementation and/or upgrading of CISs. The importance of the project's technical manager and oversight management by the project manager in keeping these tasks on the established timetable and in ensuring that the departmental and project teams are informed of the interface and conversion plans should not be underestimated.

Implementation Planning

The last step in the system design phase is to establish a detailed implementation plan. The developed functional and technical specifications define a significant amount of form and substance for the new CIS. The next step is to assess the timeframes established in the final scope document with the development timeframes established during the system design phase and the interface and conversion requirements to establish a detailed workplan. The workplan identifies a responsible party and a beginning date and end date for each phase, step, task, and subtask. This plan coordinates all tasks necessary to complete the development of new software, implement a new system, and/or upgrade a current system. Many software vendors and consultants provide an implementation workplan for their system or applications. The supplied workplans must be reviewed and revised to meet the individual needs and timetables of the institution's project (Fig. 13.6).

The workplan generally defines the project in terms of phases, steps, tasks, and subtasks. Commercially available software may be used to assist with both the development of project plans and tracking a project/implementation's progress. Through the use of this type of software, critical steps, milestone events, and project resource requirements can be managed. A milestone chart or a Gantt chart can be useful for sequentially plotting the major tasks and accomplishments required in developing or implementing the CIS. The milestone Gantt chart uses bar graphs to highlight activities and the timing of their completion. Many vendors and consultants provide an electronic copy of their developed workplan(s) utilizing these commercially available software packages.

Whether the project is software development or the implementation or upgrading of a system, the implementation workplan details the following:

- Personnel
- Timeframes
- Costs and budgets
- Facilities and equipment required
- Development or implementation tasks
- Operational considerations
- Human-computer interactions
- System test plan

These areas are detailed in an implementation workplan encompassing 14 steps. A successful implementation ensures all 14 steps are planned, executed, and tracked by the project manager and project team leaders (Fig. 13.6).

Personnel The additional staff needed to develop or implement the system may be drawn from several sources, including the nursing department, an existing information system unit, a consultant firm, or a computer vendor. Outside personnel may be considered for employment by the organization or contracted from consulting organizations to assist with an implementation; these include systems analysts, functional designers, project managers/team leaders, and a business expert (for the development of new software) (Edmunds, 1992). These personnel act as translators between the users and the programmers to ensure a detailed understanding of what the application will do and how it will work. The development or implementation team members communicate via verbal agreements, text documents, prototypes, and detailed functional specifications and through the use of models and case tools.

The project staff appointed at the beginning of the investigation should, if possible, be retained for the duration

---

14 Implementation Workplan Steps for a Clinical System

Project Planning/Administration

Hardware & Software Delivery
Application Administration

Application Verification
Team Leader Training
Conversion & Interface Planning

Building Databases (Files & Tables)

Policies and Procedures
Peripheral Device Identification

Functional Test
Integrated Test
End User Training

Live Operations

Post Implementation Evaluation

Figure 13.6
14 steps for implementation/upgrading chart.

of the project. These persons, especially the informatics nurse and the computer consultant or systems analyst, have worked closely with CIS committee members through the planning phase and the decision to proceed. In all nursing matters related to developing a CIS, the informatics nurse assumes leadership.

Human–Computer Interaction   During the design phase, the departmental teams consider the important steps of efficient implementation of a computerized system into the health care delivery system. The implementation phase focuses on experience, professional judgement, and good craftsmanship to utilize the abilities of the system for the maximum advantage of the organization. In this step, databases (tables and files, as they are sometimes called) are populated with values specific for the institution or department. The completed work flow designs are reviewed, and database entries are planned and keyed, or programmatically converted, into the system. In the course of deciding table and file (database) entries, the departmental team and project team must implement good work patterns, taking advantage of the features and functions of the new system. Implementing inefficient work patterns because they were done that way in the previous system or because they have always been done manually in a certain manner must be avoided. The work completed in the analysis phase for review of system inputs and outputs is reviewed and revised for the new system. Functional, technical, and operational issues are reviewed for the following:

- Design inputs
- Design outputs
- Design databases (files and tables)
- Design system controls

Design Inputs   The types of inputs depend largely on how data will be processed (e.g. on-line, real-time/interactive, or batch processing) and on the required outputs. Input designs require the following factors: content, data source, scope, format, medium, coding scheme, editing rules, testing, estimates of volumes, and frequency.

The contents of each input (data element) must be specified in detail to meet output requirements. The source, definitions, rules, and codes or abbreviations of the data elements must be fully spelled out. Data collected repeatedly, such as patient demographic information, should be entered into the system once and programmed to automatically populate each additional area where required.

The scope of the data inputs should be the smallest definable data elements. For example, the date of birth, as opposed to the patient's age, should be entered as an input. Each time the patient's age is required, the system should calculate the patient's age, thereby eliminating the need to ask the patient his/her age each time the patient receives care in the same health care delivery system. Each input must be in the format users will readily understand. For example, temperature, pulse, and respirations, when collected, should be entered in that order.

All types of input must be tested to ensure that essential data elements needed for outputs are logical and have been collected. Revisions and retesting, if necessary, are done to guarantee correctness. Both the estimated volume and frequency of data entry must be reviewed. The number of output forms required for patient care establishes the majority of data input requirements.

Design Outputs   Designing the CIS outputs occurs concurrently with designing the inputs. The output required by the organization or departments defines the data required as input. The system outputs are the information sought by the users and are critical to the success of the CIS. Good output design requires an understanding of users' needs. The following factors are considered in the development of output: content, format, medium, estimated volume, frequency, and distribution of information.

The content and purpose of each output must be specified in detail, and each output must be in a meaningful and easy-to-understand format. For example, the format of a report may increase its effectiveness if numbers appear with clarifying characters or colors such as percentages or symbols for "out-of-range" values. The type of medium used to present the output affects the effectiveness of the output information. An output can be a report produced on paper, microfilm, or microfiche; it can be displayed on a computer terminal or displayed as a graphic representation.

The estimated volume, frequency, and distribution of the outputs are based on the users' expected needs. Determining who the users are, what outputs they require, and at what time they are requested is accomplished through review and refinement of information gathered in the earlier phases of planning and analysis.

Design Files and Databases   File and database designs are needed to ensure efficient data processing and to help ensure prompt responses to users' informational needs. Several areas of concern must be explored: content, record format, file organization, file access, and storage requirements. The size of each file and database, including content and format of records, must be specified in detail. Both are essential to avoid data redundancy (i.e. where the same data are stored in different databases). The data elements themselves must be organized into records, files, and databases to enhance processing.

Storage requirements are affected by the volume and frequency of users' data needs. Files accessed by on-line or real-time/interactive processing will require random access storage devices. However, files accessed off-line for batch processing, for example, can use off-line storage devices. Though the cost of electronic storage has decreased dramatically in recent years, storage is affected by file size, volume, frequency, length of time for data retention, and purging capabilities of the system. Purging activity requires special rules for identifying data to be purged and determining how long to retain the data and a mechanism for either destroying data or moving it to an archival system. Data used for subsequent analysis, such as audit, quality assurance, and research, are also considered in determining storage requirements.

Design Controls   Design controls ensure that input data are duly processed, output information is complete and accurate, and data integrity has been maintained. Design controls help minimize and eliminate system errors. Adequate controls can be established through several different methods. It is possible, for example, to determine the accuracy of the source documents being input by balancing the input totals against the output totals. Controls of data input may be achieved through programmatic checking of data limits to determine if they are within normal ranges. Audit trails can check and trace transactions from input to output. The matching of computer-processed outputs with manually processed ones for a subscribed period of time may be utilized to ensure that all data are being processed correctly.

Other types of system controls utilize "back-up files" and mirrored files. These files allow the CIS to remain intact even if its current data files are damaged or destroyed. The security of the files must be maintained; every effort must be made to protect the privacy of patients' files. During the implementation phase, policies and procedures are developed to ensure system integrity and security as well as to ensure a standardized approach to utilizing the new system's functionality.

The Development Phase

When a new application is being created, all computer programs required to operate the application are coded during the development phase. Much dialog occurs between the programmers and the design team as each feature and function of the new application is developed. The programmers utilize an iterative process to ensure that the coding is to the specifications of the functional specification and to ensure that communications between the desired design, the functional specification, and the actual programming effort are working in concert. Testing at the programmer level, unit testing, is done throughout the coding effort by the programmers. Project managers and team leaders monitor progress against the workplan developed in the design phase.

In the instance where commercially available software is being considered, completion of the design phase provides the steering committee and project team with sufficient information to evaluate commercial system offerings. With the system design complete, the task of selecting a new system becomes more objective. Steps involved in a system selection are as follows:

- Request for proposal
- Evaluate responses
- Negotiate contract

Request for Proposal

The request for proposal (RFP) is derived from the work completed in the planning, analysis, and early design phases. It is developed as a tool to initiate the search for a commercially available system. The RFP summarizes the key features and functions of the new system as determined by the user requirements established in the planning and early design phase. When a system is being purchased from a vendor or outside developer, the RFP clearly spells out the objectives, functional requirements, budgetary constraints, and timelines of the project. An RFP, sometimes called a solicitation bid, is circulated among prospective bidders and establishes whether the vendor software has the ability to meet the requirements defined in the functional specifications. Some RFPs utilize weighted values assigned to key functions and establish the definition of terms for the stated requirements.

An RFP includes the following sections:

- An introduction to the organization and to the overall environment in which the system will be used.
- A description of how the general information requirements will be supplied.
- A description of any performance bond or equivalent requirement.

Reviewer Name:_____

Reviewer Name:_____ Date: _____

Application:_____

SYSTEM ATTRIBUTES	CIRCLE SCORE				
Availability of Required Features	1	2	3	4	5
Ease of Use	1	2	3	4	5
System Flexibility	1	2	3	4	5
Appearance of Screens	1	2	3	4	5
Appearance of Reports	1	2	3	4	5
Confidence That System Will Meet Expectations	1	2	3	4	5
Response Time	1	2	3	4	5
Availability of Health Features	1	2	3	4	5
Quality of Documentation	1	2	3	4	5
Impression of Vendor	1	2	3	4	5
Overall System Desirability	1	2	3	4	5
TOTAL AVERAGE RATING	1	2	3	4	5

LEGEND: POOR (1)   AVERAGE (2-3)   GOOD (4-5)

COMMENTS: _____

_____

Figure 13.7
Vendor demonstration evaluation form.

Reviewer Name:_____

Application:_____

SYSTEM ATTRIBUTES	VENDOR #1	VENDOR #2	VENDOR #3
Availability of this system to support the operation	1 2 3 4 5	1 2 3 4 5	1 2 3 4 5
Ease with which the customer learned to use the system	1 2 3 4 5	1 2 3 4 5	1 2 3 4 5
Least amount of difficulty implementing the system	1 2 3 4 5	1 2 3 4 5	1 2 3 4 5
Vendor support of the customer	1 2 3 4 5	1 2 3 4 5	1 2 3 4 5
Overall customer satisfaction with the vendor	1 2 3 4 5	1 2 3 4 5	1 2 3 4 5
Fewest resources necessary to support the system	1 2 3 4 5	1 2 3 4 5	1 2 3 4 5
Overall system desirability for hospital	1 2 3 4 5	1 2 3 4 5	1 2 3 4 5
TOTAL AVERAGE RATING	1 2	3 4	5

LEGEND:	POOR (1)	AVERAGE (2-3)	GOOD (4-5)
	Vendor #1	Vendor #2	Vendor #3
Advantages	_____	_____	_____
Disadvantages	_____	_____	_____
Critical Changes (necessary to use this system)	_____	_____	_____

Figure 13.8
Vendor site visit evaluation form.

Departmental Questions

Vendor name _____ Date____/____/____

Institution _____

Contact name _____

Contact title _____

Department director _____

Phone number/extension ( )_____

What is your length of employment with this facility? ____yrs

Were you involved in the selection of the system? _____Yes ____No

What is your opinion of the vendor personnel who assisted you in the:

Training _____
_____

Installation _____
_____

Conversion _____
_____

Support _____

Figure 13.9
Site visit questionnaire.

- A statement of the conditions for software and equipment demonstrations that will be conducted.
- An outline of the method of financing the project.
- Required training and orientation by the vendor for the system.
- An outline of the RFP evaluation criteria.
- A statement of the standards of performance used in deciding system acceptability.
- A statement of the specific hardware and software requirements.

The prospective vendors/bidders generally respond in writing according to the timeframe and format specified by the organization.

Evaluate Responses

Evaluation of the responses occurs in stages. The bidders' responses are evaluated first by the project teams and steering committee to determine the appropriateness of inclusion of the bidder for the next step of the evaluation, software demonstrations. In the software demonstration step, vendors who sufficiently meet the criteria set forth in the RFP provide a demonstration of their system's capabilities. Some organizations develop demonstration scripts outlining a scenario of events. Each vendor is evaluated on their system's ability to execute the demonstration script and the ease with which it is accomplished. The demonstration step may be an iterative process, incorporating more detailed demonstrations in subsequent rounds. Later, the financial officers, contract officers and/or legal officers of the organization review the responses for those vendors/bidders judged to most conform with the desired system requirements.

An evaluation form is used to score the vendors' capabilities for fulfilling the system requirements (Fig. 13.7). The evaluation scores help to identify the eligible system suppliers. Once a bidder's field is narrowed to no more than four vendors, the project's team is encouraged to make site visits to view the proposed system in operation. Such visits allow the committee members not only to see the system but also to directly question actual users of the system. Issues that might be addressed on a site visit are included in Fig. 13.8. Suggested questions to be asked on the site visit are included in Fig. 13.9. The vendors costs should be compared and ranked prior to negotiating the contract (Tables 13.1 and 13.2).

Negotiate Contract

The final step in the RFP process is to select the bidder/vendor and negotiate a contract. The successful bidder is contracted to develop a system, provide an already developed system, or adapt another facility's system to meet the RFP specifications. Recommended negotiation strategies include 10 principles for making the contract process less cumbersome (Ciotti and Bogutski, 1994). The principles are as follows:

- Negotiate with several "finalists"—this allows hospitals to make concessions apart from competitive negotiations.

- Include concession statements as part of the RFP, and include the RFP checklist as part of the contract in the "product definition."

- Insist on having draft copies of proposed contracts in advance of contract signing, and craft the contract language until it is acceptable to the organization

- Request staggered payments—for example, 10% with contract, 30% upon delivery of hardware and software, 20% upon successful full implementation, 20% upon the first productive use of the system, and 20% 30 days after the first month-end occurs and discrepancies are noticed.

- Understand when final acceptance of the development and implementation phases end and the maintenance phase begins.

- Extend payments of invoices beyond 45–60 days to allow sufficient time for the hospital accountants to check the invoices for accuracy.

- Negotiate the interest rate paid on payments beyond the specified due date to what Medicare, Medicaid, and Blue Cross pay in your state for remittances older than one month.

- Insist on taking several months after the system has been implemented to determine if the product is defined by the vendor's positive performance responses in the vendor's proposal.

- Insist on system response time guarantees.

- Require installers to perform a walk-through of your facility before contract negotiations are signed, and/or negotiate an install plan the same way that the system negotiations were made.

On the other hand, if the project steering committee decides to develop its own system programs, the project staff must proceed with the development phase of the system, which includes the following:

- Select hardware
- Develop software
- Test system
- Document system

Table 13.1 Worksheet Comparing Vendor Costs

Information System Application	Vendor/Supplier Costs					
	A	B	C	D	E	F
Admission/patient registration	$	$	$	$	$	$
Master patient census	$	$	$	$	$	$
Order-entry network	$	$	$	$	$	$
Patient care plans/protocols	$	$	$	$	$	$
Patient accounts	$	$	$	$	$	$
Patient classification	$	$	$	$	$	$
Nurse staffing	$	$	$	$	$	$
Nurse scheduling	$	$	$	$	$	$
Nurse personnel payroll	$	$	$	$	$	$
Total	$	$	$	$	$	$

Table 13.2   Worksheet Ranking Vendors

System Vendor/ Supplier Name	Vendor/Supplier Functional Requirements	
	Total Points (100 Maximum)	Rank
A	72	5
B	65	6
C	80	2
D	85	1
E	77	3
F	75	4

Select Hardware   Selecting the correct hardware for the system depends on its design, application, and software requirements. Technical conditions may dictate selection of a mainframe, a minicomputer, a microcomputer, or a combination of the above. Computer hardware is obtained in several different ways. Mainframes and minicomputers may be purchased or leased from a hardware vendor for in-house use. However, when cost is a significant factor, timesharing computer processing with other facilities may be considered. Since microcomputers are small, they may be the most economical for some applications. Input, output, and processing media, including secondary storage, is selected, and all hardware must be installed and able to test the computer programs at the appropriate time.

Develop Software   When a new application or system is being created, the development phase becomes an iterative process of programming sections of the design established in the functional specification, testing the design with the informatics nurse and/or design team, evaluating options suggested as a result of testing, and refining/re-evaluating the functional specification. The manager for the development project ensures the progress of the development and ensures that timelines for completion of the project are met. Business aspects are detailed and managed. These may include determination of product packaging and marketing materials, establishment of product pricing, development of system/application documentation, and the establishment of a marketing plan.

 The Testing Phase

The system, whether newly developed or commercially available, must be tested to ensure that all data are processed correctly and the desired outputs are generated. Testing verifies that the computer programs are written correctly and ensures that, when implemented in the production ("live") environment, the system will function as planned. In the development scenario, the three levels of testing are often referred to as unit testing, alpha testing, and beta testing. Unit testing, described earlier, is conducted by the individual programmers as the programs are being coded. They are tested to determine if the programming protocols are used correctly and if the programs execute correctly. Alpha testing is accomplished by a testing (system assurance) group within the development organization. Alpha testing of a system or application, done in the development lab, focuses on not only the correct execution of the programs, but on the integration of the programs with the entire application or system. Sample data mimicking true patient data are used whenever possible to test the integration of computer programs. Beta testing occurs at the first client site. Representatives of the development team assist the client in testing the programs for the first time in real-life situations.

When commercially available software is being implemented, three levels of testing are recommended. The first level is often called a functional test. During this round of testing, the departmental teams test and verify the databases (files and tables), ensuring that correct data have been entered into the files and tables. The expected departmental reports are reviewed to assure correctness and accuracy. Multiple iterations of the functional test often occur until the departmental team is confident of the system set-up and profiles. The second level of testing, integrated systems testing, begins when all departments indicate the completion of their functional testing. During integrated testing, the total system is tested; this includes interfaces between systems as well as the interplay between applications within the same system. The integrated test must mimic the production ("live") environment in terms of the volume of transactions, the number of users, the interfaced systems, and the procedures to be followed to carry out all functions of the system. It is at this point that testing of the organizationwide procedures to be instituted when the system is unavailable, downtime procedures, are thoroughly tested. Downtime procedures must be taught during end user training. The final round of testing occurs during end user training. As more users interact with the new system, previously unfound problems may surface. Evaluation of the severity of the newly discovered problems and the corrective action required is an ongoing process during implementation.

Document System

The preparation of documents to describe the system for all users is an ongoing activity, with development of the documentation occurring as the various system phases and steps are completed. Documentation should begin with the final system proposal. Several manuals are prepared: a user's manual, a reference manual, and an operator's maintenance manual. These manuals provide guides to the system components and outline how the entire system has been programmed or defined.

User's Manual

The user's manual highlights how to use the system and describes what outputs the system can produce. With commercially available software, the vendor's user's manual helps establish the organization's training manual.

Reference Manual

The reference manual is used by the project team members to understand how the system works. It describes what data are input, how the databases (files and tables) process the data, and the mechanisms used to generate outputs.

Operator's/Maintenance Manual

This manual enables operators to keep the system up and running by providing the functional and technical specifications needed to the system. Manuals must be written in sufficient detail such that system users and operators understand how the system was developed, how it operates, and how it can be maintained, updated, and repaired.

The Training Phase

It is essential to train the end users how to use the system properly. A CIS will function only as well as its users understand its operation and the operations streamline the work. Two levels of training take place for the implementation of a system. The project team and selected members of the departmental team receive training from the developers or vendor. This training details the databases (files and tables), processing logic, and outputs of all the system's features and functions. End user training, the second level of testing, takes place once the departmental and project teams have finished profiling the system to meet the functional and technical specifications developed and functional testing has been completed. End-user training stresses how the user will complete his or her work flow using the new system.

All users of the new system or application must receive training. Training on a new system should occur no more than 6 weeks prior to the activation of the new system. When training occurs more than 6 weeks before activation of the system, additional refresher training is often required by the end users. Each department must consider the following in developing their training plans:

- Total number of employees to be trained
- Number of employees that can be trained in a single day
- Whether staff will be trained during their shift or on their day off
- Whether competency requirements must be met
- Number of trainers required
- Whether training will occur on all three shifts, seven days a week

Training takes place before and during the activation of a new system. After system implementation, refresher courses as well as new employee introductory training on the use of the new system are often provided by the institution. Training of the nursing department usually requires the development of a separate training plan.

The large number of nursing staff members to be trained necessitates a significant amount of advance planning.

Training is most effective when hands-on, interactive instruction is provided. Training guides or manuals explain the system; however, retention of information is increased if the learners are able to interact with the new system in a manner simulating their work flow with the new system. Computer-assisted instruction (CAI) in a special training room or on the units can be used to provide hands-on experience. End user training is offered with two perspectives. One perspective provides a general overview of the system, and the second perspective explains how the user will interact with the system to complete his/her daily work. While a user's/training manual is developed for the training sessions, most end users express the desire to have a pocket size reminder ("cheat sheet") outlining the key functions of the new system or application. Both the user's manual and the pocket reminders should be available for departmental use. When possible, a training environment on the computer system should be established for the organization. Establishing a training lab as well as providing access to the training environment from the departments and nursing units prior to the activation of the new system provides end users the opportunity to practice at times convenient to their work requirements and reinforces the training.

The Implementation Phase

The implementation phase organizes all the steps into a detailed plan describing the series of events required to begin utilizing the system or application in the production or "live" environment and details the necessary computer and software maintenance operations required to keep the system running. This phase ensures that once the system is installed in the live environment, the system and the delivery of health care in the organization will run smoothly. The schedule of operations begun in the design phase is documented in procedures manuals for the computer operators. The "go live" workplan includes a detailed description of the preparation steps required for all facets of the system, the timing requirements to accomplish the tasks, the defining elements indicating the completion of each critical task, and the party responsible for determining if the criteria to progress in the plan have been met. The activation of interfaces, the timing of the final conversion of data (if any) into the new system, and the activation activities for each of the nursing units and departments are detailed in this plan.

Four activation approaches are possible: (1) parallel, (2) pilot, (3) phased-in, and (4) big bang theory. In the parallel approach, the new system runs parallel with the existing system until users can adjust. In the pilot approach, a few departments or units try out the new system to see how it works and then help other units or departments to use it. In the phased-in approach, the system is implemented one unit or department at a time. In the big bang approach, a cut-over date and time are established for the organization, the old system is stopped, and all units/departments begin processing on the newly installed system.

The timing of conversion activities and the activation of all interfaces requires particular coordination between the technical staff and the project teams. The project's technical manager, in conjunction with the project manager, is responsible for assuring the development of thorough "go live" plans. A command center is established to coordinate all issues, concerns and "go live" help desk functions. A sufficient number of phone lines and beepers are secured to support the move to the live production environment. Team members and trainers often serve as resources to the end users on a 24-hour basis for a period of time postimplementation. Sometimes called "super users," these team members are available in the departments and on the nursing units to proactively assist users during the first one to two weeks of productive use of the new system or application.

The coordination of all activities requires a cohesive team effort. Communication among the team members is as critical as keeping the end users informed of the sequence events, the expected time frames for each event, and the channels established for reporting and resolving issues.

The Evaluation Phase

The evaluation phase describes and assesses, in detail, the new system's performance. Utilizing the criteria established in the planning and system design phases, the evaluation process summarizes the entire system, identifying both the strengths and weaknesses of the implementation process. An evaluation study often leads to system revisions and, ultimately, a better system.

During this phase, the system is evaluated to determine whether it has accomplished the stated objectives. A system evaluation involves a comparison of a working system with its functional requirements to determine how well the requirements are met, to determine possibilities for growth and improvement, and to preserve the lessons learned from the implementation project for future efforts. The entire system operation, including end user acceptance, newly established procedures, appropriateness of equipment, scope and validity of databases, and system response times are examined. Functional performance and technical performance are evaluated thoroughly, and system costs and benefits are assessed (McCormick, 1983). Training efforts and the activation strategy utilized to bring the system live are included in the evaluation.

Evaluation of the functional performance of the system requires methods and tools that compare operations before and after system implementation. Such tools are designed to identify the effects the CIS has on the affected components of patient care. For example:

- Has patient care documentation improved through the use of a new system/application?

- Does patient care documentation take less time postimplementation than was required preimplementation?

- Does the system use increase awareness of patients' problems?

If so, the system may be considered an aid to improve the quality of patient care. In addition, "high-level" benefits identified during the feasibility study are reviewed. Examples of such benefits include nursing satisfaction (ascertained by retention data and end user questionnaires), patient satisfaction, decreased lengths of stay, reduced error of omission, and improved quality of care (Simpson, 1993b).

To evaluate an implemented hospital information system, many other principles are important for clinical information systems. One authority suggests evaluating duplication of efforts and data entry, fragmentation, misplaced work, complexity, bottlenecks, review/approval process, error reporting (or the amount of reworking of content), movement, wait time, delays, set-up, low importance outputs, and unimportant outputs (Young, 1981).

Various methods and tools used to evaluate a system's functional performance include the following:

- Record review
- Time study
- User satisfaction
- Cost-benefit analysis

Evaluating the system is the final step and ongoing step in implementation process. This evaluation component becomes a continuous phase in total quality management. The system is assessed to determine whether it

continues to meet the needs of the users. The totally implemented system will require continuous evaluation to determine if upgrading is appropriate and/or what enhancements could be added to the current system. Formal evaluations generally take place not less than 6 months and routinely every 2 to 4 years after the system has been implemented. The formal evaluation should be conducted by an outside evaluation team to increase the objectivity level of the findings. Informal evaluations are done on a weekly basis.

Record Review

A patient record review assesses how comprehensively the CIS supports patient care delivery. Departmental management reports and tracking logs supporting patient care delivery are also reviewed. Other variables can be evaluated from the patient record, such as (1) completeness of the database entries, (2) documentation of progress notes, (3) statement of types of patient problems, (4) orders, (5) listed interventions, (6) interdisciplinary communications, and (7) teaching plans.

Time Study

A time study can be conducted both before and after system implementation to compare the time staff take to provide specific patient care activities under the old and new systems. Such a study may include the time nursing staff spend in other activities required in the old versus the new system. Time studies conducted once the computer system is in place may assess the system's use by various groups of staff. For example, a time study can show how often nursing personnel access the system and for what purpose (i.e. retrieval of information, education, entry of data). It can highlight whether the system increased or decreased the time spent in providing direct patient care. Time studies may also help to estimate the cost of resources needed to run the system.

User Satisfaction

A questionnaire or a checklist can assess users' reactions and perceptions of the system as well as their satisfaction with overall system performance. It can measure whether the system improves the nurses' understanding of patient problems and thus affects patient care, and it can assess the usefulness and contributions of the system to patient care and operations. Some specific questions to assist in this evaluation and criteria for appraising the system's technical performance are listed in Table 13.3.

Other approaches to evaluating the functional performance of a system exist. Investigating such functions as administrative control, medical/nursing orders, charting and documentation, and retrieval and management reports are used to assess system benefits. Each of these areas is evaluated through time observations, work sampling, operational audits, and surveys. System functional performance can be assessed by examining nurses' morale and nursing department operations (McCormick, 1983).

Documentation of care must be assessed if patient care benefits are to be evaluated. The following questions must be answered:

- Does the system assist in improving the documentation of patient care in the patient record?

- Does the system reduce patient care costs?

- Does the system prevent errors and save lives?

To evaluate nurses' morale requires appraising nurses' satisfaction with the system. The following questions may be considered useful:

- Does the system facilitate nurses' documentation of patient care?

- Does it reduce the time spent in such documentation?

- Is it easy to use?

- Is it readily accessible?

- Are the display "screens" easy to use?

- Do the displays capture patient care?

Table 13.3 User Satisfaction Checklist

Performance area	Satisfaction Level				
	Very Satisfied	Satisfied	Neutral	Dissatisfied	Very Dissatisfied
Accuracy	1	2	3	4	5
Timeliness	1	2	3	4	5
Reliability	1	2	3	4	5
Training	1	2	3	4	5
Routine task	1	2	3	4	5
Full system potential	1	2	3	4	5
Manuals	1	2	3	4	5
Ease of use	1	2	3	4	5
Data entry	1	2	3	4	5
Information retrieval	1	2	3	4	5
Legibility	1	2	3	4	5
Completeness	1	2	3	4	5
Data entry	1	2	3	4	5
Information retrieval	1	2	3	4	5
Flexibility	1	2	3	4	5
Data entry	1	2	3	4	5
Information retrieval	1	2	3	4	5
Conciseness	1	2	3	4	5
Data entry	1	2	3	4	5
Information retrieval	1	2	3	4	5
Overall performance	1	2	3	4	5

■ Does the system enhance the work situation and contribute to work satisfaction?

To evaluate the departmental benefits requires determining if the CIS helps improve administrative activities. The following questions must be answered:

■ Does the new system enhance the goals of the department?

■ Does it improve department efficiency?

■ Does it help reduce the range of administrative activities?

■ Does it reduce clerical work?

Other criteria are necessary to evaluate technical performance; these include reliability, maintainability, use, response time, accessibility, availability, and flexibility to meet changing needs. These areas are examined from several different points—the technical performance of the software as well as hardware performance. The following questions must be answered:

■ Is the system accurate and reliable?

■ Is it easy to maintain at a reasonable cost?

■ Is it flexible?

■ Is the information consistent?

■ Is the information timely?

■ Is it responsive to users' needs?

■ Do users find interaction with the system satisfactory?

■ Are input devices accessible and generally available to users?

Cost-Benefit Analysis

A cost-benefit analysis is necessary to determine if the system is worth its price. The cost-benefit analysis relates system cost and benefits to system design, level of use, timeframe, and equipment costs. Each of these costs must be assessed in relation to benefits derived. Such an evaluation can help determine the future of the system.

■ Upgrading Clinical Information Systems

The upgrading of a system may be undertaken for a number of reasons. Software vendors often provide enhancements and upgrades to their system. New applications, features, and/or functions may be developed by the ven-

dor and become available to the organization. Upgrading a system as a result of the addition of new subsystems and technology commonly occurs. To upgrade a system, the same phases and activities described for designing and implementing must occur. However, when upgrading, dovetailing the changes into the current system will require close evaluation. New technologies are an important consideration; the following new technologies may be considered:

■ Bedside/point-of-care wireless devices

■ Workstations

■ Multimedia presentations

■ Decision support

■ Artificial intelligence

■ Neural networks

■ Integrated systems architecture

■ Interfaced networks

■ Open architecture

All of the above have been discussed within other chapters of this book, with the exception of the concepts of integrating, interfacing, or open architecture. These three important concepts are related to upgrading.

Interface Systems versus Integrated Systems

The principles of interfaced versus integrated systems need to be considered (McCormick, 1983). An interfaced system refers to a system in which each department is responsible for its own database (e.g. the laboratory, radiology, nursing, and medicine). If data are shared between departments, they are usually duplicated and transmitted to another department. The computer hardware may be shared, but the department's databases are not. These systems can run on different hardware and different operating systems that may not necessarily communicate with each other. Department heads may prefer interfaced systems. The interfaced system allows the departments more authority over the departmental application purchased and may reflect greater support for the specific needs of the individual department.

An integrated system refers to a system in which all hospital departments share common databases. Information is stored in a single file and may be accessed by all departments based on security and authority privileges. There is no need to interface departmental systems with duplicative data, since all data captured can be made available to other departments. When an integrated system is developed and implemented, decisions made by one department may affect many departments. Hardware and software become interchangeable between departments, so a large back-up inventory of equipment and software is not necessary. The major advantage of an integrated system is the ability to share common data. Most of the new large-scale CISs are examples of integrated systems. Many of the hospitals that have chosen to build their own system have chosen the integrated approach (e.g. LDS Hospital in Salt Lake City, Beth Israel Hospital in Boston, and the University of Iowa Medical Center).

Open Systems

Today, as local area networks (LANs) and wide area networks (WANs) become commonplace, the concepts of interfacing or integrating are being challenged by the open architecture (Clayton et al., 1992). The concept of open architecture for computing systems assumes a heterogeneous mixture of applications and host computers, systems, and databases. Often the systems are interfaced or are minimally interfaced with one another by means of de facto conventions and standards. As a means to integrate the systems, the network serves as an important architectural component. When all departments move onto a network, there is homogeneity in the use of the network and data transfer, but heterogeneity in the hosts and workstations is maintained. The development of national standards is a U.S. government initiative for the year 2000.

Workstations

The workstation becomes the mode to gain access to multiple applications. The user does not have to know or understand what type of hardware or software he or she is accessing, only that there is access to a broad array of information. The security and confidentiality issues raised by open architecture systems are being handled with the installation of security servers, registration centers to register use of information, and/or protocols requiring authorization.

According to Clayton et al. (1992), the advantages of updating using open architectures are modularity, rapid implementation, simultaneous existence of old and new systems running side by side, redundant pathways, and vendor and platform independence. The major disadvantage of open architecture is the lack of national standards dictating a common communication language between machines.

System Issues

As new technologies are evaluated and upgrading is considered, the design team or departmental team must reassess the original functional requirements. If the system has not been used to its limit, reserve capacity to expand the original functional requirements with the existing hardware may exist. Insofar as possible, the team needs to determine if a subsystem can be added to the working system. New functions might be required, necessitating the procurement of additional hardware. To determine if hardware or software trade-offs should be considered, the following questions might be raised:

- Which hardware subsystems will be most difficult to implement?
- Can this new function be performed with existing software?
- Is the throughput of the rate-limiting feature of the system improved by changing from software to hardware or vice versa?
- Can alterations of current hardware or software improve the feature without compromising capabilities?
- Are additional mechanical or electrical devices required to make the change?
- Are some functions better handled by remote or local processors?

Future Trends

The introduction of the computer-based patient record (CPR) has been recommended by the Institute of Medicine report. The report recommends new system designs should expand to improve the fundamental resource in health care beyond the automating of patient records (Dick and Steen, 1991).

The CPR design will be more useful if it provides practical and accurate data, practitioner reminders and alerts, clinical decision support systems, links to bodies of medical knowledge, and other aids in expanding knowledge needed in clinical decision-making. Within this definition is the concept of broadening the CPR from more than an "automated patient record" to an integral resource in the management of a lifelong health care record and in the extension of knowledge.

The fully configured workstations will require Windows applications, accelerated processors, client/server architecture, graphical user interfaces (GUI), and large storage capabilities to retrieve and process data transactionally for case management, clinical pathways, and outcomes-of-care analysis. New user-oriented interfaces provide the user with high-powered workstations; graphical, object-oriented, and metaphoric interface; and relational databases that support ad hoc querying and multiprocessing.

Summary

This chapter describes the process of designing, implementing, and/or upgrading a CIS in a patient health care facility. It outlines and describes the eight phases of the process—planning, system analysis, system design, system development, testing, training, implementation, and evaluation. The upgrading process utilizes all of the phases described.

The planning phase determines the problem scope and outlines the entire project to determine if the system is feasible and worth developing and/or implementing. The analysis phase assesses the problem being studied through extensive data gathering and analysis. The design phase produces detailed specifications of the proposed system. Development involves the actual preparation of the system. Testing is generally conducted on three levels for both the design and implementation of a commercially available system. Training includes the training of users in the use of the system for their everyday lives. Implementation outlines the detailed plans for moving the new system into the production or "live" environment. Evaluating the system determines the positive and negative results of the implementation effort and suggests ways to improve the system. Upgrading the system involves expansion or elaboration of initial functions by expanding capability or function or by adding entirely new applications. Upgrading projects require that all implementation phases be completed to assure success.

References

American Association of Nurse Executives (AONE): In Cooperation with The Center for Healthcare Information Management (CHIM). (1993). *Informatics: Issues and Strategies for the 21st Century Health Care Executive.* Resource Book and Video Set. Chicago: American Hospital Association Services, Inc.

American Nurses Association. (1994). *The Scope of Practice for Nursing Informatics.* Washington, D. C.: American Nurse Publishing.

American Society for Testing and Materials. (1993). Proposed Standards (E622). *Standard Guide for Developing Computerized Systems.* Philadelphia, PA.

Balas, E., Austin, S., Mitchell, J., et al. (1996). The clinical value of computerized information services. *Archives of Family Medicine,* 5(3), 271–278.

Ciotti, V., and Bogutski, B. (1994). 10 Commandments: Negotiating HIS contracts. *Healthcare Informatics,* 11(7), 16–20.

Clayton, P., Sideli, R., and Sengupta, S. (1992). Open architecture and integrated information at Columbia-Presbyterian Medical Center. *MD Computing,* 9(5), 297–303.

Convey, S. (1992). *The Seven Healthy Habits of Highly Effective People: Restoring the Character Ethic* (pp. 95–144). New York: Fireside.

Cook, R. (1998). Do we need this? *Modern Physician,* October 3(10), 35–58.

Dick, R., and Steen, E. (Eds.). (1991). *The Computer-Based Record: An Essential Technology for Health Care.* Washington, D. C.: National Academy Press.

Douglas, M. (1995). Butterflies, bonsai, and buonarroti: Images for the nurse analyst. In M. Ball, K. Hannah, S. Newbold, and J. Douglas (Eds.). *Nursing Informatics: Where Caring and Technology Meet* (pp. 84–94). New York: Springer-Verlag.

Edmunds, L. (1992). Methodologies for defining system requirements. Part 1. Methodology overview. *MEDINFO 92.* Unpublished report from Workshop handouts, Geneva, Switzerland.

Fitzgerald, J., Fitzgerald, A., and Satllings, W. (1981). *Fundamentals of Systems Analysis* (2nd ed.). New York: John Wiley & Sons.

Gause, D. and Weinberg, G. (1989). *Exploring Requirements: Quality before Design.* New York: Dorset House Publishing.

Ginsburg, D. A. and Browning, S. J. (1989). Selecting automated patient care systems. In V. K. Saba, K. A. Rider, and D. B. Pocklington (Eds.), *Nursing and Computers: An Anthology* (pp. 229–237). New York: Springer-Verlag.

Hendrickson, G. and Kovner, C. (1990). Effects of computers on nursing resources. *Computers in Nursing,* 8, 16–22.

Hewlett-Packard. (1993). *Choosing a Clinical Information System: A Blueprint for Your Success.* Waltham, MA: Hewlett Packard.

McCormick, K. A. (1983). Monitoring and evaluating implemented HIS. In R. E. Dayhoff (Ed.), *Proceedings of the Seventh Annual Symposium on Computer Applications in Medical Care* (pp. 507–510). New York: IEEE Computer Society Press.

Protti, D. and Peel, V. (1998). Critical success factors for evolving a hospital toward an electronic patient record system: A case study of two different sites. *Journal of Healthcare Information Management,* 12(4), 29–37.

Ritter, J. and Glaser, J. (1994). Implementing the patient care information system strategy. In E. Drazen, J. Metzger, J. Ritter, and M. Schneider (Eds.). *Patient*

Care Information Systems: Suggessful Design and Implementation (pp. 163–164). New York: Springer-Verlag.

Selker, H., Beshansky, J., Pauker, S., and Kassirer, J. (1989). The epidemiology of delays in a teaching hospital. *Medical Care, 27,* 112–129.

Simpson, R. L. (1993a). *The Nurse Executive's Guide to Directing and Managing Nurse Information Systems.*

Simpson, R. L. (1993b). Creating a paradigm shift in benefits realizations. *Nursing Management, 24*(6), 14–16.

Spillane, J., McLaughlin, M., Ellis, K. et al. (1990). Direct physician order entry and integration potential pitfalls. In *Proceedings of the 14th Annual Society for Computer Applications in Medical Care* (pp. 774–778). Washington, D. C.: IEEE Computer Society Press.

Staggers, N. (1988). Using computers in nursing: Documented benefits and needed studies. *Computers in Nursing, 6,* 164–170.

Young, E. M. (Ed.). (1981). *Automated Hospital Information,* Vol. 1: *Guide to Planning, Selecting, Acquiring, Implementing and Managing an HIS.* Los Angeles, CA: Center Publications.

Yourdon, E. (1989). *Modern Structures Analysis.* Englewood Cliffs, NJ: Yourdon Press.

Zielstorff, R. (1985). Cost effectiveness of computerization in nursing practice and administration. *Journal of Nursing Administration, 15,* 22–26.

Zielstorff, R., McHugh, M., and Clinton, J. (1988). *Computer Design Criteria for Systems that Support the Nursing Process* (pp. 1–40). Kansas City, MO: American Nurses Association.

Zinn, T.K. (1989). Automated systems selection. *Health Care,* 45–46.

Selected Readings

American Nurses Association. (1994). *The Scope of Practice for Nursing Informatics.* Washington, D. C.: American Nurse Publishing.

American Nurses Association. (1995). *The Standards of Practice for Nursing Informatics.* Washington, D. C.: American Nurse Publishing.

Anser Analytic Services. (1982). *Evaluation of the Medical Information System at the NIH Clinical Center,* Vol. 1, *Summary of the Findings and Recommendations* (contract no. NO1-CL-0-2117). Arlington, Va: Anser Analytic Services.

Arnold, J. and Pearson, G. (1992). *Computers Applications in Nursing Education and Practice* (Pub. No. 14-2406). New York: National League for Nursing.

Austin, C. J. (1983). *Information Systems for Health Services Administration.* Ann Arbor: Health Administration Press.

Axford, R. and Carter, B. (1996). Impact of clinical information systems on nursing practice: Nurses' perspective. *Computers in Nursing, 14*(3), 156–163.

Aydin, C., Rosen, P., Jewell, S., et al. (1995). Computers in the examining room: The patient's perspective. *American Medical Informatics Association Proceedings* (pp. 824–828).

Ball, M. J. and Collen, M. F. (Eds.). (1992). *Aspects of the Computer-Based Patient Record.* New York: Springer-Verlag.

Burnard, P. (1991). Computing: An aid to studying nursing. *Nursing Standard, 5*(17), 16–22.

Campbell, B. (1990). The clinical director's role in selecting a computer system. *Caring, 9*(6), 36–38.

Capron, H. L. and Williams, B. K. (1984). *Computers and Data Processing* (2nd ed.). Menlo Park, CA: Benjamin/Cummings.

Center for Healthcare Information Management (CHIM). (1991). *Guide to Making Effective H.I.S. Purchase Decisions.* Ann Arbor, MI: The Center for Healthcare Information Management.

Evans Paganelli, B. (1989). Criteria for the selection of a bedside information systems for acute care units. *Computers in Nursing, 7*(5), 214–221.

Gassert, C. A. (1989). Defining nursing information system requirements: A linked model. In L. C. Kingsland (Ed.), *Proceedings of the Thirteenth Annual Symposium on Computer Applications in Medical Care* (pp. 779–783). Washington, D. C.: IEEE Computer Society Press.

Gause, D. and Weinberg, G. (1989). *Exploring Requirements: Quality Before Design.* New York: Dorset House Publishing.

Gillis, P. A., Booth, H., Graves, J. R., et al. (1994). Translating traditional principles of system development into a process for designing clinical information systems. *International Journal of Technology Assessment in Health Care, 10*(2), 235–248.

Hendrickson, G. and Kovner, C. (1990). Effects of computers on nursing resources. *Computers in Nursing, 6,* 16–22.

HCIA. (1994). *100 Top Hospitals: Benchmarks for Success.* Baltimore, MD: HCIA Inc.

Holzemer, W. L. and Henry, S. B. (1992). Computer-supported versus manually-generated nursing care plans: A comparison of patient problems, nursing interventions and AIDS patients outcomes. *Computers in Nursing, 10*(1), 19–24.

Hopper, G. M. and Mandell, S. L. (1984). *Understanding Computers.* New York: West Publishing.

Jones, K. (1991). Computers systems in labor and delivery units: Critical issues. *Journal of Obstetric, Gynecologic and Neonatal Nursing, 20*(5), 371–375.

Kelly, P. A. and Hanchett, E. S. (1977). *The Impact of the Computerized Problem-Oriented Record on the Nursing Components of Patient Care* (contract no. NO1-NU-44126). Hyattsville, MD: Division of Nursing, PHS, US DHHS.

Mohr, D., Capenter, P., Claus, P., et al. (1995). Implementing an EMR: Paper's last hurrah. *American*

Medical Informatics Association Proceedings (pp. 157–161).

Mills, M. (1994). Nurse-computer performance considerations for the nurse administrator. *Journal of Nursing Administration, 24*(11), 30–35.

Mitchell, M. (1993). Systems design and management. *Capsules & Comments in Nursing Leadership & Management, 1*(3), 1.

Massaro, T. (1993). Introducing physician order entry at a major academic medical center. *Academic Medicine, 26*(1), 20–25.

Protti, D. and Peel, V. (1998). Critical success factors for evolving a hospital toward an electronic patient record system: A case study of two different sites. *Journal of Healthcare Information Management, 12*(4), 29–37.

Ritter, J. and Glaser, J. (1994). Implementing the patient care information system strategy. In E. Drazen, J. Metzger, J. Ritter, and M. Schneider (Eds.), *Patient Care Information Systems: Successful Design and Implementation* (pp. 163–194). New York: Springer-Verlag.

Rodnick, J. (1990). An opposing view. *Journal of Family Practice, 30*(4), 460–464.

Spann, S. (1990). Should the complete medical record be computerized in family practice? *Journal of Family Practice, 30*(4), 457–460.

Salois-Swallow, D. (1991). Formal process for the acquisition of an automated nurse scheduling system. In E. J. S. Hovenga, K. Hannah, K. A. McCormick, and J. S. Ronald. (Eds.), *Proceedings of the Fourth International Conference on Nursing Use of Computers and Information Science* (pp. 358–360). New York: Springer-Verlag.

Shelly, G. B. and Cashman, T. J. (1980). *Introduction to Computers and Data Processing*. Brea, CA: Anaheim Publishing.

Shortliffe, E. H., Tank, P. C., Amatayakul, M., et al. (1992). Future vision and dissemination of computer-based patient records. In M. J. Ball and M. F. Collen (Eds.), *Aspects of the Computer-based Patient Record* (pp. 273–293). New York: Springer-Verlag.

Silva, J. S. and Zawilski, R. J. (1992). The health care professional's workstation: Its functional components and user impact. In M. J. Ball and M. F. Collen (Eds.), *Aspects of the Computer-Based Patient Record* (pp. 102–124). New York: Springer-Verlag.

Simpson, R. (1992). What nursing leaders are saying about technology. *Nursing Management, 23*(7), 28–32.

Sorrentino, E. A. (1991). Overcoming barriers to automation. *Nursing Forum, 26*(3), 21–3.

Staggers, N. (1988). Using computers in nursing: Documented benefits and needed studies. *Computers in Nursing, 6*, 164–170.

Tierney, W., Miller, M., Overhage, J, et al. (1993). Physician inpatient order writing on microcomputer workstations: Effects on resource utilization. *Journal of the American Medical Association, 269*(3), 379–383.

Warnock-Matheron, A. and Plummer, C. (1988). Introducing nursing information systems in the clinical setting. In M. Ball, K. Hannah, U. Gerdin-Jelger, and H. Peterson. (Eds.), *Nursing Informatics: Where Caring and Technology Meet* (pp. 115–127). New York: Springer-Verlag.

Wegner, E. L. and Hayashida, C. T. (1990). Implementing a multipurpose information management system: Some lessons and a model. *Journal of Long Term Care Administration, 18*(1), 15–20.

Yourdon, E. (1989). *Modern Structures Analysis*. Englewood Cliffs, NJ: Yourdon Press.

Young, E. M. (Ed.). (1981). *Automated Hospital Information*, Vol. 2, *Guide to AHIS suppliers*. Los Angeles, CA: Center Publications.

Zielstorff, R., Grobe, S., and Hudgins, C. (1992). *Nursing Information Systems: Essential Characteristics for Professional Practice*. Kansas City, MO: American Nurses Association.

PART 5

Practice
Applications

14 Practice Applications

Patricia McCargar
Joyce E. Johnson
Molly Billingsley

OBJECTIVES

1. Review differences between nursing and health care informatics.
2. Describe the national standards of practice for nursing informatics.
3. Identify the major applications of informatics within nursing practice.
4. Describe the use of expert and decision support systems within nursing practice.
5. Define emerging technological advances in nursing practice.
6. Describe current research on the perceived benefits and barriers of information systems used in nursing practice
7. Identify some future trends in computer use in nursing practice.

KEY WORDS

information systems
clinical decision support systems
management decision support systems
patient care management
critical pathways

In the 1950s, health care agencies began using computers to process financial information. In the 1960s, the agencies expanded usage of computers to include patient data such as laboratory results. In the 1970s, the nursing profession began looking at ways in which computers could be used to support and enhance nursing practice. By the 1980s, the computer was being used for more integrated functions in practice. Applications of computers in decision support were challenged as computers were being brought to the bedside. Expanded uses of computers evolved as nurses utilized computers to improve patient care and conduct research by analyzing patient trends, variability in practice, and outcomes of care. Nursing informatics in the 1990s can be characterized by concerns about accessibility, compatibility, and overall integration of informatics efforts within nursing and the entire health care system.

This chapter focuses on the use of computers in nursing practice today. The unique contributions of nursing and the nursing process to health care informatics are highlighted, along with the standards of practice for nursing informatics that have been set forth by the American Nurses Association (ANA). Topics include the major applications of informatics within nursing practice, the use of expert and decision support systems, new technological advances, and current research on the perceived benefits and barriers of information systems used in nursing practice. The chapter concludes with some thoughts about future trends and challenges that lie ahead for the field of nursing informatics in the first decade of the new millennium.

Nursing versus Health Care Informatics

In 1995, the ANA Task Force to Develop Measurement Criteria for Standards for Nursing Informatics (American Nurses Association, 1995) defined nursing informatics as a "combination of nursing science, computer science, and information science" that is focused on the "methods and tools of information handling in nursing practice." According to the standards, nursing practice includes the following:

- Patient care
- Research
- Education
- Administration
- Informatics

Information handling includes interactions with data or information that involve the following:

- Identifying
- Naming
- Organizing
- Grouping
- Collecting
- Processing
- Analyzing
- Storing
- Retrieving
- Communicating
- Transforming

In 1998, Simpson (1998) suggested that lack of a clear definition of nursing informatics had hindered progress in this inevitable component of health care today. It was more than 14 years ago that nursing informatics was first defined, although the definition has now been expanded (National Advisory Council on Nurse Education and Practice, 1997) to define nursing informatics as the use of information technology to accomplish the functions and tasks of nursing.

What differentiates health care informatics and nursing informatics? The National Advisory Council on Nursing Education and Practice (1997) suggested that health care informatics includes the following:

- Identifying information to collect and process
- Creating databases
- Developing user-friendly data entry and retrieval screens
- Educating users to work with and maximize available information resources
- Installing and maintaining hospital information systems
- Developing distance education and telehealth systems for information exchange

The National Advisory Council on Nursing Education and Practice (1997) suggested that nursing brings a nursing perspective to health care informatics and augments it by:

- Bringing specific values and beliefs
- Bringing a specific practice base that produces unique knowledge
- Focusing attention on a specific phenomenon
- Providing a unique language and word context

Simpson, in his discussion of the technologic imperative in nursing (1998) suggests that nursing makes a unique contribution to the field of health care informatics by making it a more comprehensive, more complete discipline. This chapter on practice applications takes this theme a step further as we examine how computers assist nurses to do the actual *work* of the nursing profession—delivering quality, cost-effective patient care and advancing knowledge that improves such care at the bedside.

Standards for Practice

In 1995, the ANA Task Force to Develop Measurement Criteria for Standards for Nursing Informatics published its new set of practice standards (American Nurses Association, 1995) for nursing informatics. Two different sets of national standards guide the integration of nursing informatics—those that guide the use of information systems in nursing practice and those that determine system requirements in the clinical setting. The ANA standards include information handling that involves both patients and clients. According to the standards, a **patient** is defined as any person who is a direct recipient of clinical health services. A **client** may include the other recipients of the informatics nurse expertise such as other nurses, administrators, educators, researchers, health care practitioners, informatics professionals, other professionals, and communities. For informatics nurses, the ANA has defined six domains or foci of work: the information systems life cycle; principles and theory; information technology; communication; and databases. Databases may include but are not limited to nursing taxonomies, unified nomenclatures, and other data needed by nurses within database design.

As described in Fig. 14.1 the actual ANA practice standards include six major areas that mirror the nursing process. The first standard, assessment, focuses on information systems through which a variety of patient and client data elements are collected. The second stan-

The six practice standards for the informatics nurse

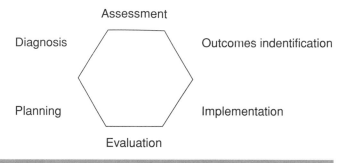

Assessment

Diagnosis

Outcomes indentification

Planning

Implementation

Evaluation

Figure 14.1
The six practice standards for the informatics nurse.
(Reproduced, with permission, from American Nurses Association (1995).)

dard revolves around information technologies that utilize the patient and client data to support ongoing and often changing decision-making requirements. The third standard includes all activities related to outcomes identification in which aggregate data reflect measurable outcomes of patient care. Planning is the focus of the fourth standard in which information-handling technologies are used to integrate and transform relevant data into the development of care plans. The fifth standard reflects the actual implementation process during which all interventions and activities are not only documented but also linked to assessment data, decisions, and identified outcomes. Finally, the sixth standard sets forth criteria to be used as the efficiency and effectiveness of decisions, plans, and activities are evaluated as a means of improving nursing practice.

In addition, the ANA standards include standards that guide the work performance of nurses who specialize in informatics. This includes the process of assuring the quality and effectiveness of nursing informatics practice; approaches for performance appraisal; and guidelines for professional development, collegiality, collaboration, research, and ethics.

The ANA's Nursing Information and Data Set Evaluation Center (NIDSEC) (American Nurses Association, 1997) has developed guidelines for composition and performance of nursing information systems. These standards, published in 1997, provide an evaluation framework for clinical nomenclature (the terms used); clinical content (the linkages between the terms); clini-

cal data repository (the storage and retrieval of data); and general system requirements such as security, confidentiality, and overall performance indicators. Standards such as these, said the ANA, guide system vendors in the development of systems that demonstrate nursing's contribution to patient outcomes. In addition, the standards serve as practical guides for nurses who make purchasing decisions.

An Array of Applications

Nursing Documentation

Historically, nursing documentation has been consistent with hospital standards, nurse practice acts, and legal definitions of clinical nursing practice. The concepts have not changed with the new computerization of nursing functions. As controls and regulations grew, the amount and quality of nursing documentation also increased. Nursing documentation in the patient record has become more complex as nursing practice has expanded to encompass care to critically ill and specialty patients. However, nursing documentation, whether manual or computerized, must adhere to certain professional standards and state laws.

Practice acts establish regulatory and statutory rules. The Joint Commission on Accreditation of Health Care Organizations (JCAHO) and the ANA set standards required for hospital accreditation and professional practice, and hospitals establish policies on which malpractice negligence rules are supported. Computer systems facilitate documentation of nurses' actions, patient's conditions, and outcomes of care planning.

Legally, an undisputed independent area of professional nursing is the recording and reporting of a nursing note. Legal definitions of nursing include necessary documentation requirements. Documentation is also clearly a nursing function recognized equally by judicial decisions (Lesnik and Anderson, 1955). Nurses can be found negligent in a malpractice case with supporting evidence from a nursing note. In a legal defense, if the hospital or staff are not legally responsible for a negligent act, conclusions may be drawn from the records. A court faced with a conflict between the record of an event made at the time and evidence of a witness relying on several years' memory is hard pressed to accept the witness's evidence. A witness is preferable only when the records are "inaccurate, illegible, or obviously unreliable" (Rozosky, 1978).

Despite legal arguments, nursing research studies have shown that nurses have not always recorded in the nursing notes. As early as the 1950s standards of recording and reporting were found wanting (Lesnik and Anderson, 1955). Even some recent studies of nurses' documentation in long-term care facilities demonstrate that manually recording patient information leads to inaccurate and incomplete information (Petrucci et al., 1992; Palmer et al., 1992).

The discrepancy between what is required by law, standards, the profession, nurse practice acts, and actual documentation can be alarmingly wide. Documentation should reflect an expanding profession's numerous independent and interdependent functions, particularly when evidence of assessment, planning, implementation, and evaluations is required by JCAHO and ANA standards.

Care Planning

Since 1980, the American Nurses Association has approved the nursing process and more recently approved nursing diagnosis as one of the classification schemes for a patient problem list. The care planning systems of today use the nursing process and are based on nursing diagnostic schemes in North America or patient problem lists in North America and Europe (Saba, 1993). These systems include assessment, diagnosis, intervention, and outcome components of care.

The computer-based patient record facilitates the automation of the nursing care planning process. Computerization can enhance the quality of information, reduce documentation, reduce errors, and increase

communication between nurses and other health care professionals within a hospital.

Components of direct patient care systems include those resulting from the process of care delivery that is interdependent with medical care, those that are independent, and those that are dependent on medical care (Romano et al., 1982). Some of the interdependent and dependent care processes that are facilitated by the computer include order entry of procedures and medications, retrieval of test results or historical information, scheduling procedures and services, tracking patients, and providing background information on patients' medical and physical conditions. The use of computers for these functions is a remarkable improvement over manual documentation because of the resulting infrastructure for hospital management and the enhanced communication within hospitals.

The components of the direct patient care system for documenting nursing practice that are independent of medical care are based on the nursing process as defined by the ANA Standards of Nursing Practice. Both in the United States and abroad, nursing documentation organization has been committed to nursing process designs since 1983 (Ashton, 1983). However, since that time, new ANA nursing standards defining the nursing process, as described below, have expanded to incorporate assessment, diagnosis, outcome identification, planning, implementation, and evaluation (American Nurses Association, 1991).

I. Nursing Process
   A. Assessment
      1. Admission assessment
         (a) Defining characteristics
         (b) Nursing examination: physiological, psychological, behavioral, functional
         (c) Vital signs, height and weight, and other flow sheets
   B. Diagnosis
         (a) Cluster defining characteristics
   C. Outcome Identification
         (a) Linkage to diagnoses
   D. Planning
         (a) Linkage between diagnoses, outcomes, and interventions
         (b) New nursing diagnosis
   E. Implementation
      1. Nursing interventions responsive to plans of care
         (a) Nursing order entry and transmission
         (b) Risk management

2. Nursing actions responsive to nurse or physician's orders and/or risk management to satisfy a diagnosis
    (a) Medication administration, intravenous medications, and blood
    (b) Vital signs and graphic flow sheets
    (c) Intake and output
    (d) Diet
3. Nursing actions responsive to procedures and unit tests and/or risk management
    (a) Automatic patient order reminders
4. Patient's actions
5. New actions

F. Evaluation
1. Patient's response and actual outcomes resulting from nursing actions in relation to the diagnoses
2. Patient's response and expected outcomes resulting from physician's orders
3. Patient's response and expected outcomes resulting from procedures and tests
4. Patient's response and expected outcomes resulting from patient's expectations
5. Patient's response and expected outcomes resulting from care delivered by other allied health professionals

II. Transfer Note

III. Discharge Care Plan and Summary

The following reports could result from a direct patient care system:

- Admission assessment

- Nursing care plan, including nursing diagnosis or KARDEX

- Daily nursing progress note, including documentation of every problem or potential problem identified in the initial admission assessment and a reassessment, analysis of new nursing diagnosis, nursing actions, and evaluations

- Medical administration sheets, including regularly scheduled medications, intravenous medications, and blood administration

- Vital signs and other flow sheets, including intake and output, height and weight, and diet

- Nursing order summary sheets

- Automatic schedule summaries for special procedures and unit tests

- Transfer note and care plan

- Discharge care plan and summary

An "ideal" computer system would document nurses' notes, care plans, and other traditional documentation requirements.

On admission, the nurse could complete a nursing assessment covering the patient's history; this includes physical characteristics, signs, and symptoms. The assessment is made 24 to 72 hours after admission depending on the hospital's policy. The nurse would enter the information into the computer through a terminal at the nursing station, a workstation at the nursing station, a pocket terminal, a notebook brought to the bedside, or a bedside terminal.

If the computer can accept order entry from the practitioner, other patient problems (e.g. allergies) could be added to the nursing assessment. Those orders for special procedures and medications may also become a part of the nursing implementation profile. The system could then prompt nurses to identify nursing care orders resulting from new practitioners' orders. The computer output generated from physicians' orders that nurses would need include medication administration sheets, vital signs and other flow sheets, and additional physician-ordered actions on the nursing order summary sheet.

Either potential or confirmed nursing diagnoses and/or patient problems are then listed by the nurse manually, or if the nurse is interacting with an expert decision support system, the computer facilitates what probable diagnoses exist. The nurse could select from predefined screens or enter these nursing and other patient problems into the computer through a terminal, or the expert system would generate a list of potential diagnoses. A selection list of outcomes related to the nursing diagnoses can be generated from the computer for the nurse to select, or in the decision support system, the known outcomes related to the particular nursing diagnoses are presented to the nurse.

The computer could then prompt the nurse to describe interventions (actions), observations, further assessments, or teaching that the nurse determines is necessary for patient care. Included in these interventions are actions that the nurse initiates because the patient has nursing care problems and actions taken in response to a physician's order. From the list of nursing actions, the computer could print automatic schedule reminders as needed. Included in these interventions are the patient's actions. However, if the nurse is interacting with a decision support system, the preprogrammed logic would list the potential nursing interventions, the expected percentage of improvement in outcomes based upon these interventions, and the side effects or complications associated with these interventions. In addition, this decision support system could display the costs of selecting alternative interventions.

The case manager or clinical nurse specialist now has the basic ingredients from the primary care nurse in order to generate an implementation strategy for the patient. The nurse can then enter evaluation information into the computer, including the patient's response to actions, expected outcomes, and dates of expected outcomes. An expected outcome can be established for every patient, every nursing or medical problem, or every action. The nurse signs his or her name and the date. If the nurse is interacting with a decision support system, a profile of other patients' responses to this same condition can be displayed to facilitate the nurse's decision. For a single patient who has a long length of stay, e.g. beyond 3 days, the computer screen can display a graphic profile of the patient's progress towards reaching the expected outcomes. This type of profile is similar to the physiologic monitoring capabilities in the current intensive care environment. However, even on acute medical wards, trends in patients' blood pressure, temperature, pulse, respirations, and other variables could be followed.

Later, the nursing progress note could contain the following:

■ New observations, signs, and symptoms.

■ Current nursing and other problems; the computer then prompts the nurse to comment if problems have changed or new problems have occurred.

■ The previously ordered actions are documented as done/not done, or given/not given, and new orders are prompted or summarized.

■ The patient's response to all actions is documented (e.g. ability to learn a certain principle of hygiene).

■ The patient's desires in selecting interventions are documented; as well as his or her preference for outcomes.

■ The patient's satisfaction with care is summarized.

The transfer note could summarize most of the above information when the patient is transferred. The nurse determines what information will be processed. The discharge care plan and summary are similar; the nurse determines the content from the patient's hospitalization—current problems, procedures, and nursing actions. In decision support systems, a profile of the patient's problems, interventions, outcomes, and satisfaction is entered into aggregate information to profile with groups of patients with the same problems.

Case Management

Case management systems include the concepts of the nursing process. If nurses are truly using the nursing process, all components of care, outcomes management, and evaluation are in place. One reason nursing personnel need to become more conscientious with their documentation of patient care is the use of documentation for case management. Within the concept of primary care, many hospitals are moving toward case management, or professional nursing network, or managed care in leveled practice (Loveridge et al., 1988; Etheridge and Lamb, 1989; DiJerome, 1992; Lamb and Stempel, 1994). This chapter discusses case management from the perspective of the nursing documentation needs.

Within case management, the level of accountability shifts from the individual patient to the management of care of entire patient caseloads, thus allowing profiles of patients and critical paths that patients take from admission to discharge to be defined. The critical path focuses on the patient outcome and/or the patient outcome timeline, rather than on the assessments and intervention strategies.

These systems provide further monitoring of the care process being completed, integration of patient care with community and home health services, and linking patterns of care and associated costs. These systems are not designed to track all patients but only (1) those with high recidivism, (2) those with medical co-morbidities, (3) the frail elderly, (4) the chronically ill, (5) the terminally ill, or (6) "outliers" of cost or length of stay. This is the demographic profile of most patients who are admitted to hospitals today.

Evaluation of the impact of the systems has suggested the following as outcomes: (1) increased client satisfaction, (2) decreased hospital admissions and ER visits, (3) decreased costs and acuity of hospital stay, (4) minimized hospital revenue loss, (5) increased job satisfaction for nurses, and (6) decreased job stress.

Care plans are integral parts of operationalizing case managed systems. In addition, patient care plans help to ensure that appropriate nursing diagnoses and interventions have been selected, admission assessment requirements are completed, discharge planning and social service needs are assessed, focused utilization/quality review is done, and patient education needs are identified. At the management level, coverage is verified, benefits are identified, certification requirements are verified, second opinion requirements are verified, and potential billing problems are identified.

These functions can occur preadmission, concurrent with care, or back-end after discharge from chart reviews. From chart reviews, the managed care coordinator must rely on expert documentation, which implies the presence of information systems to audit the occurrence of these events.

Decision-making with Administrative Data

There has been some disagreement in the nursing profession regarding the usefulness of administrative data in decision-making in nursing. Some have believed that there is little utility (Lange and Jacox, 1993), while the U.S. Office of Technology Assessment and others (Iezzoni, 1997; Diers and Bozzo, 1999) have suggested that administrative data can serve as a "gateway into more precise clinical and financial information."

A recent study from Yale illustrates ways in which data such as age, ethnicity, gender, ICD-9 coded diagnoses and procedures, and diagnosis-related groups (DRGs) can be used for "managerial epidemiology" (Fos et al., 1998), which assists nurses in better understanding clinical and management issues.

As described in Fig. 14.2, a data set of clinical descriptors can be used in a variety of ways to enhance decision-making. These include **population studies**, in which nurses must estimate the actual number of patients with certain health characteristics for research purposes or for education planning efforts; **management**

studies, in which nurses need to make management decisions based on more extensive data than census counts; and **case-mix analysis**, which can facilitate decisions that support the educational and clinical needs of nurses who care for a changing caseload of patients.

The experience at Yale suggests that administrative data that are organized into an integrated clinical/financial information system can not only enhance the problem solving skills of nurses, but also propel nurses into a wider policy role at their institutions.

Decision-making with Expert Systems

A decision support or expert system can guide, facilitate, and strengthen nursing decisions at the point of care or at the point of service. Expert systems, also known as **knowledge base systems**, process knowledge, while conventional software processes "data." According to Cullen (1998), two types of artificial intelligence—expert systems and machine learning—have been used to aid decision-making in nursing for more than a decade. Expert systems in medicine account for about 12% of those currently under development (Durkin, 1994). Both expert systems and machine learning have components that attempt to imitate human expertise by making inferences, which are defined by the Oxford Dictionary of Computing (1996) as new facts derived from a given set of facts.

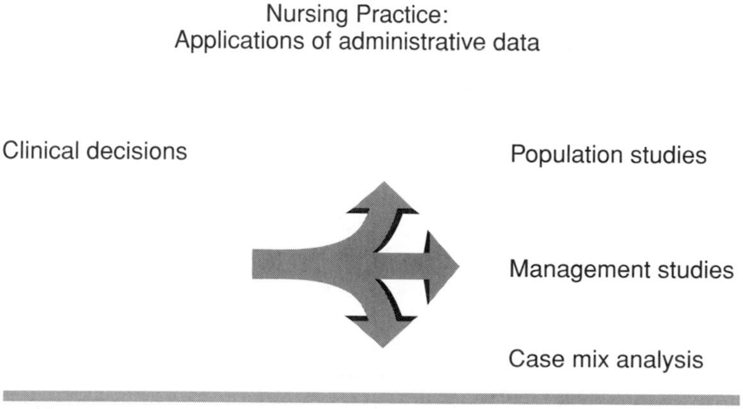

Figure 14.2
Nursing Practice: Applications of administrative data.
(Reproduced, with permission, from Diers and Bozzo (1995).)

These systems—which typically include a user interface, an inference engine, and a knowledge base—use knowledge and "thinking aloud" procedures to infer new information from what already is known about a problem and to enhance understanding, reasoning, and decision-making. Expert systems solve problems by trial and error rather than using algorithms such as those used in conventional programming to solve problems. A successful expert system has the potential to capture and preserve expertise only if the procedural knowledge of experts can be articulated.

Machine learning systems are defined (Cullen, 1998) as a "branch of artificial intelligence concerned with construction of programs that learn from experience. Learning may take many forms, ranging from learning from examples and learning by analogy to autonomous learning of concepts and learning by discovery." According to Darlington (1999), the strength of expert systems lies in their capacity to make inferences or to draw conclusions from premises. Expert systems are similar to artificial intelligence (AI) in that both technologies reproduce the human ability to select the relevant facts and draw logical conclusions. But there is an important difference between expert systems and the more experimental AI. One of the underlying principles of AI is that the system learns from previous situations. For example, if an AI system comes to a mistaken conclusion once, it can add information to its knowledge base that might help it avoid the same mistake in the future.

Nursing documentation systems that incorporate expert systems and artificial intelligence offer nurses a valuable resource—the ability to improve clinical decision-making *at the point of care in real time*. This feature substitutes retrospective and labor-intensive analysis with trend analysis. Sometimes referred to as **push technology**, this technology can recognize predictive, discriminative, or explanatory patterns in individual patients and make comparisons across groups of patients. The immediacy of such data has immediate benefits for patient care decisions and also for nursing education as students learn from the patterns that evolve within nursing practice.

A study by Petrucci et al. (1992) showed that nursing personnel improved their decision-making and the outcomes of patient care when decision support was offered to assess and intervene with patients who have urinary incontinence. The type of decision support system used in this study assisted the professional nurse and the support staff, who frequently are primary caregivers in long-term care, by describing signs and symptoms and preprogrammed nursing judgement that describe possible nursing diagnoses. Other nursing systems have been developed in the areas of computer-aided diagnosis and intervention (CANDI) (Chang et al., 1988), **AIDS** (Larson, 1988), and pain management (Heriot et al., 1988). These systems may also include such areas as nursing knowledge, reimbursement criteria, and the cost of care. Each collection of facts is arranged in a series of logical statements that reflect the thinking process of experts in the appropriate field. Depending on the application, these experts include nurses, physicians, and others in health care.

Two reviews that are focused on decision support systems in health care have been published by Miller (1994) and Johnston et al. (1994).

Outcomes Management

A chapter on the use of computers in nursing practice today would be incomplete without a description of how informatics is being used to organize and implement systems for outcomes management. A look at outcomes management provides a powerful illustration of how nurses use informatics in daily practice and thus contribute to the knowledge base in health care today.

Since 1989, there has been an emphasis on outcomes management in health care as a result of new legislation and the efforts of the Joint Commission on Accreditation of Heathcare Organizations. Outcomes management is a simple premise with complex implications for health care providers. The outcomes of health care, (i.e. both the short- and long-term results of a treatment or clinical approach, should be monitored so that the health care industry can determine and implement the best practices in medicine (Aller, 1996; Wojner and Kite-Powell, 1997). An outcomes manager, said Smith in a recent article (1998), uses information obtained by outcomes measurement to monitor and trend data and to determine the approaches for the clinical management of specific patient groups.

In his discussion about the new technologic imperative for nursing, Simpson (1998) has said that "nursing informatics makes health care informatics a more comprehensive, more inclusive discipline." Nursing's contributions to the expanding knowledge about outcomes management can be illustrated by reports in the literature that demonstrate the unique practice base of nurses and their contribution to health care informatics.

Martin (1999) and others (Martin and Scheet, 1995) have written extensively about the 20-year development of the Omaha System, with its problem classification scheme, intervention scheme, and problem rating scheme for outcomes. The outcomes capability of the system serves as a method for documentation and as a guide for nursing practice. As described in Table 14.1, the rating system was designed to measure problem-specific knowledge, behavior, and status throughout the time of service. Said Martin:

> When establishing the initial ratings for client problems, the nurse creates an independent data baseline, capturing the condition and circumstances of a client at a given point in time. This admission baseline is used to compare and contrast the client's condition and circumstances with ratings completed at later intervals and at client dismissal. The comparison or change in ratings over time can be used to assess client progress in relation to nursing intervention and thus judge the effectiveness of the plan of care.

Data are used both for individual care planning and for aggregate analysis. Such analyses are used to interface with other components of the institution's informatics systems and to evaluate the impact of patient care services, meet accreditation requirements, complete reports for third party payors, plan new programs, and ultimately advance progress in nursing.

A specific clinical example of nursing's key involvement in outcomes management was published in 1998 when Smith (1998) described a data-based system for simplifying data management for outcomes management of the mechanically ventilated patient population. In the past, the medical informatics infrastructure at this author's institution did not contain daily clinical data on this group of patients. Lack of such data made it difficult to identify trends and to identify areas for improvement in clinical practice. The author, a respiratory case manager, was then able to use the existing informatics systems at her institution and adapt them for the monitoring, storing, and retrieving of data that

could be used to determine best practices for patients who were being mechanically ventilated. This involved developing standardized criteria for such factors as reintubation rates and the starting and stopping points for weaning patients from the ventilation system. The data generated assisted the clinical staff in improving care protocols, quality improvement processes, and measurement tools.

Discharge Planning

The documentation of patient care usually begins with the admission assessment and ends with the discharge care plan. Discharge care planning systems provide for continuity of care from the home to the hospital and back to the community, another care facility, an outpatient department, or the home. The computer facilitates this communication network and can provide for this continuity when computer systems within hospitals and other care facilities can communicate with each other. An advantage of open network systems is that communication between settings can be better facilitated, and continuity of care can be improved.

Computer systems within a single hospital have been used to generate a discharge care plan for each patient. In such computerized systems, the discharge plan typically includes five components (Romano et al., 1982):

- Summary of the admission assessment
- Summary of learning needs that the patient had at discharge
- Multidisciplinary plan including problems still unresolved and outcomes not met during hospitalization

Table 14.1   Problem Rating Scale for Outcomes: The Omaha System

Concept	1	2	3	4	5
Knowledge: The ability of the client to remember and interpret information	No knowledge	Minimal knowledge	Basic knowledge	Adequate knowledge	Superior knowledge
Behavior: The observable responses, actions, or activities of the client fitting the purpose of the occasion	Not appropriate	Rarely appropriate	Inconsistently appropriate	Usually appropriate	Consistently appropriate
Status: The condition of the client in relation to objective and subjective defining characteristics	Extreme signs/ symptoms	Severe signs/ symptoms	Moderate signs/ symptoms	Minimal signs/ symptoms	No signs/ symptoms

Source: Martin and Scheet, 1995.

■ Medication and procedures that the patient must continue

■ Summary of selected patient outcomes that a multidisciplinary team desired as minimal criteria for the patient to have achieved during hospitalization

Computerized discharge care plans have the potential to be used for quality assurance, audit, research data, and information necessary for categorizing persons at discharge for prospective payment. Patients can be sent home with printed discharge plans if the content of the computerized nursing interventions or those outcomes not met while the patient was hospitalized are used. The problem list can also be sent with patients who are transferred to different institutions or to different wards within the same hospital (Wessling, 1972).

In today's managed care environment, having an availability of, and skills in using, a variety of technologic applications has become increasingly important to nurses who need to collaborate with other members of the health care team. Such technologies include but are not limited to the following:

■ E-mail

■ Listservs

■ Two-way video-conferencing

■ Web pages

■ Electronic scheduling

■ Electronic reminders

■ Remote physiologic monitoring

■ Specialty forum rooms

■ Computer-base conferencing

■ Internet relay chat

Health care professionals involved in the discharge planning process can include geographically dispersed and diverse professionals such as social workers, physicians, dieticians, occupational therapists, and physical therapists (Miller and Carlton, 1998).

Health Care Collaboration

Collaboration with other members of the health care team has always been a critical component of nursing. Advances in technology, however, have changed the ways in which members of interdisciplinary health care teams are and will be communicating with each other in the new millennium. In fact, collaboration and technology have been identified as critical elements of the

health care industry of the future (Miller and Carlton, 1998).

As primary caregivers at the bedside, nurses typically carry out the nursing process by interacting in person, in writing, or by telephone with a wide variety of health care professionals to improve patient care outcomes. Typically, these interactions include sharing information, networking, consulting, and supporting. Increasingly, as described in the sections above, this communication is being altered by the growing availability of telecommunication applications that allow asynchronous and synchronous interaction to take place (Miller and Carlton, 1998).

According to Miller and Carlton (1998), future health care practitioners such as nurses "will be active participants in collaboratively matching the wide range of telecommunications tools to the health care application need." Thus, collaboration in the years ahead will demand—for nurses and, in reality, all health care professionals—not only interpersonal skills, but also the ability to use technology as a tool to acquire and analyze information and to collaborate with others who share responsibilities for direct or indirect patient care.

■ Progress in Practice

Early in the last decade, health care researchers began assessing the value of bringing computer terminals closer to the patient and point of care, the bedside. In one study of the impact of bedside terminals on the quality of nursing documentation at New York University Medical Center, researchers differentiated the usefulness of bedside terminals from the benefit of computers in general (Marr et al., 1993). The Medical Center already had computerized documentation at the nursing terminal and added bedside terminals to measure the differences in medication administrations, daily charting (which included a record of the patient's daily functional activities and physical assessment), and admission nursing notes.

As described in Table 14.2, the variables measured were completeness of documentation measured by the presence or absence of each component of the record and timeliness of documentation as determined by comparing the time of actual entry to the time before or after the actual delivery of care. The investigators found "no significant relationship" between the presence of bedside terminals and the completeness and timeliness of medication administrations, daily charting and physical activity, or admission nursing notes. In their study, the investigators found that the bedside terminal was

Table 14.2 Qualitative Benefits of the Bedside Terminal from a Study of Nursing Use.
Difference was compared to documentation at the nursing station

- Timeliness
  a. Medication administration—No difference
  b. Daily charting—No difference
  c. Physical assessment—No difference
  d. Admission nursing notes—No difference
- Completeness of documentation
  a. Medication administration—No difference
  b. Daily charting—No difference
  c. Physical assessment—No difference
  d. Admission nursing notes—No difference

Source: Marr et al., 1993.

used less than a computer away from the patient bedside. They conclude that nursing personnel actually may need time away from the patient to collaborate with colleagues and to have thoughtful time to make substantial documentation notes. Key findings included absolutely no admission notes charted at a patient's bedside terminal and the frequency that nurses documented care for one patient at the bedside of another patient. A limitation of the study was the acknowledged placement of the bedside terminals in the patient's room. It was determined by "available space" rather than designed convenience.

Marr et al. reported other benefits from bedside terminals, which include: (1) the integration of the care plans with the nursing interventions, (2) calculation of specific acuity, and (3) automatic billing for nursing services. Other studies (Dillon, et al., 1998; Hendrickson and Kovner, 1990; Herring and Rockman, 1990; Iezzoni, 1997; Kahl, et al., 1991; Marr et al., 1993) had also demonstrated that bedside computer systems had positive effects on the efficiency, effectiveness, and satisfaction of the nursing staff.

Other issues related to bedside systems have been:

- Ergonomic design; i.e. how easy they are to use, where they are placed in the patient room, how accessible they are, how quiet they are, how unobtrusive they are to access when the patient is asleep
- Ease of use, i.e. handwriting or pen usage, finding items to chart, and time to chart

- Elimination of redundant data; i.e. does the information have to be re-entered into the main-frame or workstation
- System support for user needs at the bedside
- Availability
- Currency of data
- Access to expert systems

Given these concerns, the need for close proximity between data collection and data recording remains. As Patterson (1995) said:

The reports you get out of a system are only as good as the data you put in, and the best place and time to record a supply used, a procedure administered, a pharmaceutical issued, is where and when it happens.

Rapid advances in technology—combined with concerns about portability, accessibility, and accuracy—have now added a new feature of computer technology to informatics in nursing—the personal digital assistant (PDA)—that may make bedside terminals obsolete. This hand-held, pen-based computer—such as the Newton Message Pad or a Palm Pilot—allows data to be gathered in real time and in a variety of environments and also offers communications such as Internet access, E-mail access, and fax capabilities. This type of computer can be used at the point of care, downloaded to a workstation, and the workstation made available to an open network.

A pen is used as a pointing device to activate menu choices. Information can be entered as handwriting, printed text or hand-drawn graphics or typed with an on-screen keyboard. Handwriting is transformed into typed text through recognition software that is individualized to the user's handwriting (Donovan and Corrales, 1991). Patient data can then be downloaded to traditional computers.

According to Kasper (1996), PDA technology has resulted in a **mobile medical record**, which provides instant access to current patient charts in a wide variety of practice settings. This allows for patient records to be recorded instantly from remote settings and when nurses are at home and "on call." With PDAs, nurses and other health care providers can complete a patient record, send a prescription to a pharmacy, order follow-up clinical procedures, collect billing information, and access vast amounts of medical information. Some PDAs include built-in extensive pharmacy data and current ICD-9 codes that can assist in the billing process. Kasper (1996) reports that while few PDAs use software that is specific for nursing assessments of care plans, many are appropriate for clinical management, pharmacological reference, and patient history and physical examination data. Barcoding will also provide a means for point-of-care entry of not only supply usage but also other types of record keeping.

Patterson (1995) suggests that wireless data communication in combination with pen-based computers will be the wave of the future as the health care industry attempts to broaden usage and lower the overall costs of point-of-care computing. In 1993, for example, West Virginia University Hospital joined forces with Telxon, the world leader in wireless radio communication systems, to establish "the first totally wireless hospital." This system included a 750,000-square-foot facility, 60 hand-held, pen-based tablet-sized computers, and 32 antennas.

Patterson had predicted in 1995 that nursing homes would be "going electric" because the managed care environment was requiring electronic billing and patient records. Community, home health, and rural care agencies are increasingly using hand-held devices that can be easily carried to the point of care, where patient data can be recorded and transmitted to a central server (Kovner et al., 1997; Yancey, 1998). Whether a "computer in every hand" will become a reality in the nursing profession and in health care remains to be seen.

Benefits and Barriers

The inevitable use of computers in nursing practice has been accompanied by endless speculation about the real and future potential of using nursing information systems to improve clinical practice. Barriers and resistance can and often do accompany such technologic changes. The nursing research community has recognized the enormous importance of ending speculation and promoting quality improvements by conducting well-designed research studies on actual use versus perceptions of the realities of using computers to enhance nursing practice. Research findings are now available as a guide not only for decision-making and ongoing professional education, but also for quality improvements.

Benefits

Whether information systems actually save nurses time and improve their "efficiency" has been at the core of this debate, given the early research on the large amount of time nurses spent documenting patient information. For example, there are estimates that nurses spend between 40 and 50% of their time on paperwork (McDaniel, 1997).

Table 14.3 describes the findings from a sample of these studies. Most studies showed that using computers in nursing practice had demonstrable positive effects such as time savings, fewer errors, and more consistent documentation. There were studies, however, that did not demonstrate such results. Learning to use a computer system and completing data entry were found to be time-intensive and did not result in time savings. This was attributed to the learning curve with computers and also to differences in training techniques. Overall, however, the studies show that integrating computers into nursing practice can result in benefits in terms of time and quality of work.

Barriers

A recent review (Bowles, 1997) suggests that the barriers associated with earlier computerized systems such as lack of integration, a unified nursing language, and point-of-care terminals are slowly being resolved. According to Bowles, there are now four nursing classification systems that have been accepted by the ANA Steering Committee on Databases to Support Clinical Practice and the National Library of Medicine. Continued progress with a uniform language, as described in earlier chapters of this text, will help to resolve the lack of uniformity, which is so badly needed for data collection across practice settings on a regional and national level.

Bowles (1997) also suggested that both individual and organizational factors can present barriers to the development and use of nursing information systems. Such factors as level of education, practice setting, past work experience, age, computer anxiety, time involved in using the system, and ease of use were identified in the past, although more current research on such barriers is badly needed. A more recent study by the National Center for Nursing Research (1993) showed that organizational factors such as staffing levels, workload, communication patterns, type of unit, and administrative philosophy can also exert positive and negative influence on the success of nursing information systems.

Given the pace of change that is predicted in the information industry for the new millennium, research on the benefits and barriers of computers in nursing practice must continue as a major imperative in the nursing profession.

Summary

Although the actual components of the nursing *process* have changed little over the years, the practice environment—with its technological advances, regulatory constraints, and changing patient needs—certainly has. This chapter has described the use of the computers in the *work* of nurses within that practice environment. There are now new standards for practice in nursing informatics and a vast array of new systems for nursing documentation systems, care planning, decision-making, and outcomes management.

Maintaining the status quo with informatics in nursing practice will not be a realistic option in the rapidly changing world of the new millennium. Nurses are key contributors to patient care and, as such, must be involved in all phases of information systems development. The presence of nursing in this process will ensure that nurses contribute to technology development in every potential way that can provide strategic resources for nursing practice and ultimately for patients. The reality for the millennium may be that technology is the "tool of commonality" (Miller and Carlton, 1998) that links together the circle of health care—professionals, resources, and patients.

References

Aller, K. C. (1996). Information systems for outcomes movement. *Healthcare Information Manager, 10,* 37–53.

American Nurses Association. (1991). *Standards of Clinical Nursing Practice.* Kansas City, MO: American Nurses Association.

American Nurses Association. (1995). *Standards of Practice for Nursing Informatics.* Washington, D. C.: American Nurses Publishing.

American Nurses Association. (1997). *NIDSEC Standards and Scoring Guidelines.* Washington, D. C.: American Nurses Publishing.

Ashton, C. (1983). Nursing care plans: Aspects of computer use in nurse-to-nurse communication. In O. Fokkens et al. (Eds.), *Medinfo '83 Seminars* (pp. 332–336). Amsterdam: North-Holland.

Bowles, K. W. (1997). The benefits and barriers of nursing information systems. *Computers in Nursing, 15,* 191–196.

Chang, B. L., Roth, K., Gonzales, E., et al. (1988). CANDI: A knowledge-based system for nursing diagnosis. *Computers in Nursing, 6*(1),13–21.

Cullen, P. (1998). Gleaning patterns from practice: Intelligent systems in ambulatory care. *Nursing Economics, 16,* 133–136.

Table 14.3   Impact of computerization on nursing practice: A sample of studies

Study	Year	Findings	Impact (+ or –)
Johnson et al.	1987	Less duplication of effort; time saved; more accurate charting	+
Pierskall and Woods	1988	Decreased waiting time; elimination of unnecessary orders and services	+
Childs	1988	Reduction in telephone calls	+
Cerne and Brennan	1989	Reduction in medication errors	+
Gross	1989	Savings in overtime payments	+
Hendrickson and Kovner	1990	Time saved; less paperwork; fewer telephone calls; fewer errors; more complete documentation	+
Randall	1990	Fewer medication errors	+
Marr et al.	1993	No improvement in quality of documentation	–
Dennis et al.	1993	More efficient nursing documentation	+
Minda and Brundage	1994	Time savings	+
Pabst et al.	1996	No improvement in quality of documentation	–
McDaniel	1997	Identification of outliers; documentation of interventions	+
Kovner et al.	1997	No time savings	–
Geraci	1997	Less duplication; time savings; improved communication	+
Yancey et al.	1998	More uniform reporting	+

Darlington, K. Basic expert systems. *www.http://www.scism.sbu.ac.uk/!darlink*

Diers, D. and Bozzo, J. (1999). Using administrative data for practice and management. *Nursing Economics, 17,* 233–237.

DiJerome, L. (1992). The nursing case management computerized system: Meeting the challenge of health care delivery through technology. *Computers in Nursing, 10*(6), 250–258.

Dillon, T. W, McDowell, D., Salimian, F., and Conklin, D. (1998). Perceived ease of use and usefulness of bedside-computer systems. *Computers in Nursing, 16,* 151–156.

Donovan, W., and Corrales, S. (1991). *The Book on Bedside Computing. Inside Healthcare Computing.* Long Beach, CA: Innde Information Group.

Durkin, J. (1994). *Expert Systems: Design and Development.* New York: Macmillan.

Etheridge, P. and Lamb, G. S. (1989). Professional nursing case management improves quality, access and costs. *Nursing Management, 20*(3), 30–35.

Fos, P. J., Fine, D. J., and Zuniga, M. A. (1998). Managerial epidemiology in health administration curriculum. *Journal of Health Care Administration and Education, 16,* 1–9.

Hendrickson, G., and Kovner, C. T. (1990). Effects of computers on nursing resource use: Do computers save nurses time? *Computers in Nursing, 8*(1), 16–22.

Heriot, H., Graves, J., Bouhaddou, O., et al. (1988). Pain management decision support-system for nurses. In R. A. Greene (Ed.), *Proceedings of the Twelfth Annual Symposium on Computer Applications in Medical Care* (pp. 63–68). Washington, D. C.: IEEE Computer Society Press.

Herring, D., and Rockman, R. (1990). A closer look at bedside terminals. *Nursing Management, 21*(7), 554–61.

Iezzoni, L. (1997). Assessing quality assurance using administrative data. *Annals of Internal Medicine, 127* (8, part 2), 666–674.

Johnston, M. E., Langton, K. B., Haynes, R. B., and Mathieu, A. (1994). Effects of computer-based clinical decision support systems on clinician performance and patient outcomes. *Annals of Internal Medicine, 120,* 135–142.

Kahl, K., Ivancin, L., and Fuhrmann, M. (1991). Identifying the savings potential of bedside terminals. *Nursing Economics, 9*(6), 391–400.

Kasper, C. (1996). Personal digital assistants and clinical practice. *Western Journal of Nursing Research, 18,* 717–721.

Korpman, R., and Lincoln, A. (1988). The computer stored medical record for whom? *Journal of the American Medical Association, 259,* 3454–3456.

Korpman, R. A. (1991). Patient care automation: The future is now. Part I: Introduction and historical perspective. *Nursing Economics, 8*(3), 191–193.

Kovner, C., Schuchman, L., and Mallard, C. (1997). The application of pen-based computers technology to home health care. *Computers in Nursing, 15,* 237–244.

Lamb, G. S. and Stempel, J. E. (1994). Nurse case management from the client's view: Growing as insider-expert. *Nursing Outlook, 42*(1), 7–13.

Lange, L. L. and Jacox, A. (1993). Using large data bases in nursing and health policy research. *Journal of Professional Nursing, 9,* 204–211.

Larson, D. (1988). Development of a microcomputer-based expert system to provide support for nurses caring for AIDS patients. *Proceedings of Nursing and Computers: Third International Symposium on Nursing Use of Computers and Information Science* (pp. 682–690). St. Louis, MO: Mosby.

Lesnik, M. and Anderson, B. (1955). *Nursing Practice and the Law* (2nd ed.). Philadelphia: J.B. Lippincott.

Loveridge, C. E., Cummings, S. H., and O'Malley, J. (1988). Developing care management in a primary nursing system. *Journal of Nursing Administration, 18*(1), 36–39.

Marr, P., Duthie, E., Glassman, K., et al. (1993). Bedside terminals and quality of nursing documentation. *Computers in Nursing, 11*(4), 176–182.

Martin, K. S. (1999). The Omaha system. *On-line Journal of Nursing Informatics, 3,* 1–7.

Martin, K. S. and Scheet, N. J. (1995). The Omaha system: Nursing diagnoses, intervention and client outcomes. In ANA Database Committee, *Nursing Data Systems: the Emerging Framework.* Washington, D. C.: American Nurses Publishing.

McDaniel, A. M. (1997). Developing and testing a prototype patient care database. *Computers in Nursing, 15,* 129–135.

Miller, P. A. and Carlton, K.H. (1998). Technology as a tool for health care collaboration. *Computers in Nursing, 16,* 27–29.

Miller, R. A. (1994). Medical diagnostic decision support systems—past, present, and future. *Journal of the American Medical Informatics Association, 1*(8), 8–27.

National Advisory Council on Nurse Education and Practice. (1997). *A National Informatics Agenda for Nursing Education and Practice.* Rockville, MD: Division of Nursing, BHP, HRSA, DHHS.

National Center for Nursing Research. (1993). Using data, information, and knowledge to deliver and manage patient care. In NCNR Priority Expert Panel on Nursing Informatics (Ed.) *Nursing Informatics: Enhancing Patient Care* (pp. 21–30). Bethesda, MD: U.S. Department of Heath and Human Services.

Oxford. (1996). *Dictionary of Computing* (4th ed.). Oxford, England: Oxford University Press.

Palmer, M. H., McCormick, K. A., Langford, A., et al. (1992). Continence outcomes: Documentation on medical records in the nursing home environment. *Journal of Nursing Care Quality, 6*(3), 36–433.

Patterson, D. (1995). Bedside computing. *Nursing Homes, 44*, 16–18.

Petrucci, K. M., Jacox, A., McCormick, K. A., et al. (1992). Evaluating appropriate of a nurse expert system's patient assessment . . . Urological Nursing Information System (UNIS). *Computers in Nursing, 10*(6), 243–249.

Romano, C., McCormick, K., and McNeely, L. (1982). Nursing documentation: A model for a computerized data base. *Advances in Nursing Science, 4,* 43–56.

Rozosky, L. (1978). Medical records as evidence. *Dimensions in Health Services, 55,* 16–17.

Saba, V. (1993). Nursing diagnostic schemes. In *Papers from the Nursing Minimum Data Set Conference* (pp. 54–63). Edmonton, Alberta: The Canadian Nurses Association.

Simpson, R. (1998). The technologic imperative: A new agenda for nursing education and practice, Part 2. *Nursing Management, 29,* 24–25.

Smith. K. R. (1998). Outcomes management of mechanically ventilated patients: Utilizing informatics technology. *Critical Care Nursing Quarterly, 21,* 61–72.

Wessling, E. (1972). Automating the nursing history and care plan. *Journal of Nursing Administration, 2,* 34–38.

Wojner, A. W., Kite-Powell, D. (1997). Outcomes manager: A role for the advanced practice nurse. *Critical Care Nursing Quarterly, 19,* 16–42.

Yancey, R. Given, B., White, N. et al. (1998). Computerized documentation for a rural nursing intervention project. *Computers in Nursing, 16,* 275–284.

15

Critical Care Applications

Caroline Campbell
Susan Eckert
Kathleen Milholland Hunter

OBJECTIVES

1. Identify computer applications in critical care.
2. Understand the basic elements of arrhythmia monitors and physiologic monitors.
3. Describe how hemodynamic monitoring systems are used in critical care settings.
4. Understand the capabilities, purposes, types, benefits, and issues of critical care information systems.
5. Describe the relationship between hemodynamic monitoring systems and critical care information systems.
6. Identify trends in monitoring and computerized information management.
7. Identify special-purpose applications available.

KEY WORDS

information systems
hospital information systems
integrated information systems
critical care

Critical care nursing is the nursing specialty that deals with human responses to life-threatening problems (Kinney et al., 1988). A critically ill patient is any patient with real or potential life-threatening health problems requiring constant observation and constant intervention to prevent complications and restore health (Berg, 1981). Implied in these definitions is a technologically intense environment geared to the monitoring and support needs of the critically ill patient (Buchman, 1995). Embedded in much of that technology are microprocessors, which permit gathering, processing, and storage of large volumes of data. In 1986, Saba and McCormick estimated that the volume of data collected by nurses in critical care settings on a daily basis was as high as 1,500 data points. Much of this data originates from the machinery found in the critical care environment. As the use of technology expands, the available information expands as well, making it increasingly difficult to manage the volume of data. At the same time, the demand for cost-effective care has increased (Gardner et al., 1989). Resource shortages, both staff and time, increase the difficulty of data management. Computer technology offers solutions to these difficulties through manipulating large volumes of data and presenting them to the clinician in meaningful ways. Effective and efficient integration of information drives improvement in patient care and hence is increasingly employed in critical care settings.

Computer technology is found in many patient care units in the critical care setting. The microprocessors that are embedded in many of the devices found in the critical care setting facilitate downloading of the information that resides in the device to an information management system. Based on the sheer volume and complexity of the technology, the information management needs in the critical care area require different computer resources than those of other patient care areas. In this chapter, physiologic, arrhythmia, and hemodynamic monitors, special-purpose systems, and critical care information systems (CCISs) will be the focus of discussion. Descriptions of the specialized applications of computer technology found in the critical care area and trends toward new applications will be included in that discussion.

Developments

Developers of automated approaches to information management in critical care settings have incorporated complex formulas into physiologic monitors, rapidly analyzed small samples of gas or fluids, maintained near-normal physiologic ranges with life-supporting equipment, and stored large volumes of data that would otherwise be disorganized, lost, inaccurate, or illegible. Alarm systems have been automated so nurses can make use of each vital second.

The advantages of these automated systems resemble the advantages of computerizing nursing documentation: better control of nursing observations to promote better assessment of immediate patient needs. However, these systems focus heavily on collecting, storing, and displaying physiological data. Usually, there are modules or subsystems that address the nursing process and provide care planning and nursing documentation capabilities. The functions, purposes and benefits of these nursing process capabilities are the same as noted elsewhere in this book.

Computer Capabilities and Applications in Critical Care Settings

Computers in the critical care environment have several major capabilities:

- Process physiologic data
- Recognize deviations from preset ranges by an alarm
- File patient care documentation
- Trend data in a graphical presentation
- Regulate physiologic equipment
- Process, store, and integrate diagnostic information from various sources
- Comparatively evaluate patients with similar diagnoses

There are several data-intense information systems that exist in the critical care environment from which data can be obtained and integrated in a meaningful way. Computer applications typical in the critical care environment that will be described in this chapter include the following:

- Medical information bus
- Physiologic monitors, including arrhythmia and hemodynamic monitors
- Special-purpose systems
- Critical care information systems

Medical Information Bus

In concept, the medical information bus (MIB) is the backbone of information exchange, allowing data to be moved from device to device. The MIB eases the documentation workload generated by the proliferation of patient care devices (e.g. monitors, ventilators, infusion pumps) in the modern critical care setting. This computer-based device collects information from various sources in a standard format and supplies that information to the clinical information system. Vital information originating from the physiologic monitoring system or other special purpose system can thus be integrated by the clinical information system for use in support of patient care. Conversely, the information system can be used to control the device by reversing this flow of information across the MIB. The features of the MIB that are of most interest from a clinical user perspective are listed in Table 15.1.

Unfortunately, the concept of the MIB has not fully come to fruition. In late 1994, the Institute of Electrical

Table 15.1   Features of a Medical Information Bus

- Automatic detection of device connection
- Notification of communications failure
- Notification of disconnect
- Identification of device for host computer
- Absence of special settings on device itself
- Automatic recovery from system failure/patient transport
- Reporting of device alarm state changes
- Remote resetting of alarms
- Large device-per-bedside capacity
- Clustering of device communication cables

and Electronics Engineers' (IEEE) 1073 Medical Information Bus won industry approval. This MIB standard provides a uniform model for the method of data capture and transport as well as the language used by various bedside devices, enabling them to communicate with a central information system (Data Trap, 1997). While emerging technology begins to adopt this standard, individual interfaces must still be developed for many devices. These interfaces decode the data output from the source device, translate the output into a format that is understood by the destination clinical information system, and transport the information in an orderly fashion from the source to the destination. Such interfaces are best developed with a cooperative effort between vendors. However, it is possible for one vendor to reverse engineer an interface to be compatible with another vendor's product.

Physiologic Monitoring Systems

In the NASA programs of the 1960s, physiologic monitors were developed to oversee the vital signs of the astronauts. By the 1970s, these monitors had found their way into the hospital setting, where they replaced manual methods of gathering patient vital signs. These early monitors were large and cumbersome and had limited capabilities. In the 1980s, technology became cheaper, smaller, and significantly more powerful. These developments were used to improve overall patient monitoring capabilities (Wiggett, 1996). In the 1990s, the focus of development has shifted to integration of monitoring data into information systems. In fact, many monitoring vendors introduced clinical information systems into their standard product lines.

Most physiologic monitors consist of five basic parts as shown in Table 15.2. The sensor is the instrument

Table 15.2 Basic Components of Physiologic Monitoring Equipment

- Sensors (e.g. pressure transducer, ECG electrode)
- Signal conditioners to amplify or filter the display device (e.g. amplifier, oscilloscope, paper recorder)
- File to rank and order information (e.g. storage file, alarm signal)
- Computer processor to analyze data and direct reports (e.g. paper reports, storage for graphic files, summary reports)
- Evaluation or controlling component to regulate the equipment or alert the nurse (e.g. a notice on the display screen, alarm signal)

that is coupled to the patient and transforms the physiologic signal (e.g. temperature, pressure, ionic current) into an electrical signal that can be detected by the monitor. Careful attention to the sensor's limitations is required, since signal errors can easily originate at this point. Physiologic signals are typically of very small amplitude and must be amplified, conditioned, and digitized by the device in preparation for processing by its imbedded microprocessor. The microprocessor analyzes information, stores pertinent information in specific places, and controls the direction of reporting (e.g. a paper report, storage for graphic files, shift summary reports). The file holds the information (e.g. the storage files, signals, or alarms). The evaluation or the controlling component alerts the nursing personnel through a report, an alarm, or a visual notice (e.g. a notice on the display screen: "increase patient's oxygen or check for leaks"). Alternatively, the controlling component may regulate an external device as a result of its evaluation; e.g. drug delivery is altered via control of an infusion pump in response to a blood pressure change.

Today, most physiologic monitoring systems are available in conjunction with a clinical information system. Due to market demand, those same physiologic monitoring systems utilize open architectures, which render them capable of interfacing with clinical information systems from other vendors as long as an investment of labor and dollars is made to develop the interface. The attraction of purchasing a monitoring system that is a component of an integrated information system is that development of an interface between the monitoring system and the information system is not necessary. However, the strength of the individual monitoring and information system components must be weighed against the resources required to develop an interface when deciding to purchase an integrated system or to integrate dissimilar monitoring and information systems.

As the information from various sources is integrated into the clinical information system, the accuracy of each and every data element becomes more important. Errors that arise within the monitoring system can invade the information system, thus blurring the picture of the patient's status and making effective decisions about patient care more difficult. Regardless of the degree of sophistication of the monitoring technology, the information it processes is only as good as the input it receives. Faulty signals will continue to be processed and will result in an increase in nuisance alarms. The incidence of inaccurate information causing monitor alarms in the intensive care unit setting was studied by Tsien and Fackler. They found that 86 percent of alarms were false positive alarms resulting from, in order of incidence, bad formats or connections, poor contact of sensors, electrocardiogram (ECG) wire movement, motion artifact, measurement during arterial line clamping or flushing, and probe disconnection (Tsien and Fackler, 1997). Considerable errors can be introduced to the monitoring system at the "front end" or patient side of the monitor, and hence the sensor and patient connections to the monitor demand particular attention. For example, pressure transducers must be zeroed properly to provide accurate pressure measurements, and ECG electrodes must be periodically changed with appropriate skin preparation in order to minimize motion artifact. As information from the monitoring system is integrated into the information system, the accuracy of the monitoring data becomes increasingly important (Belzberg et al., 1996).

Monitoring systems also store various data elements with a time stamp derived from the monitoring system's internal clock. These data elements are transported with their respective time stamps to the clinical information system. If the clocks of the monitoring system or other data sources and the clock of the clinical information system are different, the effectiveness of various interventions as integrated and recorded in the patient's record may be erroneously interpreted. Therefore, attention must be given to the synchronicity of information from a variety of sources.

Physiologic monitoring systems typically have a modular platform, allowing the selection of various monitoring capabilities to match the needs of a variety of clinical settings. A careful choice of physiologic parameters will allow a critical care unit to cost-effectively offer the appropriate monitoring capabilities for its patients without offering the costly capability to monitor every conceivable parameter at every bedside. Modular formats can also facilitate data collection during transport to various diagnostic locations using a smaller transport monitor from the same manufacturer as the bedside monitor. Upon return to the patient unit, that information can be downloaded into the bedside monitor for integration into the patient's record.

More specialized monitoring capabilities such as intracranial pressure or bispectral index monitoring are also available in modular format, but modular availability is usually developed sometime after the availability as a stand-alone monitor. Typically, the patent holder of the new monitoring technology will license its software development to monitoring manufacturers for incorporation into their monitoring system. An alternative approach is to work with the monitoring vendor to develop an interface with the stand-alone monitor such that information can be exchanged between the stand-alone monitor and the physiologic monitoring system. Once information from the stand-alone monitor is imported into the physiologic monitor, that information can be passed along by the physiologic monitor to the clinical information system.

The flexibility of the modular monitoring format allows the physiologic monitor to be built around the needs of the patient found in any care setting. In the critical care setting, physiologic monitors are usually built to incorporate both arrhythmia and hemodynamic monitoring capabilities.

Hemodynamic Monitors

Advanced hemodynamic monitoring systems allow for calculation of hemodynamic indices and limited data storage. Hemodynamic monitoring can be used to (Kenner, 1990; Gardner et al., 1989; Clochesy, 1989):

- Measure hemodynamic parameters
- Closely examine cardiovascular function
- Evaluate cardiac pump output and volume status
- Recognize patterns (arrhythmia analysis) and extract features
- Assess vascular system integrity
- Evaluate the patient's physiological response to stimuli
- Continuously assess respiratory gases (capnography)
- Continuously evaluate blood gases and electrolytes
- Estimate cellular oxygenation
- Continuously evaluate glucose levels
- Store waveforms
- Automatically transmit selected data to a computerized patient database

Hemodynamic monitoring can be invasive or noninvasive. Invasive catheters are typically used to measure and monitor various pressures and cardiac output. Noninvasive monitoring methods are increasingly common and include pressure measurement using oscillometric techniques, oxygenation measurement using pulse oximetry technology, and measurement of cardiac output via doppler. A screen from a bedside hemodynamic monitoring system is shown in Fig. 15.1.

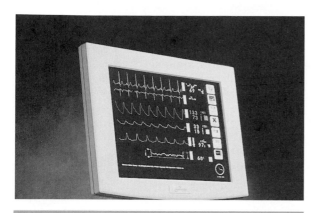

Figure 15.1
A bedside physiologic monitor: The Universal Clinical Workstation.
(Courtesy Spacelabs Medical, Inc., Redmond, WA.)

Invasive hemodynamic monitoring techniques have traditionally involved use of the pulmonary artery catheter (PAC), which was originally designed for measurement of pulmonary artery and wedge pressures. Since its inception, design modifications have been made including incorporation of a thermistor, which facilitates measurement of cardiac output and incorporation of fiber-optic technology, which facilitates measurement of mixed venous oxygen saturation (Headley, 1998). Use of the PAC has potential complications, such as infection, hemorrhage, and embolism.

With growing popularity of use, the PAC has come under recent and persistent criticism concerning its safety and appropriate use. This criticism prompted formation of the Pulmonary Artery Consensus Conference Organization (PACCO) with broad representation from professional nursing and medical societies. The PACCO determined that it is appropriate to use the pulmonary artery catheter when either conventional hemodynamic therapies have not produced desirable results or hemodynamic therapies require the monitoring provided by the pulmonary artery catheter. However, the PACCO supported further research on the impact of the pulmonary artery catheter and found that clinical knowledge of the pulmonary artery catheter, including clinical and technical aspects, probably warranted improvement (Ahrens, 1999a).

Intermittent measurement using thermodilution techniques has become the standard methodology for assessment of cardiac output. However, the accuracy of

this technique is highly user-dependent for the following reasons (Headley, 1998; Burchell et al, 1997; Von Rueden and Turner, 1999):

- The bolus must be injected within 4 seconds
- The amount of the solution must be accurate
- The temperature of the injectate must be precisely measured and accurately maintained
- The catheter must be properly placed within the heart and pulmonary artery
- The computer must have the appropriate computation constant entered
- The bolus must be injected at the appropriate time in the respiratory cycle.

The influence of these user-related issues is negated by using heating of a thermal filament embedded in the catheter to replace the injectate. The thermal filament is intermittently heated, thus sending pulses of heat energy into the right ventricle, which is then sensed by the thermistor in the pulmonary artery in much the same manner as in the traditional thermodilution technique. These measurements can be repeated at programmable intervals. The microprocessor keeps a running average of the last several minutes of values to obtain a continuously updated cardiac output measurement. Because of its more frequent measurements, this method may allow earlier detection and treatment of a change in cardiac output than conventional intermittent thermodilution. However, because this technique presents an averaged cardiac output, the response to acute changes may be considered to be slow (Headley, 1998; Mihm et al., 1998; and Burchell et al., 1997).

An alternative means of measuring cardiac output noninvasively is provided by thoracic electrical bioimpedance. Four sensors are positioned on the sides of the neck and thorax. A low-amplitude, high-frequency signal is emitted by the sensors through the thorax. The amplitude of the signal detected by the sensors is proportional to the impedance of the path traveled by the electricity through the thorax. Because electricity follows the path of least resistance and because the path through the thorax is typically composed of fluid, the measured impedance provides information about the amount of fluid in the thoracic cavity. There are three compartments in the thorax that contain fluid, namely intravascular, intraalveolar, and interstitial. Since the aorta is the largest, most distensible, blood-filled vessel in the thoracic cavity, aortic blood flow contributes significantly to the measured impedance and hence is readily tracked via this method. As the heart beats and the blood within the thorax changes, the measured thoracic impedance will change. Monitoring these changes permits measurement of stroke volume; indices of contractility such as velocity and acceleration of blood flow, supraventricular rhythm, and index; and cardiac output and index. However, in conditions that increase the fluid in nonvascular compartments of the thorax, such as pulmonary edema and pleural effusion, measurements of cardiac output using the electrical bioimpedance method are less reliable. With these exceptions, satisfactory agreement with the thermodilution technique can be obtained using thoracic bioimpedance for cardiac output measurement (Shoemaker et al., 1994; Von Reuden and Turner, 1999; Lasater, 1998). Utilizing bioimpedance as a factor integrated with analysis of the finger blood pressure waveform has also been demonstrated as a method of cardiac output measurement; however, this method has not demonstrated sufficient agreement with established technique to be of clinical value (Hirschl et al., 1997).

A critical piece of hemodynamic information involves the availability of oxygen to bodily tissues. The gold standard for measurement of the blood's oxygen saturation is co-oximetry, which is based on principles of spectrophotometry. Pulse oximetry is a noninvasive method of measuring arterial oxygen saturation that also utilizes spectrophotometry. The pulse oximeter utilizes two light-emitting diodes (LEDs), each of which emits light of different wavelengths. The light is emitted through a pulsatile arteriolar bed and then detected by a photosensor. Measurement of the amount of light detected at the photosensor and knowledge of the light absorption characteristics of oxyhemoglobin allow determination of the oxygen saturation. Because the blood volume in the arteriolar bed varies with the heartbeat, the amount of light absorbed will also vary with the pulse. This pulsatile nature allows the device to differentiate the amount of light absorbed by the venous blood and tissues from the amount of light absorbed by the arterial blood. The pulse oximeter is unable to distinguish between the various types of hemoglobin and hence the oxygen saturation is a functional saturation measurement that includes all types of hemoglobins including methemoglobin and carboxyhemoglobin.

The availability of a noninvasive oxygen saturation measurement device has resulted in widespread use of pulse oximetry in critical care environments. Unfortunately, the susceptibility of pulse oximetry to interference makes it the largest contributor to alarms in the intensive care unit (ICU). Susceptibility to motion artifact is particularly problematic. Since the technology is dependent on its ability to differentiate blood content over a pulsatile cycle, any device such as a blood pressure cuff, tourniquet, or air splint that may cause venous pulsations will limit the sensor's ability to distinguish between arterial and venous blood. Since the technology is based upon a measurement of light, any extraneous light source, including ambient light, may impact the accuracy of measurement (Ahrens and Tucker, 1999; Tsien and Fackler, 1997).

While pulse oximetry provides a measure of oxygen delivered to the tissue, mixed venous oxygen saturation (SvO_2) provides a measure of the amount of oxygen used by the patient. Normally, about 25 percent of the oxygen delivered is extracted for use. If more than 25 percent is extracted, then the body is compensating for an increased oxygen demand or a decreased oxygen delivery. Therefore, a drop in SvO_2 is a warning sign of a potential threat to tissue oxygenation. An increase in SvO_2 indicates that the tissue is not receiving oxygen perhaps because of shunting of blood from vascular collapse or obstructions. (Ahrens, 1999b; Headley, 1998).

Hemodynamic monitoring can take place at the bedside or be conducted from a remote location via telemetry. As the volume of higher acuity patients that are serviced outside of the intensive care unit increases, telemetry is more frequently utilized. Telemetry allows for the continuous monitoring of patients usually outside of the intensive care unit. Physiologic data are sent by a transmitter to an antenna system that is distributed around the nursing unit or institution (usually in the ceiling) and displayed on the monitor screen at the telemetry station (Elder, 1991). The patient wears the transmitter, which is attached to the patient via surface electrodes for monitoring of ECG. The small size and weight of the transmitter enables the patient to be mobile as long as the patient remains in the area of antenna coverage. The radio frequency (RF) signal is received by a central monitor, processed, and then displayed at the central monitors as well as at specified remote sites. Transmitters can also be attached to portable devices, which in turn are connected to the patient. This approach enables telemetric monitoring of any parameter that can be monitored by the portable monitor. An example of this approach is shown in Fig. 15.2. Through utilization of an expansive antenna system, virtually any bed in the hospital can be monitored without purchasing monitoring hardware for every bed.

Through installation of an expansive antenna system, monitoring can be made available at virtually any bed without purchasing monitoring hardware for every

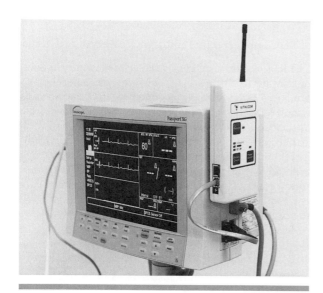

Figure 15.2
A transmitter couples to the output of a portable monitor.
(Courtesy VitalCom, Inc., Tustin, CA and Datascope Patient Monitoring, Paramus, NJ.)

bed. Use of this approach allows admission to the specialty area that best suits the patient's needs even when hemodynamic monitoring is necessary. However, it is important to remember that in that location, qualified staff members must be available to respond to alarms, attend to the patient, and make a complete assessment of the patient's cardiac condition. It is also important to remember that with telemetry, communication protocols between the central station and the bedside nurse are critically important. Pager systems that are linked to the telemetry system are now available to assist with this communication (Martin and Hendrickson, 1999).

Telemetry monitoring is susceptible to signal loss for a variety of reasons. The RF signal reception can be interrupted by obstacles in the environment including walls, furniture, and even the patient's own body. This signal loss is commonly referred to as "drop-out." Secondly, the RF signal can be interfered with by other extraneous RF signals of the same frequency. Medical telemetry is currently designated as a Part 15 or a Part 90 device by the Federal Communications Commission. According to the Part 15 and Part 90 rules, medical telemetry cannot interfere with licensed users, such as television and radio broadcasters and must endure any interference experi-

enced from these licensed users. With the conversion to digital television as mandated by Congress, the refarming of the analog stations, and the expansion of private land mobile radio use, there is diminishing airspace left for telemetry use. The Federal Communications Commission is likely to designate some portion of the frequency spectrum for use by medical telemetry under a licensed by rule status. With this allocation, telemetry manufacturers are more likely to invest in the design of more robust products using more sophisticated modulation techniques. Only then will telemetry be more immune to signal loss and interference (American Hospital Association, 1999).

Computer-based hemodynamic monitoring offers the critical care nurse a wealth of information. However, the clinicians must keep in mind that the monitor and its information do not replace clinical judgement or necessarily imply quality patient care (Macy and James, 1971; Kenner, 1990). Conversely, the critical care nurse must learn to recognize the limitations of manual estimation of physiologic parameters and not use that estimation to diagnose a monitor malfunction. For example, manual calculation of mean arterial blood pressure is based only on two discrete pressures, i.e. systolic and diastolic. The hemodynamic monitor calculates mean arterial pressure using a much larger sample of discrete pressures. Therefore, the manually calculated mean pressure is an estimate and the value calculated by the monitor is a derived measurement. The two values will not necessarily match.

Arrhythmia Monitors

Computerized monitoring and analysis of cardiac rhythm have proved reliable and effective in detecting potentially lethal heart rhythms (Widman, 1992). Standards for testing and reporting the performance of arrhythmia analysis systems have been developed by the American Heart Association. A key functional element is the system's ability to detect ventricular fibrillation and respond with an alarm. However, no standards currently specify the minimal accuracy of computerized detection systems (Mirvis et al., 1989). The basic components of arrhythmia monitors are shown in Table 15.3.

System Types There are two types of arrhythmia systems: detection surveillance and diagnostic or interpretive. In a detection system, the criteria for a normal ECG are programmed into the computer. The computer might survey the ECG for wave amplitude and duration and for the intervals between waves. The program may even include an alarm response if the R-R interval is

Table 15.3 Basic Components of Arrhythmia Monitors

- Sensor
- Signal conditioner
- Cardiograph
- Pattern recognition
- Rhythm analysis
- Diagnosis
- Written report

either less than or equal to two-thirds of the average R-R interval. Each signal may then be analyzed to determine whether the QRS duration is greater than normal.

The next programmed search may be for the presence of a compensatory pause. (i.e. a prolonged R-R interval after a premature ventricular contraction (PVC)). The computer may then be programmed to store the number of PVCs per minute and sound an alarm or alert the nurse visually (e.g. a flashing red light) and audibly (a loud sound) when more than five PVCs occur within a minute. Detection systems can even store in memory the type of arrhythmia and time of occurrence, so that the patient's arrhythmia history can be plotted and compared to medication administration and cardiopulmonary pressures as well as trended (Sorkin and Bloomfeld, 1982).

Arrhythmia systems can also be diagnostic; after the analog signals are digitized for processing, the program analyzes and diagnoses the ECG. The computer, after processing the ECG, generates an analysis report that is confirmed by a cardiologist, usually from another site. The computers that support these types of ECGs are usually dedicated systems (i.e. main memory is used only for ECG acquisition, analysis, and report generation). Diagnostic systems are usually capable of retrieving a patient's previous ECGs for comparison. Bedside monitoring capabilities are beginning to emerge that incorporate 12 lead ECG capabilities, the cornerstone of the diagnostic system.

Interpretive systems search the ECG complex for five parameters:

- Location of QRS complex
- Time from the beginning to the end of the QRS
- Comparison of amplitude, duration, and rate of QRS complex with all limb leads
- P and T waves
- Comparison of P and T waves with all limb leads

The findings are then compared to predetermined diagnostic specifications. Evaluation of these parameters are based on an arithmetic comparison of the patient's signal to a "normal" signal. Because the comparisons are arithmetic in nature, random signal noise can result in erroneous identification of arrhythmias. A purely arithmetic analysis will never replace the more discerning element of human review; therefore, arrhythmia monitors are merely another tool for use in the critical care environment, and will never replace the cognitive abilities of the caregiver.

Special Purpose Systems

Various ancillary health care groups historically have contributed information to the patient's record. As these groups begin to use information systems, the data from these systems can be incorporated into the clinical information system. Integration of these data results in a more complete representation of the patient's status and can promote efficiency in patient care (Belzberg et al., 1996). For example, interface with the admissions information system can prevent the need for redundant collection and recording of demographic data. Information from the laboratory and the radiology information systems can also be useful in developing a total picture of the patient's status, and the electronic transfer of this information is much quicker than previous manual methods. Radiology information systems are developing to include access to picture archival information as well. Ventilators may be interfaced directly with the physiologic monitoring system, or the data from the ventilators can be dumped to a respiratory therapy information system, which in turn interfaces with the critical care information system. The data elements from the various information systems will carry the time stamp of their original source information system; therefore, synchronicity of the various information system clocks is imperative.

The data management needs of radiology differ from those in the critical care area based on the need to acquire, manage, and distribute images as information. The DICOM 3.0 standard defines the uniformity issues that are technically required to achieve this data management. The benefits of a picture archiving and communications system (PACS) in the radiology area include the ability to immediately disseminate images, resulting in quicker initiation of patient interventions, and decreased loss of images, resulting in fewer repeat examinations and less radiation exposure and patient inconvenience (Esch et al., 1998).

Respiratory therapy management systems have resulted in changing documentation practices related to mechanically ventilated clinical information. Previously, this information could be found in several places such as the nurses' notes, physicians' notes, and respiratory care notes. These documentation practices resulted in difficulty in monitoring and trending mechanically ventilated clinical information. Convergence of this data in a management system has facilitated the ability to monitor, collect, enter, and retrieve data for outcomes management use. Outcomes management principles are concerned with determining short- and long-term results of treatment practices through the process of outcomes measurement in hopes of determining and implementing the best practice within a given population. The outcomes manager can use these data to monitor and trend mechanically ventilated practice patterns within and between critical care areas to focus practice improvement efforts (Smith, 1998).

Critical Care Information Systems

A CCIS is a system designed to collect, store, organize, retrieve, and manipulate all data related to the direct care of the critically ill patient. It is focused on individual patients and the information directly related to the patients' care. The primary purpose of a CCIS is the organization of a patient's clinical data for the clinician's use in patient care (Milholland and Cardona, 1983), and the power of a modern CCIS is its ability to integrate information from a variety of sources and to manipulate that information in meaningful ways. That information can then be integrated for use in outcomes management.

Most CCISs include previously developed charts that meet the basic needs of a majority of the vendor's clients. These CCISs are usually flexible and allow for customization of standard charts to fit the existing clinical practices at an individual institution. Because clinical input is essential to implementing and designing systems that reflect the reality of patient and caregiver needs, the clinician will be intimately involved in the development and implementation of the successful CCIS (Muschlitz, 1998). Although flexibility may seem a desirable trait of CCISs, the price to pay for flexibility is the very significant amount of labor required over long periods of time to customize. The degree of cus-

tomization required will be largely dependent on the level of previous clinical input used to develop the standard charts. Therefore, in addition to evaluating a CCIS's flexibility, a CCIS vendor selection criterion might be a demonstrated guidance of system development based on input from an established users' group.

Although it is possible to essentially duplicate current documentation practices using electronic format, there are disadvantages to this approach. Documentation practices will optimally be redesigned to facilitate the ability of the computer to extrapolate information across patients and across time. An example of this approach is the use of a large group of "scoring systems" which attempt to provide objective markers to describe complex and often subtle findings. One of the most widespread systems is the Glasgow Coma Scale which attempts to quantify the neurological exam in sets of reproducible observations. Validation of these scoring systems depends on showing that different observers will independently arrive at the same value, indicating that the toll has a high level of reproducibility (Belzberg et al., 1996; Teres et al., 1998).

Considerable effort is being invested in the standardization of the language used in the CCIS. Currently there are four recognized nursing nomenclatures standards: North American Nursing Diagnosis Association, Nursing Interventions Classification, the Omaha System, and the Home Health Care Classification. Additionally, the National Library of Medicine is developing a Unified Medical Language System, which contains a metathesaurus that includes information about specific concepts; a semantic network, which represents a variety of relationships among the semantic types or categories of concepts in the metathesaurus; and the UNLS Information Sources Map, which contains information about databases as a whole (Averill et al., 1998).

It seems that the task of developing the clinical information system is never complete. As new technologies are introduced or new information needs arise, changes to the CCIS become necessary. As C. Peter Waegmann, the Executive Director of the Medical Records Institute says, "Getting to the electronic patient record is a journey" (Muschlitz, 1998). The human's inherent resistance to change and the seemingly unending task of implementing change relative to the CCIS makes the role of system champion imperative to its successful implementation. The system champion is responsible for overseeing and coordinating all aspects of system development and for avoiding or overcoming obstacles with the potential to stall its ongoing development and implementation. Only an evolving CCIS will meet tomorrow's needs.

The CCIS can also support the trend of multidisciplinary documentation and multidisciplinary planning of patient care (Muschlitz, 1998). Because each of the disciplines seeks different information in often unique presentations, the ideal CCIS will allow the flexibility to meet these diversified needs (Cook, 1997).

As CCISs have matured, the functions they offer have expanded to encompass not only data collection but also functions more commonly associated with hospital information systems. Examples of these functions include order entry, results reporting, care planning, and administrative reports. CCISs offer many functions to facilitate the work of critical care nurses. Some of these functions include the following (Butler and Bender, 1999):

- Automated vital signs capture
- Cardiac rhythm analysis and dysrhythmia detection
- Reporting of laboratory results
- Calculation of medication doses, fluid infusion rates, shift, and daily intake and output volumes
- Entry and transmission of physician orders
- Admission, discharge, and transfer of patients
- Organization of patient records
- Calculation of patient nutritional requirements
- Generation of a patient plan of care
- Entry and organization of care documentation
- Prompting the caregiver for required documentation
- Provision of pop-up lists of documented choices, thereby eliminating the need for long narrative notes

The critical care flow sheet is a predominant display format for CCISs. As computer technology has advanced, the techniques for display of the flow sheet have been enhanced, but the flow sheet remains the major data interface. In most CCISs, the flow sheet display is joined by a multitude of other "charts," such as lab reports, general patient assessments, specialized assessment, and free-text notes.

Charts

The goal of a CCIS is to have as much information integrated into the system as possible so that a comprehensive picture of the patient can be obtained. As critically ill patients generate massive amounts of data, the challenge is to create logical "chunks" of information in the form of charts. Ultimately, all information pertaining to the patient should be contained in the automated record. However, it is not unusual to find only pieces of information automated due to limitations in software or interfaces.

Development of charts is a time-consuming process and requires user participation to ensure that the elements contained within the chart are appropriate for the organization and patient population(s). The selection of which chart to implement and the order of implementation should also be considered carefully to facilitate a smooth transition to an automated record. Factors such as number and type of users, frequency that the chart is accessed, impact on decreasing manual recording, and clinical utility can aid in this process.

There are a variety of chart types that can be created. Clinical charts contain patient information and are the most widely used. Many systems also have the capability of creating administrative charts that are helpful in patient care operations. Charts may also be developed to assist in assessing the quality of processes or to aid in research. Frequently, data pulled through interfaces, such as lab values or ventilator settings, are organized into a chart to display common groups of information that can be easily trended. The system may also perform calculations, e.g. hemodynamics or intravenous drip rates, which when displayed in chart format act as a ready reference for users. Charts may also be formatted to display results/reports, e.g. radiology results.

Clinical Charts

The majority of information entered or integrated in the CCIS is clinical in nature. Monitoring interfaces that contribute vital sign and hemodynamic data are invaluable tools in collecting some of this essential information. As mentioned, the need to validate the data is critical in order to ensure accurate information. For example, a stopcock turned to allow infusion through a central venous line will create falsely high pressure readings that must be corrected in order to ensure that a valid pressure reading is stored (Belzberg et al., 1996). If interfaces to the monitoring system are not readily available from the associated vendors, these interfaces can be created to facilitate this type of chart. The cardio-hemodynamics chart (Fig. 15.3) is an example of a chart that collates vital sign data, performs calculations, and summarizes critical therapies that may have influenced the patient information.

Charts may also be organized by body system. A neurologic chart (Fig. 15.4), for example, may record

	03/06/99 12:10	03/06/99 16:00	03/06/99 16:50	03/06/99 20:00	03/07/99 00:00	03/07/99 04:00	03/07/99 08:00	03/07/99 11:40
C.O. Seq. #	22	23	24	25	26	27	28	29
Temp C	37.3	37.2	37.3	37.1	37.2	37.0	37.6	37.3
Temp route	BloodTmp	BloodTmp	BloodTmp	BloodTmp	BloodTmp	BloodTmp	BloodTmp	BloodTmp
HR	95	95	104	86	86	90	101	95
Atrial Arrhythmia	A Fib	A Fib	A Fib	A Fib	A Fib	A Fib	A Fib	A Fib
Block	N/A	N/A				↑		n/a
ART SYS/M/D	139/ 82/ 72	111/ 72/ 53	107/ 72/ 47	116/ 80/ 57	106/ 76/ 53	135/ 90/ 61	157/101/ 81	146/ 94/ 80
Blood Press.Qual.	Pneum	Pneum	Pneum	Pneum	Pneum	Pneum	Pneum	Pneum
PA SYS/M/D	38/ 25/ 17	44/ 34/ 22	48/ 37/ 27	48/ 30/ 18	41/ 26/ 20	54/ 38/ 21	50/ 34/ 13	58/ 37/ 12
CVP	8	12	14	11	13	20	15	16
C.O.	4.40	4.80	5.40	5.00	4.50	5.00	4.70	4.80
C.I.	3.1	3.4	3.8	3.5	3.1	3.5	3.3	3.4
SV	46		52	58	52	56	47	51
SVR	1345	1000	859	1104	1120	1120	1464	1300
PVR	145	200	148	192	107	272	357	417
LVSWI	28	28	22	34	28	37	39	40
RVSWI	7		11	10	6	10	8	10
O2 Avail In			547					
AVDO2			3.5					
%O2 Ext			24					
O2 Cons			133					
HGB-ABG			10.5 %					
MV-O2 SAT			74					
Total PEEP	5	5	5	5	5	5	5	5
Total PBEP			5	5				
Fluid Bolus					250	250		250

Figure 15.3

A cardiohemodynamics chart.

(Courtesy GE Marquette Medical Systems, Inc., Milwaukee, WI.)

PUPILARY RESPONSE	03/08/99 08:00	03/08/99 12:00	03/08/99 16:00	03/08/99 20:30	03/09/99 00:00	03/09/99 04:00	03/09/99 08:00
R Pupil Size	Small	Small	Small		Small		Normal
R Pupil Resp	Brisk	Brisk	Brisk		Brisk		Brisk
L Pupil Size	Small	Small	Small		Small		Normal
L Pupil Resp	Brisk	Brisk	Brisk		Brisk		Brisk
GLASCOW COMA SCALE							
Eyes Open	Speech	Speech	Spont		Speech		Spont
Best Verbal Resp	None	None	Confused		None		None
Verbal Response Qualifier	Trach/ET	Trach/ET	Trach/ET		Trach/ET		Trach/ET
Best Motor Resp	Obeys	Obeys	Obeys		Obeys		Localize
GCS Qualifier	None	None	None		None		MSO4 PCA
03/08 08:00 morphine gtt							
GCS	10	10	14		10		10
ASL	2 Sedate	2 Sedate	4 Rstlss		2 Sedate		2 Sedate
Pain Rating	5	0	5	3	11	11	
03/08 08:00 pt admits to pain unable to use scale							
MOTOR STRENGTH							
R Arm Strength	VeryWeak	VeryWeak	VeryWeak		VeryWeak		Weak
L Arm Strength	VeryWeak	VeryWeak	VeryWeak		VeryWeak		Weak
R Leg Strength	VeryWeak	VeryWeak	VeryWeak		VeryWeak		Weak
L Leg Strength	VeryWeak	VeryWeak	VeryWeak		VeryWeak		Weak
MAP	93	97					

Figure 15.4
A neurologic chart.
(Courtesy GE Marquette Medical Systems, Inc., Milwaukee, WI.)

pupillary response, the Glasgow Coma Scale, sedation levels, pain ratings, motor strength, and intracranial and cerebral perfusion pressures, thus providing a comprehensive picture of a patient's neurologic status. Most systems allow annotations to the data elements so that qualifications or clarifications can be included. Noting that a patient has an endotracheal tube and cannot speak or is being heavily sedated for protection of invasive lines or to diminish intracranial pressures allows users to correctly interpret the data entered.

Patient assessment charts may be the cornerstones of the record, since they detail assessment findings that are regularly collected. As the critical care environment requires frequent assessments, these charts may be configured to ease this extensive data collection. A shift assessment chart can be created, for example, to capture more comprehensive baseline information, with a carry forward feature (data automatically "carries forward" from one time to the next) or mini assessment chart used to record assessments not required as frequently. The use of windows in charts such as these is particularly helpful in diminishing the length of the chart as well as guiding the user to the most common choices. Under pulse assessment, a window that details strength of pulse (strong/weak/thready/absent) or method of assessment (palpation/Doppler) allows the user to rapidly enter the assessment data and ensure a complete assessment is documented.

Administrative Charts

Charts may also be created to assist in unit operations. For example, designing charts to capture patients being restrained facilitates the audit process to ensure appropriate policies/procedures are being followed relative to restraints. Additionally, determining bed capacity in a system can be helpful in monitoring clinical performance or in performing operations. Admission, transfer, and discharge data can be directly entered or pulled through an interface from the admissions department's information system, thus allowing compilation of unit statistics. Based on data elements entered, any variation of key statistics can be monitored. Service, length of stay, mortality, and readmit rates are examples of data that can be formatted into a report to assist in strategic planning.

In addition to flexible charting formats and operations, current generations of CCISs offer many features to facilitate user interaction and enhance entry, retrieval, and interpretation of the clinical information within the patient database. Most of these features are available on commercial systems, although this may vary from vendor to vendor. Among the features offered by many vendors are the following:

■ Each patient's data can be accessed from any terminal or workstation. This capability can extend across units and departments or be restricted to a single unit. In some instances, an alarm on one patient can be "forwarded" to another patient location, as determined by the nurse user.

■ Admission to the CCIS database can be accomplished automatically from the hospital information system or as a manual operation on the clinical unit.

■ Graphic displays of most data in the clinical database can be constructed. These displays may be preconfigured or may be developed dynamically as needed.

■ Vital signs and other physiological data are automatically acquired from bedside instruments and incorporated into the clinical database. These data can be incorporated into flow sheets, assessments, etc.

■ Any item entered via a flow sheet can be annotated. The annotations can be viewed via the flow sheet or as a set of notes, and they can be included with free-text notes entered separately.

■ Special flow sheets incorporating required treatments and interventions may be provided. In most instances, the nurse can document the care given and not given directly on this flow sheet (on the screen). At any time, the nurse can enter an explanatory note describing the patient's response or the reasons for not delivering a specific treatment or intervention.

■ Assistance with many common clinical computations is provided. Intravenous medication dosage, intravenous flow rates, hyperalimentation, and aminoglycoside dose schedules are among the computations available. Depending on the system, these values may be part of the patient database or may be offered as an "off-line" calculator.

■ Automatic calculation of physiological indices can be perfomed. As selected data are entered into the patient database manually or directly from bedside devices, customer-specified algorithms are employed to calculate the cardiovascular, respiratory, neurological, and other indices.

■ Automatic calculation capabilities have been extended to patient acuity, patient classification, productivity measures, and other indicators.

■ Reference information is available to nurses, physicians, and other clinicians. This information may be provided by the vendor and modified by the customer, or the customer may develop all of its own materials. The information may be entered via optical scanning, direct keyboard entry, or transfer from a text file on another computer. Usually, the reference information can be printed on demand. Reference information includes specific clinical information on drugs, diseases, and patient problems as well as policies and procedures relevant to specific units.

■ Decision support features are provided, although the capabilities and operations will vary. Access to standard third-party database systems may be accomplished, and/or the vendor may supply a proprietary database management system. In all instances, these features enable the information in the CCIS to be analyzed to support research, quality improvement, outcomes, and management.

CCISs are most often used as bedside systems; i.e. there is usually access to the system at every bedside in a critical care unit as well as at the central station and various other locations. This, of course, will vary from hospital to hospital and is dependent on many factors, such as budget, space, and unit philosophy.

Personal computers (PCs) are almost universally employed in CCISs. These PCs are linked together by networks. The PCs perform data entry and screen management functions, and are frequently referred to as workstations. In addition, windows, structured lists, and icons can be used to make computer interaction easier and more meaningful to the clinical users.

Using PCs also allows access to the regular computer capabilities of the workstation. There is usually a method of exiting from the CCIS program and accessing the general computer functions of the workstation. This ability to leave the CCIS is controlled by the CCIS security system, and authorization to do so is determined by each organization. Once outside of the CCIS, the authorized user may have complete access to all computing features of the personal computer or may be restricted to a specific menu of software. Work processing, spreadsheets, and database management systems are some of the programs that could be available. In addition, if access to the full power of the computer is allowed, a user might write other programs to meet specific needs. As with central station monitors that allow the user to exit from the clinical applications, user organizations must consider the potential benefits and hazards of using this feature.

Policies, procedures, and user education programs must be developed to address concerns and issues.

Although studies show that use of bedside documentation systems result in cost reductions based on reported full-time equivalent reductions, increased revenue, better bed use, documentation that supports patient charges, and identification of best practice patterns, there are other benefits to be reaped. Other benefits include improvement in nursing productivity, quality of nursing documentation, and bed management and a decrease in patient length of stay (Butler and Bender, 1999).

Future Developments

As clinical information systems mature, their use in the patient care environment will become more pervasive. Adoption of a standard interface language will further promote the development of the medical information bus, and this will decrease the need to develop interfaces between devices. These two factors will result in a proliferation of clinical information systems across the continuum of care. As the patient moves through the ambulatory, critical care, and medical/surgical areas, patient caregivers will need easy access to secure information (Muschlitz, 1998). This necessitates thinking beyond the critical care environment in order to facilitate the integration of information between each of the patient care settings. Meaningful exchange of information will require standardized vocabularies in the various patient care settings. If this meaningful exchange can be achieved, a lifetime medical record for each patient becomes possible. A collection of these lifetime records in a clinical data repository enables trending for patient populations, comparison of an individual to that trend, and decision support for patient care strategies.

The development of clinical pathways and outcomes management are important developments in improving critical care performance. Outcomes are measurements made to determine the course of an illness and the effects of treatments on this course. CCISs can assist outcomes management by facilitating the identification and analysis of the relationships between medical interventions and outcomes as well as between outcomes and cost. Three types of data are useful in supporting outcomes analysis: input variables, which stratify patients into comparable groups, interventions, and outcomes (Dolin, 1997). In order to measure clinical outcomes without bias, the performance of critical care areas must be evaluated in meaningful ways, and this may include data following discharge of the patient from the critical care area (Teres et al., 1998). This reinforces the need to utilize standard language between patient care settings.

CCISs have recently been discussed as tools to assist in diagnosis of patient conditions through use of neural networks. Neural networks are computer simulations of the brain that are capable of converting incoming activities into an outgoing activity. The conversion includes weighting of the various inputs according to their strength of influence and then transformation of the inputs according to a predefined function (Hinton, 1992). If a set of diagnostic data could be defined as well as the relationships between those data points, the predictive ability of the neural network could be utilized to recognize patterns of symptoms, signs, and laboratory data diagnostic of a particular pathological process. Before neural networks can be used in this manner, these definitions and relationships must be defined (Armoni, 1998; Buchman, 1995).

The evolution of computer hardware is extremely rapid. The swift growth of affordable memory permits storage of information that is processed and exchanged with increasing rapidity. This evolution supports previously unimaginable innovation in the area of patient care. An example of such an innovation is the use of voice recognition in controlling technology.

There is also a growing tendency to move information utilizing wireless communications technologies (Muschlitz, 1998). As patient stays in the ICU become shorter and shorter, monitoring is going out of the intensive care unit and into other clinical care areas. Using a wireless approach, it is possible to configure a portable bedside monitor to the patient's needs without buying a monitor for every bedside. (Wiggett, 1996). Additionally, information that is collected at the bedside, e.g. admitting or registration data, can be transferred wirelessly to a remote database.

Summary

Critical care nursing has been defined as a nursing specialty dealing with human responses to life-threatening problems. Critical care nursing can be practiced in any setting but is most often found in critical care units. The complexities of patient care in these settings have resulted in the development of technology to help nurses deliver that care. In this chapter, some of those technologies have been discussed. These include arrhythmia, hemodynamic, and physiologic monitoring systems; special purpose systems; and critical care information systems. The basic functions of hemodynamic monitoring systems were described, as were the most common features that enhance their utilization. The trend towards noninvasive monitoring systems was discussed. Principal goals and purposes of critical care information systems, as well as a history of their development were presented. The most common CCIS information management features were presented. Modern CCISs incorporate personal computer technology into workstations that provide extensive computer power and many user-friendly functions. The MIB allows multiple patient care devices to communicate with a CCIS. Although not commercially available, the standards promulgated by the MIB effort are being incorporated by individual vendors. Technology continues to develop at a rapid rate, and the use of computers in critical care settings will continue to expand. Not only information systems, but specific patient care devices, will proliferate and contribute to the information flood that has generated the need for the computer systems in the first place. Coping with technology overload is an essential skill for nurses. Learning the concepts and principles of critical care computer applications presented in this chapter can be more important than focusing on a particular system or device. Understanding the basic elements will enable nurses to more easily adapt and adopt new equipment and systems.

References

Ahrens, T. (1999a). Hemodynamic monitoring. *Critical Care Nursing Clinics of North America, 11*(1), 19–31.

Ahrens, T. (1999b). Continuous mixed venous (SvO$_2$) monitoring: Too expensive or indispensible? *Critical Care Nursing Clinics of North America, 11*(1), 33–48.

Ahrens, T. and Tucker, K. (1999). Pulse oximetry. *Critical Care Nursing Clinics of North America, 11*(1), 87–98.

American Hospital Association. (April 15, 1999). Report of the American Hospital Association Task Force on Medical Telemetry. Unpublished report.

Armoni, A. (1998). Use of neural networks in medical diagnosis. *M.D. Computing, 15*(2), 100–104.

Averill, C. B., Marek, K. D., Zielstorff, R., et al. (1998). ANA standards for nursing data sets in information systems. *Computers in Nursing, 16*(3), 157–161.

Belzberg, H., Murray, J., Shoemaker, W.C., et al. (1996). Use of large databases for resolving critical care problems. *New Horizons, 4*(4), 532–540.

Berg, N. (Ed.). (1981). *Core Curriculum for Critical Care Nursing*. New York: Saunders.

Buchman, T. G. (1995). Computers in the intensive care unit: Promises yet to be fulfilled. *Journal for Intensive Care Medicine, 10*(5), 234–240.

Burchell, S. A., Yu, M., Takiguchi, S. A., Ohta, R. M., and Myers, S. A. (1997). Evaluation of a continuous cardiac output and mixed venous oxygen saturation catheter in critically ill surgical patients. *Critical Care Medicine,* 25(3), 388–391.

Butler, M. A. and Bender, A. D., (1999). Intensive care unit bedside documentation systems: realizing cost savings and quality improvements. *Computers in Nursing,* 17(1), 32–38.

Clochesy, J. M. (1989). *Advanced Technology in Critical Care Nursing.* Rockville, MD: Aspen.

Cook, B. (1997). Computerized patient records—the off-the-shelf choice. *Healthcare Technology Managment,* 8(6), 34–35.

Dolin, R. H., (1997). Outcome analysis: Considerations for an electronic health record. *M.D. Computing,* 14(1), 50–56.

Elder, A. (1991). Setting up and using a cardiac monitor. *Nursing 91,* 21(3), 58–63.

Esch, O., Burdick, T., and van Sonnenberg, E. (1998). Digital imaging and PACS: An update. *Journal of Intensive Care Medicine,* 13(6), 313–319.

Gardner, R., Bradshaw, K., and Hollingsworth, K. (1989). Computerizing the intensive care unit: Current status and future direction. *Journal of Cardiovascular Nursing,* 4(1), 68–78.

Headley, J. M. (1998). Invasive hemodynamic monitoring: Applying advanced technologies. *Critical Care Nursing Quarterly,* 21(2), 73–84.

Hinton, G. E. (1992). How neural networks learn from experience. *Scientific American,* 267(3), 145–151.

Hirschl, M. M., Binder, M., Gwenchenberger, M., et al. (1997). Noninvasive assessment of cardiac output in critically ill patients by analysis of the finger blood pressure waveform. *Critical Care Medicine,* 25,(11), 1909–1914.

Kenner, C. V. (1990). Hemodynamic monitoring. In B. Dorsey, C. Guzzetta, and C. Kenner (Eds.), *Essentials of Critical Care Nursing* (pp. 206–236). Philadelphia: Lippincott.

Kinney, M. R., Pacha, D. R., and Dunbar, S. B. (1988). *AACN's Clinical Reference for Critical Care* (2d ed.). New York: McGraw-Hill.

Lasater, M. (1998). The view within: The emerging technology of thoracic electrical bioimpedance. *Critical Care Nursing Quarterly,* 21(3), 97–101.

Macy, J. and James, T. (1971). The value and limitations of computer monitoring in myocardial infarction. *Progress in Cardiovascular Diseases,* 13, 495–505.

Martin, N. and Hendrickson, P. (1999). Telemetry monitoring in acute and critical care. *Critical Care Nursing Clinics of North America,* 11(1), 77–85.

Mihm, F. G., Geetinger, A., Hanson, C. W., et al. (1998). A multicenter evaluation of a new continuous cardiac output pulmonary artery catheter system. *Critical Care Medicine,* 26(8), 1346–1350.

Milholland, D., and Cardona, J. (1983). Computers at the bedside. *American Journal of Nursing,* 83, 1304–1307.

Mirvis, D., Benson, A., Goldberger, A., et al. (1989). Instrumentation and practice standards for electro-cardiographic monitoring in special care units: A report for health professionals by a task force of the Council on Clinical Cardiology: American Heart Association. *Circulation,* 79(2), 464–471.

Muschlitz, L. (1998). Linda Reeder, HIMSS liaison and Intesys applications specialist. *Healthcare Technology Management,* 9(4), 32–34.

Saba, V. K., and McCormick, K. A. (1996). *Essentials of Computers for Nurses* (2nd ed.). New York: McGraw-Hill.

Seyer, S., and Schroeder, L. (1997). Data trap. *Healthcare Technology Management,* 8(6), 24–27.

Shoemaker, W. C., Wo. C. C. J., Bishop, M. H., et al. (1994). Multicenter trial of a new thoracic electrical bioimpedance device for cardiac output estimation. *Critical Care Medicine,* 22(12), 1907–1912.

Smith, K. R. (1998). Outcomes management of mechanically ventilated patients: Utilizing informatics technology, *Critical Care Nursing Quarterly,* 21(3), 61–72.

Sorkin, J., and Bloomfeld, D. (1982). Computers of critical care. *Heart and Lung,* 11, 287–293.

Teres, D., Higgins, T., Steinrub, J., et al. (1998). Defining a high-performance ICU system for the 21st century: A position paper, *Journal of Intensive Care Medicine,* 13(4), 195–205.

Tsien, C. L. and Fackler, J. C. (1997). Poor prognosis for existing monitors in the intensive care unit. *Critical Care Medicine,* 25(4), 614–619.

Von Reuden, K. T. and Turner, M. A. (1999). Advances in continuous, noninvasive hemodynamic surveillance: Impedance cardiography. *Critical Care Nursing Clinics of North America,* 11(3), 63–75.

Widman, L. (1992). The Einthoven system: Toward an improved cardiac arrhythmia monitor. In P. Clayton (Ed.), *Fifteenth Annual Symposium on Computer Applications in Medical Care* (pp. 441–445). New York: McGraw-Hill.

Wiggett, J. (1996). Off the wall with patient monitors. *Healthcare Technology Management,* 7(11), 24–25.

16

Community Health Applications

Donna Ambler Peters
Virginia K. Saba

OBJECTIVES

1. Discuss the development of community health computer applications.
2. Describe management and practice applications for community and home health computer systems.
3. Discuss use of classifications/acuity.
4. Describe special purpose computer systems.
   - Outcomes (OASIS/ORYX)
   - Registration systems
   - Management information systems (MIS)
   - School health systems
   - Scheduling systems
   - Telehealth systems
   - Home technology systems

KEY WORDS

information systems
community health services
public health
home health care
home care

Community health focuses on care of all people in the community. Community health nursing, also known earlier as public health nursing, is a synthesis of nursing practice and public health practice concerned with promoting and preserving the health of populations. It is also concerned with care to noninstitutionalized clients in community settings where health care is provided as well as the care of the sick at home.

Community health nursing (CHN) is not limited to a particular age, diagnostic group, or health care facility. It focuses on the health of the well and the care of the sick using a holistic approach to the individual, family, group, and/or community. CHN focuses not only on health promotion, maintenance, and education, but also on coordinating the continuity of care across health care settings to improve the health status of all in the community. Community health nursing is practiced in public health departments; in ambulatory care settings, group practices, outpatient clinics, and free-standing community-based clinics; and in the home.

Community health computer applications and systems have been developed to support CHN, but because of the broad scope of CHN, there is a wide variance in the applications. In addition, because of the fragmentation and diversity of community health, development of computer applications has been more difficult to fund and therefore slower than in acute care. Systems have been designed for (1) specific types of CHN agencies, e.g., state and local health departments, HMOs, visiting nurse associations; (2) specific community health settings where services are provided, e.g., clinics, schools, or homes; and (3) specific types of programs, e.g., family planning or immunization. The focus of the system varies from statistical reporting, billing, and financial applications to patient care. Additionally, the systems vary depending on the specific application being addressed, e.g., classification/ acuity, computer-based patient record, managed care and home care, and educational technologies.

This chapter provides an overview of the development of computer applications in community health as well as a description of the major types of community health and home health systems, including home technology systems.

Community Health Computer Development Projects

CHN agencies have used computers since the late 1960s, when computers were introduced into the health care industry. With the enactment of the Medicare and Medicaid Legislation in 1965, reimbursement for home care services was allowed. This new legislation expanded the demand for home care services, increased the number of home health agencies (HHAs), and increased the information needs that created the need for computer systems. As a result, as early as 1969, several commercial vendors, service bureaus, and commercial companies developed billing and financial systems for visiting nurse associations (VNAs) and other HHAs. These data processing systems were primarily designed to satisfy the basic need for reporting to payers and regulators, process the information required for billing, monitor the certification requirements, and manage the home care services required by Medicare, Medicaid, and third-party payers. These systems captured patient demographics, visits, accounts payable, and journal entries for the purposes of producing canned reports, UB92s (Medicare billing forms), visit summaries, and trial balances. Although valuable, they created organizational inefficiencies, because the basic software design did not share data among applications, and thus data had to be rekeyed when used for multiple purposes (Peters and McKeon, 1998).

In the 1970s and early 1980s, many state/local official health departments developed statistical reporting systems for processing information on nursing personnel, programs, and services. Many of these reporting systems are still in use. They were primarily developed to manage the information requirements of the agency's CHN services. For example, the Florida Client Information System funded by the Division of Nursing, Public Health Service, was developed to register eligible

residents and to collect encounter information on those residents receiving community health nursing services. It was the first on-line statewide computerized community health system in the country (Florida Department of Health and Rehabilitation Services, 1983).

During the late 1980s and early 1990s, as community health nursing required information not only on payment for services, but also on the quality of care, computer applications in community health advanced. With the abrupt passage of the Balanced Budget Act of 1997, information needs for community health have catapulted beyond billing, statistical reports, and quality of care. Home health agencies, for whom prospective payment looms, now need to be able to assess the risk assumed with each patient admission, gauge the performance of staff within the agency, and compare their organization with the competition (Lee and Schaffer, 1999). To do this, the agencies need a data repository that provides them ready access to data about the types of care needed by patients, the care provided, the patient's reaction to treatments, associated outcomes, and costs. Software developers are responding by building information systems instead of data processing systems. Their emphasis is shifting from task support for caregivers to providing clinical information as a strategic resource for practice. These information systems allow for the following (Peters and McKeon, 1998):

- Relational databases that facilitate the retrieval of data for multiple purposes without rekeying
- The manipulation of data to create information and knowledge
- Point of care devices and computerized patient records (CPRs)
- Clinical repositories as a strategic resource for quality and practice
- Electronic interfacing systems to facilitate the sharing of data

The deployment of electronic information systems will greatly increase the access to detailed information regarding community health care practice. As the richness of this information grows, patients and others will also expect access to the information. It is projected that within the next five years the use of an electronic or computerized patient record will emerge that both the provider and patient will have access to. The control of information will shift from home care providers holding the bulk of patient information to patients themselves either holding the information or accessing it. While the number of patients demanding access will initially be small, these early empowered patients will have an impact far beyond their numbers (Bruegel, 1998; Reichley, 1999).

As more information about community health practice becomes available, and as it becomes more critical to the survival and success of home health agencies facing prospective payment, it will generate a greater demand for more information. For example, Shaughnessy and colleagues at the University of Colorado Center for Health Policy have developed a set of indicators needed to monitor quality of care based on medical outcomes. The preliminary design model identified a set of acute and chronic conditions as well as primary prevention screening variables that encompass broad categories and varied therapies as measurements of quality outcomes (Shaughnessy et al., 1990; Shaughnessy and Kramer, 1990). Identifying these data elements will assist in understanding more about community health and lead to the need to identify more elements, like peeling off the layers of an onion. Thus, as new systems are designed, this new information will be considered.

A critical step in this process of generating more information for community health is the definition of a data set using a consistent health vocabulary or classification that will enable the sharing of information (Bruegel, 1998). Aggregating clinical data sets of community health patients with like conditions provides the basis for standardizing and tracking processes and outcomes of care. Aggregating clinical data sets for all community health patients provides evidence to show the results of community health services in terms of value, quality, and cost-efficiency. Unfortunately, most community health agencies use data sets that are inconsistent, ill-defined, piecemeal, and/or nonreflective of community health services (Peters and McKeon, 1998). Some of the projects involved in defining a community health data set, vocabulary, and/or classification system are described below.

Data Sets

National League for Nursing   The National League for Nursing (NLN) initiated a special committee to identify the content of a database to make community health agency systems operable. They identified a basic data set for Community Health Nursing, a prototype for a basic minimum data set for CHN agencies. The basic data set was designed as a guide for establishing uniform data collection needed for statistical reporting systems that could also be linked to other agencies. It also identified statistical information needed to measure and describe services related to community needs and resources focusing on four types of data—patient, staff, agency, and community. The content was identified for computerized management information systems (MISs) developed for CHN agencies (National League for Nursing, 1977).

Uniform Data Set for Home Care and Hospice Project   In 1993, the National Association of Home Care (NAHC) Resource Committee initiated a task force to develop a Uniform Data Set for Home Care and Hospice. The need for a minimum data set was identified by NAHC as critical and was considered to be the first step toward achieving standardized, comparable home care and hospice data. NAHC determined that, in general, home care and hospice data are incomplete, in many instances inaccurate, and not uniform. The goal of the project is to identify the critical data elements and develop standardized definitions for a uniform minimum data set for home care and hospice programs. The initial data set is organized into two major categories—organizational and individual level data elements. (National Association of Home Care, 1994). Organizational data are subdivided into organization/services, utilization, financial, and personnel. Patient/client data are subdivided into demographics, clinical items, and service/utilization (Pace, 1998).

Outcome and Assessment Information Set   The Outcome and Assessment Information Set (OASIS) is a uniform data set comprised of 79 health and functional status patient assessment items that are discipline-neutral and when measured at two or more points in time serve as outcome measures. They are focused on the adult patient using Medicare services at home. They are not designed for maternity, pediatric, or hospice patients. These items are more clinically precise than most existing HHA assessment items, thereby maximizing the consistency of ratings among different caregivers collecting the same information. This allows for benchmarking data within and among HHAs. The challenge for agencies is to integrate these assessment items into their existing assessment process. OASIS items must be incorporated intact, i.e., exactly as published in the OASIS data set (Shaughnessy and Crisler, 1995) (Fig. 16.1).

The data set also consists of 10 patient-identifying information items that are used for tracking, managing, and organizing data collection and processing. Development of OASIS for home health care began in 1988 as part of a contract by the Health Care Financing Administration (HCFA) with the Center for Health Policy Research at the University of Colorado to develop, test, and improve a system of outcome measures (Shaughnessy and Crisler, 1995). HCFA's

START OF CARE ASSESSMENT (Also used for Resumption of Care Following Inpatient Stay) (Page 8 of 14)	Client's Name: Client Record No.

9. **CARDIORESPIRATORY:** Temperature ________ Respirations ________

BLOOD PRESSURE: Lying ______ Sitting ______ Standing ______

PULSE: Apical rate ______ Radial rate ______ Rhythm ______ Quality _______

CARDIOVASCULAR:

_____ Palpitations
_____ Claudication
_____ Fatigues easily
_____ Pacemaker ____________________ (Date of last battery change)
_____ Dyspnea on exertion
_____ Paroxysmal nocturnal dyspnea
_____ Orthopnea (# of pillows ______)
_____ BP problems
_____ Chest pain
_____ Cardiac problems (specify)__________
_____ Other (specify) ____________________
_____ Murmurs
_____ Edema
_____ Cyanosis
_____ Varicosities

COMMENTS:

RESPIRATORY:

History of: _____ Asthma _____ TB _____ Bronchitis _____ Pleurisy _____ Pneumonia _____ Emphysema _____ Other (specify) ____________________

Present Condition:

_____ Cough (describe) ____________________
_____ Breath sounds (describe) ____________________
_____ Sputum (character and amount) ____________________
_____ Other (specify) ____________________

(M0490) When is the patient dyspneic or noticeably **Short of Breath?**
- ☐ 0 - Never, patient is not short of breath
- ☐ 1 - When walking more than 20 feet, climbing stairs
- ☐ 2 - With moderate exertion (e.g., while dressing, using commode or bedpan, walking distances less than 20 feet)
- ☐ 3 - With minimal exertion (e.g., while eating, talking, or performing other ADLs) or with agitation
- ☐ 4 - At rest (during day or night)

(M0500) Respiratory Treatments utilized at home. **(Mark all that apply.)**
- ☐ 1 - Oxygen (intermittent or continuous)
- ☐ 2 - Ventilator (continually or at night)
- ☐ 3 - Continuous positive airway pressure
- ☐ 4 - None of the above

COMMENTS:

10. **GENITOURINARY TRACT:**

_____ Frequency
_____ Pain
_____ Hematuria
_____ Vaginal discharge/bleeding
_____ Nocturia
_____ Urgency
_____ Prostate disorder
_____ Other (specify) ____________________
_____ Dysmenorrhea
_____ Lesions
_____ Hx hysterectomy
_____ Gravida/Para
_____ Date last Pap test
_____ Contraception

(M0510) Has the patient been treated for a **Urinary Tract Infection** in the past 14 days?
- ☐ 0 - No
- ☐ 1 - Yes
- ☐ NA - Patient on prophylactic treatment
- ☐ UK - Unknown

(M0520) Urinary Incontinence or Urinary Catheter Presence:
- ☐ 0 - No incontinence or catheter (includes anuria or ostomy for urinary drainage) **[If No, go to *Section 11 - Gastrointestinal Tract*]**
- ☐ 1 - Patient is incontinent
- ☐ 2 - Patient requires a urinary catheter (i.e., external, indwelling, intermittent, suprapubic) **[Go to *Section 11 - Gastrointestinal Tract*]**

(M0530) When does Urinary Incontinence occur?
- ☐ 0 - Timed-voiding defers incontinence
- ☐ 1 - During the night only
- ☐ 2 - During the day and night

COMMENTS: (e.g., appliances & care, bladder programs, catheter type, frequency of irrigation & change)

Figure 16.1
Sample of OASIS Assessment Form.
(Courtesy Center for Health Policy Research, Colorado.)

intent was to mandate the use of this data set in Medicare certified home health care agencies as the basis for outcome-based quality improvement (OBQI) and as a case-mix adjuster for prospective payment. The regulation to mandate collection of the data set was implemented July 19, 1999.

Vocabularies

There have been several efforts in nursing to identify nursing vocabularies that would provide for unified understanding and communication among nurses. Eight vocabularies are currently recognized by the American Nurses Association (ANA), two of which are community health-specific. These are the Omaha System and the Home Health Care Classification (HHCC) System.

Classification Systems

In addition to vocabulary classifications, patient classification/intensity systems have been developed that provide information needed to measure care needs, predict resource use, and determine the requirements of home care. There are many reasons why a patient classification system is needed for home health nursing. In home health, visits are not all equal, and patients have different care needs and require different amounts of nursing care time. A classification system designed to weigh all visits by level of care could affect the practice of community health nursing by creating a quantifiable calculation of management and maintenance for a variable reimbursement system instead of a set cost per visit. This is especially valuable as the industry moves toward a prospective payment system. Such a system can also be used as the basis for the productivity measurement in quality assurance programs.

Patient classification/intensity systems developed for HHAs generally use different levels of care or client characteristics as the method for classifying patients. They are different from the acuity classification methods, based on workload measurements, developed for predicting nurse staffing levels in hospitals. Generally, hospitals' methods predict hours of patient care required based on a list of patient care activities weighted by predetermined workload measures.

Omaha System   A nursing diagnosis vocabulary for community health nursing was developed back in the 1970s by the Visiting Nurse Association of Omaha. This vocabulary is consistent with the general and comprehensive practice of community health nursing (Simmons,

1980). Included in the system are 44 nursing diagnoses that were arrived at empirically from the practice of the community health nurses employed by the visiting nurse agency. The diagnoses are organized by the four broad domains addressed by community health nurses: environmental, psychosocial, physiological, and health-related behaviors. Each diagnosis is described by a list of signs and symptoms. The problem may be referenced as health promotion, potential, or deficit/impairment/actual. The patient may be defined as an individual or family (Martin and Scheet, 1992, 1995).

The Omaha System also includes terms for interventions. The intervention scheme is an organized framework of community nursing activities designed to address specific nursing diagnoses using four broad categories of interventions: health teaching, treatments, case management, and surveillance. There is also a five-point Likert type outcome rating scale that measures the concepts of knowledge, behavior, and status for each identified nursing diagnosis (Martin and Scheet, 1992, 1995).

Home Health Care Classification System   The HHCC System was developed from the Home Care Project conducted at the Georgetown University School of Nursing. The HHCC consists of the Saba HHCC of Nursing Diagnoses and Nursing Interventions. They were designed so that both vocabularies—HHCC of Nursing Diagnoses and the HHCC of Nursing Interventions—could be classified and encoded. The two vocabularies consist of four sets of nursing parameters: (1) 145 nursing diagnoses, (2) three expected outcomes (axes) ("improved," "stabilized," and "deteriorated"), (3) 160 nursing interventions, and (4) four types of intervention actions ("assess," "direct care," "teach," and "manage"). The HHCC of Nursing Diagnoses and the HHCC of Nursing Interventions are both classified according to 20 home health care components: (1) activity, (2) bowel elimination, (3) cardiac, (4) cognitive, (5) coping, (6) fluid volume, (7) health behavior, (8) medication, (9) metabolic, (10) nutritional, (11) physical regulation, (12) role relationship, (13) respiratory, (14) safety, (15) self-care, (16) self-concept, (17) sensory, (18) skin integrity, (19) tissue perfusion, and (20) urinary elimination. The HHCC also includes 20 medical diagnosis and surgical procedure groups, and 10 socio-demographic data elements. (See Appendix A for HHCC of Nursing Diagnoses and Nursing Interventions).

HHCC System Description   The HHCC System was described under "Vocabularies." It is designed to predict home health care needs and resource use for the Medicare and elderly populations (Saba, 1991). The HHCC System translates clinical nursing parameters, medical parameters, and socio-demographic data into a clinical case-mix classification for home health patients according to their expected care needs and utilization of home health resources. Resources are predicted in terms of home visits by nurses and all other disciplines for a specific time period within an episode of home health care. Actual client outcomes are also evaluated (Saba, 1992a; Saba, 1992b; Saba and Zuckerman, 1992) (Fig. 16.2).

The HHCC System is based on a conceptual framework using the six phases of the nursing process to assess patients in a holistic manner: (1) assessment, (2) diagnosis, (3) outcome identification, (4) planning, (5) implementation, and (6) evaluation (American Nurses Association, 1991) (Fig. 16.3).

Patient assessment data are correlated, using the 20 home health care components, with the four sets of nursing parameters, as well as the medical and socio-demographic variables. The HHCC System's 20 home health care components provide the framework for assessing the functional, psychological, physiological, and behavioral patterns of home health care, but also for measuring and/or evaluating their actual outcomes. The correlations are used to derive a score that is used to predict (1) care needs in terms of home health components and their respective nursing diagnoses and interventions and (2) resource use for a specified time, e.g., 30-day intervals, in terms of nursing and all discipline visits (nursing, physical therapy, occupational therapy, speech therapy, medical social work, and home health aide).

The HHCC System identifies the relationships between medical and nursing diagnoses in predicting resource use. It can differentiate between the type of case and the length of service. The HHCC System's 20 home health care components classify the clinical care process for an entire episode of home health care by extending the clinical assessment parameters into care pathways. The HHCC System provides HHAs with an innovative clinical classification method for predicting and allocating resources and determining staffing needs and costs. The HHCC System can run on a microcomputer using a portable notebook to facilitate ease of use for data collection.

Community Health Intensity Rating Scale   Another patient intensity classification system is the Community Health Intensity Rating Scale (CHIRS). The CHIRS is also predicated on the nursing process. The original CHIRS was a prototype classification tool that included 15 parameters that represented the same four home

health domains as the Omaha System—environment, psychosocial, physiological, and health behaviors.

Each of the 15 parameters included patient profiles to illustrate the extent of nursing input required for patient care for four levels of care contained within each parameter, for a total of 60 profiles (Table 16.1). A profile was selected for each parameter, and then the rater implicitly integrated these into a categorical rating for the patient's resource requirements. These ratings were as follows: level 1, minimum requirements; level 2, moderate requirements; level 3, major requirements; and level 4, extreme requirements (Peters, 1988). Unfortunately, this format was challenging to apply in the workplace setting, so CHIRS has been reformatted into a comprehensive patient assessment form divided into the original 15 parameters. The responses for each of the assessment questions are weighted, producing a score for each parameter from 0 to 4 and a final intensity score between 15 and 60. Thus, a nurse can now get an intensity rating for a patient while at the same time doing a comprehensive assessment (Table 16.2).

The CHIRS concept of patient need incorporates not only the physiological aspects of care, but also the context of patient need within a patient's support system (e.g., family, home environment, and community resources). All of these areas are especially important as home care moves into managed care, where the goal of care is to educate and empower patients toward long-term independent management of their own health status and health problems. The CHIRS has been applied to several different community populations in addition to home health. These populations include maternal and child health, frail elderly, HIV/AIDS patients, patients using high technologies in the community, and substance-abusing homeless families. It is currently being adapted for school use as the School Health Intensity Rating Scale (SHIRS). It is anticipated that SHIRS will provide the foundation for determining school nurse staffing based on the quantified students' health needs determination.

Community Health Systems

"Community health systems" connotes those computerized information systems specifically developed and designed for use by community health agencies, programs, and services. Community health systems address the broad areas of (1) health care programs, (2) agencies, and (3) settings. They support health promotion and disease-preventive programs; statistical information required by state/local health department programs; and funding

Home Health Care Classification System
Patient Assessment Form

NOTE: DO NOT CODE a Nsg DX if a Nsg RX not identified & Vice Versa
1.   CODE ALL Nursing Diagnoses, Use Coding Scheme, that will be addressed in the care process.
2.   ENTER Expected Outcome for Each Nursing Diagnosis as Improved, Stabilized, or Maintained.
3.   CODE ALL nursing interventions, Use Coding Scheme, ordered by the Nurse or Physician to be provided during Episode of Care.
4.   ENTER Type of Intervention Action for Each Nursing Intervention as : Assess, Care, Teach, or Manage.

Home Health Component	Nursing Diagnosis	Expected Outcome			Nursing Intervention	Type of Action			
		I	S	D		A	C	T	M
BEHAVIORAL COMPONENTS									
1. Medications									
2. Safety									
3. Health Behavior									
PSYCHOLOGICAL COMPONENTS									
4. Cognitive									
5. Coping									
6. Self-Concept									
7. Role Relationship									
PHYSIOLOGICAL COMPONENTS									
8. Cardiac									
9. Respiratory									

I = Improved, S = Stabilized, D = Deteriorated	A = Assess, C = Care, T = Teach, M = Manage

Figure 16.2
Home Health Care Classification (HHCC) System Patient Assessment Form.
(Courtesy Virginia K. Saba, Ph.D., developer.)

Home Health Care Classification System (Continued)

Home Health Component	Nursing Diagnosis	Expected Outcome			Nursing Intervention	Type of Action			
		I	S	D		A	C	T	M
10. Metabolic									
11. Bowel Elimination									
12. Urinary Elimination									
13. Physical Regulation									
14. Skin Integrity									
15. Tissue Perfusion									
FUNCTIONAL COMPONENTS									
16. Activity									
17. Nutrition									
18. Fluid									
19. Sensory									
20. Self-Care									

I=Improved, S=Stabilized, D=Deteriorated	A=Assess, C=Care, T=Teach, M=Manage

*Virginia K. Saba, 4/95

Figure 16.2 *(continued)*

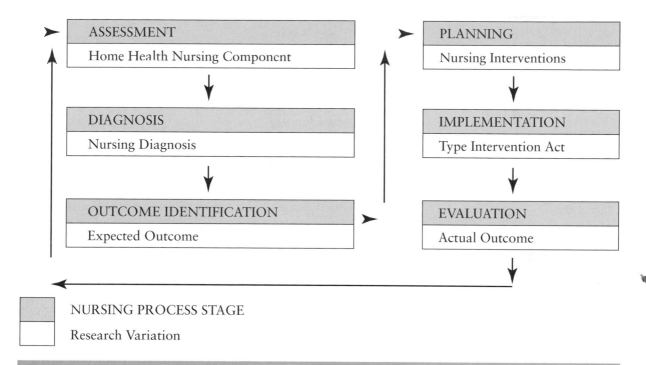

NURSING PROCESS STAGE

Research Variation

Figure 16.3
Home Health Care Classification (HHCC) using the nursing process.

information for federal block grants, categorical grants, or other grant programs. They also assist community health agencies in the decision-making processes for the management of nursing facilities. Community health systems are also used to evaluate the impact of noninstitutional nursing services on patients, families, and community health conditions. Other systems have been developed as standalone/turnkey systems specifically designed for special programs, projects, and studies.

State/Local Health Department Systems

The information systems for state/local health departments have traditionally been statistical reporting systems. They were specifically designed to collect the information requirements needed to satisfy various funding sources. Other systems have been developed that have other applications and are used to support and manage nursing services. For example, a patient registration can provide data not only on caseload and census, but also home, clinic, and school visit services. On the other hand, personnel and management systems

are used for preparing personnel payrolls and management data. The major ones include:

- Statistical reporting systems
- Registration systems
- Management information systems
- Personal/client management systems

Statistical Reporting Systems   Statistical reporting systems are community health computer systems that have been developed to collect and process statistical information primarily for state/local health departments. They emerged as the need for uniform information from all official state and local health departments became a national initiative. Because the federal government has not mandated or provided reimbursement for health promotion and disease prevention services, the government has not been able to require official state and local community health agencies to collect standardized data sets. Furthermore, the government is still dealing with the issues of privacy and confidentiality. These systems

Table 16.1   Community Health Intensity Rating Scale Parameter Definitions

Environmental Domain

Finances	Available financial resources, including employment status, of an individual/family reflecting the adequacy/availability of income related to financial obligations.
Physical environment/safety	Condition of client's home/neighborhood, including safety factors and availability of necessary facilities and transportation to those facilities.

Psychosocial Domain

Community networking	Individual family's knowledge and use of community resources/services, including their plan to deal with emergencies, and the availability and accessibility of the community resources.
Family system	Interpersonal relationships within the household (primary unit) and/or with relatives, friends, and significant others outside the household such as church members, social group members, and fellow employees. It includes the sufficiency of the family care-giving system.
Emotional/mental response	Mental status and the expression of feelings, including cheerfulness, grief, depression, anxiety, and coping behaviors that arise from an individual's/family's perception of self, considering their spiritual beliefs and cultural background, as it relates to current change.
Individual growth and development	Life development and maturation of cognitive, physical, and social tasks including ability to speak, read, and write as an individual moves from infancy to old age.

Psychosocial Domain

Sensory function	The body functions concerned with the use of senses to include vision, hearing, taste, touch, smell, proprioception, and an individual's perception of pain.
Respiratory/circulatory function	The body functions concerned with (1) the transfer of gases to meet ventilatory needs, and (2) the supply of blood tissues via the cardiovascular system.
Neuromusculoskeletal function	The body functions concerned with the integration and direction of regulatory processes related to gross and fine body movements including level of consciousness, speech patterns, muscle strength, coordination, skeletal integrity, and degree of physical independence/mobility.
Reproductive/sexual function	The body functions concerned with menstruation, pregnancy, lactation, and sexual practices. Included are sexual organs and secondary sexual characteristics.
Digestion/elimination	The ability to ingest food and fluids, utilize nutrients, and excrete waste products from the body.
Structural integrity	The character and intactness of the body's protective mechanisms, including skin and/or the immunological system.

Health Behaviors Domain

Nutrition	An individual's/family's selection, preparation, and consumption of nutrients according to a prescribed diet that considers cultural and health factorrs.
Personal habits	An individual's/family's management of personal health habits. It includes sleep activity patterns, personal hygiene, and avoidance of harmful substances. It addresses client/family habits or preferences, not ability to perform activities of daily life.
Health management	An individual's/family's management of their own health status including a measure of their involvement, their technical abilities, and their ability to self-medicate.

Modified, with permission, from Iyer and Camp (1999, p. 311).

Table 16.2 Community Health Intensity Rating Scale Nutritional Assessment

Prescribed Diet

_regular	_fluid restriction	_formula and breast
_established	_TPN	_baby solids
_new	_feeding problems	_infant formula
_tube feeding	for infant	_breast feeding

Appetite

_good	_too good	_unable to eat
_sufficient	_poor	

Compromised Nutritional Status

_yes	_no	_refuses to eat

Dietary Intake

_satisfactory reflects Rx		_does not reflect Rx
_modified re: preferences		_not modified re: preferences

Protein Intake

_sufficient		_good
_compromises condition		_poor

Nutrition Support System Status

_none	_self-care	_problem w/system
_functional	_new	

Able to Shop for Food

_yes	_food brought in	_no
_shop with relative/friend		

Food Selection

_N/A	_can't afford adequate food	_jeopardizes health
_healthy selections		
_satisfactory		

Able to Prepare Meals

_N/A	_yes	_no
_only with outside help		

Food Preparation

_healthy preparation	_N/A	_jeopardizes health
_satisfactory	_prepares inappropriate meals	

Weight

_within normal limits	_greater or less than 10% ideal
_greater or less than 25% ideal weight	_morbid obesity/severe emaciation
_recent weight loss	

vary from state to state and agency to agency, and as a result, there is no uniform means of comparing state programs and services at a national level and no reliable method of developing trends on the effectiveness and efficiencies of state/local health department programs.

Several state health departments are developing new systems for collecting community health statistics. They are implementing communication networks that link state and local community health agencies together. Many states, such as Michigan, Missouri, Florida, and Kentucky, have implemented computer networks. They are primarily statistical reporting systems designed to collect and process on-line data required for federal, state, and local community health programs. An example of a community care network is shown in the initial trial sites of the system being implemented in West Virginia (Fig. 16.4).

The Missouri Health Strategic Architectures and Information Cooperative (MOHSAIC) is an example of a state project designed to collect client centered data

including services performed by providers. Clusters of data would also be aggregated for evaluating program-specific reporting requirements (Hoffman, 1993). Texas is linking 400 public health clinics via a new Health Integrated Client Encounter System (ICES). It was designed to meet prevention as well as outcome goals. It is used to log in all assessment data and track preventive services such as tuberculosis care, immunizations, and other preventive measures. Kansas and North Carolina are also developing similar systems that focus on community health assessment and preventive services (Clinical Data Management, 1994).

A national information system is being proposed by the Centers for Disease Control (CDC) for collecting federal program data from state/local community health agencies. CDC is the federal agency mandated to collect all state data required for statistical reporting and funding of all federal programs, such as the immunization program. In mid-1993, CDC identified not only huge data gaps, but also the lack of coordination in the existing federally

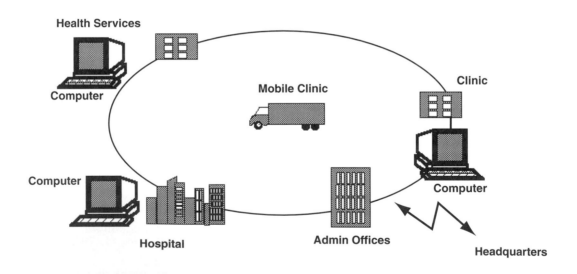

Figure 16.4
Community care network example.

funded public health, surveillance, information, and other data systems. CDC proposed that these statistical reporting systems should use not only a common classification scheme, but also the same data standards. They proposed that these existing systems should be integrated into one national information system, which should collect data on all enrolled/registered state/local clients and their encounters with community health services (National Center for Health Statistics, 1994).

Registration Systems   Client registration information systems (CISs) are designed to identify state/local residents/clients eligible for CHN services in clinics and homes. These systems generally consist of an on-line communication network, with terminals located in each of the local/district offices that are linked to the central computer facility and used to collect, store, and process all data. The centralized registry can then be accessed from the local/district units prior to providing services.

Management Information Systems   Many state/local health departments have also developed management information systems (MISs), which focus on the management of statistical and operational needs of the agency and the professionals. An example of a state/local health department MIS is B.E.S.T. (Barry-Eaton Software Technologies), which supports the environmental, financial, personal health activities, and requirements for the Barry-Eaton Health Department, Charlotte, Michigan. This system captures a variety of professional activities that focus on patient and environmental health services. This MIS is run on a microcomputer using pull-down menus, on-line documentation, and a database management software package. This system is used to capture and query the databases, which represent a mix of computer modules and/or special subsystems (Barry-Eaton Software Technologies, 1992).

Client/Personal Management Systems   A client/personal management system is another type of system that provides the framework for collecting and reporting statistical as well as financial data needed for the management of health personal/client and programs (Michigan Health Department, 1988). The State of Michigan Personal Health: Nursing Information System (PH-NIS) is an example of such a system. It was designed to be a "road map" and not a "blueprint" for the overall management of the personal/client health program and is designed to collect, organize, and standardize minimal statistical and financial information for the management and administration of the program activities.

This system consists of two major types of data: (1) provider information and (2) client information. The provider information consists of a registry of all personnel regardless of position and/or title including type, category, and program, (e.g., staff nurse, full time, immunization program). The personal/client health information includes demographics, patient history, and care activities.

Special Purpose Systems

Special purpose systems have been developed to collect statistical data for administering a specific program (rather than an agency), regardless of what type of agency offers the program. Stand-alone systems are designed to collect and summarize management data on services in clinics, schools, and homes. These systems provide the statistics needed to obtain funds from federal, state, or local units for categorical programs and/or block grants. Programs such as family planning, infant immunizations, early periodic screening and testing (EPST), maternal and infant (MI), children and youth (C/Y), crippled children, tuberculosis, drug abuse, or HIV have statistical reporting requirements that can be met by these systems.

Many other activities conducted in the CHN field require special-purpose systems designed for health surveillance programs, screening clinics, immunization clinics, and special statistical studies designed to collect large databases. The screening programs are used for early detection and prevention of diseases, epidemiological activities, and health promotion. Many such studies, programs, and projects have been described in the literature, each of which required a computer system or application specifically designed to process the data.

The major computer systems developed for special programs, studies, and projects can be described as follows:

- Categorical program systems
- Special study systems
- Screening program systems
- Epidemiologic program systems
- School health systems

Categorical Program Systems

Categorical program systems have been designed to support data processing and tracking for specific programs such as cancer detection; the women, infant, children's food program (WIC), maternal and child health (MCH) immunization, or family planning. Other systems have been designed to collect uniform longitudinal data for a specific disease condition, such as rheumatic diseases, that can be used as national databases. Categorical program systems generally count, track, and identify the health status of registered clients. For example, the WIC system is designed to process on-line certification and to generate food vouchers. Such systems are used to prepare billing information as well as comprehensive statistical reports. They generate all data required for cost reporting and the preparation of any customized reports needed to meet a user's unique reporting requirements. An example of a computer screen from a cancer control program is illustrated in Fig.16.5.

Special Study Systems

Special study systems generally require a specially designed computer application. Studies that collect large volumes of data require computer processing using standard statistical software programs and/or specially designed computer-processing models. Generally, large databases are collected for surveys, clinical trials, research studies, health policy, and other projects requiring volumes of data to resolve a problem. Many research studies analyze federal databases to develop outcome measures. Other studies requiring special stand-alone systems are national surveys of nurses and/or CHN agencies.

One of the major obstacles in developing special study systems is the management of large databases that are complex and create time-consuming data entry tasks. The introduction of point-of-service on-line data entry terminals has replaced data collection forms, making it easier to develop special studies systems. With this approach, these systems can process the data in an ongoing mode that reduces the time to process the study findings and generate reports.

Screening Programs

Screening programs illustrate another type of special-purpose computer application. Screening programs are used to detect individuals afflicted with a specific disease or predisposing health condition. Such programs generally use a computer system to collect important health information that may be mandated by federal, state, or local regulations. The computer system monitors and evaluates the results of screening tests. The data collected are transferred to a large computer facility and are aggregated for program analysis. Such

applications allow retrospective analysis of a large database that can be used to measure the effectiveness of the screening program.

Epidemiological Program Systems

Epidemiological program systems focus on the assessment of a population group with special health conditions. The results of such computerized assessments, such as audiovisual testing, immunization profiling, health appraisals, or dental checkups assist in identifying health care needs. Computer applications can be customized for other epidemiological prevention programs. They can be used to conduct standardized interviewing, by telephone, of clients who call a health care facility for assistance or information. These systems can summarize patient interviews, select care plans, and assess client problems.

School Health Systems

School health systems have emerged as computerized school-based record systems designed to improve data collection and monitor and evaluate health of school age students. These systems can be school building-based or district-based, meaning that the software may capture information about the students in one building only, or it may be capable of rolling up student data electronically to the district level from each school building, avoiding manual consolidation. The statistical advantage to the roll-up capability is obvious.

Commercial software options for school nursing take two basic forms. One form is to use a PC-based, stand-alone software product; the second form is to work with the health module that comes with the administrative software package used by the school district. The specialized, PC-based software is more comprehensive, but using the health module of the school administrative package allows for integrating the health components with the financial, human resource, and broader student management modules, thus eliminating duplicate data entry (Hedberg, 1997b). Table 16.3 lists common capabilities of school nursing programs. Additional capabilities that vary among products include health care plans, student activity records, medication logs, appointment scheduling, and referral/tracking (Hedberg, 1997a).

The need to introduce computerized health care programs is becoming increasingly important in school nursing in order to provide an opportunity for collecting health-related data on the students and employees in the school and communicating that data in a meaningful

Breast & Cervical Cancer Control Program
Screening Form

Health Dept. ID ⌣⌣   Clinic ID ⌣⌣   Date of Birth ⌣⌣⌣⌣⌣⌣   Client Identification ⌣⌣⌣⌣⌣⌣⌣⌣⌣⌣⌣⌣
                                mo   day   yr

Last Name	First Name	Middle Initial

Provider Name

Type of File Maintenance Action:

1 ☐ First reporting of this screening

2 ☐ Additional data for previously reported screening

3 ☐ Delete this screening record

Which Title XV Screening Year? ⌣⌣

01 First screening by HD (Yr. 1)

02 Screening anniversary of Yr. 1 (Yr. 2)

03 Screening anniversary of Yr. 2 (Yr. 3)

etc. (NOTE: A woman may visit the HD many times for follow-up during any screening year, *but* year remains constant)

CLINICAL BREAST EXAM:

Date First Scheduled	Actual Date of Exam	
Mo Day Yr	Mo Day Yr	Provider Notified?
___/___/___	___/___/___	☐ No ☐ Yes ☐ NA

Clinical Breast Exam Results: (Check all that apply)

RIGHT		LEFT
1 ☐	No mass present	1 ☐
2 ☐	Breast removed	2 ☐
3 ☐	Symmetrical thickening present	3 ☐
4 ☐	Asymmetrical thickening present	4 ☐
5 ☐	Smooth, mobile round/oval mass	5 ☐
6 ☐	Irregular, firm, mobile mass - indeterminate	6 ☐
7 ☐	Irregular, hard, fixed mass	7 ☐
8 ☐	Examination refused	8 ☐
9 ☐	Examination omitted	9 ☐
10 ☐	Other Abnormal Findings	10 ☐
	Specify _____	
11 ☐	No change from previous exam	11 ☐

Based on the Clinical Breast Exam, is Follow-up Required?   ☐ No   ☐ Yes (If yes, go to Breast Follow-up Form)

Figure 16.5
Cancer control program screen.
(Courtesy Michigan Department of Public Health, Cancer Section.)

Table 16.3   School Nursing Product Capabilities Common to All Software Packages

Product Capability	Capability Description
Individual student records	Individual files that contain each student's health record. Entering the student's name, a portion of the name, and/or an identifier can usually access this file.
Immunization records	The individual student record contains a special section for recording student immunizations. The programs that have this option allow for recording the date the immunization was given; some allow for dosage, lot number, etc.
Dental records	The individual student record contains a special section for the student's dental health records.
Other health screenings	The individual student record contains a special section for the student's other health screenings such as vision and hearing, heights and weights, postural screening.
Family history	A section of the student health record that focuses on family history and/or diagnoses
Multiple record diagnoses	Several diagnoses may be entered for one visit. Each diagnosis that is entered may be used to generate reports or lists.
Injury/incident reports	A section of the individual student record that focuses on incidents. In the case of injuries, this may include the type of injury, what the student was doing at the time of injury, and the place where the injury occurred.
Special emergency comment fields	This is a quick and easy-to-access file outside of the student record. The file contains emergency information such as the phone numbers of the student's parents and primary care physician and any student allergies.
Create reports and lists	This option allows the user to create a list or report based on individual student records such as those who have had chicken pox, injuries in specific areas of the school, or those behind in their immunizations.
Multiple school use	This function refers to situations in which one school nurse is servicing and collecting data on students from multiple school buildings using the same computer.
Daily log	The nurse's daily log keeps a record of the events for each day. This allows for easy review of trends or numbers of visits by a specific student without requiring a review of individual student records.
End-of-year processing	This function allows for the generation of annual reports as well as programming students to the next grade.

Modified, with permission, from Hedberg (1997b).

way. These systems need to address the same problems as the computer-based patient record regarding data security and ensuring the privacy and confidentiality of the individual's (student) data.

 Home Health Care Systems

Home health systems are information systems designed to support home health care nursing also called care of the sick at home. Home health systems support home care and hospice programs provided by HHAs, such as VNAs, hospital-based programs, proprietary agencies, and other not-for-profit HHAs. Home health systems to date have been primarily designed to collect and process data in order to prepare the documents required by HCFA and third-party payers for payment of home care services. However, the majority of vendors have already introduced, or are planning to introduce software with expanded clinical functions. In 1996, seven new vendors offered clinically oriented products at the NAHC annual meeting (Williams, 1997). The financial, managerial, and clinical applications are used for efficient management of an HHA. Other vendors offer applications that focus on scheduling, cost statistics, patient census, utilization reports, visit tracking, accounting reports, and discharge summaries. Patient outcomes are an important development area receiving attention from vendors, although development is hampered by the limited clinical expertise of the vendors that design and develop such programs (Williams, 1997).

Because back office systems were developed first and remain the legacy systems of most national vendors, and because many of the specialized programs, such as outcomes, are being developed by companies as stand alone products, there is an issue of separate databases and the inability to appropriately merge administrative and clinical data. This situation affects the ability of an HHA to make informed choices about resource allocations, care quality issues, and pricing of services (Bender, 1998).

Both the home care industry and information technology are changing rapidly. Just a few years ago, computing choices were limited to time-sharing systems, microcomputers, and stand-alone systems. The two changing markets have brought together both changing needs and changing products. Examples include clinical support and networked system products, client/server computing, and a conversion to Windows-based products.

Time sharing systems are computer-based systems developed by service bureaus that are shared by many HHAs. The service bureau purchases its own mainframe computer (hardware) large enough to be shared with many HHAs, determines the hardware architecture, and develops its own proprietary computer programs (software) to process the HHA data. The service bureau designs the data collection forms or methods for collecting data, determines the data needed for preparing the billing and financial requirements, and develops the required reports. The bureau also develops user's manuals, provides training sessions, and supports any other technological needs for their users.

The HHAs that use these service bureaus use microcomputers with fixed menus to collect, store, and batch data and then transmit the batches on-line to the service bureau's central computer. However, the agency only collects and enters data into the computer system and may not have real-time access to patient information stored in the patient's database.

Stand-alone systems (turnkey systems) are commercial systems developed for direct installation and implementation in an HHA. With this type of system, the HHA buys the computer system as configured by the vendor. The HHA buys the hardware and software and uses the computer system to collect, store, process, and control its own patient and visit data. The vendor, on the other hand, usually provides the HHA with all of the necessary equipment: hardware (a mainframe, minicomputer, or microcomputer) and any other required peripheral equipment as well as the software (computer programs) needed to run the system, including all forms and standardized reports for that specific agency.

In this type of system, the commercial vendor generally maintains, updates, and supports all software programs as well as ensures that the software programs meet state and federal regulations. The vendor generally offers training courses to the HHAs on how to run the system. The major advantage of this option is that the agency owns its own equipment (hardware), system (software), and patient data (databases). The agency can utilize the computer system for other applications such as word processing and E-mail.

With the introduction of computer networks as a means of sharing and communicating data among users, both local area networks (LANs) and wide area networks (WANs) have been introduced. Network configurations efficiently utilize the latest technology as well as reduce costs. Local area networks link units within the HHA, whereas wide area networks share data among agencies to establish continuity of care services across settings.

LANs are used to link units within an HHA as well as link subunits with each other and with a central office. Many state and large community health agencies are using LANs to link and integrate the service units of their health services. LANs allow the HHAs to share hardware and software for their individual computer system while still using the network to communicate with each other.

The WANs as well as the Internet are also used to communicate and transmit data across settings, i.e., to communicate and transmit data from one system in one institution to another system in another community agency or another HHA and then back to the institution. In this instance, the WAN requires a standardized data format (such as Health Level 7) so that data can be communicated across settings using different brands of computers.

Another means of communicating data is with the client/server. Client/server computing came into use in the early 1990s. Clients are the single-user workstations that provide individuals with their needed computing power and connectivity to other users and databases. The servers are the multi-user processors with shared memory that provide common services to the clients, such as communications and database access. The key to successful client/server computing is openness. Openness allows the data to move freely between applications, such as clinical and financial, without reliance on proprietary technologies. Although there is much confusion about the use of the label client/server, vendors are moving in that direction (Williams, 1997).

Vendors are also adapting their home care products to the Windows technology. Reasons include customer familiarity with Windows functionality and the fact that the new specialized applications have been developed utilizing Windows, particularly those where graphic interface is most appropriate, such as scheduling and outcomes tracking (Williams, 1997).

Systems that will be examined further include:

- Financial and billing systems
- Scheduling systems
- Point-of-care clinical systems
- Computer-based patient record systems

Financial and Billing Systems

Financial and billing systems are data processing systems that were built around the Medicare cost-reimbursement model for home health agencies. They are primarily designed to furnish information essential for reimbursement of services provided to patients eligible for Medicare, Medicaid, and other third-party payers. These systems use a variety of input forms or data entry screens—admission data, assessment data, and plan of treatment data—to collect the required information. The data are needed to obtain approval for a patient to receive reimbursable services, as well as to obtain payment for visits and services provided by all types of disciplines. Services are billed for each specific patient, and payment is received based on the current Medicare regulations. Revenue and cost data are periodically reconciled in order to determine the agency's position under/over the Medicare cost caps, not to evaluate profitability (Williams, 1997). These systems generally include the applications listed below:

- General ledger
- Accounts receivable
- Accounts payable
- Billing
- Reimbursement management
- Cash management

Additionally, they generate financial reports such as:

- Costs per visit
- Personnel costs
- Payroll information

- Budget projections
- Patient census
- Patient daily visits
- Patient services
- Patient supply lists (Fig. 16.6)

As was mentioned, the billing and financial systems have been developed specifically for certified HHAs that provide Medicare and Medicaid program services. The systems have changed as the Medicare program payment requirements changed. In the late 1960s, the initial Medicare program required that a Medicare eligible request for payment be completed to justify care. At that time, the goal of many large HHAs was to have these new forms completed by computer in order to bring about a faster cash flow, produce detailed patient accounts receivable, and capture statistical data to meet other reporting needs (Health Care Financing Administration, 1980).

In 1985, HCFA mandated a more comprehensive and complex method for certifying Medicare eligibility of patients, billing, and payment for services and for determining the costs of care. HCFA initiated several forms for the Medicare program: *HCFA Form 485 Plan of Treatment* (Fig. 16.7) to be completed by a physician; *HCFA Form 486 Medical Update* to be completed by a nurse or therapist; and *HCFA Form 487 Addendum, HCFA UB-92 Claims Form*, and the *HCFA Form 1728 Cost Reporting.*

These forms, which are updated periodically, are required to collect data for Medicare claims and for third-party payers. The forms, once completed, are used by an HHA to obtain the certification of eligibility for the patient to receive reimbursable home visits for a period of 60 days. The HCFA forms provide the basis for the HHA billing and financial computer systems. They are used to collect a variety of variables including medical diagnoses, functional limitations, goals of care, activities permitted, and other variables. They also collect data on allowable services provided by the six disciplines—skilled nursing, physical therapy, occupational therapy, speech therapy, medical social work, and home health aide.

The increase of managed care in the home health arena and the impending prospective payment system for home care services will have an impact on these financial and billing systems. Most vendors are responding by expanding the back-end financial reporting capabilities and emphasizing reports that will help agencies identify the factors that impact delivery cost

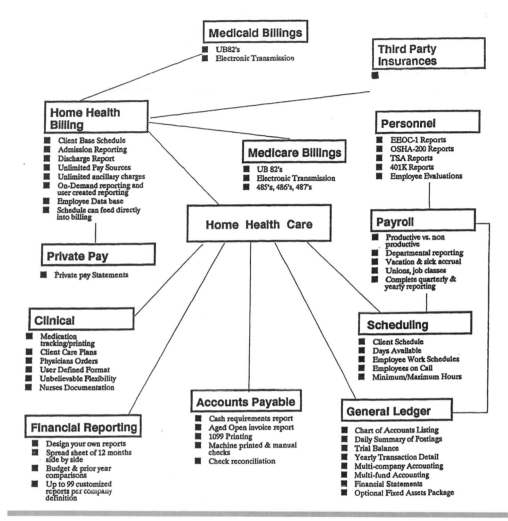

Figure 16.6
Home health care applications.
(Courtesy Advanced Information Management, Inc., Neenah, WI.)

and profitability. Vendors are being more cautious about fundamental changes to the systems that would accommodate discounted fee-for-service billing, capitated reimbursement, and other scenarios different from the cost-reimbursement model (Williams, 1997).

One area where significant changes are expected is with the electronic data interchange (EDI), moving data between payers and providers. EDI was introduced to home care in the early 1990s, 10 years after it was introduced in the acute care arena. Several states implemented laws or instituted new programs that focused on

cutting administrative health care costs by using EDI to transmit Medicare/Medicaid claims data. New York led the way, followed by Arizona, by passing a law mandating health care providers to use EDI. Iowa passed legislation for the development of a community health management system (CHMIS) to transmit not only claims data, but also clinical health care transactions data (Goedert, 1994). Today, both managed care payers and providers are seeking "paperless processing" for transactions including enrollment, eligibility verification, inquiry, and payment (Williams, 1997). Specification of

Department of Health and Human Services
Health Care Financing Administration

Form Approved
OMB No. 0938-0357

HOME HEALTH CERTIFICATION AND PLAN OF TREATMENT

1. Patient's HI Claim No.	2. SOC Date	3. Certification Period From: To:	4. Medical Record No.	5. Provider No.

6. Patient's Name and Address	7. Provider's Name and Address

8. Date of Birth:	9. Sex [ ] M [ ] F	10. Medications: Dose/Frequency/Route (N)ew (C)hanged

11. ICD-9-CM	Principal Diagnosis	Date

12. ICD-9-CM	Surgical Procedure	Date

13. ICD-9-CM	Other Pertinent Diagnoses	Date

14. DME and Supplies	15. Safety Measures:

16. Nutritional Req.	17. Allergies:

18.A. Functional Limitations

1 [ ] Amputation	5 [ ] Paralysis	9 [ ] Legally Blind
2 [ ] Bowel/Bladder (Incontinence)	6 [ ] Endurance	A [ ] Dyspnea With Minimal Exertion
3 [ ] Contracture	7 [ ] Ambulation	B [ ] Other (Specify)
4 [ ] Hearing	8 [ ] Speech	

18.B. Activities Permitted

1 [ ] Complete Bedrest	6 [ ] Partial Weight Bearing	A [ ] Wheelchair
2 [ ] Bedrest BRP	7 [ ] Independent At Home	B [ ] Walker
3 [ ] Up As Tolerated	8 [ ] Crutches	C [ ] No Restrictions
4 [ ] Transfer Bed/Chair	9 [ ] Cane	D [ ] Other (Specify)
5 [ ] Exercises Prescribed		

19. Mental Status:

1 [ ] Oriented	3 [ ] Forgetful	5 [ ] Disoriented	7 [ ] Agitated
2 [ ] Comatose	4 [ ] Depressed	6 [ ] Lethargic	8 [ ] Other

20. Prognosis:

1 [ ] Poor	2 [ ] Guarded	3 [ ] Fair	4 [ ] Good	5 [ ] Excellent

21. Orders for Discipline and Treatments (Specify Amount/Frequency/Duration)

22. Goals/Rehabilitation Potential/Discharge Plans

23. Verbal Start of Care and Nurse's Signature and Date Where Applicable:

24. Physician's Name and Address	25. Date HHA Received Signed POT	26. I [ ] certify [ ] recertify that the above home health services are required and are authorized by me with a written plan for treatment which will be periodically reviewed by me. This patient is under my care, is confined to his home, and is in need of intermittent skilled nursing care and/or physical or speech thera‐py or has been furnished home health services based on such a need and no longer has a need for such care or therapy, but continues to need occupational therapy.
27. Attending Physician's Signature (Required on 485 Kept of File in Medical Records of HHA)	Date Signed	

FORM HCFA-485 (C4) (4-87)

PROVIDER

Figure 16.7
Health Care Financing Administration (HCFA) Form 485.

standards for system-level EDI is part of a national effort known as Health Level 7 (HL7). In home care, initial attention seems to be focusing on admission, discharge, and transfer (ADT) data between referral sources such as hospitals and home care.

Scheduling Systems

Scheduling systems are also being used to enhance home health systems. They are designed to schedule the care-givers providing services with the patients requiring the visit, at the same time matching the caregiver capacity with the required patient care. Some systems use graphical scheduling calendars and others provide road maps on how to travel to a location in the shortest distance (Fig. 16.8). These systems can also track personnel by scheduling on- and off-duty time as well as generate their payroll. Since these systems are interactive, schedules can be adjusted daily on-line, making edits and revisions to existing schedules more efficient. Schedules can be done for a month or more in advance, thus ensuring that patients receive the same staff for each home visit. This consistency in staff usually increases patient satisfaction. In general, scheduling systems reduce schedule conflicts, improve financial control, enhance productivity, reduce administrative costs, and decrease travel time.

Point-of-Care Clinical Systems

Clinical systems began as extensions of the billing and financial systems designed for HHAs to include all aspects of patient care. These systems focus on patient/professional encounters and episodes of care. Many of the newer systems collect information needed to document the patient care process. These systems allow for the data to be entered at the office by a data processor or at the point of care using laptops or pen-based computers. Such systems generally contain a patient database that includes demographic information, health history, initial nursing assessment, and patient care services information. They document and track ongoing patient care data. Even though they document the care, they are not the legal patient record, and the patient data must be printed out to maintain a legal record.

Point-of-care systems are also beginning to include software-aided care planning. Some are including critical pathways that have been developed by other, non-computer-based companies. Critical pathways provide a new approach to documentation in the home care setting. The critical pathway has been defined as a diagram of the sequence of events leading to a desired clinical outcome (Goodwin, 1992). This differs from the traditional care planning process by outlining a systematic plan for interventions and teaching by diagnostic categories. Figure 16.9 illustrates a pathway and provides a clear definition of patient outcomes and the time frame to meet the outcomes.

The laptop systems are being designed to collect and transmit patient data and messages to and from the agency's main computer. Many architectural designs using this new technology are being developed for nurses to chart visit details, patient care services, and clinical assessment information collected at points of service such as at the patients' home; these data can be downloaded to the HHAs at a convenient time. The care provider can query, collect, and retrieve data from the computer system. These systems generally use menu-driven software, which prompts users through every step. Windows versions of the software are now appearing on the market.

Using the point of care technology provides an agency with more than just a means of documenting care. It is a means to accomplish the following.

1. Organize work for maximum efficiency. The system allows clinicians to have all the data in front of them and integrates scheduling, billing, payroll, and patient care documentation into one easy process. These systems, for example, generate an HCFA Form 485 Plan of Treatment as a by-product of care assessment. Work flow is therefore more logical and timely.

2. Stop errors before they occur. These systems provide interaction with the caregiver and often have error messages for incorrect data. For example, the system may prompt the clinician if the blood pressure data entered was too high or if a mandatory assessment field was left blank. Documentation is therefore more consistent, accurate, and accessible.

3. Enforce policy to ensure quality. Agency policy is part of the system content. Therefore, interaction of the clinician with the system ensures policy compliance. For example, if it is agency policy to take the blood pressure on all patients, the blood pressure will be part of the assessment on the system that the clinician needs to complete. On most systems, the agency could make this a mandatory field, and the clinician would not be able to exit the record until the blood pressure reading was entered.

4. Define and present best practices to the clinicians. The master libraries containing the clinical content are customizable by the agency. Therefore, once best practices are determined they can be entered into the master libraries and instantly be available to the staff in the field as soon as they log on.

The real value of point-of-care systems lies in the data itself. With the right point-of-care system, individual patient care data can be aggregated, making it possible to identify trends in care, utilization, and outcomes. These trends can help an agency determine its case-mix. They can also generate information for managed care contracts, new business models, new services, and new organizational policies. These data can also quantify outcomes, thereby providing proof of the value of the services rendered (Harrell, 1999).

Computer-Based Patient Record Systems

The next generation of clinical systems will be the computer-based patient record systems, also known as the (CPR) and/or the electronic patient record (EPR) system.

A CPR is a compilation of medical information regarding an individual patient within a given agency that resides within the electronic information system. Used more broadly, a CPR can become a "virtual" medical record that resides in different information systems and locations at the same time and, once collected, can reflect the current health status and lifetime medical history of an individual. Concerns about CPRs include privacy, confidentiality, and data security (Remington, 1998). Another issue that needs to be addressed is use and acceptance of the electronic signature.

In 1991, the Computer-Based Patient Record Institute (CPRI) was established and committed to initiate and coordinate activities urgently needed to facilitate and promote the routine use of CPRs. The CPRI defined the CPR as "an electronic patient record that resides in a system specifically designed to support users through the availability of complete and accurate data, practitioner reminders and alerts, clinical decision support systems, links to bodies of medical knowledge and other aids" (Dick and Steen, 1991, p. 167) A national information infrastructure is being developed for health and

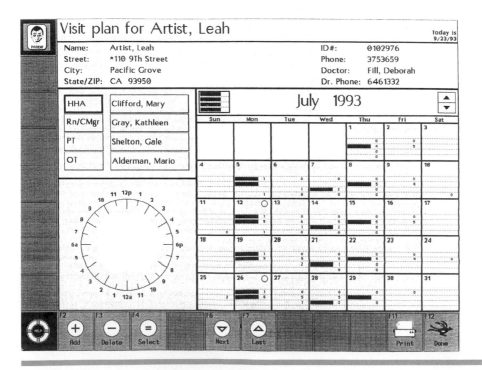

Figure 16.8
Home visit scheduling calendar.
(Courtesy Road Runner Technologies, Inc., Pleasanton, CA.)

NURSING CRITICAL PATHWAY FOR INSULIN DEPENDENT DIABETES MELLITUS

Patient's Name _____ LAST _____ FIRST _____ Pt. No. _____ SPECIAL INSTRUCTIONS

☐ Type I ☐ Type II   Date Initiated _____

PROBLEM LIST

NO. | Knowledge Deficit Re: Self-Care

	WEEK 1	WEEK 2	WEEK 3	WEEK 4	WEEK 5
CONSULTS/ COORDINATION OF CARE	Assess need for HHA, MSW, Rehab., Vol. Referrals completed as needed. I___ R		Interdisciplinary coordination/ communication. R		
SKILLED EVALUATION/ TREATMENT	Admission assessment. Assess peripheral circulation. Assess s/sx hypo/hyperglycemia. Assess diabetes complications. Glucometer testing. I			R	Blood glucose stable. No s/sx acute episode.
MEDICATION *Evaluate*	Evaluate medication regime and response. Assess insulin administration skills. I				No medication changes within last 2 weeks. No untoward S/E's. R
Instruct	Instruct in medication name, dose, schedule, purpose, action. Instruct in preparation and administration of insulin. Instruct in site rotation, storage of insulin and disposal of equipment. I	Patient/caregiver verbalize medication name, dose, schedule, purpose. Patient/caregiver demonstrate correct administration, site rotation, storage of insulin and equipment disposal. R	Patient/caregiver verbalize action time of medication. R	Continue to evaluate knowledge and teaching needs.	Patient/caregiver independent in medication regime. R
DIET/ NUTRITION *Evaluate*	Assess diet understanding and compliance. I			Continue to evaluate knowledge and teaching needs. R	
Instruct	Begin instruction in prescribed diet and/or food exchange system. I	Instruct in meal planning. I	Patient begins to follow prescribed diet. Continue instruction. R		Patient follows prescribed diet. R

Codes: I = Initiated   R = Resolved

©VNANV 710p1 (8/94)

Figure 16.9
Critical pathway chart.
(Courtesy Visiting Nurse Association of Northern Virginia, Inc.)

NURSING CRITICAL PATHWAY FOR INSULIN DEPENDENT DIABETES MELLITUS

Patient's Name _____ LAST _____ FIRST

Pt. No. _____   Date Initiated ___ / ___ / ___

		WEEK 1	WEEK 2	WEEK 3	WEEK 4	WEEK 5
ACTIVITY	Evaluate	Assess level of activity.	→	→	Assess effects of exercise on BG levels.	→
	Instruct		Instruct in benefits of exercise on BG control. Instruct in interaction of activity, diet and insulin. Instruct in appropriate adjustments of each.	Instruct in safe exercise regimen.	Patient implements exercise safely.	Patient verbalizes understanding of interaction of diet, medication and exercises. Patient verbalizes benefits of exercise.
		I	R	I	R	R
SYMPTOM MANAGEMENT		Instruct in s/sx of hypoglycemia. Instruct in blood glucose testing. For Type I DM: Instruct in urine testing for ketones.	Patient/caregiver identify s/sx of hypoglycemia, means to prevent and action to take. Patient/caregiver demonstrate blood glucose monitoring and understand when to notify MD. Instruct in s/sx of hyperglycemia. Instruct in disease process and BG control goals.	Patient/caregiver identify s/sx of hyperglycemia, means to prevent and action to take. Instruct in foot/skin care. Instruct in sick day care.	Patient/caregiver demonstrate foot/skin care. Patient/caregiver verbalize understanding of sick day care. Instruct in chronic complications and prevention.	Patient/caregiver verbalize s/sx requiring medical attention. Patient/caregiver verbalize importance of dietary and exercise consistency.
		I	I R	I R	I R	R
PSYCHOSOCIAL/ DISCHARGE PLANNING		Discuss care plan, goals and discharge plans with patient/caregiver. Assess support systems.	Assess adjustment of diagnosis and treatment regimen. Patient ventilates feelings.	Instruct in need for routine medical, dental, and ophthalmologic exams. Instruct in need for diabetic ID. Reinforce positive results of good DM management.	Preparation for discharge.	Patient has follow-up medical appointment. Patient has diabetic ID ordered. Patient has references for continuing education.
		I	I R	I	I R	R

Date Resolved/Initials

Codes:
I = Initiated
R = Resolved

Initials/Staff Signature and Title:

___ / ___
___ / ___
___ / ___

©VNANV 710p2 (9/94)

Figure 16.9 (continued)

health care that is centered around the CPR (Computer-Based Patient Record Institute, 1992).

CPRI initiated five work groups to work on CPR activities. The Codes and Structures Work Group delineated their activities into two subcommittees: (1) Structures Concept Model and (2) Codes. The Structures Concept Model Subcommittee described the CPRS as the functions and characteristics that support the CPR: (1) information content, (2) time, and (3) information representation. The Codes Subcommittee is involved with the development and use of CPR messages, communications, codes, and identifiers. The CPRS is also concerned with data security, availability, reliability, integrity, and persistence.

The CPRSs will be designed to capture, transmit, store, manipulate, and retrieve patient-specific health care-related data. The systems will contain comprehensive longitudinal patient record data designed to provide clinical, financial, and research data. They will be linked through high-speed communication information highways capable of transmitting text, voice, and images. CPRI is working with all the organizations involved in developing standards and is focusing on coordination and consolidating what other groups are doing. They are not developing the data elements themselves (Fig. 16.10).

Home Technology Systems

As home care has evolved and technology has advanced, innovative home technology systems are emerging. The extension of technology systems into the home allows working people to save time, travel, and workdays that would have been consumed by medical and other health care services. These systems maintain continuity of care from hospital to home as well as keep the family together. This technology allows the patient to view and participate interactively in his or her health care via the Internet or some other remote communication network.

Furthermore, of the top 10 diagnosis related groups (DRGs) in home care, seven allow for the inclusion of telehealth as part of the clinician's visit pattern: CHF, CVA, pneumonia, COPD, postoperative coronary bypass, circulatory disorders, and diabetes. With respect to these conditions, nurses can use electronic methods to ensure medication compliance, obtain vital signs, follow up on patient teaching, obtain nutritional information, and provide family support. Physical therapists can use the system to ensure the patient's ability to perform therapeutic exercises. Speech therapists can follow-up on speech and swallowing instructions through telehealth. Occupational therapists can gauge the patient's ability to follow safety instructions or to apply positional devices. Home health aide visits can be supervised at least in part through telehealth. The nurse will also be able to update the plan of care with the aide when on-line. Future systems may include the ability to case conference with all disciplines including the physician (Warner, 1998). Unfortunately, there are two problems preventing the rapid use of telehealth in home care. One is the fact that it is not reimbursable under home care Medicare payments; only actual visits are reimbursable. However, this will change under the pending

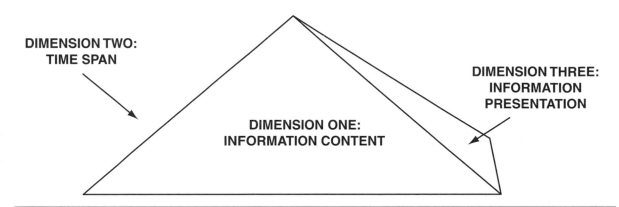

Figure 16.10
Computer-based patient record model.

Prospective Payment System (PPS). Second, there isn't enough data to demonstrate its efficiency. The biggest home care studies have typically had only a 100 or fewer patients, and there are seven million people using home care services (Lewis, 1999)!

Beyond organized home care, however, the introduction of on-line home-based computer terminal communication links brings health care information to the home from a variety of information providers. Technological applications support several innovative home technological advances:

- Home care communication systems
- Home high-tech electronic monitoring systems
- Home educational technology systems

Home Care Communication Systems

Communication systems link patients' homes to health care facilities and health care professionals; home care workers to their supervisors; and patients and families with community resources. Communication systems make it possible for patients to communicate with providers or other resources to get health care advice, avoid inconvenient and expensive visits to health care providers, and omit unnecessary visits to health care facilities.

The computer terminal in a patient's home can be used to (1) assist in self-diagnosis and preventive medicine; (2) reduce unnecessary outpatient visits; (3) provide self-directed triage; and (4) eliminate the "worried well" aspects of many patient-provider interactions. This leads to the following benefits:

- Improved patient and provider satisfaction
- Patient time savings in tracking and receiving information
- Reduced need to see a health care provider
- Increased reliance on computer-based information
- Reduced information calls
- More cost-effective home care

These terminals can also streamline administrative requirements such as obtaining physician orders and confirming appointments due to improved communications with the physicians and other health care professionals. Queries regarding immunizations for travel, flu vaccines, side effects of medications, nonprescription medications, and school and work health forms can increase early detection and reduce visits to health professional offices and hospitals.

Home health care is increasingly using devices that allow health care providers to communicate with patients in their homes. For example, the Texas Telemedicine Project in Austin, Texas is using two-way interactive video to connect specialists in major urban centers with health professionals in rural areas for diagnosis and consultation. The communication technology is used to transmit x-rays, electrocardiograms, and other clinical data for analysis by the specialists. Electronic health care allows rural professionals to "see," via the two-way interactive video, more clients without having to make "home visits," thus saving travel time and ultimately cost.

The Home Assisted Nursing Care Network (HANC) is a system produced by HealthTech Services of Northbrook, IL. HANC is a programmed computer stationed in the patient's home. The unit is a voice-activated, 3.5-foot-tall robot with a video screen. A central nursing station is linked to the home system by telephone lines. HANC can walk patients through a dressing change, assess the condition of an intravenous (IV) site, or provide reminders for taking medications. HANC is FDA-approved and can be programmed in multiple languages (Warner, 1998).

The University of Iowa is conducting a study of rural telemedicine that is designed to determine how to improve academic-rural partnerships and increase collaboration between the University of Iowa and community-based health care providers. Another project is being conducted by the Concurrent Engineering Research Center, West Virginia University. They are also studying the use of real-time technology for the collaboration, treatment, and longitudinal coordination of care of patients in a rural state.

Telecommunications will never replace the practitioner or direct patient-provider relationships, but will ensure more prudent use of health care services. Voice recognition will further enhance these efforts. Programs already exist where voice recognition technology is used to supplement practitioners in extracting patient satisfaction surveys and in eliciting behavior modification by use of phone dial-ups and reminders. This same technology can also be used for education for specific ailments.

Community Health Networks A community health network is an innovative ambulatory care system specially developed to provide services by computer. Computer terminals are placed in homes of "heavy users of health care" such as the family with young children, pregnant women, disabled, and the elderly. The system allows the subscribers to telephone for assistance and guidance on services offered via the terminal. The system performs a triage of actions but not necessarily diagnoses. They include the following:

- Download the patient record from hospital to the home database.
- Enter a series of questions about symptoms using expert system logic until the pathways are concluded.
- Track self-care and, depending on the responses to questions, call or make an appointment with a clinician.
- Provide additional information on the condition if self-care is chosen to assist the client to resolve the problem.

Community health networks appear to increase client satisfaction, and it is anticipated that they will reduce telephone calls and unnecessary trips to the emergency room or physician offices for the "worried well." For example, ComputerLink was a project conducted by Case Western Reserve University (Cleveland, OH) that offered programs and services to support self-care in the home. They were primarily designed to support AIDS, as well as the caregivers of Alzheimer's Disease patients living in their homes. ComputerLink ran within the Cleveland Free Net, a public access computer network. Computer terminals were placed in the homes of the patients using standard telephone lines to allow the patients and/or their caregivers to communicate with the Information Network Services staff at Case Western. ComputerLink offered home care users information, communication, and decision support to enhance self-care and promote home-based treatment of their study patients. It served as a "support group without walls" (Brennan, 1993).

Home High-Tech Monitoring Systems

Home high-tech monitoring systems are using computers to link patients at home to health care facilities. Monitoring devices that transmit vital signs and other critical data are used in the home to conduct postsurgical checkups, for example. They allow health care providers to monitor the progress of their patients. Monitoring technology permits the transmission of health care information both to and from the home. Monitoring systems are being used not only for diagnosis and treatment but also for prevention. Monitoring devices will be increasingly miniaturized and made portable. They will be linked to home information systems and providers via cellular telephones.

The Visiting Nurse Service of New York is using glucometers fitted with modems for many of its diabetic patients. A patient's blood sugar level is tested at intervals during the day and called into a data center. Then a weekly report is generated showing the highs and lows. Multiple admission heart failure patients get machines that measure pulse, weight, and oxygen saturation. When one of the measurements goes beyond an acceptable range, an alarm on the computer goes off. This allows for early intervention that could prevent complications and/or a hospital readmission (Lewis, 1999).

Another monitoring device is a remote defibrillator that allows hospitals to diagnose and resuscitate a homebound patient who has suffered a cardiac arrest. A transtelephonic defibrillator device located in the home, called a "briefcase," is linked to a hospital base unit. When a client feels that he or she is having a heart attack, a caregiver in the home opens the "briefcase," activates the transmitter, and places the electrode pads on the client's chest. An EKG is immediately transmitted to the hospital, and the interactive speaker phone is activated. If the hospital base unit determines that the client is having a heart attack, the device triggers an electronic shock to the patient to stimulate the heart.

Sophisticated telemetry devices such as digitized x-rays and EKG, electronic stethoscopes, and interactive video equipment are using telecommunications technology to enable specialists at a teaching hospital to examine patients in a remote clinic. The clinicians can examine patients, hear heartbeats, study x-rays and laboratory results, and perform other critical assessments with these devices. Two monitors are used to communicate between the two locations. One monitor is used to interact with the rural physician and patient, and the other is used to view the images close up from cameras attached to the biomedical devices.

Another type of monitoring device is the alert systems that are the emergency systems widely used in home settings. Alert systems are primarily communication devices that allow the homebound to signal for help in an emergency. A one-way signaling device that is worn around the neck allows a patient, by pressing on a button, to signal for help to a friend, hospital emergency room coordinator, fire department, etc. Another communication device being researched is a two-way communication device that allows the health care provider in a hospital to communicate with a patient in distress. Other "telemonitoring" devices have been invented that allow patients to administer tests such as vital signs and transmit them to a health care provider (Little, 1992). There are even programs that have been developed to monitor prescription medication consumption.

Home Educational Technology Systems

Home educational technology systems require communication linkages, information access, and educational materials. These technologies meet the need for clients to reach beyond their environment to "see" and "hear," i.e., to experience, view, and visualize situations and communicate educational information. Information access provides the network to access distant databases. There is a growing use of user-friendly technologies that make it possible to interact via on-line computer terminals using handwriting or voice (Olsen et al., 1992).

Educational systems offer advanced learning applications. They use technological media to interact with and educate patients in the home and the community. The types of learning that can be communicated into the home are still being researched. However, the developed home teaching strategies using information technologies include active learning, personalization, individualization, cooperative learning, improving learning strategies and thinking skills, contextual learning, and sophisticated evaluation strategies.

A critical component of home educational technologies is in bringing effective self-care and health promotion into the home. Home computers offer this information as an essential commodity. As new knowledge bases on treatments and alternate therapies, as well as prevention and handling of chronic disabilities, are developed, they will allow health care consumers to assume more responsibility for their self-care, wellness, and prevention of disease.

Patients using communication systems will have not only Internet access to clinical information about specific diseases on the World Wide Web (WWW), but also advice about an individual's health status and self-care, access to their own health care records, and evaluations of providers and therapies. Through interactive learning, communication, and Internet technologies in the home, patients will become active participants in health care decisions.

Home consultation is now available in the home via computer-based stand-alone software programs that do not require a communication network. The use of computer-assisted instruction (CAI), and interactive video (IV) program tapes are available for the personal computer.

Databases systems are being developed, whereby consumers can be linked to a "smart database" with answers and health care advice for minor requirements such as a

rash or a temperature. Once the two-way video networks are in place, clients will be able to consult with health care providers without making a physical visit to a clinician. Clinicians can then provide consultation, observe their patients, and feel connected. Visual and graphic interactive communications are far more effective in educating patients than pamphlets on topics such as nutrition. Clinicians can observe their patients and guide home health workers to use monitoring equipment, or view a specific part of the body, or teach a worker to conduct an examination for viewing. Additionally, the technology can enhance the use of electronic services to schedule health care appointments, automate insurance claims filing, and provide information on eligibility benefits and costs.

Video-conferencing includes the transmission of a video image with a voice in real time and visual, interactive discussion between two or more parties in different locations (Little, 1992; Preston et al., 1992). A benefit of this technology is that it can reduce health care costs in three ways by reducing:

- Time discussing normal test results
- Time spent monitoring chronic patients
- Time spent on information-related calls

Remote interactive video consultation will reduce the need for patients to travel to specialists or for specialists to travel to rural hospitals (Fig. 16.11). Other benefits are that video consultation can:

- Increase timeliness of professional consultation
- Improve access to care
- Increase patient compliance with a recommended course of treatment due to increased patient convenience.

Once in place, the broadband networks can reach into the home through telephone or cable TV networks. They are able to offer video consultations and video instructions, support home care services for homebound patients, and allow clinicians to provide remote diagnostic evaluations and consultations (see Fig. 16.11).

Future Trends

In the future, the technology revolution will take place in the home. This is already happening in homes that have a personal computer and modem. The implementation of technology use in organized home care has been somewhat slow; however, the implementation of PPS and managed care payments in addition to the lowering costs of hardware will increase the rate of growth in the near future. Home health care is becoming

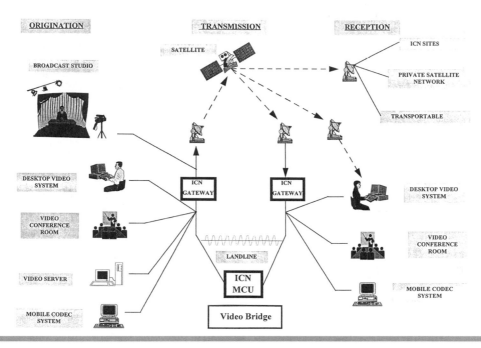

Figure 16.11
Video-conferencing model example.

high-tech as well as high-touch. Community health information networks will link claims, outcomes, billing, utilization review, and patient records on a single system. Shift claims and eligibility data will be transmitted over electronic highways, building databases to track clinical outcomes.

The CPR is a reality; health information consultation and monitoring systems are appearing in the home, and the impact on health care and health providers is revolutionary. These systems are putting more science into the art of nursing and medicine and affect not only home care itself but also national health care policy. The systems as envisioned can facilitate disease prevention and health promotion and allow outcome measures to influence effectiveness and contain health care costs (Little, 1992).

Through the use of the Internet, such systems are possible. Such technology will be implemented and allow the information revolution to expand from hospital to the home and, more importantly, to the clients themselves. As clients increasingly join the communication stream in regard to their health, many of the barriers that have prevented their increased involvement and

empowerment will disappear. For example, as clients retrieve and review their medical records at home at their leisure without distractions, they will have the time and the ability to check reference sources, post questions on the Internet, and ask questions of friends and family. This will most likely impact the quality and content of the information clinicians will include on the health care record (Bruegel, 1998).

The national information infrastructure (NII) using the Internet will be used to communicate provider-to-provider regardless of location; physician-to-patient/family; patient-to-provider/family-to-provider; and patients-to-families and truly will provide "health care without walls."

Summary

This chapter described the various computer applications found in community health. It presented an overview of the beginnings and development of community health computer systems. Several of the development projects were discussed including the data sets projects, prospective payment projects, and OASIS.

An overview of the different types of community health systems was presented, including statistical reporting, registration, management information systems, personal/client management, and special programs. Home health systems were also presented, which included a review of their financial and billing systems, scheduling systems, point-of-care systems, and electronic patient records.

The last section focused on home technology systems that include a wide range of home communication Internet systems, monitoring equipment, devices, and alert systems. A presentation was also provided on the use of home educational technologies for education and teaching health care in the home setting.

References

Bender, A. (1998). Management information systems: A required tool for survival. *Home Health Care Management and Practice, 10*(2), 37–42.

Barry-Eaton Software Technologies. (1992). *Healthy People 2000.* Charlotte, MI.

Brennan, P. F. (1993). ComputerLink: Computer networks and community health connections. *Nursing Dynamics, 2*(1), 9–15.

Bruegel, R.B. (1998). The increasing importance of patient empowerment and its potential effects on home health care information systems and technology. *Home Health Care Management and Practice, 10*(2), 69–75.

Dick, R. S., and Steen, E. B. (Eds). (1991). *The Computer-Based Patient Record: An Essential Technology for Health Care.* Washington, D. C.: National Academy Press.

Florida Department of Health and Rehabilitative Services (1983). *HRS Manual: Systems Management: Client Information System: Personal Health.* Tallahassee, FL.

Goedert, J. (1994). More states turn to EDI as a way to cut expenses. *Health Data Management,* 35–38.

Goodwin, D. R. (1992). Critical pathways in home healthcare. *Journal of Nursing Administration, 22*(2), 35–40.

Harrell, J. (1999). The future of point of care technology. *The Remington Report, 7*(2), 12–14.

Health Care Financing Administration. (1980). *Medicare: Provider Reimbursement Manual: Part II-Provider Cost Reporting Forms and Instructions.* Baltimore, MD:HCFA (1728), DHHS.

Hedberg, S. (1997a). Administrative student information management software (AS/IMS) for school nurse record keeping and reporting. *Journal of School Nursing, 13*(2), 40–48.

Hedberg, S. (1997b). A comparative analysis of PC-based school health software. *Journal of School Nursing, 13*(1), 30–38.

Hoffman, N. L. (1993). *Missouri Health Strategic Architectures and Information Cooperative.* Project Report.

Iyer, P. W., and Camp, N. H. (1999). *Nursing Documentation,* 3rd ed. St. Louis, MO: Mosby.

Lee, S. S. and Schaffer, C. (1999). Ten emerging trends in home care and technology. *The Remington Report, 7*(2), 24–25.

Lewis, A. (1999). Tough times for home care are better times for telemedicine. *The Remington Report, 7*(2), 4–6.

Little, A. D. (1992). *Telecommunications: Can It Help Solve America's Health Care Problems?* Cambridge, MA.

Martin, K. S., and Scheet, N. J. (1992). *The Omaha System: Applications for Community Health Nursing.* Philadelphia, PA: W.B. Saunders.

Martin, K. S., and Scheet, N. J. (1995). *The Omaha System: Applications for Community Health Nursing,* (2nd ed.). Philadelphia, PA: W.B. Saunders.

McDonald, F. (1987). Computer applications in Diabetes management and education. *Computers in Nursing, 5*(5), 181

Michigan Health Department, Nursing Administration's Forum. (1988). *PH-NIS: Personal Health-Nursing Information System.* Michigan.

National Association for Home Care. (1994). *Progress Toward a Uniform Minimum Data Set for Home Care and Hospice.* Washington, D. C.

National Center for Health Statistics. (1994). *Subcommittee on State and Community Health Statistics: Minutes of Meeting.* Washington, D.C.: NCHS, National Committee on Vital and Health Statistics.

National League for Nursing. (1977). *Statistical Reporting in Home and Community Health Services* (pub. no. 21-1652). New York.

Olsen, R., Jones, M. G., and Bezold, C. (1992). *21st Century Learning and Health Care in the Home: Creating a National Telecommunications Network.* Alexandria, VA: Institute for Alternative Futures, Washington, DC: Consumer Interest Research Institute.

Pace, K. (1998). The information challenge. Unpublished manuscript.

Peters, D. A. (1988). The development of a community health intensity rating scale. *Nursing Research, 37*(4), 202–207.

Peters, D. A., and McKeon, T. (1998). *Transforming Home Care: Quality, Cost, and Data Management.* Gaithersburg, MD: Aspen Publishers.

Preston, J., Brown, F., and Hartley, B. (1992). Using telemedicine to improve health care in distant areas. *Hospitals and Community Psychiatry, 43*(1), 25–32.

Reichley, M. (1999). Automation for the 21st century. *Success in Home Care,* 12–16.

Remington, L. (1998). The mouse that roared help! *The Remington Report, Supplement 6*(5), 9–11.

Saba, V. K. (1991). *Home Health Care Classification Project* (NTIS #PB92-177013/AS). Washington, DC: Georgetown University School of Nursing.

Saba, V. K. (1992a). Home health care classification. *Caring, 10*(5), 58–60.

Saba, V. K. (1992b). The classification of home health care nursing diagnoses and interventions. *Caring, 10*(3), 50–57.

Saba, V. K., and Zuckerman, A. E. (1992). A new home health care classification method. *Caring, 10*(10), 27–34.

Shaughnessy, P. W., Bauman, M. K., and Kramer, A. M. (1990). Measuring the quality of home health care. *Caring, 9*(2), 4–6.

Shaughnessy, P. W., and Crisler, K. S. (1995). *Outcome-based Quality Improvement*. Denver, CO: Colorado Center for Health Policy and Services Research.

Shaughnessy, P. W., and Kramer, A. M. (1990). The increased needs of patients in nursing homes and patients receiving home health care. *New England Journal of Medicine, 332*(1), 21–27.

Simmons, D. A. (1980). *A Classification Scheme for Client Problems in Community Health Nursing* (DHHS Publication No. 80-16). Washington, D.C.: Government Printing Office.

Warner, I. (1998). Telemedicine in home health care: The current status of practice. *Home Health Care Management and Practice, 10*(2), 62–68.

Williams, T. (1997). *Guide to Successfully Automating Your Home Health Organization* (2nd ed.). Los Altos, CA: Home Health Business Resources.

Selected Readings

Clinical Data Management. (1994). Texas links 400 public health clinics. *Clinical Data Management, 1*(5), 1.

Community Nursing Organizations' Consortium. (1993). *Community Nursing Organizations National Demonstration: Mission Statement*. VA: Project Hope.

Computer-Based Patient Record Institute, Inc. (1992). *Newsletters*. Chicago, IL.

Custom Data Processing, Inc. (1992). *On-line Software Solutions for Local Health Departments and State Government Organizations*. La Grange, IL.

National League for Nursing. (1978). *Selected Management Information Systems for Public Health/Community Health Agencies*. New York.

New Jersey State Department of Health. (1977). *Home Health Agencies Management Information System*. Washington, D. C.: DN, HRA, DHHS.

Saba, V. K. (1982). The computer in public health: Today and tomorrow. *Nursing Outlook, 30*(9), 510–514.

Saba, V. K. (1983). How Computers Influence Nursing Activities in Community Health. In NIH (Ed.) *First National Conference: Computer Technology and Nursing* (pp. 7–11). (NIH pub. No. 83-2142). Bethesda, MD: National Institutes of Health.

CHAPTER **17**

Ambulatory Care Systems

Susan K. Newbold

OBJECTIVES

1. Identify treatment areas included in the ambulatory arena.
2. Understand information issues in ambulatory care.
3. Delineate functions for information systems, regulatory requirements, and sources for further information.

KEY WORDS

information systems
community health services
regulatory requirements
reimbursement

As a response to increasing costs of providing health care, the health care industry has moved away from the expensive inpatient, acute care environment to caring for clients in various ambulatory care settings. There are numerous organizations that fit within the umbrella of ambulatory health care. They include ambulatory clinics and surgery centers, single- and multi-specialty group practices, diagnostic laboratories, health maintenance organizations, independent physician associations, birthing centers, and college and university health services. Other organizations that serve the ambulatory population are faculty medical practices, community health centers, Indian health centers, hospital-sponsored ambulatory health services, urgent and immediate care centers, office-based surgery centers and practices, pain management clinics, podiatry offices, networks, mobile clinics, and groups of ambulatory care organizations.

A unique facility designed to reach ambulatory clients is a "wellmobile"—a recreational vehicle transformed into a clinic on wheels. Brocht et al. (1999) discuss the information management needs for this setting and the challenges of capturing and organizing data for client care. The workspace is minimal necessitating hardware solutions smaller than a laptop computer, the caregiver population changes requiring an intuitive system interface, the clients are diverse, multilingual and high-risk, and the documentation requirements are complex.

Issues surrounding those who work in ambulatory care are similar across the health care enterprise including increased accountability, the need for continuous and documented service improvements, and pressures to control utilization. Effective reimbursement of services is paramount for continued operation. The ambulatory care arena, just like other health care sectors, require data in order to manage care.

Applications

The applications needed in the ambulatory environment are similar to those required in the in-patient arena. Registration, billing, accounts receivable, accounts payable, patient and staff scheduling, and managed care functionality are the major application areas. The emphasis in the past has been on financial and administrative applications, but some organizations are now adding automated clinical applications.

The benefits that can be achieved by utilizing electronic records encompass the financial, administrative, and clinical areas. Financial benefits include a cost-effective and timely bill submission process. Administrative benefits include a reduction in the size of the record room, increase in the privacy of data, availability of the chart, formats that are legible and comply with legal regulations, and the promotion of quality assurance. Additional administrative benefits for automated ambulatory care records are the ability for home access by physicians and nurse practitioners, alerts for incomplete data, and the integration of clinical data. Clinically, the automated record can provide a problem list, a medication record, vital signs, progress notes, results from the laboratory and radiology, flow sheets, growth charts, immunization records, medication allergies, profiles, alerts and reminders and a follow-up system (Benson and Rcimlinger, 1991).

A patient master index is the basis for collection of all patient related data. If the ambulatory care organization is part of a greater health care enterprise then this master patient index must be integrated into an enterprise-wide index. A master patient index is a central repository for patient/member information across the enterprise including sophisticated tools for querying, updating, and managing the index. It must be able to accommodate multiple patient identifiers so that different locations can maintain their current medical record identification system. The registration system collects patient demographics and insurance information.

The patient scheduling system must link existing scheduling systems so that scheduled activities are coordinated across locations to schedule appointment times, providers, resources, and locations throughout the hospital or organization. The patient needs to be seen at the appropriate time with the proper personnel, equipment, supplies, and chart information.

In the financial arena, client benefits need to be verified and accurate insurance information obtained. A correct bill needs to be submitted to the proper payor. Larger ambulatory care organizations utilize electronic data interchange (EDI) to automate the exchange of data (typically between providers and payors) such as claims, submittals and remittances and health plan eligibility information. Some organizations also provide integrated credit card payment applications so that patients may utilize credit cards which are processed immediately. Payments when received, electronically or manually, must be posted to the proper account. If the payor or the client does not pay the bill within a pre-defined time period, a collections process must be instituted. The electronic or manual system must support adjudication which is the process of determining which payor pays which portion of the bill. The eligibility process needs to be conducted with each instance of service as clients may have changed insurance plans since the last contact with the healthcare organization. Claims submitted to the payor may be either electronic or paper. In the ideal electronic system, claims are edited prior to submission so that charges are paid and not rejected which necessitates further processing, costing time and money.

Other functions of the ambulatory care environment can be enhanced by electronic information technology for data collection and management. Referrals are required by many health plans when a patient is to be seen (or referred) to another healthcare provider. Automatic transfer of these requests will aid patient care and payment of the bill. The multitude of contracts between the health care facility and the payor need to be documented and managed through a contract administration function. Reports must be included in any information technology application. Beyond standard reports, the user must be able to generate user-specified reports. Medical record location can be tracked automatically with an automated system.

The physicians and nurse practitioners must be credentialed in order to provide services. Credentialing is the exhaustive verification of the medical licenses and qualifications. Health care providers must be recredentialed on a regular basis. An automated system can enhance lookup and maintenance of this data.

Accounting for costs can be aided by information technology. Systems must support the Resource Based Relative Value Scale (RBRVS) and the Relative Value Unit (RVU). The RBRVS procedure fee pricing is a model designed by the Department of Health and Human Services (DHHS). In this system, each Physicians' Current Procedural Terminology (CPT) code has a relative value associated with it. The payor will pay the physician on the basis of a monetary multiplier for the RVS value.

Behind the scenes, a database must be maintained of all the current coding schemes utilized for the ambulatory environment. These include CPT (AMA, 2000), the Ninth Revision of the International Classification of Diseases (ICD-9-CM) (HCFA, 1991), the HCFA Common Procedure Coding System (HCPCS) (HCFA, 1998), and the National Drug Code (NDC), managed by the FDA (1995).

Regulatory Requirements

CPT Codes describe medical procedures performed by physicians and other health providers. The codes were developed by the AMA to assist in the assignment of reimbursement amounts to providers by Medicare carriers. A growing number of managed care and other insurance companies, however, base their reimbursements on the values established by HCFA. The most recent version is CPT 2000, which contains 7,755 codes and descriptors (AMA, 2000).

The ICD-9-CM (HCFA, 1991) is based on the official version of the World Health Organization's ICD-9 (1992). It is designed for the classification of morbidity and mortality information for statistical purposes, for the indexing of hospital records by disease and operations, and for data storage and retrieval. Diagnoses and procedures coded in ICD-9-CM determine the diagnosis related group (DRG) that controls reimbursement by HCFA programs, and most other payors. The U.S. is currently using the 9th revision although other countries are using the tenth version (*http://www.cdc.gov/nchs/about/ otheract/icd9/abticd9.htm*; Brown, 1999).

The HCFA HPCS (1998) is a collection of codes that represent procedures, supplies, products, and services which may be provided to Medicare beneficiaries and to individuals enrolled in private health insurance programs. The codes are designed to promote uniform reporting and statistical data collection of medical procedures, supplies, products and services.

The NDC system identifies pharmaceuticals in detail including the packaging. Its use is required by the FDA for reporting and it is used in many healthcare information systems to aid in reimbursement. At the end of 1995 there were over 170,000 NDC codes. The current edition of the NDC Directory is limited to prescription drugs and a few selected over-the-counter products (FDA, 1995). The directory is available on the Internet at: *www.fda.gov/cder/ndc/index.htm*.

Regulatory requirements for the ambulatory setting include the Ambulatory Payment Groups (APGs) classification system mandated by Congress as part of the Balanced Budget Act of 1997 (Public Law 105-32). Software is available to help ambulatory care organizations determine outpatient payment and verify payment received. It also makes it possible for outpatient managers to determine patterns, to predict cost of resource use and to evaluate managed care and physician contracts.

There are a multitude of other federal, state, and local regulations including those from HCFA. Among these are the Health Plan Employer Data and Information Set (HEDIS®) (National Committee for Quality Assurance, 1997). HEDIS® is a standardized, comprehensive set of indicators used to measure the performance of a health plan. Another is Outcome and Assessment Information Set (OASIS) regulations for the home care industry (Shaughnessy, Crisler, and Schlenker, 1997). OASIS is a data set for use in home health agencies and is an initiative from the Health Care Financing Administration. The purpose is to provide a comprehensive assessment for an adult home care patient; and measure patient outcomes for purposes of outcome-based quality improvement.

In the ambulatory care environment there is much emphasis on data at the individual patient level. Also, it is important to aggregate data to view patient care and payment trends.

Member Associations Involved in Ambulatory Care

As varied as the types of organizations that serve the ambulatory populations are, so are the organizations which serve the professionals that work in those organizations. Some ambulatory care organizations will be highlighted.

The American Academy of Ambulatory Care Nursing (AAACN) is a member organization specifically for nurses. The AAACN offers networking opportunities for the membership by geographic location through local networking groups and by specialty practice through special interest groups (SIGs). One SIG for informatics, is working to develop an ambulatory care data set for nursing. The organization also represents ambulatory practice to other political advocacy organizations, to government and quasi-government agencies, and in the federal and state legislative arena. They offer education through publications, electronic media, and conferences (*http://www.aaacn.inurse.com/*).

The Medical Group Management Association (MGMA), founded in 1926 and based in California, is a major organization in the United States representing medical group practice nationwide. About 8,300 health care organizations and 21,000 individuals are MGMA members, representing more than 209,000 physicians (*http://www.mgma.org*). The organization supports education, networking, job recruitment, research, and political action.

The Society for Ambulatory Care Professionals (*http://www.sacp-net.org/*) is associated with the American Hospital Association. It is an organization of management professionals across the continuum of health care services, including, outpatient, ambulatory, and home health care in hospital and freestanding settings. They offer networking opportunities, education, publications, and legislative advocacy.

The Federated Ambulatory Surgery Association (FASA) is a nonprofit association representing the interests of ambulatory surgery centers in the United States. FASA represents the physicians, nurses, administrative staff, and owners industry before the media, Congress, state legislatures, and regulatory bodies. FASA publishes a bimonthly journal and other publications to inform its members and the public. Also FASA conducts educational programs on a variety of topics (*http://www. fasa.org/about.html*).

The American Association of Ambulatory Surgery Centers (AAASC) is a member organization that promotes advocacy at the national level through relationships with the HCFA and Congress, networking and educational opportunities (*http://www.amainc.com/aaasc/aaasc.html*).

The Association for Ambulatory Behavioral Healthcare is an international organization of ambulatory mental health care providers dedicated to the delivery of high-quality psychiatric and chemical dependency treatment within a continuum of care. This membership association which started about 1975 is based in Alexandria, Virginia (*http://www.aabh.org/*).

American Health Information Management Association with over 38,000 members, is a membership organization of health information management professionals. The purpose is to foster the professional development of its members through education, certification, and lifelong learning thereby promoting quality information to benefit the public, the healthcare consumer, providers, and other users of clinical data in any healthcare setting (*http://www.ahima.org*).

There are local groups to support the ambulatory care information systems specialist professionals such as AIM—the Ambulatory Information Management association. It is a specialty organization of the California Health Information Association (CHIA).

Accreditation Organizations

Accrediting organizations validate standards of practice and promote quality care. A private, not-for-profit organization was formed in 1979 called the Accreditation Association for Ambulatory Health Care (AAAHC). Their mission is to develop standards, and conduct a survey and accreditation program (*http://www.aaahc.org*).

COLA, headquartered in Columbia, Maryland, is a non-profit, physician-directed, national accrediting organization. The purpose of COLA is to promote excellence in medicine and patient care through programs of voluntary education, achievement, and accreditation (*http://www.cola.org*).

The National Committee for Quality Assurance (NCQA) is a private, not-for-profit organization dedicated to assessing and reporting on the quality of managed care plans. They are governed by a board of directors that includes employers, consumer and labor representatives, health plans, quality experts, policy makers, and representatives from organized medicine (*http://www.ncqa.org/Pages/Main/index.htm*).

Healthcare professionals that work in the ambulatory care arena need to keep up with regulatory changes in the environment. Among the ways to obtain an education include journals and conferences, as well as membership in organizations.

Journals and Courses

The *Journal of Ambulatory Care Management* by Aspen Publications (Gaithersburg, MD), is a quarterly publication. Each issue focuses on one topic of interest related to ambulatory care. The *Journal of The Ambulatory Pediatric Association* is a publication of the Ambulatory Pediatric Association. The journal, started in 1999, is available both on the world wide web and in hardcopy. The *Journal for Healthcare Quality* is a publication started in 1979 by the National Association for Healthcare Quality. The articles in the journal are refereed.

The Joint Commission on Accreditation of Healthcare Organizations (JCAHO) offers several courses related to ambulatory care. Among the titles are "Freestanding Ambulatory Care Accreditation" and "Pharmacy for Home Care, Long Term Care and Ambulatory Infusion." (*http://www.jcaho.org*).

Ambulatory care takes place in a multitude of settings, all requiring data. Various applications in the ambulatory arena are similar to those in the inpatient settings. Regulator requirements include APGS, HEDIS, and OASIS. Data is collected on an individual consumer and also on a population. There are several member organizations, accreditation organizations, journals, and conferences which focus on ambulatory care.

References

American Medical Association. (2000). *Current Procedural Terminology: CPT 2000*. Chicago, IL: AMA.

Benson, D., and Reimlinger, G. (1991). Electronic medical records in the ambulatory setting: The quality edge. *Ambulatory Care Management 14*, 78–87.

Brocht, D.F., Abbott, P.A., Smith, C.A., Valus, K.A., and Berry, S.J. (1999). A clinic on wheels: A paradigm shift in the provision of care and the challenges of information infrastructure. *Computers in Nursing 17*(3), 109–113.

Brown, F. (1999). *The ICD-9-CM Coding Handbook*. Chicago, IL: American Hospital Association.

FDA. (1995). *National Drug Code Directory*. Washington, D.C.

HCFA. (1998). *HCFA HCPCS 1998*. Washington, D.C.

HCFA. (1991). *ICD-9-CM*, vols. 1–3 (4th edition). Washington, D.C.

National Committee for Quality Assurance. (1997). *HEDIS® 3.0*. Washington, D.C.

Shaughnessy, P.W., Crisler, K.S., and Schlenker, R.E. (1997). *Medicare's OASIS: Standardized Outcome and Assessment Information Set for Home Care*. Denver, CO: Center for Health Policy and Services Research.

WHO. (1992). *ICD-10*. Geneva.

PART **6**

Administrative Applications

18

Administrative Applications of Information Technology for Nursing Managers

Roy L. Simpson
Kathleen A. McCormick

OBJECTIVES

1. Provide an overview of applications/implications—current and future—of information technology (IT) for nursing management.
2. Outline the factors that determine system cost.
3. Discuss the need for nursing data standards.
4. Describe the benefits for nursing of administrative information technology.
5. Delineate specific computer applications for nursing administration.

KEY WORDS

organization and administration
information systems
hospital information systems
manpower
management information systems
personnel management
patient care management
quality assurance

The combination of managed care and the exponential growth of technology has created a wealth of opportunity for nursing in terms of IT. At the same time, it has created a challenge: When faced with limited time, personnel, and financial resources, should nursing pursue its mission to provide care, or should it concentrate on mastering emerging technologies? The answer is both, given today's industrywide demands to increase the quality of care while decreasing its cost.

Currently, very little patient information and data needed to make care decisions is gathered or stored in digital form. Nurses rely on handwritten notes—both their own and those of physicians. Caregivers spend as much as 40 percent of their time on paperwork, much of it spent looking for a critical piece of information (United States Advisory Council on the National Information

Infrastructure, Undated). As a result, nurses must often make care decisions without the benefit of real-time access to critical information, which reduces quality, and sacrifice productivity and accuracy, which increases costs.

One of the most effective ways to balance the cost/quality issues is by embracing information technology, specifically those applications aimed at streamlining and eliminating manual administrative tasks.

This chapter describes how computerized nursing systems—specifically, administrative applications—can help nursing manage and use information to enhance and improve:

■ Individual patient care
■ Organizational performance
■ Staff productivity

- Governance
- Management
- Support processes

Since this chapter focuses on administrative applications rather than clinical ones, it also focuses on applications of IT for the two levels of nursing that use administrative applications most often. These levels and their administrative information requirements include the following.

- Nursing administration. The nurse administrator manages and influences environmental practice. Typically, nursing administration assumes judicial responsibility for managing patient care and budget, and overseeing nursing managers. The nurse administrator's role is to provide leadership in setting goals for the effective and efficient care for patients and for evaluating the quality of nursing services that are provided. Furthermore, the administrator is responsible to the organization as a whole, the community, the nursing profession, and the health care delivery system (American Nurses Association, 1988). Specifically, nursing administrators report to the organizational "C" level (i.e., CEO, CFO, or COO). Nursing administration requires information from and about nursing services in order to run nursing departments.

- Nursing services management. The nurse manager's role is to control nursing services and report back to nursing administration. Primarily, nurse managers coordinate nursing activities, participate in resource utilization decisions, and serve as the link between nursing services staff—both internal and external to the organization. Nurse managers implement strategic plans (developed by nursing administration) and participate in forming policy and developing staffing, scheduling, and evaluation performance standards. Nursing management requires information from and about patient care services/staff nursing in order to run individual nursing units.

Applications/Implications of Information Technology for Nursing Management

Both nurse administrators and nurse managers are required to collect and analyze large amounts of data—which it has become impossible to do effectively without

computerized management information systems. In general, nursing "systems" are actually an aggregation of six types of applications, including:

1. Bibliographic databases
2. Word processing applications
3. Database programs
4. Decision analysis programs
5. Spreadsheets
6. Project management programs (Anderson et al., 1992)

Together, these applications form systems that satisfy the four essential information needs of nursing administration and nursing management, which are:

1. Measuring patient dependence and patient classification schemes
2. Managing nursing workload
3. Scheduling
4. Executing business and accounting tasks

All of these needs—even more imperative in today's cost-controlled, quality-focused health care environment—require data. Ultimately, they all serve to help nursing measure, monitor, and manage services, which requires answering several key questions:

- Rates of occurrence: How often and when are services provided?
- Cost: What is the financial impact of services?
- Intensity: What level of service is required?
- Resource utilization: What resources are required to provide specific levels of service?
- Outcomes of care: What is the result of services performed?

In addition to managing services, nursing management is also increasingly responsible for effective management of financial and patient care data to:

- Demonstrate compliance with standards set by the Joint Commission on Accreditation of Healthcare Organizations (JCAHO) and other standard-setting organizations
- Document conformity to state and federal government regulations
- Manage credentialing
- Develop risk management programs to reduce organizational liabilities, identify legal risks, and minimize financial liability in legal matters

- Recruiting and retaining qualified staff

- Support the personnel, information, and technologic infrastructure necessary to further organizational goals

- Assure customer (patient) satisfaction

- Establish patterns of care, benchmarks, and outcomes necessary for evaluating past and forecasting future patient care quality

- Ensure effective and efficient use of facility, equipment, service, and financial resources

- Determine case-mix in terms of patient diagnosis, age, and other variables to optimize third-party payer reimbursement

- Assure follow-up care of chronic patients and assess efficiency of that care

- Satisfy data requirements of managed care contracts

- Demonstrate organizational efficiency, effectiveness, and performance to optimize competitive position

Increasingly, nurse administrators are also being asked to focus on outcomes of care (Ullian, 1992). While clinical systems collect the clinical data used to measure outcomes, administrative systems play a key role in interpreting that data. In the future, nursing administration can look forward to enterprise-wide administrative systems that marry clinical and financial data and lay the groundwork for comprehensive data collection. These value-added systems will provide the necessary data for in-depth analysis and continuous quality improvement.

The "Real" Cost of Administrative Systems

What Does It Cost to Automate?

To determine the true cost of automation, one must take three things into account:

1. Cost of the hardware and software. While hardware and software are often the only thing considered when determining cost, they are, today, perhaps the least costly element given the constantly declining cost of technology. The administrative system that cost $4 million dollars in 1972 now costs less than $250,000. But today's $4 million system would be worth that much. The value of technology has caught up with its price.

2. Cost of education. A system is only effective if nurses use it, and nurses cannot use a system unless they get the necessary training. Training costs can comprise everything from instruction fees to travel expenses and the cost for temporary staffing during training.

3. Intellectual resources. Nursing management should serve as advisors, directors, and influencers of the technology that nursing uses. In fact, in the selection of patient care systems, the JCAHO now mandates nursing involvement. And for good reason. This is the only way we can ensure that technology is applied to meeting nursing's information needs, advancing nursing practice, and, realistically, ensuring nursing's continued viability (Simpson, 1999). Any system cost estimate should include the necessary resources for nursing management to be actively involved in system selection and evaluation.

To determine these costs, it's helpful to start with a model, either clinical or financial.

How much can automation save?

Health care organizations create, move, store, and retrieve billions of patient records every year. While managed health care has increased health care's information requirements, advancing technology has increased the availability—and therefore the demand—that that information be in electronic form. The only way for nursing management to effectively control this amount of information is through computerization.

Continued reliance on manual data collection is having and will continue to have serious implications, including:

- Increased administrative cost. National health expenditures are projected to total $2.2 trillion and reach 16.2 percent of the gross domestic product (GDP) by 2008 (Office of the Actuary, Health Care Financing Administration, Undated). Controlling administrative data and documenting practice to monitor quality and assess cost and value consume as much as 20 percent of that total U.S. health care bill. This is at least twice and as much as 10 times what other countries—including those with national healthcare—expend.

- Compromised quality. At least 30 percent of the information required to make diagnosis and treatment decisions is unavailable at the time the decision needs to be made (Dick and Steen, 1991). Much of this information is nursing information.

For example, inadequate documentation of medication administration has led to adverse drug events that add roughly $3 billion per year to hospital bills (Melmon, 1971).

The potential savings of automation are significant. Health care administrators can help reduce health care costs a total of $36.8 billion per year through four applications of computers:

- Patient information management and transfer, $30 billion
- Electronic claims processing, $6 billion
- Electronic inventory management, $600 million
- Video-conferencing for professional training, $200 million

Automation will allow nursing management—specifically—to reduce annual costs to hospitals by at least $12.7 billion. This will be accomplished by:

- Reducing costs associated with adverse medical reactions
- Decreasing nursing clerical time
- Reducing costs associated with record maintenance
- Curtailing malpractice costs
- Hastening retrieval of valid and reliable information
- Easing aggregation of medical information for research
- Improving internal and external review of records (Little, 1992)

The Need for Nursing Data Standards

For some time, there have been standards motivating nursing to focus on effective and efficient administration. Established by the American Nurses Association (ANA) in 1988, these standards remain the prevailing measures by which professional nurses evaluate practice.

Several years after developing practice standards, the ANA established the Nursing Information and Data Set Evaluation Center (NIDSEC) to create and disseminate standards for information systems. These standards were designed to ensure complete, accurate documentation of nursing practice and to serve as a guide by which to evaluate information systems. The ultimate goal of these standards is to expedite the evolution of large, accessible pools of patient data that reflect the true nature, cost, and effects of nursing practice.

The NIDSEC standards apply to four aspects of nursing data sets and the systems that contain them—nomenclature, clinical content, clinical data repository, and general system characteristics. Though most often applied in the selection of clinical systems, these standards could serve as an equally good model for evaluating administrative systems for nursing.

In addition, thanks to JCAHO initiatives that have shifted the orientation of health care information systems from monitoring processes to measuring outcomes, there is also a need for standards to facilitate:

- Combining data from different sources in new ways
- Linking clinical and administrative data
- Using external databases to monitor hospital performance (American Association of Nurse Executives, 1993)

Specifically, the JCAHO's initiatives have created an additional need for standards to (Porter, 1994):

- Support access to external comparison databases
- Ensure data security and confidentiality
- Promote the development of knowledge-based systems
- Provide a link to physicians' information systems
- Support continuous quality improvement projects
- Ensure data integrity
- Integrate with existing standards and procedures related to documentation requirements
- Support needs assessments

Moreover, the lack of standards has become a key obstacle to the development of universal computer-based medical records, as recommended by the Institute of Medicine more than a decade ago (Simpson, 1991a–d).

Benefits for Nursing of Administrative Information Technology

Nursing administrative systems fall into three basic categories of use:

1. Strategic
2. Operational
3. Tactical

In general, they help nursing:

- Improve communication
- Improve order entry
- Improve continuity of care
- Spend more time on patient care
- Guide critical thinking
- Tap into expert resources
- Evaluate care

In addition, nurse administrators have identified several other specific benefits of using information technology (American Association of Nurse Executives, 1993), including:

- Expanded utilization of nursing staff resources
- Improved quality of patient care monitoring
- Improved documentation
- Improved communication
- Improved planning
- Increased standardization of nursing practice
- Ability to define nursing practice and associated problems/issues
- Ability to define methods to track patient care delivered, outcomes achieved, and revenue generated
- Enhanced recruitment and retention
- Improved evaluation of care provided
- Support for the dynamic organization, capable of change

While benefits come at the end of a successful system installation, the time to ensure their realization is at the beginning, during system implementation. As early as system selection and no later than initial planning, organizations should outline desired benefits and then manage system implementation to those benefits via weekly updates, scorecards, and other evaluation/measurement methods.

 ## Specific Computer Applications for Nursing Administration

Approximately 26 administrative applications are available on computers for nurse administrators and managers. Table 18.1 summarizes them.

Nursing Administrators' Data Needs

In general, nursing administrators uses computer systems to collect data needed for planning, budgeting, and reporting, which ensure quality care. The major applications they use are for:

- Quality assurance
- Personnel files
- Communication networks
- Budgeting and payrolls
- Census
- Regulatory reporting
- Forecasting and planning
- Claims processing and reimbursement
- Risk pooling
- Costing nursing care
- Case-mix
- Consumer surveys

 ## Quality Assurance

The key words for measuring quality in the decade ahead are effectiveness, efficiency, and outcomes.

Nursing is increasingly accountable for the care it delivers. But health care encompasses many variables and a myriad of assessment methods for evaluating structure, actions, outcomes, and processes. Nursing has dedicated more than a decade to the issue of quality assurance, developing a host of frameworks and methods in the process. Ultimately, all of the resultant quality assurance worksheet forms should be computerized.

In 1989, the ANA, the National Commission on Nursing Implementation Project (NCNIP), and the National League for Nursing (NLN) sponsored an invitational conference to identify what was needed to assess quality of nursing care. Participants agreed that establishing nursing information systems (NISs) would facilitate a quality assurance system and that establishing a taxonomy or classification nomenclature system—such as nursing diagnosis—would facilitate development of a standardized nursing database. Also deemed necessary were continued studies on nursing's impact on patient outcomes and the structural variables affecting the nursing process.

However, computer systems have not yet risen to the information needs of nursing. The reason for this is that they cannot identify valid and reliable criteria upon which to input information. That is nursing's job. As a

Table 18.1   Computer applications for administrative information management

- Quality assurance
- Personnel files
- Communication networks within the nursing department and outside the nursing department
- Budgeting and payrolls
- Census
- Summary reports for state, federal, and hospital regulations
- Forecasting and planning
- Claims processing (reimbursement)
- Risk pooling
- Costing nursing care
- Case-mix management
- Consumer surveys
- Nursing intensity
- Patient classification
- Acuity systems
- Staffing and scheduling
- Inventory
- Patient billing
- Incident and other reports
- Poison control
- Allergy and drug reactions
- Error reports
- Infection control
- Unit reports
- Utilization review
- Shift summary reports

result, many of today's systems do little more than automate the same information and problems that exist in the manual methods of monitoring quality assurance.

The JCAHO also uses computers to monitor adherence to its quality assurance standards, but only to analyze the volumes of data accumulated annually from standard compliance reviews. In the future, the JCAHO aims to make these databases available to the public, which can then use them to compare quality among institutions.

Ensuring quality care that is efficient and cost-effective is of importance in today's health care environment. The goal of 21st century system designers will be the creation of decision support systems that can support clinical management, utilization review credentialing,

and quality assurance, including clinical indicators and peer review criteria, and report adherence to professional/hospital standards and performance measures (Simpson, 1992). Critical to their development will be complete information on national and local recommendations. Hospitals will need to report on individual provider policies and guidance. As a result of such systems, resource allocations—previously based on best guesses—will be derived from quantitative data and profiles of professional performance and utilization of resources (Silva and Zawilski, 1992).

Increasingly, the decade ahead will require quality management that ensures the value of purchased care (Sennett, 1992). Computer support attempts to identify care that is inappropriate or inefficient or excessive or to identify low-cost care alternatives. Such applications are marketed as health care management systems.

In evaluating care, computerized patient record documentation is used to understand the logic of diagnosis, planning, interventions, and outcomes achieved. Trends toward prospective management or point-of-service management are emerging, since retrospective management offers less opportunity to rationally manage care.

Identifying patterns of care and high- or low-performance providers requires data over time and based on outcomes of care. The medical record becomes the repository of clinically relevant events divided into units of analysis to describe the persons served and to summarize these events. This type of analysis is becoming especially important to profile or case managers. To satisfy all monitors of quality in the patient record, the record must be accessible, standardized, simplified, accurate, complete, and cost-effective.

For nursing administrators, the computer-based patient record offers the ability to:

- Provide accessible clinical data that characterizes patients' conditions, prior management, and current treatment.
- Provide clear and defined databases to permit epidemiological assessment of patient outcomes and patterns of practice, revealing best and worst practice management strategies.
- Provide interactive decision support tools on information derived from large groups of patients.
- Decrease administrative record keeping and standardize forms for reimbursement.

Figure 18.1 is a model for computerization of quality assurance with expanded nursing input and new outputs,

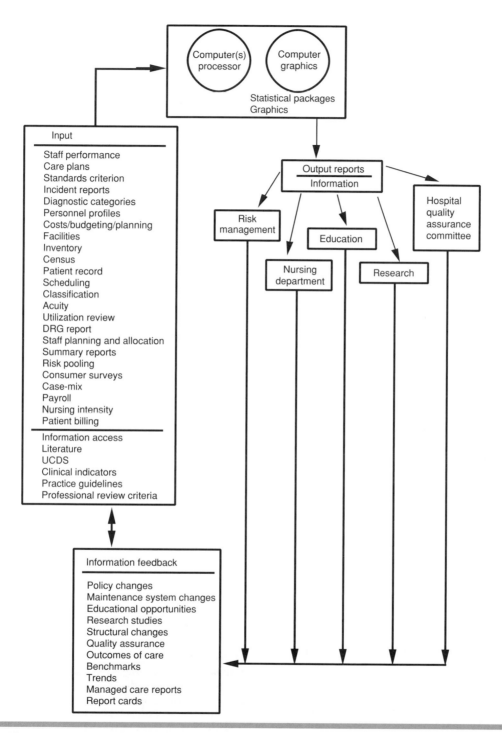

Figure 18.1
A model for computerization of quality assurance.

for the total information management of quality in a nursing department.

Personnel Files

Because computers can help organize information, they are being used to assist administrators in personnel planning and productivity analysis. Such systems maintain and update employees' permanent files, provide ready access to personnel profiles, and support employee quality control. These systems generate reminders for various personnel actions, such as license renewal or position change, and they produce reports on labor costs, employee analysis, and forecast requirements (Austin, 1979).

A personnel file can be used to:

- Generate mailing lists
- Plan educational programs
- Determine eligibility for promotion
- Provide a personnel census
- Generate budget expenditures
- Identify personnel with special skills
- Validate registered licenses
- Validate certification updates
- Prepare profile analyses

A relatively new system is the "recruitment manager" for nurse administrators (Garre, 1990). This software accurately and rapidly tracks and monitors recruiting efforts. It will increasingly become necessary to maintaining competitive advantage, facilitating policy development, and enhancing predictability in the market.

Communication Networks

Computer systems that facilitate communication are designed to transmit information from point to point in a computer terminal network. In these systems, called local area networks (LANs), messages are not usually processed but are transmitted from one terminal (entry) to another (receiver).

When networked, computers serve as data integrators. Networks—essentially computerized communication systems—affect work patterns by reducing nurses' clerical functions. These systems also enhance enterprisewide communications (Schmitz et al., 1976).

Networks have many functions. Some of the more typical functions include (Filosa, 1978):

- Sending notices of patient appointments, admissions notification, discharges, and hospital census

- Providing summary information on laboratory tests, medications, and other orders
- Locating patients
- Identifying current charges and patient needs
- Ensuring accurate billing

Computer networks eliminate searches through procedure manuals and expedite delivery service and procedure requisitions, thus reducing clerical tasks. Networks reduce the need for couriers to hand-carry reports and forms from the nursing department to the nursing unit, further reducing nursing time spent on administration.

Wide-area networks (WANs) link nurse administrators through to nursing departments outside the hospital or agency, broadening information access considerably.

Budgeting and Payroll

One of the greatest advantages of computers for nursing administrators is in budgeting, a complex process that includes many layers of cost analysis. Included below is a list of financial functions that computer systems provide for nursing administrators. They can be derived from the hospital cost accounting systems or "downloaded" from spreadsheet software into nursing administration systems.

- Accounts receivable
- Patient accounts
- Accounts payable
- General ledger
- Property ledger accounting
- Debts
- Collections
- Preventive maintenance costs
- Medicare/Medicaid patient profiles
- Private insurance profiles
- Cost allocation
- Cash control

Equally important to specific functionality are the information reports that come from payroll systems, inventory records, incident reports, length-of-stay reports, the nursing record, and quality care information.

Because nursing is central to health care delivery, it is critical that organizations be able to assess the adequacy of nursing care and determine its cost. To evaluate nursing productivity, organizations frequently use such criteria as nursing hours per patient day, staff-to-patient ratios, the number of full-time and part-time employees, and cost per patient day. Formulas for analyzing the cost of nursing care have also been developed. Since these reports require information, computers have been used to process summary reports.

Computer systems can adjust to several types of budgeting, the three most common being:

1. A fixed budget where an absolute dollar amount is needed and no provision of variance is allowed because it presumes an absolute volume throughout the year.

2. A flexible budget that assumes the expected procedures with monthly variance reports adjusted to reflect actual volume, since the manager cannot control volume.

3. Case-based budgets that are built around product-line structures and assume that department managers control neither the volume, procedures, nor revenue. Budget assumptions flow from demand forecasts by product, bill of sources by product, and case-based reimbursement. Variance reports are adjusted for variations in actual versus expected volume.

Census

A census is a registration of inpatients and the beds they occupy. Census systems allow users to enter information on patient admission, discharge, birth, death, or transfers. They maintain a master file of available beds and bassinets, along with appropriate legal information on occupancy. The census application is also the heart of most HISs, most of which allow on-line control of the census function. Organizations need current reports at all times to account for patients in the hospital, emergency room, or outpatient clinics. All hospital areas must have continuous access to the computer system in order to determine patient status, from preadmission to admission, transfer, discharge, or death. The census system usually provides immediate information on bed availability. Standard reports can provide statistical analysis and forecasting information, such as which units have reduced census between April and July or September and December.

The census system is the cornerstone of administrative systems. It provides daily, weekly, or monthly statistical analysis of patient admission by hospital service, gender, and age. Detailed census statistics include patient days for each gender and age category within

hospital services and are used to analyze hospital services and to determine variations in time and patient mix for each hospital service.

Regulatory Reporting

There are several types of summary reports required to satisfy state and federal requirements and meet JCAHO accreditation standards. These reports might include:

- Incident reports
- Poison control
- Allergy and drug reactions
- Error reports
- Infection control reports
- Unit reports including census
- Patient status
- Activities
- Procedures
- Patients at risk
- Utilization review information

Most of these reports originate on the nursing unit and are filled out by staff nurses, head nurses, unit managers, or supervisors. If a nursing service administrator neglects to include the summary reports in nursing service information, however, this important information may not receive adequate attention.

Forecasting and Planning

There are systems that can predict staffing requirements, determine trends in patients' nursing care needs, and forecast departmental budgetary compliance. They can also project staffing needs to support effective management of float personnel and interunit personnel exchange. Nurse administrators can use computers to define monitoring tasks and to establish which variables patient care personnel must monitor for inpatients who require atypical care patterns.

Many types of systems are available for planning schedules, hospital expansions, finances, and preventive maintenance. On-line patient scheduling systems provide accuracy, flexibility, and timeliness for outpatient and inpatient scheduling. Users can delineate visit codes and control length of visit and numbers of assigned professional staff. Summary reports help with clinic and inpatient staffing plans.

Hospital Expansion

Many systems provide the census, staffing, scheduling, and financial data organizations need to manage expansion. Systems can help organizations do everything from identifying programs for elimination to enhancing financial planning. Indeed, prospective financial information has replaced retrospective planning.

Preventive Maintenance

Preventive maintenance planning requires systems that help organize and schedule maintenance. Automated planning ensures more reliable equipment and reduces equipment failure. Even the computer needs a maintenance planning system—to determine both beneficial "downtime" and scheduled maintenance.

Planning Systems

Organizations can use planning systems to determine what information is needed for what services. Periodic audits can uncover unnecessary services or those that need to be used by different groups of patients. For example, an audit of lodging use by parents of pediatric patients with terminal cancer may show that the services are underused. However, if spouses and relatives of geriatric patients need such a facility, this insight could help the organization reallocate resources for optimum benefit. Computerized planning systems can provide the information to accommodate such decisions.

Planning systems can also help administrators determine available space both within the hospital and on hospital grounds, categorizing that space by such criteria as type, location, and amount, among others.

To direct a service, administrators must be able to define the service's mission and scope, and the objectives that follow the mission and specify the desired departmental outcomes. Another important resource for today's administrator is a business plan that includes the following:

1. Organization plan
2. Market/competition analysis
3. Production or operations plan
4. Marketing/distribution plan
5. Management/personnel organizational plan
6. Development timeline or schedule
7. Financial plan

Computer software can help create and develop each of these plans. For example, graphics software packages that allow the development of flowcharts are valuable for creating organizational plans. Spread sheets are good for developing schedules.

Gantt charts can be used to graphically depict blocks of time, representing the number of weeks, months, or years required to complete tasks. They are also useful for displaying critical and noncritical tasks. There are several software products that are now available to prepare Gantt charts. Figure 18.2 shows how a Gantt chart can be used to develop schedules and monitor projects. This example was developed by an administrator proposing a new outpatient clinic (Johnson, 1988).

Another planning tool, the Program Evaluation Review Technique (PERT), is used to analyze operations and describe and schedule project tasks. Projects with "critical paths" can be monitored using PERT charts. Figure 18.3 illustrates a simple critical path.

Financial Plan

The financial plan should include at least two levels of planning, strategic and operational. Strategic-level timeframes may range from 5 to 10 years. Operational timeframes are shorter, often no more than a year, with periods broken down into quarters or months. Projections included in operational plans include volume, revenue, rates, expenses, inflation, growth, assets required, capital structure, net income, and cash flow. Most applications allow the user to identify three basic content reports: income statement, cash flow statement, and balance sheet. Tables 18.2, 18.3, and 18.4, respectively, show examples of each of these types of statements.

The income statement was generated from a data sheet specifying the charge units, payer mix, reimbursement type, expenses, profit margin, revenues/rates, and market limits for prices.

Cash flow statements can be generated after defining all of the above data sheets plus cash sources. The balance sheet defines the equipment, cash, and other assets as well as the business liabilities and financing structure. This balance sheet depends on viable definitions of cash, accounts receivable, inventory, capital assets, accumulated depreciation, accounts payable, long-term debts and equity, which may require consultation with financial specialists.

Tables 18.5, 18.6, and 18.7 illustrate how to put the financial plans in place. They outline the income statement, revenue projections, and salary projections involved

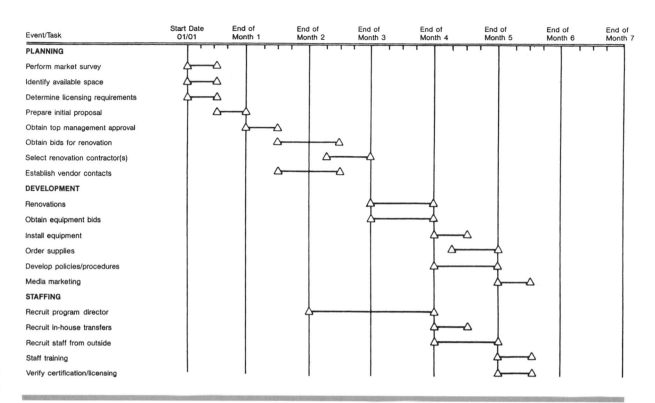

Figure 18.2
Gantt chart.
Reproduced, with permission, from Johnson (1988).

in establishing a gerontology care unit. The break-even analyses predicting different occupancy rates over two different years are depicted in Figs. 18.4 and 18.5. These analyses show that a unit would be profitable at a minimum of 56.3 percent occupancy for the first year and 70 percent occupancy in later years.

 Claims Processing and Reimbursement

Third-party payer claims information relies on accurate and reliable documentation. The most important information to capture includes

- Types of services provided
- The agent, or provider, to be reimbursed for those services
- The amount charged for the services

- Sufficient information about the patient to permit linkage to the health insurance policy reimbursing the patient

The patient record could become the source of this information provided that the information is accurate, accessible at low cost and timely, capable of extracting the critical review criteria or indicators, and in sufficient detail to capture the medical and nursing elements.

Risk Pooling

Risk pooling, or risk adjustment, involves describing the relative risks associated with populations of a specific age, gender, race, and/or clinical condition. The goal of risk adjustment is to effectively manage and appropriately apply resources for each group. To minimize the

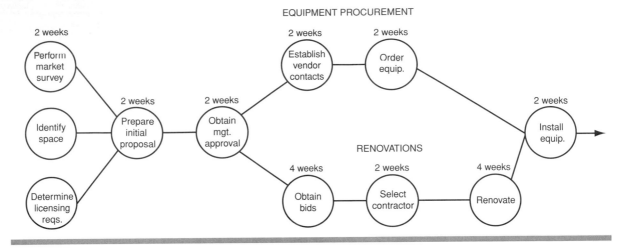

Figure 18.3
PERT chart showing a critical path.
Reproduced, with permission, from Johnson (1988).

Table 18.2	Example of an income statement

Business ABC Income Statement	
Gross revenues	$XXX,XXX.XX
Less: allowances and bad debts	XX,XXX.XX
Net revenues	$XXX,XXX.XX
Other revenues	X,XXX.XX
Operating expenses	$XXX,XXX.XX
Interest expenses	XX,XXX.XX
Depreciation and amortization	XX,XXX.XX
Total expenses	$XXX,XXX.XX
Net income (loss) pre-tax	$ X,XXX.XX
Taxes	XXX.XX
Net income (loss)	$ X,XXX.XX

Reproduced, with permission, from Johnson (1988).

Table 18.3	Example of a cash flow statement

Business ABC Statement of Cash Flows	
Beginning cash balance	$XXX,XXX.XX
Net income	X,XXX.XX
Depreciation and amortization	XX,XXX.XX
Increase to debt	XX,XXX.XX
Accounts payable: Current	X,XXX.XX
Accounts payable: Prior	(X,XXX.XX)
Total cash sources	$XXX,XXX.XX
Uses of cash	
Accounts receivable: Current	$ X,XXX.XX
Accounts receivable: Prior	(X,XXX.XX)
Inventory: Current	X,XXX.XX
Inventory: Prior	X,XXX.XX
Payment of debt	XX,XXX.XX
Capital expenditures	XX,XXX.XX
Total uses of funds	$ XX,XXX.XX
Ending cash balance	$XXX,XXX.XX

Reproduced, with permission, from Johnson (1988).

Table 18.4   Example of a balance sheet

Business ABC Example of a Balance Sheet	
Assets	
Cash	$XXX,XXX.XX
Accounts receivable	XX,XXX.XX
Inventory	XX,XXX.XX
Total current assets	$XXX,XXX.XX
Capital equipment	XXX,XXX.XX
Less accumulated depreciation	XX,XXX.XX
Net fixed assets	XXX,XXX.XX
Total assets	$XXX,XXX.XX
Liabilities and equity	
Accounts payable	$XXX,XXX.XX
Long-term debt	XX,XXX,XX
Equity	
Paid-in capital	XXX,XXX.XX
Retained earnings	XX,XXX.XX
Total equity	XXX,XXX.XX
Total liabilities and equity	$XXX,XXX.XX

Reproduced, with permission, from Johnson (1988).

risks of population differences, most administrators focus on the process of care delivery (e.g., number of pregnant women seen during their first trimester) rather than the outcomes (number of low birth weight infants, hospital readmission rates), because outcomes can be skewed patient population characteristics.

Risk pooling also depends on the ability to aggregate data on expected health care costs of distinct populations. It can be based upon individual risks or group risks. The patient record can provide this information if the data stored expand morbidity and mortality and address functional status, health status, satisfactions, and other quality indicators of care. Current patient records have too much superfluous information to contain specific risk factors but could include those data elements. Many of the indicators of complications of care, safety, and incidents will be found within the nursing record and should be considered a source of those data elements.

According to Sennett (1992), an impediment to risk pooling is the lack of standardization and vocabulary within current patient records. Similarly, confidentiality requirements of data must be assured. Finally, explicit guidelines for use to describe the specific data elements

Table 18.5   Income Statement for GCU

Category	Sept-Dec			
	1987	1988	1989	1990
Gross patient revenue	$410,200	$1,328,600	$1,560,375	$1,799,450
Deductions from revenue	75,800	245,800	288,700	332,900
Net patient revenue	334,400	1,082,800	1,271,675	1,466,550
Direct expenses				
Salaries	148,909	459,777	548,444	647,959
Benefits-15% salaries	22,336	68,967	82,267	97,197
Office supplies	735	2,205	2,293	2,408
Medical supplies	2,435	7,305	7,670	8,130
Equipment depreciation	4,367	13,100	13,100	500
Misc. expense	625	1,875	1,931	1,989
Renovation	5,375			
Totals	184,782	553,229	655,705	758,203
Indirect expense	146,329	438,102	519,253	600,421
Total expense	331,111	991,331	1,173,958	1,358,624
Gain/loss	3,289	91,469	96,717	107,926
Statistics				
Patient days	1,465	4,745	5,475	6,205
% of occupancy	57.2	61.9	71.4	81.0
Break-even patient days	1,439	4,071	4,763	5,372
Break-even % occupancy	56.2	53.1	62.1	70.1

Reproduced, with permission, from Johnson (1988).

Table 18.6   Revenue projections for GCU

Source	1987	1988	1989	1990
Patient service revenues*	280	280	285	290
Charge per patient day	57.2%	61.9%	71.4%	81.0%
Projected occupancy	1,465	4,745	5,475	6,205
Patient days	410,200	1,328,600	1,560,375	1,799,450
Gross revenue				

*Expressed as a percentage of gross revenue; calculated using appropriate patient mix and payer reimbursement methods: prospective payment system (PPS) for Medicare, per diem for Medicaid, and percentage of charges for Blue Cross, HMOs, and commercial insurers.
Note: Patient day charges will increase in 1989 and 1990 based upon hospital rate increases.
Reproduced, with permission, from Johnson (1988).

Table 18.7   Salary projections for GCU

RNs	1987	1988	1989	1990
Patient days	1,465	4,745	5,475	6,205
Standard	6.2	6.2	6.2	6.2
Man hours	9,083	29,419	33,945	38,471
Average hourly rate	12.46	13.08	13.81	14.64
Salaries	$113,174	$384,801	$468,780	$563,215
Unit secretaries				
Man hours	1,738	5,200	5,200	5,200
Average hourly rate	7.50	7.88	8.32	8.32
Salaries	$13,035	$40,976	$43,264	$45,864
Coordinator				
Man hours	1,396	2,080	2,080	2,080
Salaries	$22,700	$34,000	$36,400	$38,900
Total man hours	12,217	36,699	41,225	45,751
FTEs	16.23	15.39	19.82	22.00
Total salaries 166	$148,909	$459,777	$548,444	$647,979
Increases				
RN and unit secretary	0	5%	5.6%	6%
Coordinator	0	0	7%	7%

Reproduced, with permission, from Johnson (1988).

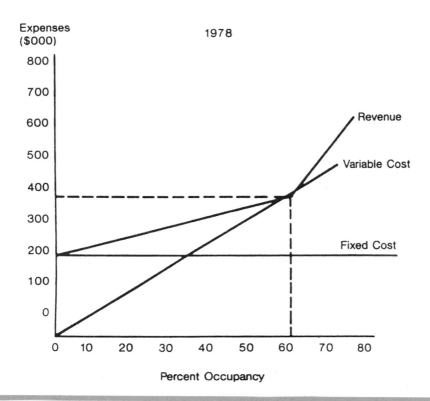

Figure 18.4
Break-even analysis for GCU Occupancy.
Reproduced, with permission, from Johnson (1988).

need to be specified, as well as systems developed to assure compliance with those guidelines (Sennett, 1992).

Costing Nursing Care

In 1981, Thompson estimated that nursing services accounted for 35 percent of total hospital costs (Thompson, 1981). In a country with national health care, like Australia, where costs have been examined, nursing service has been determined to be the largest single component of a hospital's expenditures (Picone, 1991). In the United States, Halloran estimates that nursing averages 25 percent of total hospital costs, ranging between 20 percent in large hospitals and 50 percent in smaller ones (Halloran, 1994).

With hospital costs at 40 percent of health care costs, U.S. citizens pay about $100 billion dollars per year for hospital nursing. However, room and board rates—

rather than service rates—have traditionally been used to calculate costs. In order to cost out nursing services today, a logical and sequential series of activities needs to occur, and each requires specific systems, from classification to staffing.

The cost identification of nursing services is but one system in a series of systems (Van Slyck, 1991a–g). In order to accurately cost out nursing services, Van Slyck states that organizations must identify a series of independent and interrelated systems and subsystems, including:

1. A belief system that identifies the organization's statements on patient cost identification, pricing policy, and nursing care.

2. A patient classification system that categorizes patients into distinct groups based on pre-established criteria.

3. A staffing system that identifies patients, nursing staff requirements, and allocation based on the quantifiable needs (acuity) of the patients.

4. A costing system or method that can identify nursing care costs within a facility for each patient for each hospital day.

5. An audit system for formal and systematic verification of patient acuity levels.

In addition to patient dependence, Halloran identifies other factors that contribute to the cost of nursing (Halloran, 1994), including tradition, budgetary constraints, the effects of physical facilities, and the staff nurse organization. Tradition involves how nurses perceive their jobs, as procedural or helping doctors cure patients, for example. Budgetary constraints are inherent in hospital organization, since fundamental changes in budget are, at best, difficult to make. The effect of

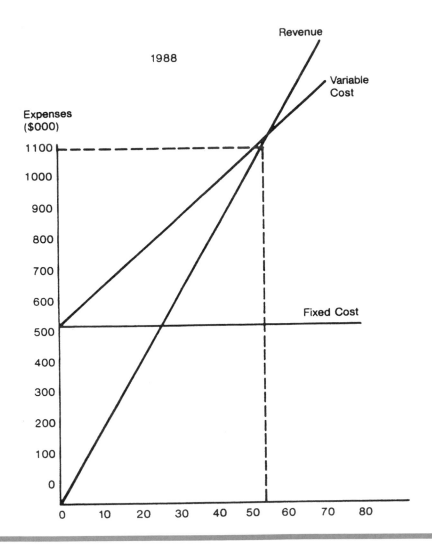

Figure 18.5
Break-even analysis for GCU Occupancy.
Reproduced, with permission, from Johnson (1988).

physical size and layout is important because some ward sizes may be inefficient. And nursing costs can be skewed by nurses' perception of their roles, say, as professional or technical.

Inherent in the above systems is the need to explore a number of other premises, including the ideas that:

- Patient charges should be based on the cost of providing the services.

- Patients should pay for the services they receive and not for that of other patients or other services.

- Organizations can identify, define, measure, and assign revenue to departments, service centers, or product lines that incur the costs for providing the service.

- Hospitals believe patients have a right to know what they are paying for.

- Charges make a contribution to the organization.

Inherent in a costing system is a classification system as a method of sorting the patient population within a given hospital into homogenous groups based on established criteria. To be used for costing, a patient classification system needs to be simple and practical at the staff-nurse level. It would have to include any of the patient's family that nurses teach and/or counsel. The system could not use zeros, because even if the patient does not require a procedure (e.g., ambulation), the nurse is still accountable for monitoring and evaluating the appropriateness of that decision (to ambulate or not to ambulate). The system would emphasize processes instead of tasks and would focus on assessment, planning, intervention, and evaluation of outcomes.

The classification system should be integrated with the patient record, which typically has more accurate data. The value of a classification system lies in its ability to keep outlier patients to a minimum. Moreover, including a classification system in the patient record also allows for archival retrieval of critical information. The system would be based on services delivered instead of perceived patient need.

Staffing systems identify and allocate nursing resources. As such, they need to be flexible enough to include direct care, indirect care, and general unit activities.

Costing systems convert data from classification, staffing, and belief systems to information for identifying the cost of delivering nursing services. In order to accomplish this, nursing and the financial management systems must be integrated, and costs and cost accounting methodologies must be defined similarly.

The final system is the audit system. The audit system verifies the patient acuity level and is most important for the long-term integrity of the data. Since patient acuity drives nursing staffing and thus directly impacts on the costs of nursing, the design and implementation of the audit is critical to the overall success.

The three current models used for costing nursing include:

1. Charge codes specified for services or track (e.g., nursing education, third-party coverage for nursing care).

2. Acuity-based cost on the patient bill without an associated charge.

3. Separating nursing and non-nursing components of room and bed charges using acuity-based nursing costs.

Nursing Resource Use

A study of nursing resource usage and costs in Australia defined the elements of a valid and reliable workload measurement in the acute-care environment (Hovenga, 1994). The workload is necessary as an indicator of resource usage and how nursing service costs can be captured. The many variables that go into determining case mix, resource usage, and inpatient costs are shown in Fig. 18.6. Hovenga suggests that workload monitoring involves using either individual activities or a patient classification method (patient groups).

Nursing classification schemes are needed to classify nursing resource usage for patients in defined groups in order to cost out nursing services. Three ways of classifying patient groups have been defined: patient nurse dependency, diagnosis-related groups (DRGs), and severity of illness.

The problem with classifying patients to determine costs is that different people in the health care environment require different views of patient care and resources. For example, the nursing administrator needs to know the amount and type of nursing services required to care for patients. The health provider is more interested in defining the health care condition with its concurrent diagnoses and therapeutic procedures, whereas the hospital administrator wants to identify patients in classes in terms of total resources to be provided to meet requirements of the patient episode.

In an unpublished study of predicting nursing care costs with nursing diagnoses, Halloran predicts that the

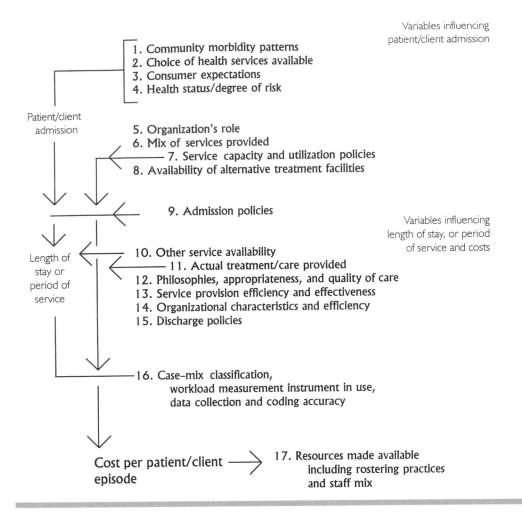

Figure 18.6
Conceptual framework of variables influencing case-mix, resource usage, and inpatient costs.
Reproduced, with permission, from Hovenga (1994).

cost for caring for one nursing diagnosis in a large University Hospital in the United States is $8.90 (based upon 1987 dollars). This figure comes from calculated hours of nursing care to take care of a patient with one nursing diagnosis. To cost out nursing diagnoses, Halloran did not distinguish one nursing diagnosis as more costly than another. He used nursing diagnoses to cost out nursing instead of classification instruments alone, since nursing diagnoses include the physical and functional status of patients in addition to their psychological and social characteristics.

On average, in the acute-care hospital, a patient averages between 13 and 22 nursing diagnoses during a typical hospital stay. In examining the relationship between nursing diagnoses and DRGs and nursing time, Halloran found that 45 percent of the variation in time nurses spent with patients related to their nursing diagnoses; 15 percent to their DRGs; and less than 2 percent to demographics. In addition, in previous publications, he found that nursing diagnoses explained 50–60 percent of the variation in length of stay, except in maternity and newborn nursery environments (Halloran et al., 1988). In this study, the nursing staff manually entered the nursing diagnoses at 3 p.m. each day for each patient. These data were entered into the hospital information system. When aggregated nursing diagnoses were examined, the nurses' management of patient discomfort was the most frequently found nursing diagnosis (altered comfort: discomfort) (Table 18.8).

 ## Case-Mix Management

Case-mix management involves several applications of several systems integrated to determine the patient's demographics, financial payers with cost and charges, and general administrative information including:

- Discharge status
- Length of stay
- DRG classification
- Department usage
- Utilization of services
- Severity of illness
- International Classification of Diseases: Diagnoses and Procedures
- Nursing diagnoses and procedures
- Attending doctor and primary nurse
- Readmission status

Additional nursing-specific data include the acuity of nursing hours and patient classification to determine the patient intensity.

In 1987, Halloran described a nursing management information system based on case-mix and nurse capability. This nursing case-mix complemented the DRG medical system and the social data system. Together they were found to be highly predictive of patient resource use, cost, and length of stay. The cost implications were derived from patient classification (patient demand) and nurse assignment (capability). Patient dependency was examined using nursing diagnoses (Halloran, 1987).

Tong and Jones (1990) described the advantages of case-mix management on patient care, analyzing differences in case-mix managed care versus usual care. The differences in tracking patient care in terms of patient outcomes, length of stay, and costs are shown in Table 18.9. They concluded that case-mix management—designed to maintain optimum quality while conserving resources—is more cost effective in profiling patient care, practice patterns, and budgeting product lines.

 ## Consumer Surveys

Today's administrative applications require more information on performance measures. Performance measures include surveys on the elements of health care, health care providers, and the consumers—or purchasers—of health care services. These measures are important to better

understanding health care services and to improving the health care services provided.

One element of performance measures consumer satisfaction with care. Managed care systems include patient survey information in the minimum data standards, since consumer satisfaction can be used to market the services of an organization. However, the variability in tools to collect satisfaction information limits the ability to compare data from health plans. The principal advantage of standardizing consumer response is the ability to make comparisons among the multiple sites of hospital chains. Standardization may also benefit aggregating data to develop state-of-the-art survey instruments.

 ## Patient Satisfaction

Patient satisfaction information becomes more important to today's outcomes-oriented health care. After all, it's possible to have positive outcomes with negative patient satisfaction, as well as the opposite situation, in which despite a negative outcome, the consumer or significant other was very satisfied with the care. In addition to satisfaction surveys, consumers must be queried regarding their decisions about purchasing health care, their attitudes toward products, and their perceptions of convenience, location, price, reputation, and quality. Demographic patient data—socioeconomic level, age, gender, race, and address—need to be collected in relation to the survey.

 ## Access to Care

Another element of consumer surveys is access to care. The Institute of Medicine defines access as "a shorthand term for a broad set of concerns that center on the degree to which individuals and groups are able to obtain needed services from the medical care system" (Millman, 1993). This same report describes specific indicators to measure access, including prenatal care and breast and cervical cancer screening. The number of patients who have encounters with the health care system, the amount of time they wait, the availability of primary care or specialty physicians, and the availability of nurse practitioners to triage patients become more important in managed care computer systems.

Nursing Unit Management's Data Needs

Like those for nursing administration, the essential applications for nursing unit management systems have also expanded. Today, they include:

Table 18.8   Nursing hours and cost per patient condition by division using nursing diagnoses

Areas	Nursing Diagnoses		Total Number Nsg. Dx for Time Interval	Nursing Hours (a) Worked per Nursing Dx			Nursing Hours (b) Paid per Nursing Dx			Cost (c) Worked Hours per Nursing Dx			Cost (d) Paid Hours per Nursing Dx		
	Total Patient Days Reported	Mean Number Nsg. Dx for Patient Day		*	**	***	*	**	***	*	**	***	*	**	***
MATERNITY/PERINATAL NURSING															
M4	4,685	8.807	41,263	0.99	1.60	1.60	1.60	1.82	1.82	13.95	20.02	20.02	16.37	23.47	23.47
MA5	8,476	13.379	188,643 (e)	0.33	0.59	0.59	0.37	0.67	0.67	4.34	7.27	7.27	5.09	8.49	8.49
MN5	6,017	12.505													
MA6	1,709	12.852	26,010 (e)	2.32	3.43	3.43	2.60	3.91	3.91	30.98	41.01	41.01	35.71	47.83	47.83
MN6	438	9.2371													
Total & Mean MacDonald	21,325	12.001	255,916	.063	1.04	1.04	0.72	1.19	1.19	8.60	12.76	12.76	10.02	14.91	14.91

(a) Total nursing hours worked for time interval - total number of nursing diagnoses for time interval.
(b) Total nursing hours paid for time interval including benefits - total number of nursing diagnoses for time interval.
(c) Total nursing dollars paid for worked hours for time interval - total number of nursing diagnoses for time interval.
(d) Total nursing dollars paid for time interval including benefits - total number of nursing diagnoses for time interval.
*   Category of worker includes head nurse, assistant head nurse, advanced clinical nurse, staff nurse I & II, PRN nurse, LPN I & II, or tech I & II.
**   All categories of workers.
*** All categories of workers except for Hemo, PES, AES, and OR/RR.
Reproduced, with permission, from Halloran (1994).

Table 18.9   Financial effects of two treatment plans

Case as Managed	Alternate Treatment
Tuesday	**Tuesday**
Admission for severe anemia, chronic rectal bleeding, lower abdominal pain	Admission for severe anemia, chronic rectal bleeding, lower abdominal cramps
Workup for anemia	Consultation by gastroenterologist
Transfusions	Workup for anemia
	Transfusions
Wednesday	
Consultation by gastroenterologist	**Wednesday**
	Upper endoscopy of stomach and duodenum
Thursday	
Upper endoscopy of stomach and duodenum	**Thursday**
	Barum enema (large bowel X-ray study)
Friday	Attending physician checks results; cancer of the cecum
Barium enema (Large bowel X-ray study)	Call surgeon
	Coordinate colonoscopy and surgery
Saturday	
Attending physician checks results: cancer of the cecum	**Friday and Saturday (Sunday)**
	Bowel preparation with laxatives and antibiotics
Monday	
Surgical consult	**Monday**
	Colonoscopy followed by resection of right colon
Tuesday	Eight-day postoperative management
Colonoscopy	
Wednesday	
Bowel preparation with laxatives and antibiotics	**Total length of stay:** 14 days
	Cost savings:
Friday	Four hospital days $2,180.00
Resection of right colon	One bowel preparation 11.17
Eight-day postoperative management	**Total savings:** $2,191.17
Total length of stay: 14 Days	18 percent of total cost
Total cost: $12,405	

Reproduced, with permission, from Tong and Jones (1990).

- ■ Nursing intensity
- ■ Patient classification systems
- ■ Acuity systems
- ■ Staffing and scheduling systems
- ■ Inventory
- ■ Patient billing
- ■ Incident reports
- ■ Poison control
- ■ Allergy and drug reactions
- ■ Error reports
- ■ Infection control
- ■ Unit activity reports
- ■ Utilization review
- ■ Shift summary reports

Nursing Intensity

Nursing intensity includes measures of nursing hours per patient day derived from census data, cost data, and patient classification or workload measures. It comprises patient acuity and patient classification or workload measurement and helps determine required nursing resources (Thompson and Diers, 1991). To date, there is no single system that provides unit-to-unit or hospital-to-hospital comparisons. As a result, an administrator comparing intensity per case could not determine if variances are due to differences in patient acuity or to bias introduced by using different classification or workload measurements. Comparing hospitals, one could not determine if the intensity is due to different levels of personnel, sicker patients, or poor administrative management. Until systems that weight or risk-adjust the many variables involved in assessing intensity, cross-site comparisons will be based upon several underlying assumptions.

Nursing intensity refers to the amount and type of nursing resources used to care for an individual patient over the entire hospital stay or episode of care (O'Brien-Pallas and Giovanetti, 1993). Further, nursing resources are defined as the nursing care time (in hours) required to deliver both direct and indirect care and the mix or level of nursing staff involved in the delivery of that care (Giovanetti, 1978).

The Patient Intensity of Nursing Index (PINI) includes the amount of care measured in hours. It includes complexity of care, the clinical judgement necessary to care for patients in specific clinical settings, and medical severity (Prescott, 1991). This is one of the models that includes a risk adjustment in the acquisition of data.

Recently, intensity has been expanded to include hours of care, complexity of patient conditions, medical severity, and the environment (O'Brien-Pallas et al., 1994).

Halloran (1985) and Reitz (1985) have also developed patient classification measures that incorporate nursing's critical thinking associated with assessment and management of patient care. These systems have been developed and tested mostly in adult medical and surgical patients.

In a recent validation study of nursing intensity measures, Rosenthal et al. (1992) described the use of a nursing severity index based on nursing diagnoses. The finding that the nursing severity index was related to mortality rates and had other prognostic accuracy similar to other nursing intensity scores validates this tool as potentially useful in case-mix, outcomes assessment, quality assurance, and care management. Though the prognostic accuracy of this system was similar to commercially available and widely used severity-of-illness measures (Medigroups), the system needs to be tested in a variety of hospitals to determine if hospital comparability and variance can be explained by nursing diagnoses.

Patient Classification Systems

An approach to management efficiency is the patient classification system, a scheme by which patients' needs for nursing services can be assessed (Jelinek et al., 1973; Jelinek et al.,1974)

Patient classification is defined as the "identification and classification of patients into groups or categories and the quantification of these categories as a measure of the nursing effort required [in care giving]" (Giovanetti, 1979). Such systems are ultimately used to plan nurse staffing assignments based on patient needs. Hundreds of such systems exist, their development stimulated by JCAHO recommendations in the 1980s that all hospitals use a documented method to allocate and distribute nurses based on patient care requirements.

JCAHO standards (Joint Commission on Accreditation of Healthcare Organizations, 1993, 1999) include: "The nurse executive and other appropriate registered nurses develop hospital-wide patient care programs, policies, and procedures that describe how the nursing care needs of patients or patient populations are assessed, evaluated, and met. . . . The hospital's plan for providing nursing care is designed to support improvement and innovations in nursing practice and is based on both the needs of the patients to be served and the hospital's mission."

There are three types of patient classification systems that rely on task determinations:

1. Those that use a system to identify patient profiles and predict the need for nursing,

2. Those that identify all nursing care tasks associated with patient care and standard times used to conduct each task, then sum the tasks to produce hours of care needed, and

3. Those that use a critical indicator approach, basing total nursing care time on a few indicators of care which are weighted to reflect relative nursing effort.

In 1978, the federal government published reports on methods for studying nurse staffing in a patient unit. The report recommended establishing staffing needs by comparing the service level with care estimates based on patient classification and the head nurse's perception of adequate care. The model also provided a conceptual framework for evaluating personnel skills or different staffing patterns (Division of Nursing, DHHS, 1978).

Today, however, many issues still exist in choosing a patient classification system, including whether a staffing formula based on patient classification is reliable and which method of patient classification is best for a particular institution.

A stated aim of patient classification and its methodology is to match staffing to patient requirements in order to:

■ Optimize personnel use

■ Improve the quality of care

■ Reduce costs engendered by overstaffing

Furthermore, patient classification systems represent a methodological approach unique to the nursing profession. By devising a method to assess patients' needs for nursing care—and thus the hours of care required during each 24-hour period and the category of personnel needed—a quantitative statement of patients' requirements for nursing care can be established. Better classification systems include measures of functional status, patterns of dependency, and quality-of-life measures to support clinical nursing decisions.

Today, computers are used administratively not only in hospitals but also in long-term care facilities, community and home health agencies, ambulatory care centers, and independent nursing practices—the entire continuum of care (Sennett, 1992). These settings also require quality management to ensure the value of purchased care. Information Technology (IT) will allow organizations to identify inappropriate care or inefficient and excessive care, as well as low-cost alternatives. Such programs are marketed as health care management systems.

With hundreds of classification systems available, it is impossible to estimate overall time, complexity of patient care, and nursing contribution to outcomes. Unless one classification system is used, it is impossible to compare nursing's use of time, skills, and complexities from setting to setting.

There are three possible solutions:

1. Develop a national model for a patient classification system that all hospitals would use

2. Allow each site to use its own system and never use classification in outcomes research

3. Reduce all systems to a common denominator that then could be used to study variability of nursing time, complexity, and costs across different patient conditions.

The third approach was used by Thompson and Diers (1988), who described nursing care costs across different DRGs in an eight-hospital study with different patient classification systems. They converted all classification systems to the common denominator of time of patient care. Adding some form of hours of nursing care to a national database would allow one to see trends in nursing care per patient condition (Prescott, 1994). According to Prescott, the major disadvantage to using hours of nursing care as a measure of nursing intensity is the lack of inclusion of complexity in the definition and the fact that many hospitals do not store patient classifications electronically.

One of the disadvantages of using current classification systems is that no one has developed efficient ways to adjust risk for patients' age, gender, socioeconomic status, and numbers of conditions or for nursing skill levels (e.g., MSN, BNS, ADN, or diploma, licensed or not licensed assistive personnel). Nursing skill levels also confound measurement of hours of care given (McHugh, 1994). Therefore, aggregating one hospital against another does not reflect the sicker, older, or more disadvantaged patients compared with another group or the level and/or experience of the nurse provider.

Since most measures arrive at a number of nurses per patient or per medical or nursing diagnosis, current systems account for the role of clinical nurse specialists, case managers, or consultants. With the move away from acute-care environments, and with patients receiving care in day care centers or urgent-care environments, it is difficult to resolve the concept of unit of time versus episode of care. Should the classification include the concept of time per day, episode of care, or encounter of care? Nurse administrators should understand these basic limitations when interpreting and comparing certain outcome measures.

Decision Support System

A patient classification decision support system should include more than patient classification for nursing staffing. An example of a variance report based on acuity level derived from a decision support system is shown in Table 18.10. It should integrate costing of nursing services, budgeting, program assessment, quality screens, activity tracking, communication with departments, and development of nursing charges per patient. The reports needed in today's environment are average value per patient, per-skill mix per shift, and hours or units of classification by day or stay. The decision support systems that produce such information are the engines needed by the critical path manager or the case manager to integrate costs with resources and outcomes of care.

The advantage to these systems is that they can:

- Identify high volume cases
- Develop treatment profiles
- Build profiles of baseline data for usual lengths of stay, costs, outcomes, and staffing requirements
- Review the patient distribution across nursing units
- Identify providers associated with high or low outcomes for special patient conditions

Nurse case managers can build treatment profiles by day or stay; separate normative patients from outliers; pick out model providers who attain outcomes; compare alternate patterns with outcomes and between nursing services, skill mix, experience mix, or units; and identify the cost per case.

In 1983, many Australian hospitals began using a classification scheme developed there by Hovenga (1994), the Patient Assessment and Information System (PAIS). The system's use has been extended to allocating nursing services and costing nursing services per DRG. One of the difficulties in adapting PAIS for many hospitals in Australia was the lack of a uniform nursing language system to classify and describe consistently how nurses describe their practice and what they do. When examining nursing work, Hovenga finds the elements in Table 18.11 important to analyzing nursing

work. She further classifies nursing work in terms of direct patient/nurse interactions (medication administration), indirect patient related interactions (documentation), and indirect non–patient-related interactions (education and committee attendance).

Acuity Systems

Acuity reflects the relative proportion of nursing time required for each classified patient type. Classification translated into workload equals acuity. Staffing is based on patient types. Newer computer systems integrate acuity with nursing care planning or cost out nursing based on acuity needs.

Software programs, interchangeable with programmable calculators, can compute staffing needs, allocate staff, and construct management reports. In addition, they provide a unit profile that adjusts for staff illness and absences, overtime, and other factors.

In 1989, Weitzman and Clapham described Northwestern University Hospital's use of the HBO (now McKesson HBOC) clinical cost accounting system to integrate acuity into a clinical cost accounting-decision support system. Relying on the system developed at Northwestern that classifies patients into five levels of acuity, the combined decision analysis system incorporates 60 other factors divided among 14 categories to classify patients into groups according to level of illness and nursing care requirements.

The two major components are patient attributes and nursing staffing data. The 14 categories of nursing activities assign a weight to care, patient status, medication and IV, irrigation, special treatments, emotional support, diet, hygienic needs, and observations. The system is only useful if the patient has at least one overnight stay. Data are entered for days, evenings, and nights. A clinical nurse manager, who is not included in the staffing score, oversees the validity of the scores. The system identifies three levels of nursing skills: registered, licensed, or graduate, and nursing assistants in 2-, 4-, and 8-hour timeframes. Nursing acuity scores reflect charge codes that are unit- and acuity-level-specific.

A study by Kuhn (1980) stated that one could predict 69 percent of variation in nursing activity and staffing by assessing hygiene, nutrition, elimination, body fluids, patient gender, and whether the patient was quadriplegic, paraplegic, or terminally ill. Halloran (1985) found that the patient's ability to perform activities of daily living (ADL), degree of mobility, and the presence of pain were predictive of the nursing care needs.

Table 18.10   Variance report based on acuity level

	Actual Cost (1)	Budget Cost (2)	Total Variance (3)	% Total Variance (4)	% Volume Variance (5)	% Rate Variance (6)	% Efficiency Variance (7)
CCU							
Acuity Level 1	40,887.57	39,535.62	1,351.95	3.42	−0.87	4.09	0.20
Acuity Level 2	7,237.07	7,141.22	99.85	1.34	2.15	0.40	−1.21
Acuity Level 3	19,600.79	20,217.24	−616.45	−3.05	1.01	−1.61	−2.45
Acuity Level 4	34,559.73	35,323.17	−763.44	−2.16	−1.58	4.65	−5.23
Acuity Level 5	21,548.42	21,175.61	372.81	1.76	0.00	12.36	−10.60
Total CCU	123,833.59	123,392.87	440.72	0.36	-0.33	19.53	−18.85

Reproduced, with permission, from HBOC, Star Product. Unpublished internal user document, 1992, Atlanta, GA.

Table 18.11   Elements important when analyzing nursing work

- Time required to perform the job
- Organization and methods employed, including the availability and use of labor saving devices
- Cost of providing the nursing service
- Numbers of patients cared for
- Education, skills, experience, and physical attributes required to perform the job
- Boundaries of nursing practice and relationship with other health professionals
- Philosophical basis of work performed and its relationship to objectives to be achieved
- Working conditions relative to award requirements or other health workers
- The value of the job
- Level of agreement of actual job to job description
- Level of job satisfaction
- Opportunity for staff development and career advancement
- The quality of the product in terms of:
    - Meeting organizational objectives
    - Meeting professional standards of practice
    - Compliance with legal and statutory regulations
    - Meeting consumer expectations
    - Meeting other health workers' expectations
    - Meeting accreditation requirements

Reproduced, with permission, from Hovenga (1994).

Finnegan et al. (1993) describes the need to link acuity systems with cost, care, and quality measurement to determine patient outcomes. The resultant system produces a more complete picture of nursing's role in outcomes.

 ## Staffing and Scheduling Systems

Computer systems for staffing and scheduling have existed for more than 3 decades. Staff rosters and scheduling systems are available on a variety of platforms, from mainframes to PCs. They can operate on the hospital's patient acuity system or census, and they provide daily staffing worksheets, productivity sheets, and assignments based on qualifications, unit preference, and skills. Scheduler systems create customized schedules and automatically incorporate workload, work preferences in nursing, special requisitions, and assignments to continuing education programs.

The success of a nurse scheduling system depends on being able to accommodate many of the constraints involved in adequately staffing a hospital (Okada, 1992), including:

- Recognizing day-to-day sequencing of the varied roles a nurse may assume. For example, the system may include hospital policy describing how many consecutive days a person must remain on the night shift.

- Satisfying individual preferences for days off or particular tasks. For example, some nurses need every Monday off for childcare, or they prefer to staff only patients with particular conditions.

- Requiring an equality of workload. For example, weekend/holiday services must be distributed equally among nurses, monthly or annually.

- Constraining team member composition. For example, nurses have special skills, and a hospital requirement may be that at least two leadership nurses must be available on each shift. Another example is that the team must be composed of one nurse from each skill category.

Administrative systems help nursing managers manage patient data, staff data, and financial data. A comprehensive system includes acuity, staffing, scheduling, staff profiles, assignments, and management reports.

McHugh (1987) focused on studying four staffing patterns using computer simulation to examine differences in wage costs and in over- and understaffing produced by these patterns. The patterns that she studied include fixed distributed, float pool, controlled variable, and skill center staffing.

The study modeled three types of hospitals: a small community hospital, a large community hospital and a large Veterans Affairs hospital. She found that fixed variable staffing produced the highest wage costs, followed by float pool staffing. There were no differences between controlled variable and skill staffing for mean yearly wage costs. With regard to the incidence of overstaffing, fixed distributed staffing performed poorly compared with the other three staffing patterns.

 ## Inventory

An inventory is a record of pharmacy items and other supplies that are received and disbursed; it shows what is in stock on nursing units. These applications provide necessary information for auditing and analyzing use of unit stock and maintenance files on unit stock activity. Nursing unit managers are often accountable for records related to storeroom and sterile supplies. Computerized supply inventories give them the capability to account for stock items, track expired lots, and bill patients for supplies used.

A special type of inventory is the narcotic usage inventory, which produces special records describing the receipt, disbursement, and amount of narcotic drugs on a nursing unit. These systems can produce summary reports acceptable for legal documentation of narcotic usage.

The inventory that utilizes bar codes has become the primary foundation for billing patients, the mechanism to measure utilization, and an automated tracking system of resource consumption.

Patient Billing

Computers allow nurse managers to enter charges for services rendered or supplies used. More important, computers can record charges and transmit them to patient files to be compiled and entered into the patient's overall bill. Two stages of compilers are common:

1. Those that record charges for compilations and correct incorrect charges.

2. Those that transmit unit charges to a central automated record compiled with the patient's total hospital bill.

Other Unit Management Reports

Many nursing unit management reports can be recorded and transmitted to the appropriate hospital department. Such reports cover the following:

- Incident reports
- Poison control
- Allergy and drug reactions
- Error reports
- Infection control
- Unit activity reports
- Utilization review
- Shift summary reports

Incident Reports

Incident reports identify patient, visitor, or personnel accidents. With documented records of incidents, an organization can initiate corrective policies, education, or research programs. When incident reports are printed in the risk management office as they occur, corrective actions may be taken. For example, if a nurse receives a needle puncture, the nurse administrator might inform that nurse to seek corrective treatment immediately, assign a float nurse to cover, and inform the head nurse of an emergency sick leave request.

When incident report summaries indicate statistically significant occurrences of particular problems (e.g., patient falls and medication errors), the incidents may precipitate policy changes, new documentation requirements, or in-service education programs. If patients fall frequently on geriatric services, nurse administrators may want to determine if the nursing assessment for documentation on the computer includes a category for "mobility" or "potential for trauma." If nursing personnel are not using that category either before or after an incident, in-service education, policy changes, and documentation requirements might be considered.

Poison Control

Poison control report systems can maintain files of accidental poisonings and include information on the most common toxic substances and appropriate antidotes or therapy.

Allergy and Drug Reactions

Allergy and drug reaction reports include not only patients with particular allergies but also those patients receiving medications known to have incompatibilities. These lists can be produced regularly, and logs can be compiled indicating the number of patients who have come in contact with drugs they are allergic to or medications that are incompatible with other drugs.

Error Reports

Error reports may include medication or documentation errors. They can be summarized and transmitted to a nurse administrator for review on a regular basis. Some error systems track errors on-line, alerting nurse managers to take quick corrective action. Today's error systems flag the inappropriate assignment of DRG codes to patients, inappropriate use of procedures and tests, undocumented follow-up on abnormal procedures, and delays in scheduling tests and procedures and provide closer monitoring of errors related to the achievement of outcomes.

Infection Control

Infection control reports recognize patterns of bacterial or viral spread throughout a hospital or nursing unit. These systems integrate infection reports, incident reports, and laboratory culture, screening reports over time to describe patterns of probable infection in the hospital. Often areas of contamination can be recognized from these reports. Computerized monitoring provides summary information.

The HELP system has an automated antibiotic consultant that chooses the appropriate antibiotic regimen for a patient when pathogens are reported (Evans et al., 1993). The antibiotic assistant also helps identify patients receiving inappropriate antibiotic therapy as soon as the antibiotic susceptibility tests are known.

Unit Activity Reports

Unit activity reports include census, patient status, shift reports, other unit activities, procedures, and identification of patients at risk. Widely computerized, they provide timely information that the unit nurse can input and send to the nursing administrator. In some hospitals, evening and night supervisors no longer collect, photocopy, and distribute shift reports, causing many hospitals to eliminate this level of supervision.

Patients at risk can be automatically and rapidly identified through computer systems. In addition, when special procedures or medications are ordered for patients at risk, alert notices are printed at the nursing station. If emergencies occur, emergency procedures can be printed on the unit.

Utilization Review

Utilization review summary reports include information on the concurrent review of all patients. Information is available to certify each patient for admission and length of stay. Patient demographics information is combined with the diagnosis and operative information to determine length-of-stay data. Daily summary reports may then be produced for utilization review. The summary report lists all patients who must be reviewed for admission certification and extension of length of stay.

Utilization review subsystems are available. Reports are available 5 days a week to identify patients who are near the end of their certified stays and those who need continued stay review. The report includes up-to-date patient information, including diagnoses, procedures, previous certification detail, and reviewer comments.

The utilization review is sequenced by the nursing station, identified hospital service and bed, or last review coordinator and bed review. Daily summaries are provided when needed, and current and future review loads are predicted. To indicate future staffing needs, the system provides summaries of future patient loads. Each month, the summary reports review each patient's admitting diagnosis to:

- Provide information to establish cost rates for each diagnosis
- Examine the effectiveness of review mechanism
- Support more effective discharge scheduling

These systems can provide either diagnosis or procedure reviews.

Newer utilization review applications pool successful procedures and tests to attain outcomes, document and reference literature that supports the appropriate use of the procedures and tests, and provide boundaries of practice for the health care provider.

Shift Summary Reports

Shift summary reports computerize summaries of patient classifications, acuity/staffing information, and nursing personnel information. These cumulative shift reports integrate the information of other nursing unit reports and are then transmitted to the nursing administrator to integrate with nursing service information. These records are also integrated with the hospital or nursing department budgeting system.

The Future of Computerized Nursing Administrative Systems

Several critical trends—from globalization to the culture of change and the rise of the information age—will fuel development and deployment of future information technology.

Because each technological advance spawns another, no one can predict the tools health care will have at its disposal in the 21st century. What is reasonably certain, however, is that there are many tools that promise to improve patient care, reduce its cost, and make it easier to provide. Table 18.12 (Simpson, 1999) lists some of the more promising developments with their applications and implications for nursing.

Summary

This chapter presented a broadened description of the expanded responsibilities of today's nurse administrator. Because of these increased responsibilities, this chapter also described the expanded systems that serve as tools for nursing services administration and nursing unit management. Because nursing administration has more obligations, there has been an increase in the number and depth of computer applications that facilitate efficient capture of financial data. Today's nurse administrator has moved into the role of corporate executive officer with obligations to report to the institution, to society, and to national accrediting bodies. These responsibilities are also imposed by the professional practice of nursing. Today's nurse administrator needs more than a basic understanding of word-processing and E-mail systems. Today's nurse administrator has a moral obligation to help improve health care costs by better managing nursing information.

Table 18.12 Emerging Technologies for Nursing

The Technology	What It Is or What It Does	How Nursing Can Use It	What It Means for Nursing
Internet	The vast collection of interconnected networks that all use the TCP/IP protocols and that evolved from the *ARPANET* of the late 1960s and early 1970s.[a]	Distance learning, research clinical decision-making, wellness models, telemedicine	• Better information and much more of it can improve patient care • Patient education can enhance wellness • Degree of access/experience becoming a critical professional differentiator
Continuous speech recognition (CSR)	Natural or conversational speech is recorded, and phoneme recognition is used to recognize streams of speech sounds. Phonemes are the smallest units of speech sounds, similar to "atoms" of speech.[b]	Charting	• Reduces time spent on administration so that more can be spent on patient care • Lack of accepted nursing vocabulary limits data retrievability
Wireless computing	Any mobile terminal, mobile station, personal station, or personal terminal using nonfixed access to the network.	Point-of-care data collection/retrieval	• Improved patient care
Thin-client computing	A "stripped down" personal computer designed specifically to be a client in a client/server network.	Home care, ambulatory care, nursing/health care corporations	• Cheaper technology; thin clients tend to cost less than fully equipped models, since they don't need full software or internal devices of their own. • Easier to learn/maintain
Data warehouses, data marts, and data mining	• A data warehouse is a central repository for data collected by various business systems across the enterprise. • A data mart is a subset of the data warehouse, designed to serve a particular community of knowledge workers (e.g., nurses). • Data mining is the analysis of data for new relationships.	Research; clinical decision-making; patient education	• Improves clinical decision-making by providing access to data from all parts of the enterprise that can be drilled down for nursing specificity • Lack of defined nursing vocabulary limits data mart utility

Reproduced, with permission, from Simpson (1999).
[a]Glossary of Internet Terms, *http://www.matisse.net/files/glossary.html#Internet.*
[b]Clark, Holly, "Continuous Speech Recognition: What You Should Know," *Journal of AHIMA*, October 1998, *http://www.ahima.org/publications/2f/focus.3.1098.html.*

References

American Association of Nurse Executives (The AONE) in Cooperation with the Center for Healthcare Information Management (CHIM). (1993). *Informatics: Issues and Strategies for the 21st Century Health Care Executive. Resource Book and Video Set.* Chicago: American Hospital Association Services, Inc.

American Nurses' Association Task Force on Standards for Organized Nursing Services. (1988). *Standards for Organized Nursing Services and Responsibilities of Nurse Administrators Across all Settings.* Kansas City, MO: American Nurses' Association.

Anderson, R. A., Dobal, M. T., and Blessing, B. B. (1992). Theory-based approach to skill development in nursing administration. *Computers in Nursing, 10*(4), 152–157.

Austin, C. (1979). *Information Systems for Hospital Administration.* Ann Arbor, MI: Health Administration Press.

Dick, R. S., and Steen, E. B. (Eds.). (1991). *The Computer-Based Patient Record: An Essential Technology for Health Care.* Institute of Medicine, Washington, D. C.: National Academy Press.

Division of Nursing, DHHS. (1978). *Methods for Studying Nurse Staffing in a Patient Unit: A Manual to Aid Hospitals in Making Use of Personnel,* (DHHS pub. no. 78-3). Washington, D.C.: U.S. Government Printing Office.

Evans, R. S., Pestotnik, S. L., Classen, D. C., and Burke, J. P. (1993). Development of an automated antibiotic consultant. *M.D. Computing, 10*(10), 17–22.

Filosa, L. (1970). Automated communication saves time, money. *Hospital Progress, 49,* 115–118.

Finnegan, S. A., Abel, M., Dobler, T., et al. (1993). Automated patient acuity: linking nursing systems and quality measurement with patient outcomes. *Journal of Nursing Administration, 23*(5), 62–71.

Garre, P. P. (1990). A computerized recruitment program. *Journal of Nursing Administration, 20*(1), 24–7.

Giovanetti, P. (1978). *Patient Classification Systems in Nursing: A Description and Analysis* (DHEW, Publ. No. HRA 78–22). Hyattsville, MD: Government Printing Office.

Giovanetti, P. (1979). Understanding patient classification systems. *Journal of Nursing Management, 15*(8), 31–34.

Halloran, E. (1985). Nursing workload, medical diagnosis related groups, and nursing diagnoses. *Research in Nursing & Health, 8,* 421–433.

Halloran, E. (1987). Case-Mix: Matching patient need with nursing resource. *Nursing Management, 18*(3), 27–42.

Halloran, E., Kiley, M. L., and England, M. (1988). Nursing diagnosis, DRGs and length of stay. *Applied Nursing Research, 18*(3), 27–39.

HBOC. (1992). Star Product. Unpublished internal user document. Atlanta, GA.

Hovenga, E. (1994). *Casemix, Hospital Nursing Resource Usage and Costs: The Basis for a Nursing Utilization Review System.* Doctoral Dissertation.

Jelinek, R., Zinn, T., and Brya, J. (1973). Tell the computer how sick the patients are and it will tell how many nurses they need. *Modern Hospital, 121,* 81–85.

Jelinek, R., Haussman, D., Hegyvary, S., and Newman, J. (1974). *A Methodology for Monitoring Quality of Nursing Care,* (DHEW pub. no. HRA 74-25). Washington, D. C: U.S. Government Printing Office.

Johnson, J. (Ed.). (1988). *The Nurse Executive's Business Plan.* Rockville, MD: Aspen Publishers, Inc.

Joint Commission on Accreditation of Healthcare Organizations. (1993). *Accreditation Manual for Hospitals* (AMH).Oakbrook Terrace, IL.

Joint Commission on Accreditation of Healthcare Organizations. (1999). *HAS 1999 Hospital Accreditation Standards.* Oakbrook Terrace, IL.

Kuhn, B. G. (1980). Prediction of nursing requirements from patient characteristics. Parts I & II. *International Journal of Nursing Studies, 17,* 5–12; 69–78.

Little, A. D. (1992). *Telecommunications: Can It Help Solve America's Health Care Problems* (Reference No. 91810-98).

McHugh, M. (1987). *Comparison of Four Nurse Staffing Patterns for Wage Costs and Staffing Adequacy Using Computer Simulation.* Doctoral Dissertation. Ann Arbor, MI: The University of Michigan.

McHugh, M. (1994). Issues in defining "intensity of nursing care": as an element of the nursing minimum dataset (unpublished). *Report to the Database Steering Committee,* March 12. American Nurses Association.

Melmon, K. (1971). Preventable drug reaction- causes and cures. *New England Journal of Medicine, 284*(24), 1, 361.

Millman, M. (Ed.). (1993). *Access to Health Care in America.* Institute of Medicine Report. Washington, D. C.: National Academy Press.

O'Brien-Pallas, L. and Giovanetti, P. (1993). Nursing intensity. In M. Ogilvie and E. Sawyer (Eds.). *Managing Information in Canadian Health Care Facilities.* Ottawa, Canada: Canadian Hospital Association Press.

O'Brien-Pallas, L., Giovanetti, P, and Peerboom, E. (1994). *Care Costing and Nursing Workload: Past, Present and Future, A Review of the Literature.* University of Toronto: Quality of Nursing Worklife Monograph Series.

Office of the Actuary, Health Care Financing Administration. National Health Expenditures Projections: 1998-2008. *http://www.hcfa.gov/stats/NHE-Proj/proj 1998/hilites.htm*

Okada, M. (1992). An approach to the generalized nurse scheduling problem-generation of a declarative program to represent institution-specific knowledge.

Computers and Biomedical Research, 25(5), 417–434.

Picone, D. M. (1991). *Casemix Funding: Professional and Industrial Impacts on Nursing*. National Casemix Conference.

Porter, S. (1994). Complying with JCAHO's IM Standards. *Healthcare Informatics, 11*(7), 62, 64, 66.

Prescott, P. (1991). Nursing intensity: Needed today for more than nurse staffing. *Nursing Economics, 9*(6), 409–414.

Reitz, J. (1985). Toward a comprehensive nursing intensity index. Part I, Development, and Part II Testing. *Nursing Management, 16*, 21–42.

Rosenthal, G. E., Halloran, E. J, Kiley, M. et al. (1992). Development and validation of the nursing severity index: A new method for measuring severity of illness using nursing diagnoses. *Medical Care, 30*(12), 1127–1141.

Schmitz, H., Ellerbrake, R., and Williams, T. (1976). Study evaluates effects of new communication system. *Hospitals, 50*, 129.

Sennett, C. (1992). The computer-based patient record: The third party payer's perspective. In M. J. Ball, and M. F. Morris (Eds.), *Aspects of the Computer-based Patient Record* (pp. 40–45). New York: Springer-Verlag.

Silva, J. S., and Zawilski, A. J. (1992). The health care professional's workstation: Its functional components and user impacts. In M.J. Ball, and M.F. Collen. (Eds.), *Aspects of the Computer-based Patient Record* (pp.102–124). New York: Springer-Verlag.

Simpson, R. (1991a). The role of the clinical nurse specialist in information systems selection. *Clinical Nurse Specialist, 5*(3), 159–163.

Simpson, R. (1991b). The Joint Commission did what you wouldn't. *Nursing Management, 22*(1), 26–27.

Simpson, R. (1991c). Technology: Nursing the system, computer-based patient records. Part I: The Institute of Medicine's Vision. *Nursing Management, 22*(10), 24–25.

Simpson, R. (1991d). Technology: Nursing the system, computer-based patient records, Part II: IOM's 12 Requisites. *Nursing Management, 22*(11), 26–27.

Simpson, R. (1992). *Decision Support for Product Line Management in Technology: Nursing the System*. Atlanta, GA: HBO.

Simpson, R. (1999). Toward a new millennium: outlook and obligations for 21st century health care technology. *Nursing Administration Quarterly, 24*(1), 1–2.

Thompson, J. D. (1981). Prediction of nurse resource use in treatment of diagnosis related groups. In H. Werley, and M. R. Grier (Eds.), *Nursing Information Systems* (pp. 60–75). New York: Springer.

Thompson, J. D., and Diers, D. (1988). Management of nursing intensity. *Nursing Clinics of North America, 23*(2), 473–491.

Thompson, J. D., and Diers, D. (1991). *Nursing Resources: DRG Their Design and Development* (pp. 121–122). Ann Arbor, MI: Health Administration Press.

Tong, D. A., Jones, P. L. (1990). Physicians, financial managers join forces to control costs. *Healthcare Financial Management*.

Ullian, E. (1992). Hospital administrators' needs for computer-based patient records. In M. J. Ball and M. F. Collen (Eds.), *Aspects of the Computer-based Patient Record* (pp. 30–35). New York: Springer-Verlag.

United States Advisory Council on the National Information Infrastructure. A Nation of Opportunity: A Final Report of the United States Advisory Council on the National Information Infrastructure. *http://www.ed. psu. edu/INSYS/ESD/tech/Highway/nation.impact.html#health*

Van Slyck, A. (1991a). A systems approach to the management of nursing services. Part I: Introduction. *Nursing Management, 22*(3), 16–19.

Van Slyck, A. (1991b). A systems approach to the management of nursing services. Part II: Patient classification system. *Nursing Management, 22*(4), 23–25.

Van Slyck, A. (1991c). A systems approach to the management of nursing services. Part III: Staffing system. *Nursing Management, 22*(5), 30–34.

Van Slyck, A. (1991d). A systems approach to the management of nursing services. Part IV: Productivity monitoring system. *Nursing Management, 22*(6), 18–20.

Van Slyck, A. (1991e). A systems approach to the management of nursing services. Part V: The audit system. *Nursing Management, 22*(7), 14–15.

Van Slyck, A. (1991f). A systems approach to the management of nursing services, Part VI: Costing system. *Nursing Management, 22*(8), 14–16.

Van Slyck, A. (1991g). A systems approach to the management of nursing services. Part VII: Billing system. *Nursing Management, 22*(9), 18–21.

Weitzman, L. J., and Clapham, K. T. (1989). Nursing acuity sensitive decision support system. In L. Kingsland (Ed.). *Proceedings from the Thirteenth Annual Symposium on Computer Applications in Medical Care* (pp. 844–847). Washington, DC: IEEE Computer Society Press.

Selected Readings

Ball, M. J., and Collen, M. F. (Eds.). (1992). *Aspects of the Computer-based Patient Record*. New York: Springer-Verlag.

Connor, R. et al. (1961). Effective use of nursing resources: A research report. *Hospital, 35*, 30–39.

Davies, A. R. (1992). Health care researchers' needs for computer-based patient records. In M. J. Ball and M. F. Collen (Eds.), *Aspects of the Computer-based Patient Record* (pp.46–56). New York: Springer-Verlag.

Diers, D. (1992). Diagnosis related groups and the measurement of nursing. In L. Aiken, and C. Fagin (Eds.), *Charting Nursing's Future*. Philadelphia, PA: J.B. Lippincott.

Finkler, S. A. (1991). Variance analysis: Extending flexible budget variance analysis to acuity. Part I and II. *Journal of Nursing Administration, 21*(7–8), 19–25.

Fralic, M. F. (1992). Into the Future: Nurse executives and the world of information technology. *The Journal of Nursing Administration, 22*(4), 111–112.

Giovanetti, P. and Mayer, G. (1984). Building confidences in patient classification systems. *Nursing Management, 15*(8),31–34.

Halloran, E. (1988). Nursing workload, medical diagnosis related groups, and nursing diagnosis. *Research Nursing Management, 18*(3), 27–30, 32–36.

Health Department of Western Australia. (1991). *Nursing Staffing Methodology.* Report, 1–86.

Health Management Technology. (1994). Market Directory: More than 600 information technology company listings. *Health Management Technology,* 15–81.

Lewis, E. N. (1988). *Manual of Patient Classification.* Rockville, MD: Aspen Publishers, Inc.

O'Connor, F. (1983). Nurse management systems and budget control. In O. Fokkens, A. Haro, and A. Vanderwerff et al. (Eds.), *MEDINFO 83 Seminars.* Amsterdam: North-Holland.

Prescott, P. A. (1986). DRG prospective reimbursement: The nursing intensity factor. *Nursing Management, 17*(1), 43–48.

Prescott, P. and Phillips, C. (1988). Gauging nursing intensity to bring costs to light. *Nursing and Health Care, 9*(1), 17–22.

Prescott, P. A., Ryan, J. A., Soeken, K. L, et al. (1991). The patient intensity for nursing index: A validity assessment. *Research in Nursing and Health, 14,* 213–221.

Saba, V., Reider, K., and Pocklington, D. (Eds.). *Nursing and Computers: An Anthology.* New York: Springer-Verlag.

Saba, V. (1988). Classification schemes for nursing information systems. In N. Daly and K. Hannah (Eds.), *Proceedings of Nursing Computers. Third International Symposium on Nursing's Use of Computers in Information Science* (pp. 184–193). St. Louis, MO: Mosby.

Saba, V., Johnson, J., Halloran, E., and Simpson, R. (1994). *Computers in Nursing Management.* Washington, D. C: American Nurses Publishing.

Simpson, R. and Waite, R. (1989). NCNIP's system for the future: A call for accountability, revenue control, and national data sets. *Nursing Administration Quarterly, 14*(1), 72–77.

Software Guide. (1993). *Nursing Management 24*(7), 70–98.

Sovie, M. D. Tarcunale, M. A., Vanputte, A. W. and Stunden, A. E. (1985). Amalgam of nursing acuity, DRGs and costs. *Nursing Management,* 16(3), 22–42.

Thibault, C., David, N., O'Brien-Pallas, L., and Vinet, A. (1990). *Workload Measurement Systems in Nursing.* Montreal: Quebec Hospital Association.

Thompson, J. D. (1984). The measurement of nursing intensity. *Health Care Review, 53.*

19

Translating Evidence into Practice: Guidelines and Automated Implementation Tools

Lynn McQueen
Kathleen A. McCormick

OBJECTIVES

1. Define clinical practice guidelines and explain their use.
2. Discuss how guidelines promote effective and efficient care.
3. Describe how to evaluate the quality of a guideline.
4. Identify a three-pronged approach to implementation decisions.
5. Discuss how specific implementation tools can be selected.
6. Identify two nursing roles relevant to guideline implementation.
7. Discuss policy issues related to guidelines.

KEY WORDS

information systems
health services administration
health care
practice patterns
quality of health care
quality assurance
guidelines
practice guidelines

This chapter contains two major sections, which discuss (1) fundamentals of clinical practice guideline use and (2) computerized tools to support guideline implementation. The first part provides fundamental information about clinical practice guidelines and their use. Guideline development methods, evaluation, limitations, and implementation issues are discussed. The second part deals with issues relevant to informatics and guideline use. A multipronged, active, theory-based approach to implementation is advocated, and specific strategies for selecting tools for a guideline implementation tool kit are presented. The importance of being able to manage change is central to both sections, and suggestions for further research are interspersed throughout.

Fundamentals of Clinical Practice

It is said that "Life belongs to the living, and he who lives must be prepared for changes" (Johann Wolfgang von Goethe, 1749–1832). The current pace of change only foreshadows what is to come. As the pace accelerates, providers seek ways to adapt to the unprecedented transformations occurring as technology spreads through health care settings and society at large.

At the start of a new millennium, quality and cost issues drive the direction of change in health care. As policy makers, providers, researchers, and consumers simultaneously demand both high quality care and controlled health-related spending, population-based approaches to health promotion and disease management, such as evidence-based health, focus on twin goals: efficiency and effectiveness. Both are linchpins of quality. But tools are needed in order to make evidence-based health a reality. Computers house potentially the most powerful tools available. As computers facilitate the organization of meaningful information about patients, providers, and organizations, the availability of this information makes it far easier to focus on efficiency and effectiveness. But integrated computer and decision support systems are in their infancy. Although the benefits of simply linking clinical and administrative databases have yet to be reached, market trends and commercial forces, including the rise of health maintenance organizations (HMOs) and relentless struggles to reduce fragmentation, increase the pressure to develop dynamic, powerful, and flexible automated systems.

We are heading towards diffuse information networks and infrastructures (Shortell et al., 1996). With these systems in place, providers will have the support needed for seamless translation of evidence into high-quality patient care and ongoing system-wide changes. Output will come from diverse, integrated quality tools (such as computerized guidelines with automated reminders) accessible within integrated clinical workstations. Once quality tools are automated and timely information is readily available across disciplines, continuous quality improvement (CQI), utilization management, and patient-centered care will be systematized (Institute of Medicine, 1992) and the delivery of effective and efficient care will be transparent. It will be built into what we do every day.

Clinical Practice Guidelines

Defined by the Institute of Medicine as "systematically developed statements to assist practitioner and patient decisions about appropriate health care or specific clinical circumstances" (Institute of Medicine, 1990) evidence-based (scientifically grounded) clinical practice guidelines (also known simply as "guidelines" or "practice parameters") are gaining favor as instruments for promoting quality care. Guidelines provide a convenient way to present vast, complex data about outcomes, efficiency, effectiveness, patient preferences, policy, and costs as meaningful information (Cook et al., 1997). Guidelines present this diverse information in useful formats—thereby supporting informed decision-making for providers and patients (McCormick, 1998; McGlynn, 1996). Guidelines are defined as quality tools because, when implemented effectively, they promote improved patient outcomes and reduce the outcome variations documented over the past 2 decades (Wennberg and Fowler,

1977; Wennberg et al., 1989; 1990; Wennberg, 1996; Ashton et al., 1998). Effectiveness and efficiency are thus enhanced.

A guideline is composed of multiple recommendations. Each recommendation links practice to supporting evidence for a specific intervention. For example, within a guideline about diabetes, there will be many individual recommendations concerning various aspects of prevention, diagnosis, and treatment. One recommendation might address foot assessment to prevent amputation, and another might involve patient education about glycemic control. In a high-quality guideline (evidence-based and developed using rigorous methods), the strength of the available evidence is explicitly stated for each recommendation so that clinicians and patients can judge for themselves (Eddy, 1990; Hadorn et al., 1996; Woolf et al., 1996).

Despite growing popularity, the "guidelines movement" has only become potent during the 1990s. Much is still being learned. Additional evidence is needed regarding the impact of guidelines on costs and the extent to which guidelines contribute to improved outcomes. Grimshaw and Russell (1993) found that 55 out of 59 published evaluations of guideline effectiveness report statistically significant improvements in professional performance, and 9 out of 11 outcomes studies report significant improvement. However, there is little standardization between existing studies, sources of bias are sometimes ignored, and the methods used to measure outcomes are not consistently rigorous. Although the impact of guidelines requires much further investigation, optimism persists regarding their potential contributions to quality.

Since guidelines are not directives, flexibility and discretion in application are needed. A guideline can be used as is, adapted for use based on local circumstances, and/or used as a basis for developing algorithms, critical paths, and other ("spin-off") quality tools (Anders et al., 1997; Gates, 1995; Gottlieb et al., 1992). Not all guideline recommendations fit every clinical circumstance nor every patient. In addition, the provider must generally trust that compliance will ultimately improve outcomes, or the guideline should not be used. Trust is especially important when deciding to computerize a guideline. Computerizing quality tools, such as guidelines, is resource-intensive and should not be started until credibility of the guideline content has been established.

Guideline Evaluation: Establishing Information Credibility

Prior to using or computerizing a guideline, critical appraisal is needed (Sackett and Parkes, 1998). For many reasons, such as widespread gaps in the available evidence, many guidelines have limitations. These limitations need to be understood, and efforts should be made to minimize their effects (Anders et al., 1997). Again, this is especially important if computerization is being considered.

The first questions to ask are "who developed this guideline" and "what was their motive?" Providers are more likely to use a guideline when they trust the credibility of the sponsor and do not suspect a serious political or financial agenda that would compromise objectivity (McQueen, 1998). The composition of the guideline panel is also significant. While a multidisciplinary panel is sought, the appropriate make-up of the panel depends on the topic. Nursing representation is relevant for most health topics, but especially for topics like pressure ulcer treatment that require significant nursing involvement.

The scientific rigor of the development methods is key to the quality of the guideline (Sackett and Parkes, 1998; Woolf et al., 1996) and needs to be evaluated carefully. A central issue is whether or not the methods and the strength of evidence for each recommendation are plainly discussed so that providers can evaluate guideline credibility. A methods section will be part of a quality guideline and should clearly explain how the guideline was developed. It is particularly important to consider the data sources that were used, the inclusion/exclusion criteria used to select this data, and the currency of the information.

Evaluations of the methods used to analyze the data are critical. Who served as the methodologist? Were meta-analysis and other sophisticated statistical techniques used? Is the strength of the evidence explicitly stated? Strong evidence is not needed for each recommendation. This is unrealistic. Even in a quality, evidence-based guideline, the strength of the evidence will vary between recommendations, since there will typically be strong evidence for one intervention and missing or inconsistent evidence (uncertainty) for another. But the strength of the evidence for each recommendation should be presented clearly. The use of expert opinion should also be considered. While expert opinion may be necessary to fill in gaps in the evidence, over-reliance on expert opinion at the expense of the statistical analysis of data potentially compromises credibility.

Another guideline limitation is that patient preferences are often not adequately addressed (Bastian, 1996). Patient participation in decision-making contributes to improved patient satisfaction and other positive outcomes (Deber, 1996; Hagen and Whylie, 1998; Kasper et al.,

1992). The needs of patients are especially important if the condition is a chronic and non-life-threatening condition, such as benign prostatic hyperplasia (Roberts, 1994). In these instances, the patient's preferences become the focus of the decision, and flexibility is needed to assure that personal choices are prioritized.

The absence of cost information is a common guideline limitation. Ideally, enough data about costs and outcomes are available so that the harms and benefits of different interventions can be easily compared and contrasted. Unfortunately, adequate cost information is rarely available or is outdated. However, strides are being made in this area, and rapid progress is expected over the next 5 years (Edinger and McCormick, 1998; Grady and Weis, 1995).

In summary, "guidelines are only as good as the evidence on which they are based" (Management Decision Research Center, 1998). Providers need to assess the quality of a guideline and evaluate whether or not it will contribute to improved patient outcomes. If the guideline was developed and/or endorsed by trusted stakeholders and if it is deemed quality- and evidence-based, providers are much more likely to trust and use it. Key questions to ask are:

- Who developed this guideline, and why did they do it?
- Is the guideline developed using an evidence-based approach (is it grounded in science and is evidence prioritized over expert opinion)?
- Is the guideline current (when was it last updated)?
- Is it presented in a flexible format (are patient preferences taken into account? Is there a capability for shared decision-making with patients, and is individual clinical judgement possible?)?
- Are the benefits and harms presented to support sound decision-making?
- Are costs considered? Is this important for this specific topic?

Overview of Guideline Implementation Issues

Guideline implementation involves applying textual information to real situations. Successful implementation implies compliance and the ability to manage change. Because real situations are fluid, implementation is a dynamic process that is by nature complex and multifaceted.

Implementation is the *active* employment of a guideline to promote effective and efficient care in order to improve patient outcomes. Although much additional study is needed, reports of guideline implementation have risen sharply over the past 2 decades. To date, the use of guidelines has been studied and described in a wide variety of settings (Anderson, 1993; Aucott et al., 1999; Brown et al., 1995; Brox, 1996; Brunt, 1993; Buss et al., 1999; Carey, 1995; Crist, 1997; Dalton et al., 1999; Deyo, 1994; Duncan, 1995; Emslie et al., 1993; Fang et al., 1996; Duncan and Otto, 1995; Hetlevik et al., 1999; Hunsicker et al., 1998; Institute of Medicine, 1992; Kaegi, 1995; Lawler and Viviani, 1997; McCaffery and Ferrell, 1994; Mitchell, 1999; Newman et al., 1993; Newman, 1994; Rischer and Childress, 1996; Schmidt et al., 1994; Schriger, 1996; Schriger et al., 1997; Solberg et al., 1997; Steffensen et al., 1995; Steven and Fraser, 1996; Van Rijswijk, 1999; Wakefield et al., 1998; Weingarten et al., 1995; Woolf et al., 1996; Yawn et al., 1999).

Evaluation of the effects of clinical practice guideline use has lagged in published research (Fang et al., 1996). Due to the myriad of complex factors that impact outcomes, there is a lack of conclusive evidence about what works and does not work when using guidelines in real situations. Little is also known about how to manage diversity across settings. Instead, publications relevant to guideline implementation cover a diverse range of topics, and the meaning of the cumulative literature is elusive. While effective implementation of guidelines has been associated with quality improvements (Aucott, 1999; O'Connor et al., 1996) and while Brook (1996), Davis and Taylor-Vaisey (1997), Feder et al. (1999), and others report a positive association between guideline use and patient outcomes, additional hard evidence of consistent, measurable improvement is needed. This is especially true, since some research conducted during the late 1980s and early 1990s on the effects of guidelines was not promising. For example, even when providers self-report adherence to guideline recommendations, evidence suggests that the guidelines were not always used (Lawler and Viviani, 1997; Steffensen et al., 1995; Weingarten et al., 1995).

The nature of implementation studies is shifting. Early investigations of guideline implementation typically focused on strategies designed to change physician practice. Donabedian's measurement of treatment structures, processes, and outcomes (1980) was the theoretical basis for many studies, but processes—not outcomes—were typically the focus. The processes studied included provider processes, such as "buy-in," as well as patient/provider-influenced factors, such as compliance.

Although processes are still studied, reports of appropriateness from Brook (1996), McGlynn and Asch (1998), and others at RAND heightened awareness of the need to focus also on *outcomes*. During the 1990s, it became obvious that the amount of work needed to improve outcomes had been consistently underestimated (Forrest et al., 1996). For example, the effort required to implement guidelines and other quality tools effectively—let alone efficiently—is now the focus of many studies. But the field is young. Issues relevant to the translation of evidence into practice (including the use of guidelines as a tool for this purpose) are only starting to be adequately addressed.

Active Guideline Implementation: Finding What Works

The lessons learned from nursing care plans are applicable: guidelines that sit on a shelf will collect dust and not contribute to improved outcomes. Quality improvement using guidelines and other quality tools is most likely achieved and sustained over a long period when there is ongoing commitment from leaders to manage change proactively. Strong leadership promotes an active, multipronged, theory-based approach (Lee, 1995; Davis et al., 1995; Schriger et al., 1997). But there is no "magic bullet." Quality improvement is painstaking (Rolnick and O'Connor, 1997). Long gone are notions that distributing a guideline to providers ("throwing it over the wall") will ultimately improve the health of a patient or make a provider's job easier. Grimshaw and Russell (1993) are among those to caution against any expectation that "passive dissemination" alone will ultimately help patients.

Guideline implementation is now recognized as a social process that is best promoted when users have time to gain awareness of the guideline content, develop a favorable attitude, and make a choice to adopt (Mittman et al., 1992; Rogers, 1995; Rubinstein et al., 2000; VanAmringe and Shannon, 1992). The ability to manage change is at the center of this process. After initial, active/multipronged/theory-based dissemination and implementation efforts are completed, reinforcement and confirmation are needed indefinitely in order to sustain any quality improvements. But these social processes are strengthened when implementation decisions are grounded in science and mandated by organizational leaders and guideline champions (Gates, 1995; Rubenstein et al., 2000; Mittman et al., 1999).

As awareness of the significance of social factors grows, increased attention is being paid to the organizational barriers and facilitating factors associated with the use of guidelines. For example, De Rosario (1998), Newcomer (1994), Rolnick and O'Connor (1997), and Choddoff and Crowley (1995) report common roadblocks to successful implementation. The need for strong collaborative teamwork is a common theme across organizational studies. Some studies consider general organizational factors, while others focus on specific disciplines or settings. For example, Funk et al. (1991a, 1991b, 1995) have considered barriers specific to nursing, and Schriger (1996) has explored "what it would take" to overcome barriers and make implementation successful in emergency room settings.

Review articles by Davis and Taylor-Vaisey (1997), Grimshaw and Russell (1993), Grimshaw et al. (1994), Greco and Eisenberg (1993), Oxman (1995), Worral et al. (1997), and others report that no one implementation strategy works consistently across settings. For this reason, increased attention is now directed towards organizational strategies designed to promote best practices rather than trying to change providers. Organizational strategies are typically tailored to matching implementation goals to real world circumstances. Kaluzny et al. (1995) emphasized the importance of implementing guidelines in stages, providing "small wins," and building on existing governing mechanisms already in place within the institution. Goldberg et al. (1998) conducted a clinical trial to determine the effectiveness of "academic detailing" (AD; a form of individualized, targeted education [Soumerai, 1990]) and CQI on increasing guideline compliance. Positive results were found when AD and CQI were used together. From these and other studies, evidence is accumulating regarding effectiveness of strategies and tools, but far more research is needed. Ultimately, whatever strategies and tools are chosen to facilitate guideline implementation, a systematic approach is beneficial. The next section describes one organization using such an approach.

■ Translating Evidence Into Practice: The Department of Veteran's Affairs Model

The Department of Veteran's Affairs (VA) provides an example of a large organization that uses a systematic approach to implement multiple guidelines across facilities and integrate these guidelines into system-wide quality improvement efforts. The VA is an ideal organization to study guideline implementation, and specifically to study the computerization of guidelines, because administrative and data systems are centralized and because

implementation strategies and tools can be tested in the VA facilities that provide care to 3.5 million veterans (Hynes et al., 2000; Kizer et al., 2000).

The VA goes beyond simply implementing guidelines; the effect of guidelines on patient outcomes and system-wide change is systematically studied, and the information gained from research is fed back to providers. With strong leadership, the organization is committed to a rational, evidence-based approach to systematizing quality improvement. Researchers collaborate with administrators, clinicians, and others to assure that the approach is rigorous and promotes both critical thinking and organizational learning. Through the Quality Enhancement Research Initiative (QUERI) and other efforts, knowledge is evolving about what is needed for successful guideline implementation and how the guidelines generally promote improved patient outcomes and system efficiency (Kizer, 1998; Rubenstein et al., 2000; Mittman et al., 1999; Tomich, 1999; Demakis et al., 2000; Kizer et al., 2000; and Feussner et al., 2000).

For example, in order to promote guideline compliance, the VA classified four types of implementation tools but encouraged local facilities to decide which tools best suit their needs (Management Decision Research Center, 1998). The four basic categories of tools are:

- ■ **Knowledge-based tools:** designed to make providers, patients, and other decision-makers aware of a guideline(s). Knowledge-based tools include continuing education materials and guideline documents in various formats, such as laminated pocket-cards and electronic text disseminated over the Internet or an intranct.

- ■ **Attitude-based tools:** designed to promote agreement with a guideline. These tools include academic detailing materials, endorsements by professional organizations/societies or formal statements by opinion leaders. Professional listservs that facilitate interactive discussion about guideline implementation, such as an informatics listserv and an evidence-based health listserv, are also attitude-based tools.

- ■ **Behavior-based tools:** promote change management generally and specifically promote provider compliance with guidelines. These tools are associated with resources, such as time, financial incentives, skill and staffing mix, and patient acceptance. Examples of behavior-based tools are skill-building classes or programs, decision-support systems, and electronic or paper patient education information.

■ **Maintenance tools:** reinforce the continued use of guidelines after initial implementation. The benefits of adhering to best practices can then be sustained over time. These tools include computerized reminder systems, audit and feedback programs, standing orders, computerized checksheets, and chart shingles (laminated kardex-like pages with the guideline recommendations printed on them).

A "tool kit" is one way to assemble a variety of tools from each of the above categories. A tool kit is customized to the needs of the local facility and contains several tools—each of which can be used independently or together to leverage guidelines (Griffith et al., 1995). An implementation team would typically use a systematic approach to consider various tools and strategies, select specific tools for the tool kit, prepare and test user documentation and support materials, and then educate clinicians and others about how to choose and use the tools they need.

Tools are selected for inclusion in the tool kit based on the culture and goals of the organization. For example, if a computer-literate staff is already using an integrated information system, automated tools will be a natural choice. Given the potential power of computers, automated tools should be considered early. However, organizational and individual readiness needs to be assessed, and user support should be planned carefully. This involves assessing past implementation issues, motivation, and organizational climate—including commitment.

Whenever possible, the impact of each tool should be evaluated, and the data should be used to promote ongoing improvement. Evaluation plans ideally begin prior to use of the tool so that pre/post analysis is an option. Barriers and facilitators for using each tool need to be identified as part of the evaluation. Ultimately, optimal outcomes will be achieved and sustained most easily when the tools used to promote guideline implementation are integrated with other quality improvement tools and become a natural part of the clinical routine (McCormick, 1998).

The VA is promoting the use and evaluation of tool kits and other customized products designed to assure that accurate, current evidence is in the hands of clinical decision-makers when needed (Demakis et al., 2000). Through QUERI and other initiatives, VA investigators evaluate the impact of specific implementation approaches, strategies, and tools. QUERI, therefore, artfully links research to clinical interactions, thus promoting a rational approach to decision-making. This type of creativity underlies the systematic

integration of research and quality improvement while also maximizing the unique strengths of local facilities.

Computers as a Tool to Facilitate Guideline Implementation

This section presents information for providers seeking computerized tools to promote guideline implementation. The majority of this section discusses the selection of automated tools for inclusion in an implementation tool kit. An active, multipronged, theory-based approach to tool kit development is described followed by a discussion of strategies for choosing specific tools for the tool kit. The Department of Veterans Affairs is again used as a model. Evolving roles for nurses are discussed, and policy implications are explored.

Computers and Guidelines

At their best, automated tools are the most powerful resource available to facilitate guideline implementation. For many reasons, computers are potentially an ideal match for guidelines: (1) computers permit centralized storage and retrieval of guidelines; (2) computers facilitate communication between different providers or between providers and patients; (3) computers enhance the speed, timeliness and presentation of feedback and other reports; (4) computers expand the accessibility of guidelines and related decision analysis tools; (5) computers make decision analysis infinitely easier and more powerful; and (6) computers provide a means for integrating guidelines with clinical information about effectiveness and outcomes. In short, computers make it easier for providers and patients to access, use, and communicate guideline-related information. This promotes sound decision-making and facilitates change.

Evidence to support the benefits of using computers as a guideline implementation tool is growing. Shiffman et al. (1999b) provides the most comprehensive review of computer-based guideline implementation systems published to date. In a systematic review of 25 studies (including nine randomized controlled trials) published between 1992 and January 1998, the authors found that guideline compliance improved in 14 out of 18 systems and that documentation improved in 4 out of 4 studies. Shiffman and colleagues identified numerous, diverse factors (such as the provision of a wide array of information management services) that potentially influence the success or failure of computerized guideline systems. The authors warn that this area of research is very young and that confounding variables and publication bias prohibit final conclusions.

Research relevant to the intersection of guideline implementation and informatics becomes increasingly technical as issues relevant to technology transfer are prioritized. For example, work relevant to unified language and coding is proliferating. Extensive work is currently under way by InterMed that studies the cognitive processes relevant to computerized guideline encoding. The InterMed collaboration is a partnership between Columbia, Harvard, Stanford, and McGill universities. Investigators from these diverse institutions collaborate in the development and testing of software, tools, and system components that facilitate and support the standardized implementation and sharing of guidelines (Patel et al., 1998). Figure 19.1 is a model of the process envisioned by the InterMed collaboratory.

In order to pursue their goals, InterMed collaborators developed a standardized, common language to represent guidelines. This language is called the GuideLine Interchange Format (GLIF) and has been studied as a vehicle for disseminating guideline text (Ohno-Machado et al., 1998). This is landmark work, since integration demands that culturally diverse and geographically separated organizations standardize computer applications. While this area of research carries obvious complexity

and is resource-intensive, it will ultimately advance guideline implementation efforts dramatically.

The advantages of using a common format such as GLIF are to (Patel et al., 1998):

- Support multidisciplinary teams developing guidelines
- Reduce the duplication efforts in guideline development
- Provide feedback mechanisms to update guidelines concurrent with advances in medical and nursing knowledge.

Other systems have been developed to allow local variation of guidelines. Fridsma et al. (1996) proposed a simple prompted diskette that allows the user to convert guideline recommendations into locally useful applications. Lobach (1995) has described a model of local adaptation using five national guidelines implemented at Duke University.

In summary, computers can be used as quality implementation tools in a variety of ways depending on creativity, resources, and the organizational culture present (Harvey and Kitson, 1996). The technological sophistication of automated tools crosses a spectrum. Some computerized guideline tools, such as those using artificial

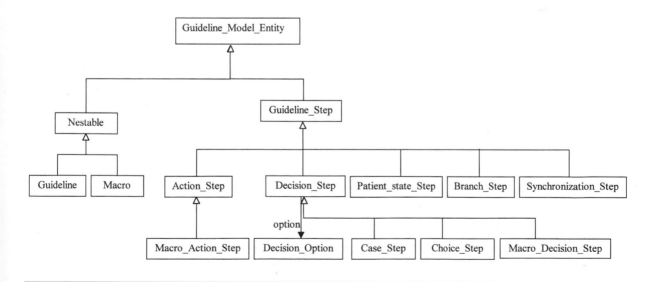

Figure 19.1
GLIF Model version 3.0.
Reproduced, with permission, from Aziz A. Boxwala, 2000 (in press).

intelligence, are complex, while others, such as the dissemination of text using the Internet or an intranet, are relatively simple and easily created. Regardless of the level of sophistication, opportunities to use computers as tools to improve patient outcomes are expanding quickly. The field is wide open.

Using a Three-Pronged Approach to Consider Various Automated Tools: Theory-Based, Active, Multipronged

The consideration of automated tools for a guideline implementation tool kit requires a thoughtful, systematic approach. In this section, approaches used by guideline implementation teams are discussed. Specific strategies to guide the selection and customization of tools for the tool kit are then explored.

As recommended by Mittman et al. (1999) and others, a *theory-based* approach to considering tools helps to assure that implementation decisions are rational and grounded in science. Evidence summarized in review articles also suggests that an *active* and *mutlipronged* approach is also beneficial (Davis and Taylor-Vaisey, 1997; Davis et al., 1995; Grimshaw and Russell 1993; Grimshaw et al., 1994; Greco and Eisenberg 1993; Mittman et al., 1992; Oxman, 1995; Worral et al., 1997). An "active" approach discourages use of only passive dissemination and implementation methods—such as merely handing out a guideline to providers and assuming that it will be read and followed. A multipronged approach means that several diverse guideline implementation tools will be used simultaneously and supported by leaders from the top down (e.g., by policies issued by leaders) and from the bottom up (e.g., by staff at all levels and across disciplines serving as champions and guideline promoters). The goals of this combined approach are: (1) rational choices and (2) change management. Discussions of several computerized tools to consider are listed below. Using a theory-based, active, multipronged approach, nurses must consider which of the following tools best fit local needs.

Decision Support Systems   Decision analysis offers a way to link the probability of a clinical course to the likelihood of specific outcomes. The results of clinical decisions can then be predicted, and the probability of alternative strategies can be quantified. Decision models, data, and complex analyses are required. There are many ways in which these systems can be applied to guideline implementation. For example, providers could learn about, test, and improve a new guideline using a decision support sys-

tem. But there are potential limitations. Invalid or conflicting evidence is sometimes used in analyses. In addition, coding is complex, and lack of expertise and resources currently prohibit widespread use. But this is changing as applications become more powerful and integrated systems are capable of capturing performance information and linking it concurrently with outcomes.

Computerized Reminder Systems   Many common reminder systems are not automated. Laminated cards, posters, preprinted forms within charts, and pocket guides are all reminders familiar to most providers. Automated reminders are infinitely more powerful, especially when they cannot be ignored or turned off easily. Whatever their form, reminders are most useful when used in "real time" (at the point of patient contact). Both automated and paper reminders are ideal for health promotion and preventive care. For example, a computer can be programmed to analyze a patient's age, risk factors, and other data in order to generate a screening reminder at the appropriate time. Although they are still being studied, automated reminders may be the most promising guideline implementation tools now available—particularly when the reminders are integrated within decision support programs or other integrated systems during real time.

Profiling or Auditing Used with Provider Feedback   When information is fed back to providers and facilities, quantitative performance data are linked to social processes such as peer influence. For example, data collected about the interventions of a group of providers can be linked to outcomes and fed back. In some instances, benchmarks are used; other times, provider performance is compared to colleague performance. As accountability is increasingly demanded of all professions, nurses can expect wider use of feedback and profiling. Since computers can readily be programmed to feed back the vast quantity of clinical and administrative data now being collected by many organizations, these applications will proliferate. Audit and feedback of information are generally most useful when provided at the time of the patient encounter or soon after and when the feedback is stimulating and interactive. Delayed or disconnected feedback is less useful or counterproductive, and over-auditing may contribute to inappropriate use (Robinson et al., 1996).

On-line Communication Strategies   On-line communication provides a convenient, cost-effective vehicle for information dissemination and exchange. On-line

Table 19.1   A listing of URLs in the U.S. to obtain full texts of clinical practice guidelines on-line

http://www.ahcpr.gov

http://text.nlm.nih.gov

http://www.ngc.gov

tools are more powerful when integrated within an overall communication strategy and targeted to the specific information needs of each stakeholder. Soon it will be hard to imagine guideline implementation without the World Wide Web.

The United States government has provided valuable access to guidelines on the Internet since the early 1990s. The National Library of Medicine (NLM) and the Agency for Healthcare Research and Quality (AHRQ) have full text and abstracted versions of guidelines available. The latest access to guidelines is a cosponsored U.S. Guideline Clearinghouse that involves the government and private sector resources. Table 19.1 provides the key URLs to access valuable guideline content on-line.

The potential uses are unlimited. Listservs, such as one on evidence-based nursing organized in the United Kingdom, are used to discuss guideline recommendations and other relevant topics (to access this, E-mail *mailbase@mailbase.ac.uk*, and in the text type :"join nurse-decision" followed by your_firstname your_surname). Patients search on-line guideline-derived patient brochures and discuss guideline recommendations with on-line providers. Guideline text is easily downloaded by patients and providers, rural clinics gain access to the latest update of a guideline, and facilities within large organizations use the Intranet to exchange information about compliance. As the "digital age" promotes Web applications, their influence on clinical decision-making and outcomes will expand rapidly but remain difficult to measure. Zielstorff (1998) has studied the issue and obstacles associated with on-line practice guidelines and provides specific suggestions for overcoming barriers, including better accommodation of imprecise knowledge in clinical algorithms using fuzzy logic. Dugas (1998) reported the use of intranet-based information systems specifically for nurses. Additional research on this topic is needed soon.

Automated Flow Sheets as Part of an Electronic Patient Record   As the level of integration described by Shortell et al. (1996) becomes a reality, electronic patient records (EPR), also known as electronic medical records, are gaining popularity as a way to combine stored data

repositories with information management tools. For example, computerized records provide a practical way to use guidelines to support creation of clinical protocols (Bazzoli, 1995). This allows knowledge to be represented in various formats so that it is available to facilitate accurate and timely decisions. Tang et al. (1999) also reports use of EPR for evaluating interventions designed to improve guideline compliance. As EPR evolves, mechanisms for recording data will improve so that the frequency of events within specified time periods can more easily be analyzed. These data can then be linked to a variety of computerized tools relevant to guidelines. For example, automated flow sheets used to collect patient information relevant to guideline compliance will become more sophisticated. Flow sheets can then be easily transferred to the paper record, torn off, and used by providers at the bedside or linked to patient education information.

Computers Used to Facilitate Academic Detailing (AD) is an acronym used to describe customized "educational outreach." Individual providers are targeted for education. Computers can supplement AD in a variety of ways. For example, computer-assisted instruction or videodisc technology can be used to convey information about a guideline and allow the provider to explore this information safely prior to applying it to real patients. Unlike conferences or workshops, which are often passive, computerized academic detailing provides focused, individualized education that can be highly interactive. The stimulating, engaging nature of computer-facilitated AD promotes success.

Choosing Computerized Tools

Although a theory-based, active, multipronged approach aids in the initial consideration of appropriate tools, the unique needs of each health care setting also guide implementation decisions about tools. Once a systematic approach has been used to consider various options, multidisciplinary guideline implementation teams can identify strategies to guide their selection of specific tools for a guideline implementation tool kit. The team will also need to address how tools can best be combined with each other and integrated into system-wide quality improvement initiatives (Kinney and Gift, 1997; Levknecht et al., 1997; Aucott et al., 1995). Decisions can then be made about how best to customize tools to fit the local environment (Gates, 1995).

Numerous strategies directly linked to informatics are available to facilitate guideline implementation. Duff and Casey (1998) describe strategies for using informatics to promote access, communication, and evaluation of guidelines. Shiffman et al. (1999a) stress the importance of implementation strategies that promote workflow integration and describe an information services model designed to maximize such integration. The authors provide a checklist for those using computers as an implementation tool and also describe a model for evaluating computerized guideline implementation tools.

Davis et al. (1995) is another author who suggests a useful strategy designed to facilitate selection of specific tools. Davis' strategy helps providers identify gaps between ideal and actual performance. To assist providers in selecting the right tools to fill these gaps, Davis categorizes electronic and other tools as *weak, moderately effective*, and *relatively potent*. It may be helpful for an implementation team to use Davis' strategy to walk themselves through real examples. Early questions are: under usual clinical circumstances, which tools would promote guideline compliance? What factors would most likely contribute to provider use of a guideline? What barriers can be expected?

The team might, for example, consider which tools would facilitate implementation of a diabetes guideline. The adoption of such a guideline might start when providers review patient outcomes (for example, amputation rates) and recognize that their facility has a higher amputation rate than expected given their population. In other words, a gap between ideal and actual performance is identified. Guidelines designed to prevent amputation might then be adopted, and an active, multipronged, theory-based approach might be employed by a guideline implementation team. In order to promote compliance with the guideline recommendations, the team considers which tools would encourage use of the guideline (thereby closing the gap between existing and ideal practice). Electronic tools, such as automated reminders that alert providers that a patient is at high risk might be employed. An automated phone reminder system or electronic E-mail reminders can be used to remind the patient to take off his or her shoes in the waiting room. An outcomes monitoring system might be used to link interventions to amputation rates and then provide feedback to providers about the impact of their care. These and other electronic and paper options can be deemed weak, moderately effective, or relatively potent depending on the resources, creativity, and organizational culture of the unit.

The previously described VA taxonomy (Management Decision Research Center, 1998) can also guide selection of tools for a guideline implementation tool kit. Computerized tools from all four categories can be considered: knowledge-based tools, attitude-based tools, behavior-based tools, and maintenance-based tools.

Knowledge-based tools will sometimes be the top priority depending on the culture. For example, computers can be used to provide diabetes guideline text to providers or patients or to forward algorithms to providers showing the logic of the guideline. Providers may also want to consider attitude-based tools. For example, computers can be used by professional organizations or specialty groups associated with diabetes to convey their endorsement of the guideline to providers and patients. When seeking behavior-based tools, administrative systems can be used to determine staffing needs after a guideline is implemented, or to calculate the resource changes associated with guideline implementation. For example, perhaps implementation of the diabetes guideline leads to increased patient education. Additional staff time may be needed and there may be financial implications. Computers can track this information over time. Perhaps computers contribute most to system-wide quality improvement when used as maintenance-based tools. Used in this capacity, computerized reminder systems, computerized standing orders, and automated audit/feedback systems can be integrated to assure that the quality improvement gains (such as decreased amputation rates) associated with guideline implementation are sustained over time. Maintenance is an important, sometimes neglected, priority when implementing guidelines.

Once the tools have been selected and the tool kit is being used to facilitate implementation, the work is just starting. Change management principles suggest that use must be encouraged over time and that each tool be evaluated. Information about what works in a specific environment is gained through iterative processes. Barriers to implementation as well as facilitating factors are revealed as each tool is used in various situations; adjustments are then made accordingly. Cumulative information from the evaluation is also fed back to providers and facilities on an ongoing basis. As information is gained over time, a culture of critical thinking and organizational learning is fostered, and guideline use becomes part of the daily routine.

Nursing Roles

As computer applications in quality improvement expand, so do nursing roles. These roles increasingly appear in published literature, and it is obvious that many new roles are evolving. While many guideline-related studies focus on nursing and the use of specific guidelines (Dalton, 1996; Dalton et al., 1999; Duncan and Otto, 1995; Franck, 1992; McCaffery and Ferrell, 1994; Rischer and Childress, 1996; Wakefield et al., 1998; Miaskowski et al., 1999; Buss et al., 1999; Hall, 1999; Van Rijswijk and Braden, 1999), studies relevant to the computerization of guidelines and nursing are less common and are diffuse. Existing publications cover a diverse range of topics: the integration of information technology with outcomes management (Cole and Houston, 1997); coding and taxonomy issues relevant to outcomes—including standardized language and other issues tied to the nursing minimum data set (Moorhead et al., 1998; Blewitt and Jones, 1996; Timm and Behrenbeck, 1998; Brazile and Hettinger, 1995; Prophet and Delaney, 1998; Crist, 1997; Lowe and Baker, 1997); and the development of nurse-sensitive outcome measures (Pierce, 1997).

While some publications, such as Summers' (1987), describe nurses serving as information managers, others emphasize specific nursing roles relevant to guideline computerization. Studies also describe participatory roles as nurses collaborate on teams. It is important for the profession that nurses serve on multidisciplinary teams and develop team-building and leadership skills. These teams are becoming increasingly popular as integration is used to improve organizational learning and quality (Alemi et al., 1998; Heil et al., 1997; Kaluzny et al., 1995; Kasper et al., 1992; McLaughlin and Kaluzny, 1994; Mittman et al., 1999; Newcomer, 1994).

There are numerous rapidly evolving roles for nurses relevant to guideline computerization. As nurses increasingly serve as the architects and designers of integrated infrastructures and other computerized systems (Zielstorff, 1995), the needs of providers will increasingly be prioritized. As this occurs, guidelines and other clinical documents will be included and customized within systems. This trend can be expected to contribute to improved patient outcomes, but this area warrants further study.

Among the most exciting evolving roles for nurses is that of facilitator. Nurse facilitators are used by large organizations to assist providers with guideline implementation. For example, nurse facilitators explain the guideline recommendations, find both automated and paper tools to ease the implementation process, and assist with practical problems (Forrest et al., 1995). The Mayo Clinic has been a leader in using nurse facilitators to promote change at the systems level. Solberg et al.

(1997b) describe how nurse facilitators have contributed to quality improvement at HealthPartners, an affiliate of the Mayo Clinic in Minnesota.

Policy Implications

Guideline implementation and informatics are best understood within the broader context of health care policy. Guidelines and other knowledge tools are gaining popularity at the same time that technology expands and concerns for quality compete with resource allocation. For example, computerized guidelines that increase staffing requirements are implemented just as providers are told to increase the number of patients seen per hour and also reduce expenditures. These trends influence attitudes and the decisions made about guideline use and guideline implementation. Those implementing guidelines can promote their use by assuring that staff needs are considered on an ongoing basis.

In order to adapt to the unrelenting pace of change, providers must manage the trade-offs that underlie operation amidst conflicting demands. As organizational integration and re-engineering spreads, providers increasingly will be required to actively promote organizational goals (such as cost containment) while simultaneously serving as patient advocates. They will be asked to eliminate staffing just as they are asked to assure patient safety, ethical quality care, and a reasonable degree of organizational stability. How can conflicting demands such as these be satisfied? While there are no easy answers, the use of accurate, timely information to support rational decisions is the best hope. Quality, evidence-based guidelines are one potential resource. Computers can facilitate the availability of this information for decision-makers.

Even the best guidelines carry political and other controversy. It is unavoidable. As the new millennium begins, loud questions about the legal and ethical implications associated with guidelines will continue to be asked. For example, is a provider protected from litigation if a guideline is followed? Is the guideline developer liable when guideline use is linked to a poor outcome? Once again, quick, easy answers are not forthcoming. However, it is beneficial to address these issues directly as soon as guideline implementation begins and encourage ongoing discussion and negotiation.

A policy issue of specific relevance to nursing relates to the composition of guideline development panels and the critical appraisal of guidelines. There is currently no national professional or academic group with overall responsibility for assessing nursing content within guidelines or for suggesting appropriate representation of nurses on multidisciplinary panels. This activity occurs, but it is sporadic and unorganized. Guideline developers do not readily know where to turn when seeking to involve nurses. For example, while the Agency for Healthcare Research and Quality (AHRQ) and the U.S. Preventive Services Task Force (now combined) have strong records of appointing highly qualified nurse experts to their panels, it cannot be assumed that the quality of nursing input is optimal in the absence of centralized professional guidance (Griffith, 1993).

Summary

As quality and cost issues drive the explosive pace of change in modern health care organizations, issues related to the provision of effective and efficient care come into focus. Clinical practice guidelines are fast becoming a primary quality improvement tool for promoting efficiency and effectiveness. But not all guidelines are created equal. Since providers are held accountable for their decisions, it is important to know how to evaluate a guideline, adapt it to an individual patient, and promote its use throughout the organization. An active, multipronged, theory-based approach combined with judgement about the needs of the specific organization can be helpful when seeking tools to leverage guideline use. Computerized tools should be considered carefully because they are potentially so powerful. Computerized tools come in many forms, including decision support systems and automated reminders. Development of a tool kit composed of several electronic and paper tools is helpful. The tools can be used together or in isolation, but their use should be evaluated over time. Policy and ethical concerns should be addressed early and on an ongoing basis.

References

Alemi, F., Moore, S., Headrick, L., et al. (1998). Rapid improvement teams. *Joint Commission Journal on Quality Improvement, 24*(3), 119–129.

American Institutes for Research. (1995). Users' perceptions of four clinical practice guidelines and their development. Presentation, October 30.

American Public Health Association. (1990). Public health policy-making in the presence of incomplete evidence. *American Journal of Public Health, 90,* 746–750.

Anders, R. L., Tomai, J. S., Clute, R. M., and Olson, T. (1997). Development of a scientifically valid coordinated care path. *Journal of Nursing Administration, 27*(5), 45–52.

Anderson, G. (1993). Implementing practice guidelines. *Canadian Medical Association Journal, 148*(5), 753–755.

Anderson, R. M. (1995). Patient empowerment and the traditional medical model: A case of irreconcilable differences. *Diabetes Care, 18,* 412–415.

Armstrong, D. (1977). Clinical sense and clinical science. *Social Science and Medicine, 11,* 599–601.

Ashton, C. M., Petersen, N. J., Souchek, J., et al. (1998). Geographic variation in utilization rates in Department of Veterans Affairs Hospitals and clinics. *New England Journal of Medicine, 340*(1), 32.

Aucott, J. N., Pelecanos, E., Dombrowski, R., et al. (1999). Implementation of local guidelines for cost-effective management of hypertension. A trial of the firm system. *Journal of General Internal Medicine, 11*(3), 139–146.

Augustine, N. R. (1999). When politics interferes with science. *The Washington Post*, Wednesday Ed, August 6.

Austin, S. M., Balas, E. A., Mitchell, J. A., and Ewigman, B. G. (1994). Effect of physician reminders on preventive care: Meta-analysis of randomized clinical trials. *Proceedings of the Annual Symposium on Computer Applications in Medical Care,* 121–124.

Backer, T. E. (1995). Integrating behavioral and systems strategies to change clinical practice. *The Joint Commission Journal on Quality Improvement, 21*(7), 351–366.

Balas, E. A., Boren, S. A., Brown, G. D., et al. (1996). Effect of physician profiling on utilization. Meta-analysis of randomized controlled trials. *Journal of General Internal Medicine, 11*(10), 584–590.

Balas, E. A., Austin, S. M., Mitchell, J. A., et al. (1996). The clinical value of computerized information services. A review of 98 randomized clinical trials. *Archives of Family Medicine, 5*(5), 271–278.

Balas, E. A., Stockham, M. G., Mitchell, J. A., et al. (1997). In search of controlled evidence for health care quality. *Journal of Medical Systems, 21*(1), 21–32.

Balas, E. A., Boren, S. A., and Griffing G. (1998). Computerized management of diabetes: A synthesis of controlled trials. *Proceedings of the American Medical Informatics Association,* 295–299.

Basinski, A. S. (1995). Evaluation of clinical practice guidelines. *Canadian Medical Association Journal, 153,* 1575–1581.

Bastian, H. (1996). Raising the standard: Practice guidelines and consumer participation. *International Journal for Quality in Health Care, 85*(5), 485–490.

Batalden, P. B., Nelson, E. C., and Roberts, J. S. (1994). Linking outcomes measurement to continual improvement: The serial "V" way of thinking about improving clinical care. *Joint Commission Journal on Quality Improvement, 20*(4), 167–180.

Bazzoli, F. (1995). Clinical protocols: The next automation frontier. Computerized records will play a key role in the implementation of clinical guidelines. *Health Data Management, 3*(2), 30–32, 34–46, 38.

Beed, G. (1995). Implementing outcomes research: When theory meets reality. *Managed Care Medicine,* April, *18*(12), 27–31.

Beresford, E. B. (1991). Uncertainty and the shaping of medical decisions. Washington, D. C.: *Hastings Center Report,* July–August.

Bergman, D. A. (1995). Thriving in the 21st Century: Outcome assessment, practice parameters, and accountability. *Pediatrics, 96(Supplement),* 831–5.

Berlowitz, D. R. (1998). Inadequate management of blood pressure in a hypertensive population. *New England Journal of Medicine, 339,* 1957–1963.

Bero, L. A. (1998). Closing the gap between research and practice: An overview of systematic reviews of interventions to promote implementation of research findings. *British Medical Journal, 317,* 465–468.

Berwick, D. M. (1989). Continuous improvement as an ideal in health care. *The New England Journal of Medicine, 320*(1), 53–56.

Berwick, D. M. (1994). Eleven worthy aims for clinical leadership in health system reform. *Journal of the American Medical Association, 272*(10), 797–802.

Blewitt, D. K., and Jones, K. R. (1996). Using elements of the nursing minimum data set for determining outcomes. *Journal of Nursing Administration, 26*(6), 48–56.

Bodenheimer, T. (1999). Disease management—promises and pitfalls. *The New England Journal of Medicine (Sounding Board), 340*(15), 1202–1204.

Bourdieu, P., and Coleman, J. S. (Eds.). (1991). *Social Theory for a Changing Society.* Boulder, CO: Westview Press.

Brazile, R. P., and Hettinger, B. J. (1995). A clinical information system for ambulatory care. *Computers in Nursing, 13*(4), 151–158.

Brennan, T. A. (1991). Practice guidelines and malpractice litigation: Collision or cohesion? *Journal of Health Politics, Policy, and Law, 16*(1), 67–85.

Brook, R.H. (1996). Practice guidelines: To be or not to be? *The Lancet, 348*(9033), 1005–1006.

Brown, J. L., Shye, D., and McFarland, B. (1995). The paradox of guideline implementation: How AHCPR's depression guidelines was adapted at Kaiser Permanente Northwest Region. *Joint Commission Journal on Quality Improvement, 21*(1), 5–21.

Brox, W. T. (1996). Implementation of guidelines for prevention of deep vein thrombosis in a managed care environment. *Orthopedics, August 19(Supplement),* 12–14.

Broxman, G. P., Levine, M. N., Mohide, E. A., et al. (1995). The practice guidelines development cycle: A conceptual tool for practice guidelines development and implementation. *Journal of Clinical Oncology, 13,* 5025.

Brunt, B. (1993). Clinical practice guidelines. *Journal of the Ohio Nurses Association, 23*(9), 35–37.

Burack, R. C., and Gimotty, P. A. (1997). Promoting screening mammography in inner-city settings. The sustained effectiveness of computerized reminders in a randomized controlled trial. *Medical Care, 35*(9), 921–931.

Buss, I. C., Halfens, R. J., Abu-Saad, H. H., Kok, G. (1999). Evidence-based nursing practice: Both state of the art in general and specific to pressure ulcers. *Journal of Professional Nursing, 15*(2), 73–83.

Button, P., Androwich, I., Hibben, L., et al. (1998). Challenges and issues related to implementation of nursing vocabularies in computer-based systems. *Journal of the American Medical Informatics Association, 5*(4), 332–4.

Calloway, S. D., and Kelly, J. (1996). Preconference workshop materials: The Zitter Group Conference on Implementing Practice Guidelines. San Francisco. January 21–23.

Camp, V. (1994). Computers. Better data + critical thinking = improved care. *Nursing Staff Development Insider, 3*(5), 2–5.

Canadian Medical Association. (1999). Clinical Practice Guideline Infobase. *http://www.cma.ca/cpgs/handbook/*

Canfield, K., Silva, M., and Petrucci, K. (1994). The standard data model approach to patient record transfer. *Proceedings of the Annual Symposium for Computer Applications in Medical Care,* 478–482.

Carey, M. (1995). Diabetes guidelines, outcomes, and cost-effectiveness study: A protocol, prototype and paradigm. *Journal of the American Dietetic Association, 95*(9), 976–978.

Cassarad, S. D., Wesman, C. S., Gordon, D. L. and Wong, R. (1994). The impact of unit-based self-management by nurses on patient outcomes. *Health Services Research, 29*(4), 415–433.

Cassens, B. J. (1992). *Preventive medicine and public health* (2nd ed.). Baltimore: Halwal Publishers.

Chang, B. L. (1991). Computerized nursing information in eastern Europe. *Western Journal of Nursing Research, 13*(4), 537–538.

Chatellier, G., Colombet, I., and Degoulet, P. (1998). An overview of the effect of computer-assisted management of anticoagulant therapy on the quality of anticoagulation. *International Journal of Medical Informatics, 49*(3), 311–320.

Choddoff, P., and Crowley, K. (1995). Clinical practice guidelines: Roadblocks to their acceptance and implementation. *The Journal of Outcomes Management, 2*(2), 5–10.

Cleary, P. D., and Edgman-Levitan, S. (1997). Health care quality: Incorporating consumer perspectives. *Journal of the American Medical Association, 278*(19), 1608–1612.

Cole, L., and Houston, S. (1997). Integrating information technology with an outcomes management program. *Critical Care Nursing, 19*(4), 71–79.

Cook, D. J., Mulrow, C. D., and Haynes, R. B. (1997). Systematic reviews: Synthesis of best evidence for clinical decisions. *Annals of Internal Medicine, 126,* 364–371.

Coyle, M. (1997). The health of the public: Moving towards consumer driven health improvement. *Medical Outcomes Trust Monitor, 2*(3), 18–19.

Crist, L. (1997). Outcomes system implementation for subacute care. *Nursing Care Management, 2*(1), 33–41.

Cudworth, A. (1998). Quality and Standards. *Nurse Manager, 5*(8), 10.

Dalton, J. A., Blau, W., Lindley, C., et al. (1999). Changing acute pain management to improve patient outcomes: An educational approach. *Journal of Pain Symptom Management, 17*(4), 277–287.

Dalton, J. A. (1996). Outcomes that provide evidence of change in cancer pain management. *Nursing Clinics of North America, 30*(4), 683–695.

Daley, J., Dhuri, S. F., Henderson, W., et al. (1997). Risk adjustment of the postoperative morbidity rate for the comparative assessment of the quality of surgical care: Results of the national veterans affairs surgical risk study. *Journal of the American College of Surgeons, 185*(4), 328–340.

Davis, D. A., Thomson, M. A., Ocman, A. D., and Haynes, R. B. (1995). Changing physician performance: A systematic review of the effect of continuing medical education strategies. *Journal of the American Medical Association, 274,* 700–705.

Davis, D. A., and Taylor-Vaisey, A. (1997). Translating guidelines into practice: A systematic review of the theoretic concepts, practical experience and research evidence in the adoption of clinical practice guidelines. *Canadian Medical Association Journal, 157*(4), 406–416.

Dawson, S. (1995). Never mind solutions: What are the issues? Lessons of industrial technology transfer for quality in health care. *Quality in Health Care, 4*(3), 197–203.

Deber, R. B. (1996). Shared decision making in the real world. *Journal of General Internal Medicine, 11,* 377–378.

Delaney, C., Mehmert, P. A., Prophet, C. M., et al. (1992). Standardized nursing language for healthcare information systems. *Journal of Medical Systems, 16*(4), 145–159.

Demakis, J.G., McQueen, L., Kizer, K., and Feussner, J.R. (2000, June). Quality enhancement research initiative (QUERI): A collaboration between research and clinical practice. *Medical Care, 38*(Suppl 6), 17–25.

DeRosario, J. M. (1998). Overcoming 10 roadblocks to initiating practice guidelines. *Journal for Healthcare Quality, 20*(2), 23–24.

Dexter, P. R., Wolinsky, F. D., Gramelspacher, G. P., et al. (1998). Effectiveness of computer-generated reminders for increasing discussions about advance directives and completion of advance directive forms: A randomized, controlled trial. *Annals of Internal Medicine, 128*(2), 102–110.

Deyo, R. A., Andersson, G., Bombardier, C., et al. (1994). Outcome measures for studying patients with low back pain. *Spine, 19(18 Supplement),* 2032S–2036S.

Donabedian, A. (1980). *Explorations in quality assessment and monitoring. Volume 1: The definition of quality and approaches to its assessment.* Ann Arbor: Health Administration Press.

Donahue, D. C., Lewis, B. E., Ockene, I. S., and Saperia, G. (1996). Research collaboration between an HMO and an academic medical center: Lessons learned. *Academic Medicine, 71*(2), 126–32.

Dowie, R. (1998). A review of research in the United Kingdom to evaluate the implementation of clinical practice guidelines in general practice. *Family Practitioner, 15*(5), 462–70.

Drucker, P. F. (1994). The age of social transformation. *The Atlantic Monthly, 274*(5), 53–80.

Duff, L., and Casey, A. (1998). Implementing clinical guidelines: How can informatics help? *Journal of the American Medical Informatics Association, 5*(3), 225–226.

Duff, L. (1998). The RCN strategy on clinical guidelines. *Nursing Standard, 13*(8), 33–34.

Duck, J. D. (1993). Managing change: The art of balancing. *Harvard Business Review,* November–December, 109–130.

Dugas, M. (1998). An intranet-based information system for nurses. *MD Computing, 15*(3), 158–61.

Duncan, S. D., and Otto, S. E. (1995). Implementing guidelines for acute pain management. *Nursing Management, 26*(5), 40, 44–47.

Eastwood, A. F., and Sheldon, T. A. (1996). Organization of asthma care: What difference does it make? A systematic review of the literature. *Quality in Health Care, 5,* 134–143.

Eddy, D. M. (1990). Guidelines for policy statements: The explicit approach. *Journal of the American Medical Association, 263,* 3077–84.

Edgman-Levitan, S., and Cleary, P. D. (1996). What information do consumers want and need? *Health Affairs, 15*(4), 42–56.

Edinger, S., and McCormick, K. A. (1998). Databases—their use in developing clinical practice guidelines and estimating the cost impact of guideline implementation. *Journal of the American Health Informatics Association, 67*(4), 52–60.

Eisenberg, J. (1998). Clinical economics: A guide to the economic analysis of clinical practices. *Journal of the American Medical Association, 262*(20), 2879–86.

Ellrodt, A. G., Conner, L., Riedinger, M. S., and Weingarten, S. (1992). Implementing practice guidelines through a utilization management strategy: The potential and challenges. *Quality Review Bulletin, 18*(12), 456–460.

Ellrodt, G., Cook, D. J., Lee, J., et al. (1997). Evidence-based disease management. *Journal of the American Medical Association, 278*(20), 1687–1692.

Emslie, C., Grimshaw, J., and Templeton, A. (1993). Do clinical guidelines improve general practice management and referral of infertile couples? *British Medical Journal, 306*(June), 1728–1731.

Epstein, R. S., and Sherwood, L. M. (1996). From outcomes research to disease management: A guide for the perplexed. *Annals of Internal Medicine, 124,* 832–837.

Fang, E., Mittman, B. S., and Weingarten, S. (1996). Use of clinical practice guidelines in managed care physician groups. *Archives in Family Medicine, 5,* 528–531.

Faller, H. S., Dowell, M. A., and Jackson, M. A. (1995). Bridges to the future: Nontraditional clinical settings, concepts, and issues. *Journal of Nursing Education, 34*(8), 344–349.

Feder, G., Exxles, M., Grol, R., et al. (1999). Clinical guidelines: Using clinical guidelines. *British Medical Journal, 318*(7185), 728–730.

Fennessy, G. (1998). What's the evidence? Clinical effectiveness. *Nursing Standard, 13,* 1–13.

Ferguson, T. (1997). Health online and the empowered medical consumer. *Joint Commission Journal on Quality Improvement, 23*(5), 251–257.

Feussner, J.R., Kizer, K.W., and Demakis, J.G. (2000, June). The quality enhancement research initiative (QUERI): From evidence to action. *Medical Care, 38*(Suppl 1), 1–6.

Flower, J. (1995). Collaboration: The new leadership. *Healthcare Forum Journal, 38*(6), 20–26.

Fonteyn, M. (1998). The Agency for Health Care Policy and Research guidelines: Implications for home health care providers. *American Association of Clinical Nursing, 9*(3), 338–354.

Forrest, D., Hoskins, A., and Hussey, R. (1996). Clinical guidelines and their implementation. *Postgraduate Medical Journal, 72,* 19–22.

Fox, R. C. (1980). The evolution of medical uncertainty. *The Millbank Quarterly, 58*(1), 1–49.

Franck, L. S. (1992). The influence of sociopolitical, scientific, and technological forces on the study and treatment of neonatal pain. *Advances in Nursing Science, 15*(1), 11–20.

Fridsma, D. B., Gennari, H. J., and Musen, M. A. (1996). Making generic guidelines specific. *Proceedings of the American Medical Informatics Association Annual Fall Symposium,* 597–561.

Funk, S. G., Champagne, M. T., Wiese, R. A., and Tomquist, E. M. (1991a). Barriers: The barriers to research utilization scale. *Applied Nursing Research, 4,* 39–45.

Funk, S. G., Champagne, M. T. Wiese, R. A., and Tomquist, E. M. (1991b). Barriers to using research findings in practice: The clinicians perspective. *Applied Nursing Research, 4,* 90–95.

Funk, S. G., Champagne, M. T., Wiese, R. A., and Tomquist, E. M. (1995). Administrators views on barriers to research utilization. *Applied Nursing Research, 8,* 44–49.

Gates, P. E. (1995). Think globally, act locally: An approach to implementation of clinical practice guidelines. *Joint Commission Journal on Quality Improvement, 21*(2), 71–85.

Goldberg, H. I., Wagner, E. H., Fihn, S. D., et al. (1998). A randomized controlled trial of CQI teams and academic detailing: Can they alter compliance with guidelines? *Joint Commission Journal on Quality Improvement, 24*(3), 130–142.

Gottlieb, L. K., Sokol, H. N., Murrey, K. O., and Schoenbaum, S. C. (1992). Algorithm-based clinical quality improvement. Clinical guidelines and continuous quality improvement. *HMO Practice, 6*(1), 5–12.

Grady, M. I., and Weis, K. A. (Eds.). (1995). *Cost Analysis Methodology for Clinical Practice Guidelines.* Rockville, MD: U.S. Department of Health and Human Services, Agency for Health Care Policy and Research, AHCPR Publication No. 95-0001.

Gray, J. A., Haynes, R. B., Sackett, D. L., et al. (1997). Transferring evidence from research into practice 3: Developing evidence-based clinical policy. *Evidence Based Medicine, 2*(2), 36–38.

Greco, P. J., and Eisenberg, J. M. (1993). Changing physician's practice. *New England Journal of Medicine, 329,* 1271–1273.

Greenberg, G. T. (1990). The pitfalls of meta-analysis. *Journal of the American Geriatrics Society, 38,* 607.

Greengold, N. L., and Weingarten, S. R. (1996). Developing evidence-based practice guidelines: The experience at the local hospital level. *Journal on Quality Improvement, 22*(6), 391–402.

Greer, A. L. (1995). The shape of resistance . . . the shapers of change. *The Joint Commission Journal on Quality Improvement, 21*(7), 328–332.

Greer, J., and Hexum, J. (1987). Dimensions of computerized quality assurance systems. *Journal of Nursing Quality Assurance, 1*(4), 9–14.

Greer, A. L., Wolff, M., and Dettman, F. G. (1995). Emerging themes in efforts to improve the quality of care: Overview. *Joint Commission Journal on Quality Improvement, 21*(7), 319–324.

Griffith, H. M., and DiGuiseppi, C. (1994). Guidelines for clinical preventive services. Essential for nurse practitioners in practice, education and research. *Nurse Practitioner, 19*(9), 25–28, 31, 35.

Griffith, H. M. (1993). Needed—A strong nursing position on prevention services. *Image: Journal of Nursing Scholarship, 25*(4), 272.

Griffith, H. M., Dickey, L., and Kamerow, D. B. (1995). Put prevention into practice: A systematic approach.

Journal of Public Health Management and Practice, 1(3), 9–15.

Grilli, R., and Lomas, J. (1994). Evaluating the message: The relationship between compliance rate and the subject of a practice guideline. *Medical Care, 32*(3), 202–213.

Grimshaw, J. M. (1996). Towards effective professional practice. *Therapie, 51*(3), 233–236.

Grimshaw, J., Freemantle, N., Wallace, S., et al. (1994). Developing and implementing clinical practice guidelines. *Effective Health Care Bulletin No. 8: Implementing clinical guidelines: Can guidelines improve clinical practice?* Leeds UK: The University of Leeds.

Grimshaw, J. M., and Russell, J. T. (1993). Effect of clinical guidelines on medical practice: A systematic review of rigorous evaluations. *The Lancet, 342,* 1317–1322.

Grindel, C. G., and McGuffin, B. (1992). Standards of clinical nursing practice: A link to quality of care. *Medsurg Nursing, 1*(2), 23–28.

Grogan, C. M., Feldman, R. D., Nyman, J. A., and Shapiro, J. (1994). How will we use clinical guidelines? The experience of medicare carriers. *Journal of Politics, Policy and Law, 19*(1), 7–26.

Guidotti, T. L. (1996). Preventive medicine: Notes toward an agenda for change. *American Journal of Preventive Medicine, 12*(3), 165–171.

Hadjipavlou, A. G., Simmons, J. W., and Pope, M. H. (1998). An algorithmic approach to the investigation, treatment and complications of surgery for low back pain. *Seminars in Spine Surgery, 10*(2), 193–218.

Hadom, D. C., Baker, D., Hodges, J. S., and Hicks, N. (1996). Rating the quality of evidence for clinical practice guidelines. *Journal of Clinical Epidemiology, 49*(7), 749–754.

Hagen, N. A., and Whylie, B. (1998). Putting clinical practice guidelines into the hands of cancer patients. Editorial. *Canadian Medical Association Journal, 158*(3), 347–348.

Hagland, M. (1997). Putting a new spin on information systems. *Trustee,* March, *50*(3), 14–17, 28.

Haines, A., and Donald, A. (1998). Making better use of research findings. *British Medical Journal, 317,* 72–75.

Hall, C. M. (1999). Pressure ulcers: Are you aware? *Journal of Nursing Administration, 29*(4), 17–32.

Handley, M. R., Stuart, M. E., and Kirz, H. L. (1994). An evidence-based approach to evaluating and improving clinical practice: Implementing practice guidelines. *HMO Practice, 8*(2), 75–82.

Harr, D. S., Balas, A., and Mitchell, J.(1996). Developing quality indicators as educational tools to measure the implementation of clinical practice guidelines. *American Journal of Medical Quality, 11*(4), 179–185.

Harvey, G., and Kitson, A. (1996). Achieving improvement through quality: An evaluation of key factors in the implementation process. *Journal of Advanced Nursing, 24,* 185–195.

Haynes, R. B., Sackett, D. L., Gray, J. A., et al. (1996). Transferring evidence from research into practice: The role of clinical care research in decision making. *Evidence-Based Medicine, 1*(7), 196–199.

Headrick, L., Katcher, W., Neuhauser, D., and McEachem, E. (1994). Continuous quality improvement and knowledge for improvement applied to asthma care. *Joint Commission Journal on Quality Improvement, 20*(10), 562–568.

Hefferin, E. A., Horsley, J. A., and Venturna, M. R. (1982). Promoting research-based nursing: The administrator's role. *Journal of Nursing Administration, 12*(5), 34–41.

Heil, R., Lane, S., Maahs, D., et al. (1997). Using a performance improvement team to reinvent a mandatory education program. *Joint Commission Journal on Quality Improvement, 23*(2), 103–116.

Heller, C. (1996). Leveraging information technology for quality improvement. *Healthcare Information Management, 10*(1), 53–59.

Henry, S. B., Douglas, K., Galzagorry, G., et al. (1998). A template-based approach to support utilization of clinical practice guidelines within an electronic health record. *Journal of the American Medical Association, 5*(3), 237–244.

Hetlevik, I., Holmen, J., and Kruger, O. (1999). Implementing clinical guidelines in the treatment of hypertension in general practice: Evaluation of patient outcome related to implementation of computer-based clinical decision support system. *Scandinavian Journal of Primary Health Care, 17*(1), 35–40.

Hooker, R. C. (1997). The rise and rise of evidence-based medicine. *The Lancet, 349,* 1329–1330.

Horwitz, R. I., and Horwitz, S. M. (1993). Adherence to treatment and health outcomes. *Archives of Internal Medicine, 153*(August 23), 1863–1868.

Huber, D. (1996). *Leadership and Nursing Care Management.* Philadelphia: WB Saunders & Co.

Hunsicker, K., Fuss, M. A., Shollenberger, D., and Pasquale, M. D. (1998). A fever workup guideline. *International Journal of Trauma Nursing, 4*(3), 85–93.

Hunt, D. L., Haynes, R. B., Hanna, S. E., and Smith, K. (1998). Effects of computer-based clinical decision support systems on physician performance and patient outcomes: A systematic review. *Journal of the American Medical Association, 280*(15), 1339–1346.

Hynes, M., Cowper, D., Kerr, M., Kubal, J., and Murphy, P.A. (2000, June). Database and informatics support for QUERI. *Medical Care,* Supplement, *38*(Suppl. 6), 114–128.

Institute of Medicine. Field, M. J., and Lorh, K. N. (Eds.). (1990). *Clinical Practice Guidelines: Directions for a New Program.* Washington, D. C.: National Academy Press.

Institute of Medicine. Field, M. J., and Lohr, K. N. (Eds.). (1992). *Guidelines for Clinical Practice: From*

Development to Use. Washington, D. C.: National Academy Press.

Institute of Medicine. Field, M. J. (Ed.). (1995). *Setting Priorities for Clinical Practice Guidelines*. Washington, D. C.: National Academy Press.

James, P. A., Cowen, T. M., and Graham, R. P. (1998). Patient-centered clinical decisions and their impact on physician adherence to clinical guidelines. *Journal of Family Practice, 46*(4), 311–318.

Janarkar, S. (1996). Editorial page. Telemedicine's economies win supporters. *The New York Times*, November 26.

Kaegi, L. (1995). Nurses leading the change to take national AHCPR guidelines into local settings. *Joint Commission Journal on Quality Improvement, 21*(1), 45–49.

Kaegi, L. (1995). From paper to practice to point of care: Reports from a Zitter group conference on implementing practice guidelines. *The Joint Commission Journal on Quality Improvement, 22*(8), 551–589.

Kahan, J. P., Bernstein, S. J., Leape, L. L., et al. (1994). Measuring the necessity of medical procedures. *Medical Care, 32*(4), 357–365.

Kaluzny, A. D., Konrad, T. R., and McLaughlin, C. P. (1995). Organizational strategies for implementing clinical guidelines. *Joint Commission Journal on Quality Improvement, 21*(7), 347–351.

Karp, H. B. (1996). *The change leader*. San Diego: Pfeiffer Publishers.

Kasper, J., Mulley, A., and Wennberg, J. (1992). Developing shared decision-making programs to improve the quality of health care. *Quality Review Bulletin, 18*, 183–190.

Keller, L. S., McDermott, S., and Alt-White, A. (1991). Effects of computerized nurse care planning on selected health care effectiveness measures. *Procedures from the Annual Symposium of Applied Medical Care, 1991*, 38–42.

Khuri, S. E., Daley, J., Henderson, W., et al. (1998). The Department of Veterans Affairs' NSQIP: The first national, validated, outcome-based, risk-adjusted, and peer-controlled program for the measurement and enhancement of the quality of surgical care. National VA surgical quality improvement program. *Annals of Surgery, 228*(4), 491–507.

Kibbe, D. C., Kaluzny, A. D., and McLaughlin, C. P. (1994). Integrating guidelines with continuous quality improvement: Doing the right thing the right way to achieve the right goals. *Joint Commission Journal on Quality Improvement, 20*(4), 181–191.

Kinney, C. F., and Gift, R. G. (1997). Building a framework for multiple improvement initiatives. *Joint Commission Journal of Quality Improvement, 23*(8), 407–423.

Kirchner, M. (1991). Who pays for new technology? *Business & Health, 9*(11), 20–110.

Kitchiner, D., Davidson, D., and Bundred, P. (1996). Integrated care pathways: Effective tools for continuous evaluation of clinical practice. *Journal of Evaluation in Clinical Practices, 2*(1), 65–69.

Kizer, K. W. (1998). Clinical practice guidelines. *Federal Practitioner*, 52–58.

Kizer, K. W., Demakis, J. G., and Feussner, J. R. (2000, June). Reinventing VA health care: Systematizing quality improvement and quality innovation. *Medical Care, 38*(Suppl 6), 129–141.

Kleinpell, R. M. (1997). Whose outcomes. Patients, providers, or payers? *Nursing Clinics of North America, 32*(3), 513–520.

Klunk, S. W. (1997). Conflict and the dynamic organization. *Hospital Materials Management Quarterly, 19*(2), 37–44.

Knickman, J. R., Hughes, R. G., Taylor, H., et al. (1996). Tracking consumers' reactions to the changing health care system: Early indicators. *Health Affairs, 15*(2), 21–32.

Kotter, J. P. (1995). Leading change: Why transformation efforts fail. *Harvard Business Review*, March/April, 59–67.

Krieglestein, C. F., Schall, R., Runkel, M., and Herfarth, C. (1997). Using of information systems for direct surgical patient management. *Langenbecks Archives, 114*, 656–659.

Krishna, S., Balas, E. A., Spencer, D. C., et al. (1997). Clinical trials of interactive computerized patient education: Implications for family practice. *Journal of Family Practice, 45*(1), 25–33.

Lawler, F. H., and Viviani, N. (1997). Patient and physician perspectives regarding treatment of diabetes: Compliance with practice guidelines. *Journal of Family Practice, 44*, 369–373.

Lee, T. H., Pearson, S. D., Johanson, P. A., et al. (1995). Failure of information as an intervention to modify clinical management: A time-series trial in patients with acute chest pain. *Annals of Internal Medicine, 122*, 434–437.

Levinson, E. A. (1996). The politics of interpretation. *Contemporary Psychoanalysis, 32*(4), 631–648.

Levknecht, L., Schriefer, J., Schriefer, J., and Maconis, B. (1997). Combining case management, pathways, and report cards for secondary cardiac prevention. *Joint Commission, 23*(3), 162–174, Washington, D.C.

Lobach, D. F. (1995). A model for adapting clinical practice guidelines for electronic implementation in primary care. *Proceedings of the 19th Annual Symposium on Computer Applications in Medical Care*, 581–585.

Lomas, J. (1991). Words without action? The production, dissemination, and impact of consensus recommendations. *Annual Review of Public Health, 12*, 41–65.

Lomas, J. (1993). Diffusion, dissemination, and implementation: Who should do what? *Annals of the New York Academy of Sciences, 703*, 226–235.

Lomas, J. (1993). Making clinical policy explicit. Legislative policy making and the lessons learned from practice guidelines. *International Journal of Technology Assessment in Health Care,* 9(1), 11–25.

Lomas, J., Anderson, G. M., Komnick-Pierre, K., et al. (1989). Do practice guidelines guide practice? *The New England Journal of Medicine,* 321(19), 1306–1311.

Lomas, J., Enkin, M., Anderson, G. M., et al. (1991). Opinion leaders vs. audit and feedback to implement practice guidelines. *Journal of the American Medical Association,* 265(17), 2202–2217.

Lomas, J., and Haynes, R. B. (1988). A taxonomy and critical review of tested strategies for the application of clinical practice recommendations: From "official" to "individual" clinical policy. *American Journal of Preventive Medicine, 4(Supplement),* 77–94.

Lomas, J., Sisk, J. E., and Stocking, B. (1993). From evidence to practice in the United States, the United Kingdom, and Canada. *Millbank Quarterly,* 71(3), 405–410.

Love, R. R. (1995). Changing the health promotion behaviors of primary care physicians: Lessons from two projects. *Joint Commission Journal for Quality Improvement,* 21(7), 339–343.

Lowe, A., and Baker, J. K. (1997). Measuring outcomes: A nursing report card. *Nurse Manager,* 28(11), 38–41.

Lowry, M. (1998). Working in syndicate groups towards the development of clinical care protocols: A study into the professional learning of undergraduate nursing students. *Nurse Education Today,* 18(6), 470–476.

Lusk, R., and Herrmann, K. (1998). The computerized patient record. *Otolaryngol Clinics of North America,* 31(12), 289–300.

Madigan, E. A. (1998). Evidence-based practice in home healthcare. A springboard for discussion. *Home Health Nursing,* 16(6), 411–415.

Management Decision Research Center. (1998). *Clinical Practice Guidelines.* Boston: VA Health Services Research and Development Service, in collaboration with the Association for Health Services Research.

Marin, L., Lacalle, J. R., Briones, E., et al. (1996). Change in physicians' behavior after implementation of guidelines together with feedback assessment of their practice. *Annual Meeting of the International Society for Technology Assessment in Health Care,* 12, 52.

McCaffery, M., and Ferrell, B. (1994). How to use the new AHCPR cancer pain guidelines. *American Journal of Nursing,* 94, 42–47.

McCormick, K., Moore, S. R., and Siegel, R. A. (1994). *Clinical Practice Guideline Development: Methodology Perspectives.* AHCPR No. 95-0009. Washington, D. C.: US Public Health Service.

McCormick, K. A. (1995). Including oncology outcomes of care in the computer-based patient record. *Oncology,* 9(11) (Supplement), 161–167.

McCormick, K. A. (1998). New tools—new models to integrate outcomes into quality measurement. *Seminars in Nursing Management,* 6(3), 119–125.

McGlynn, E. A. (1996). Setting the context for measuring patient outcomes. *New Directions in Mental Health Services,* 71, 19–32.

McGlynn, E. A., and Asch, S. M. (1998). Developing a clinical performance measure. *American Journal of Preventive Medicine,* 14(3 Supplement), 14 21.

McHolm, G., and Greenes, R. A. (1997). Locating physicians on the World Wide Web: Managed and unmanaged health care delivery. *Medical Practices Management,* November–December, 138–143.

McLaughlin, C. P., and Kaluzny, A. D. (1994). *Continuous Quality Improvement in Health Care.* Gaithersburg, MD: Aspen Publishers.

McQueen, M. L. (1998). Interests in Evidence: Politicians' Involvement in Developing Evidence-Based Policies. Ann Arbor, MI: UMI Services of The Bell & Howell Publishing Company.

Miaskowski, V., Crews, J., Ready, L. B., et al. (1999). Anesthesia-based pain services improve the quality of postoperative pain management. *Pain,* 80(1–2), 23–29.

Mitchell, P. H. (1999). Outcomes research and the neuroscience nurse: What's in it for clinical practice? *Journal of Neuroscientific Nursing,* 30(5), 318–321.

Mittman, B. S., Pugh, J. A. Rubenstein, L. V., and Charns, M. P. (1999). Making ongoing improvement a reality. *Presentation at the Second Annual Meeting for the Quality Enhancement Review Initiative.* Reston, VA: Department of Veterans Affairs, Health Service Research and Development.

Mittman, B. S., Tonesk, X., and Jacobson, P. D. (1992). Implementing clinical practice guidelines: Social influence strategies and practitioner behavior change. *Quality Review Bulletin, December,* 18(12), 413–422.

Montgomery, A. A., and Fahey, T. (1998). A systematic review of the use of computers in the management of hypertension. *Journal of Epidemiological Community Health,* 52(8), 520–525.

Moorhead, S., Clarke, M., Willits, M., and Tomsha, K. A. (1998). Nursing outcomes classification implementation projects across the care continuum. *Journal of Nursing Care Quality,* 12(5), 52–63.

Moorhead, S., Head, B., Johnson, M., and Maas, M. (1998). The nursing outcomes taxonomy: Development and coding. *Journal of Nursing Care Quality,* 12(6), 56–63.

Morgan, M. M., Goodson, J., and Barnett, G. O. (1998). Long-term changes in compliance with clinical guidelines through computer-based reminders. *Proceedings of the American Medical Informatics Association,* 493–497.

Mosser, G. (1996). Clinical process improvement: Engage first, measure later. *Quality Management in Health Care,* 4(4), 11–20.

Murrey, K. O., Gottlieb, L. K., and Schoenbaum S. C. (1992). Implementing clinical guidelines: A quality management approach to reminder systems. *Quality Review Bulletin,* December, 18(12), 423–433.

Nardella, A., Pechel, L., and Snyder, L. M. (1995). Continuous improvement, quality control, and cost containment in clinical laboratory testing. Effects of establishing and implementing guidelines for preoperative tests. *Archives in Pathology and Laboratory Medicine, 119*(6), 518–522.

National Library of Medicine. (1994). Vocabularies for computer-based patient records: Identifying candidates for large scale testing. Minutes of a meeting sponsored by the NLM and the Agency for Health Care Policy and Research. *http://medlineplus.nlm.nih.gov.lo/mincocab/html*

National Library of Medicine. (1999a). Fact Sheet: Partners in information access for public health professionals. *http://.www.nim.nih.gov/nno/partners.html*

National Library of Medicine. (1999b). Fact Sheet: Unified Medical Language System. *http://www.nim.nih.gov/pubs/factsheets/umls.html*

Newcomer, L. N. (1994). Leading clinical quality improvement. Six pointers for implementing guidelines. *Healthcare Forum Journal, 37*(4), 31–33.

Newman, D. D., McCormick, K. A., Colling, J., and Pearson, B. (1993). A guideline for the nation: Managing urinary incontinence. *Journal of Home Health Care Practice, 5*(3), 33–44.

Newman, D. K. (1994). Strategies for managing urinary incontinence in homebound patients. *ADVANCE for nurse practitioners, August,* 11–14.

Nichols, N. A. (1994). Medicine, management, and mergers: An interview with Merck's P. Roy Vagelos. *Harvard Business Review,* November–December, 105–114.

O'Connor, M. P. (1999). Implementing change in the organization of nursing care. *New Zealand Nursing Journal, 69*(4), 8–11.

O'Connor, P. J., Solberg, L. I., Christianson, J., et al. (1996). Mechanism of action and impact of a cystitis clinical practice guideline on outcomes and costs of care in an HMO. *Joint Commission Journal on Quality Improvement, 22*(10), 673–682.

Ohm, B., and Brown, J. (1997). Quality improvement pitfalls and how to overcome them. *Journal for Healthcare Quality, 19*(3), 16–20.

Ohno-Machado, L., Gennari, H. J., Murphy, S. N., et al. (1998). The guideline interchange format: A model for representing guidelines. *Journal of the American Medical Informatics Association, 5*(4), 357–372.

Ornstein, S. M., Jenkins, R. G., Lee, F. W., et al. (1997). The computer-based patient record as a CQI tool in a family medicine center. *Joint Commission Journal on Quality Improvement, 23*(7), 347–361.

Oxman, A. D. (1995). No magic bullet: A systematic review of 102 trials of interventions to improve professionals practice. *Canadian Medical Association Journal, 153,* 1423–1431.

Pare, G., and Elam, J. J. (1998). Introducing information technology in the clinical setting. Lessons learned in a trauma center. *Internal Journal of Technology Assessment in Health Care, 14*(2), 331–343.

Pascale, R., Millemann, M., and Gioja, L. (1997). Changing the way we change. *Harvard Business Review, 75*(6), 126–139.

Patel, V. L., Allen, V.G., Arocha, J. F., and Shortliffe, E. H. (1998). Representing clinical guidelines in GLIF: Individual and collaborative expertise. *Journal of the American Medical Informatics Association, 5*(5), 467–483.

Pauly, M. V. (1995). Practice guidelines: Can they save money? Should they? *Journal of Law, Medicine, and Ethics, 23*(1), 65–74.

Petrucci, K. E., Jacox, A., McCormick, K., et al. (1992). Evaluating the appropriateness of a nurse expert system's patient assessment. *Computers in Nursing, 10*(6), 243–249.

Petrucci, K. E., Petrucci, P., and Canfield, K. (1991). Evaluation of UNIS: Urological nursing information system. *Proceedings of the Annual Symposium for Computer Applications in Medical Care,* 43–47.

Petrucci, K. E., McCormick, K. A., and Scheve, A. A. (1987). Documenting patient care needs: Do nurses do it? *Journal of Gerontological Nursing, 13*(11), 34–38.

Pierce, S. F. (1997). Nurse-sensitive health care outcomes in acute care settings: An integrative analysis of the literature. *Journal of Nursing Care Quality, 11*(4), 60–72.

Prophct, C. M., and Delaney, C. W. (1998). Nursing outcomes classification: Implications for nursing information systems and the computer-based patient record. *Journal of Nursing Care Quality, 12*(5), 21–29.

Quigley, P., Mathis, A., and Nodhturft, V. (1994). Improving clinical documentation quality. *Journal of Nursing Care Quality, 8*(4), 66–73.

Renvoize, E. G., Hampshaw, S. M., Pinder, J. M., and Ayres, P. (1997). What are hospitals doing about clinical guidelines? *Quality Health Care, 6*(4), 187–191.

Regan, J. A. (1998). Will current clinical effectiveness initiatives encourage and facilitate practitioners to use evidence-based practice for the benefit of their clients? *Journal of Clinical Nursing, 7*(3), 244–250.

Rich, M. W., Beckham, V., Wittenberg, C., et al. (1995). A multidisciplinary intervention to prevent the readmission of elderly patients with congestive heart failure. *New England Journal of Medicine, 333,* 1190–1195.

Rischer, J. B., and Childress, S. B. (1996). Cancer pain management: Pilot implementation of the AHCPR guideline in Utah. *Joint Commission Journal on Quality Improvement, 22*(10), 683–700.

Roberts, R. G. (1994). New guidelines based on symptoms and patient preferences. *Geriatrics, 49*(7), 24–31.

Robinson, M. B., Thompson, E., and Black, N. A. (1996). Evaluation of the effectiveness of guidelines, audit and feedback: Improving the use of intravenous thrombolysis in patients with suspected acute myocardial infarction. *International Journal of Quality in Health Care, 8*(3), 211–222.

Rogers, E. M. (1995). Lessons for guidelines from the diffusion of innovations. *Joint Commission Journal on Quality Improvement, 21*(7), 324–328.

Rolnick, S. F., and O'Connor, P. J. (1997). Assessing the impact of clinical guidelines: Research lessons learned. *Journal of Ambulatory Care Management, 20*(4), 47–55.

Rosser, W. W., McDowell, I., and Newell, C. (1991). Use of reminders for preventive procedures in family medicine. *Canadian Medical Association Journal, 145*(7), 807–813.

Rubenstein, L. V., Mittman, B. S., Yano, E. M. and Mulrow, C. D. (2000, June). From understanding health care provider behavior to improving health care: The QUERI framework for quality improvement. *Medical Care 38*(Suppl 6), 129–141.

Sackett, D. L., and Parkes, J. (1998). Teaching critical appraisal: No quick fixes. Editorial. *Canadian Medical Association Journal, 158*(2), 203–204.

Safran, C., Rind, D. M., Davis, R. M., et al. (1995). An electronic medical record that helps care for patients with HIV infection. *Proceedings of the Annual Symposium of Computer Applications in Medical Care*, 224–228.

Schafer, J. (1995). Battle over practice guidelines leaves future of AHCPR hanging in the outcome. *Journal of Investigative Medicine, 43*(6), 495–500.

Schmidt, K., Holida, D., Kleiber, C., et al. (1994). Implementation of the AHCPR guidelines for children. *Journal of Nursing Care Quality, 8*(3), 68–74.

Schriger, D. L. (1996). Emergency medicine clinical guidelines: We can make them, but will we use them? (Editorial). *Annals of Emergency Medicine, 27*(5), 655–657.

Schriger, D. L., Baraff, L. J., Rogers, W. H., and Cretin, S. (1997). Implementation of clinical guidelines using a computer charting system. Effect on the initial care of health care workers exposed to body fluids. *Journal of the American Medical Association, 278*(19), 1585–1590.

Shea, S., DuMouchel, W., and Bahamonde, L. (1996). A meta-analysis of 16 randomized controlled trials to evaluate computer-based clinical reminder systems for preventive care in the ambulatory setting. *Journal of the American Medical Informatics Association, 3*(6), 399–409.

Shiffman, R. N., Brandt, C. A., Liaw, Y., and Corb, G. J. (1999a). A design model for computer-based guideline implementation based on information management services. *Journal of the American Medical Informatics Association, 6*(2), 99–103.

Shiffman, R. N., Liaw, Y., Brandt, C. A., and Corb, G. J. (1999b). Computer-based guideline implementation systems: A systematic review of functionality and effectiveness. *Journal of the American Medical Informatics Association, 6*(2), 104–114.

Shortell, S. M., Gillies, R. R., Anderson, D. A., et al. (1996). *Remaking Health Care in America*. San Francisco, CA: Jossey-Bass Publishers.

Shortell, S. M., and Kaluzny, A. D. (1994). *Health Care Management: Organizational Design and Behavior*. (3rd ed.). Albany, NY: Delmar Publications.

Simpson, R. L. (1999). Changing world, changing systems: Why managed health care demands information technology. *Nursing Administration Quarterly, 23*(2), 86–88.

Sisk, J. E. (1998). How are health organizations using clinical guidelines? *Health Affairs, 17*(5), 91–109.

Sisk, J. E. (1995). Promises and hazards of strategies to implement change. *Joint Commission Journal for Quality Improvement, 21*(7), 357–360.

Smith, J. A., Scammon, D. L., and Beck, S. L. (1995). Using patient focus groups for new patient services. *The Joint Commission Journal on Quality Improvement, 21*(1), 22–31.

Smith, M. (1998). Researching integrative therapies: Guidelines and application. *Journal of Emergency Nursing, 24*(6), 609–613.

Snyder, C. R. (1995). Reflections on human nature. Book Review. *Journal of Social and Clinical Psychology, 14*(4), 409–412.

Solberg, L. I., Brekke, L. M., Kottke, T. E., and Steel, R. P. (1998). Continuous quality improvement in primary care: What's happening? *Medical Care, 36*(5), 625–635.

Solberg, L. I., Kottke, T. E., and Brekke, M. L. (1996). Using continuous quality improvement to increase preventive services in clinical practice—going beyond guidelines. *Preventive Medicine, 25*, 259–267.

Solberg, L. I., Mosser, G., and McDonald, S. (1997a). The three faces of performance measurement: Improvement accountability and research. *Joint Commission Journal on Quality Improvement, 23*(3), 135–147.

Solberg, L. I., Reger, L. A., Pearson, T. L., et al. (1997b). Using continuous quality improvement to improve diabetes care in populations: The IDEAL model. Improving care for diabetics through empowerment active collaboration and leadership. *Joint Commission Journal for Quality Improvement, 23*(11), 581–592.

Soumerai, S. B., and Avorn, J. (1990). Principles of educational outreach ('academic detailing') to improve clinical decision making. *Journal of the American Medical Association, 263*(4), 549–556.

Spernak, S. M., Budetti, P. P., and Zweig, F. (1992). *Use of Language in Clinical Practice Guideline*. Washington, D.C. Center for Health Policy Research, George Washington University; and Rockville, MD: The Agency for Health Care Policy and Research under Contract No. 282-87-0049.

Staples, L. H. (1990). Powerful ideas about empowerment. *Administration in Social Work, 14*(2), 29–33.

Steffensen, F. H., Olesen, F., and Sorensen, H. T. (1995). Implementation of guidelines on stroke prevention. *Family Practice, 12*, 269–273.

Steven, I. D., and Fraser, R. D. (1996). Clinical practice guidelines. Particular reference to the management of pain in the lumbosacral spine. *Spine, 21*(13), 1593–1596.

Stonestreet, J. S., and Prevost, S. S. (1999). A focused strategic plan for outcomes evaluation. *Nursing Clinics of North America, 32*(3), 615–631.

Straus, S. E., and Sackett, D. L. (1998). Using research findings in clinical practice. *British Medical Journal, 317*, 339–342.

Strohschein, S., Schaffer, M. A., and Lia-Hoagberg, B. (1999). Evidence-based guidelines for public health nursing practice. *Nursing Outlook, 47*(2), 84–89.

Summers, S. (1987). The nurse as an information manager. *Kansas Nurse, 62*(4), 2.

Swanson, G. M. (1994). May we agree to disagree or how do we develop guidelines for breast cancer screening in women? *Journal of the National Cancer Institute, 86*(12), 903–906.

Tang, P. C., LaRosa, M. P., Newcomb, C., and Gorden, S. M. (1999). Measuring the effects of reminders for outpatient influenza immunizations at the point of clinical opportunity. *Journal of the American Medical Informatics Association, 6*(2), 115–121.

Tatalovitch, R., Smith, T. A., and Bobic, M. P. (1994). Moral conflicts and the policy process. *Policy Currents, 14*(4).

Thombury, J. R. (1994). Why should radiologists be interested in technology assessment and outcomes research? *American Journal of Radiology, 163*, 1027–1030.

Timm, J. A., and Behrenbeck, J. G. (1998). Implementing the Nursing Outcomes Classification in a clinical information system in a tertiary care setting. *Journal of Nursing Care Quality, 12*(5), 62–72.

Todd, W. E., and Nash, D. (Eds.). (1997). *Disease Management: A Systems Approach to Improving Patient Outcomes.* Chicago: American Hospital Association.

Tonges, M. C., and Madden, M. J. (1993). Running the vicious cycle backward and other systems solutions to nursing problems. *Journal of Nursing Administration, 23*(1), 39–44.

Tomich N. (1999). QUERI: Putting evidence into medical practice. *U. S. Medicine, 35*(7), 3, 12, 15.

Trabin, T., and Freeman, M. A. (Eds.). (1996). *The Computerization of Behavioral Healthcare.* San Francisco: Jossey-Bass.

Trafford, A. (1997). In evaluating the data, Scientists are only human. *The Washington Post*, Editorial page, June 10.

Turner, B.J., Day, S. C., and Borenstein, B. (1989). A controlled trial to improve delivery of preventive care: Physician or patient reminders? *Journal of General Internal Medicine, 4*(5), 403–409.

University of Alberta. (1999). How to use a clinical practice guideline. *http://www.med.ualberta.ca/ebm/clinprac.htm*

U.S. Preventive Services Task Force. (1996). *Guideline to clinical preventive services.* 2nd ed. Baltimore: Williams & Wilkins Publishing Company.

VanAmringe, M., and Shannon, T. (1992). Awareness, assimilation and adoption: The challenge of effective dissemination and the first AHCPR-sponsored guidelines. *Quality Review Bulletin, 18*(12), 397–404.

Van Rijswijk, L. (1999). Clinical practice guidelines: Moving into the 21st Century. *Ostomy Wound Care, January(Supplement)*, 47S–53S.

Van Rijswijk, L., and Braden, B. J. (1999). Pressure ulcer patient and wound assessment: An AHCPR clinical practice guideline update. *Ostomy Wound Management, 45*(1A Supplement), 56S–67S.

Veney, J. E., and Kaluzny, A. D. (1991). *Evaluation and Decision Making for Health Services* (2nd ed). Ann Arbor, MI: Health Administration Press.

Wagner, E.H., Austin, B. T., and Von Korff, M. (1996). Organizing care for patients with chronic illness. *Millbank Quarterly, 74*, 511–544.

Wagner, E. H. (1997). Managed care and chronic illness: Health services research needs. *Health Services Research, 32*, 710–714.

Wakefield, B., Johnson, J. A., Kron-Chalupa, J., and Paulsen, L. (1998). A research based guideline for appropriate use of transdermal fentanyl to treat chronic pain. *Oncological Nursing Forum, 25*(9), 1505–1513.

Walker, K. (1994). Confronting "reality": Nursing, science, and the micro-politics of representation. *Nursing Inquiry, 1*(2), 46–56.

Weingarten, S., Riedinger, M., Conner, L., et al. (1994). Reducing lengths of stay in the coronary care unit with a practice guideline for patients with congestive heart failure. *Medical Care, 32*(12), 1232–1243.

Weingarten, S., Stone, E., Hayward, R., et al. (1995). The adoption of preventive care practice guidelines by primary care physicians: Do actions match intentions? *Journal of General Internal Medicine, 10*, 138–144.

Weingarten, S., and Ellrodt, A. G. (1992). The case for intensive dissemination: Adoption of practice guidelines in the coronary care unit. *Quality Review Bulletin, 18*(12), 449–455.

Wennberg, J. E., and Fowler, F. J. (1977). A test of consumer contribution to small area variations in health care delivery. *Journal of the Maine Medical Association, 68*(8), 275–279.

Wennberg, J. E., Freeman, J. L., Shelton, R. M., and Bubolz, T. A. (1989). Hospital use and mortality among Medicare beneficiaries in Boston and New Haven. *New England Journal of Medicine, 321*(17), 1168–1173.

Wennberg, J. E. (1990). Better policy to promote the evaluative clinical sciences. *Spine, 2*(1), 21–29.

Wennberg, J. E. (1996). Practice variations and the challenge of leadership. *Spine, 21*(12), 1472–1478.

Woolery, L. K. (1990). Professional standards and ethical dilemmas in using information systems. *Journal of Nursing Administration, 20*(10), 50–53.

Woolf, S. H. (1990). Practice guidelines: A new reality in medicine I. Recent developments. *Archives in Internal Medicine, 150,* 1811–1818.

Woolf, S. H., DiGuiseppi, C.G., Atkins, D., and Kamerow, D. B. (1996). Developing evidence-based clinical practice guidelines: Lessons learned by the US Preventive Services Task Force. *Annual Review of Public Health, 17,* 511–538.

Woolf, S. H., Grol, R., and Hutchinson, A. (1999). Clinical guidelines: Potential benefits, limitations, and harms of clinical guidelines. *British Medical Journal, 318*(7182), 527–530.

Woolf, S. H., and Lawrence, R. S. (1997). When politicians play doctor. *The Washington Post,* Editorial page, Sunday, May 4.

Wong, E. T., and Abendroth, T. W. (1996). Reaping the benefits of medical information systems. *Academic Medicine, 71*(4), 353–357.

Worrall, G., Chaulk, P., and Freake, D. (1997). The effects of clinical practice guidelines on patient outcomes in primary care: A systematic review. *Canadian Medical Association Journal, 156*(12), 1705–1712.

Yawn, B. P., Casey, M., and Hebert, P. (1999). The rural health care workforce implications of practice guideline implementation. *Medical Care, 37*(3), 259–269.

Zielstorff, R. D. (1995). Capturing and using clinical outcome data: Implications of information systems design. *Journal of the American Medical Informatics Association, 2*(3), 191–196.

Zielstorff, R. D. (1998). Online practice guidelines: Issues, obstacles, and future prospects. *Journal of the American Medical Informatics Association, 5*(3), 227–236.

20

Challenges for Data Management in Long-Term Care

Patricia A. Abbott
David Brocht

OBJECTIVES

1. Define knowledge discovery in large datasets (KDD).
2. Differentiate between verification and discovery based approaches to hypothesis testing.
3. Outline the KDD process.
4. Discuss challenges inherent in long-term care and other health care data sets.
5. Discuss the potential of KDD for use in analysis of large health care data sets.

KEY WORDS

information systems
computer science
knowledge management
knowledge discovery in databases (KDD)
data mining
analytical techniques

The use of information systems in health care has evolved into the study of "biomedical data, knowledge, and information, including their proper use for healthcare, biomedical research, and problem solving" (Shortliffe, 1991). The challenges of problem solving and decision-making in health care has led to the investigation and development of knowledge-based systems that enhance the human ability to analyze, problem-solve, treat, diagnose, and estimate prognoses of health-related conditions (Peng and Reggia, 1990).

Decision-making in health care is a knowledge-intensive activity that may surpass the ability of the human cognitive processor to manage. The impact of disease processes, care processes, and environmental influences all combine to present a continually shifting target for decision-makers in health care. Interestingly, Pauker, Gorry, Kassier, and Schwartz (1976) assert that clinicians make clinical decisions on "guesses" of initial hypotheses, which are based on minimal amounts of data. The difficulties inherent in clinical decision-making

are now further compounded by the rapid proliferation of massive and distributed health care data warehouses that are unwieldy for purposes of analysis. Factors that contribute to patient outcomes can be related to specific patient characteristics; external forces such as facility ownership, reimbursement patterns, and regulatory agencies; and internal forces such as case-mix and staffing ratios. These data points are captured and stored in a variety of systems, both internal and external to the agency and/or enterprise. Correlations and patterns that may emerge when integrated are trapped in these disparate data silos, termed by McCormick (1981) as "data cemeteries." The challenge facing information technologists is how to unlock the information trapped in these massive and fragmented sets to determine causation or look for predictors of untoward outcomes and then to incorporate such findings into systems that support decision-makers. The webs of causality in health care are exceedingly complex, requiring new approaches to knowledge discovery and application.

The purpose of this chapter is to introduce and detail a method known as "knowledge discovery in datasets" (KDD) and to discuss its applicability for use in large collections of data such as those associated with long-term care (LTC). It is critically important that readers are aware that the *tools* of KDD are totally independent from the *data* upon which they operate. Therefore, KDD utility is domain-independent and can be used in any large collection of data. It has been noted that the value of KDD as an approach is often confused with the character of the data, which in health care, has a tendency to be "noisy" or dirty. One should never confuse the validity of the tools and approaches of KDD with the characteristics of the data.

Innovative Approaches to Information Management in Health Care

The move towards integrated health systems and the tracking of data from "cradle to grave" has highlighted the need for a method by which the vast amounts of data being collected can be analyzed and visualized. The need for automated and intelligent database analysis is receiving increasing levels of attention as health care enterprises and payers struggle to make sense of the data that tremendous amounts of resources are being spent to capture. As noted earlier, the problem arises in the intensive multidimensionality, fragmentation, and distribution of health care data that can overload human cognition as well as traditional methods of aggregation and analysis.

This problem is very evident in LTC facilities, where the integration of automation is low, the population health status is very complex, and the factors that contribute to health status and outcomes are fragmented and distributed. The availability of clinically usable knowledge bases that incorporate and provide not only patient/environment-specific factors but knowledge based on previously validated studies in long-term care is practically nonexistent. While the mission of LTC facilities is to maintain dignity and optimal levels of health for chronically ill persons, it is very difficult to do so when health data are limited, unmanageable, and inaccessible. Increasing public and governmental attention is being focused on the quality and effectiveness of care in LTC, giving impetus to efforts to improve patient outcomes. Outcomes management is most effective when the actions and impacts can be measured and analyzed. Management is impaired when the foundation of measurement is not in place.

The question becomes, therefore, how can we begin to harness the data that are being collected, how can

we turn the data into information, and how can we use the information to generate new knowledge? Discovery-based approaches such as KDD—sometimes referred to as "data mining"—may be one method of working with massive, distributed, and multidimensional health care data.

Knowledge Discovery in Large Data Sets

KDD is defined by Abbott (2000) as the "melding of human expertise with statistical and machine learning techniques to identify features, patterns, and underlying rules in large collections of healthcare data." Fayyad et al. (1989, p. 6) define KDD as the "non-trivial process of identifying valid, novel, potentially useful, and ultimately understandable patterns in data." According to Goodwin et al. (1997, p. 22) data mining and KDD in health care uses a "combination of artificial intelligence and computer science techniques to help build knowledge in complex health care domains." In essence, KDD can be viewed as extracting high-level knowledge from low level data (Fayyad et al., 1989). KDD uses discovery-based approaches in which pattern recognition and matching, classification or clustering schemas, and other algorithms are used to detect key relationships in the data.

The techniques used in KDD and data mining are not new, having been discovered in the field of artificial intelligence (AI) research in the 1980s. The finance and banking industry have a strong history in the utilization of KDD approaches. Data mining has been used extensively in business to predict future customer markets and current customer behavior (Moriarty, 1997). Future customer characteristics are predicted based upon past behavior and strategies are implemented based upon the projected future characteristics (Saarenvita, 1999). For example, "market-basket analysis" is a type of KDD where large databases containing customer buying patterns are examined for purchases that cluster together. A market-basket analysis may demonstrate that the purchase of a man's suit is closely linked with the purchase of a new shirt and tie. The business manager would then use this information prospectively to enhance the probability of the sale of a new shirt and tie by offering an incentive to the customer to purchase the additional pieces at the same time as the new suit. Other common applications of KDD include predicting loan default by identifying factors that contribute to this negative outcome and applying them prospectively in loan approval systems. The use of KDD in health care has been primarily focused on fraud detection in health care claims processing and for cost analysis. However, the success of KDD as evidenced in industries other than health care highlights tremendous potential for use in clinically related sets.

Aside from the logistic challenges, substantial work is needed to influence a movement beyond traditional and comfortable approaches to data analysis in health care. This is not to imply that standard approaches to analysis are no longer of value. However, one size does not and cannot fit all. In light of the challenges of terabytes of data and market-driven, rapid competition for resources and customer bases, innovative approaches to data analysis in health care warrant further attention. Munhall (1997, p. 203) asserts that

> Manuals and methods are the antithesis of creative thought. They mobilize behavioral assumptions and prescribe consistency of presentation and forbid wandering to a different form of rhetoric and discourse that is "out of the box." . . . unless he or she already knows that living knowledge and discovery lies outside the box.

The push is on for innovative discovery-based approaches to data analysis—looking for the living discovery and knowledge outside the comfort range of traditional approaches.

Differentiation of Verification versus Discovery Approaches

How are traditional approaches different from KDD? Current statistical models based on regression offer the possibility of in-depth analysis but may require unrealistic assumptions about the distribution and interdependence of data or errors. Traditional analysis supports a *verification-based approach* to hypothesis testing. A specific hypothesis is made, variables suspected to be contributors to the phenomenon of study are isolated, and analytic tools are used to either refute or prove the original postulate. This requires that the investigator have a detailed understanding of all (obvious and nonobvious) elements that could affect the outcome and then complete complex iterative queries of the data to further refine the analysis. The effectiveness of this approach can be limited by a variety of issues including the knowledge base of the investigator, the ability of the investigator to detect trends in the data and to pose proper questions, the ability to compose the complex queries required, the character and quality of multivariate data, and the ability to work with constrained or artificially imposed constructs. Most statistical models focus on the values that are expected—those elements that appear as the unexpected (outliers) are those that invalidate the model.

In contrast, KDD is based on *discovery-driven approaches* to hypothesis testing, where the unexpected is valued. This technique can be used to sift through large repositories to "discover" trends, predictive patterns, or correlations in data; confirm hypotheses; and highlight exceptions. KDD is particularly valuable for use in nonlinear, combinatorially explosive, and nonmonotonic problems. The two primary goals of KDD lie within prediction and description. Description in KDD deals with the discovery of patterns interpretable by humans, which are used to describe the data. Prediction focuses upon using variables within the data set to predict future or unknown values of other variables of interest. In working with large health care data sets, the discovery of interpretable patterns that illuminate the phenomenon under study in concert with the discovery of information that can be used to predict such phenomena could be incorporated into automated systems, leveraging the value of the data that we are spending thousands of dollars to collect.

It is important to emphasize KDD as a *process* is different from (but complementary to) the frequently applied term of "data mining." KDD focuses upon the overall process of discovering useful knowledge from data and is composed of several steps (Fig. 20.1), while "data mining" generally refers solely to the use of algorithms for extracting patterns from the data. KDD is interactive and iterative, involving the application of the algorithms to extract the patterns and then a concerted effort to *interpret* the patterns that have been presented. It could be said then that the application of the techniques without a matching strong understanding of the problem domain is not evidence of the application of KDD as a process. Work with data mining algorithms, however, is one of the most active research areas in KDD.

Background of Knowledge Discovery in Large Data Sets

Analyzing large data sets in the quest to find "nuggets" of useful and interesting patterns of information has been labeled with many different titles. The terms, such as knowledge extraction, data mining, data pattern processing, data archaeology, and information discovery, can be found in much of the literature. The term "knowledge discovery in databases" (KDD) was coined in 1989 to "refer to the broad process of finding knowledge in data, and to emphasize the 'high-level' application of particular data mining methods" (Fayyad et al., 1989). These authors assert that the term "data mining"

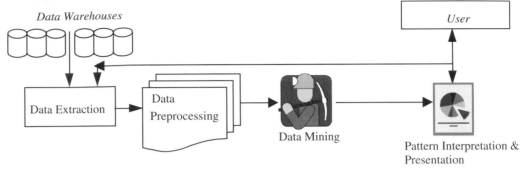

Data Extraction: Searching for and choosing data

Data Preprocessing: Choosing variables, dealing with noise and multidimensionality

Data Mining: Analysis of data using association, clustering, modeling, classification, etc.

Pattern Interpretation & Presentation: Interpretation, evaluation, and presentation of patterns

Figure 20.1
KDD process. (Abbott, 2000.)

has traditionally been used by the management information systems (MIS) community, while AI and machine learning researchers have adopted KDD.

As noted earlier, the use of KDD in the truest form is the application of the techniques of KDD to discover useful knowledge from data. This is in contrast to the term "data mining," which refers to the application of algorithms to extract patterns without the further use of the additional steps critical to KDD (such as interpreting the results and the requisite understanding of the problem domain). The additional steps of KDD are what differentiates the technique from data mining in the singular sense. The application of data mining techniques without a firm understanding of the problem domain has been labeled as "fishing" or "dredging" in the statistical literature (Keppel, 1991). These terms refer to the improper discovery of erroneous patterns that may be elicited and presented without understanding the spurious nature of the results and the consequential negative impact on statistical conclusion validity.

Broad outlines of the nine steps in KDD are presented here, based on the work of Fayyad et al. (1989). This practical overview demonstrates the interactive and iterative nature of the KDD process.

The initial step of KDD involves obtaining an in-depth understanding of the application domain via

experience and examination of prior knowledge generated in the domain. It also involves in-depth work with the end-user to obtain an understanding of the needs and or goals of the persons that the application of KDD will serve. Brachman and Anand (1996, p. 40) believe that for the development of successful KDD applications, it is critical that the developer "understands the exact nature of the interactions between humans and data that leads to the discovery of knowledge." The secondary step involves creating a target data set, which involves selecting the warehouse or data set upon which KDD is to be tested. At this point, the data subselection process has not begun. The third step involves subselection, preprocessing, and cleaning of the data to examine the impact of outliers and noise on the data set. It is during this step that decisions related to missing or "dirty" data are made. Wreden (1997, p. 47) refers to this step as "Purgatory before Nirvana." Brachman and Anand (1996) make the point that caution in "scrubbing" away anomalies in the data is warranted, since these could be crucial indicators of interesting domain phenomena.

The fourth step involves feature or dimension reduction. As is often the case, the number of variables that are gleaned in the second step are highly dimensional, and frequently there are certain dimensions that can be used to identify the factor structure and then model for the set of variables (Stevens, 1996). The use of dimensionality reduction or transformation methods is applied in this phase. Brachman and Anand (1996) label this reduction as parameter restriction and suggest it as a way to deal with massively overwhelming amounts of data. These authors state that not all variables will have utility in an analysis and believe that parameter shrinkage makes a model more robust. A commonly used approach is called a principal components analysis (PCA).

The fifth step involves choosing the data mining task. The selection of the data mining approach is based on a goal of the KDD process such as summarization, dependency modeling, classification, regression, or others (Fayyad, 1989). Each of these approaches has strengths and weaknesses, and the decision of what method to use is dependent upon the task at hand and the inclination of the modeler. Brachman and Anand (1996) assert that the choice of approach can be determined as data sets are being investigated, a point that emphasizes the intertwining of data analysis and model creation in the KDD approach. These authors frame the model selection process in a "human-centered" approach, asserting that when completing the knowledge engineering that is required for model selection "background knowledge of the domain expert is crucial" (Brachman and Anand, 1996, p. 47).

Subsequent to step five is the selection of the data mining algorithm, once again based on the overall goal of the KDD process. The selection of the best method to search for patterns in data is made. In addition, considerations of the needs of the end-user are included here, for example, making the determination if the system is to be used to explain the patterns or to use the patterns for prediction purposes.

The seventh step involves the actual data mining, which is the active investigation of the transformed data set for interesting patterns, frequently via the use of neural networks (NN). The final two steps involve the interpretation of the output of the data mining and finally the incorporation and/or dissemination of the knowledge out to the users. Generally, output involves the analysis of results and can be represented in many different formats such as reports of goodness of fit, outliers, scatterplots, graphical representations, and alarming (or monitoring) functions. The type of output and dissemination is once again based on the needs of the user and the type of problem. The final step also involves reconciling new findings with previously known facts, a point of particular importance in clinical situations.

Work involving prediction of hospital mortality (such as the APACHE system) and multiple citations of data mining instances can be found in the literature. However, evidence of KDD use as a *process* in health care is very sparse. The majority of applications of KDD are found in the finance and banking domains. One exception involves the Key Findings Reporter (KEFIR) system (Matheus et al., 1997). The KEFIR system was designed to discover, explain, and report on key findings in large databases. This system was tested in a large health care database, renamed HEALTH-KEFIR, and was used primarily in the analysis of cost data. An interesting point made by these authors is that when examining health-related data, it is not effective to look only at retrospective changes in data over time but to look prospectively to determine how actions can be taken to reduce further expenditures. In discussing potential savings achievable in the future in health care by analyzing large data sets, these authors assert that "we need to 1) forecast the measure's future deviation from the norm, 2) translate that deviation into impact on the bottom line, and 3) determine how much of that amount we can expect to save by intervening with an appropriate action" (Matheus, et al., 1997, p. 501).

In taking the statements made by Matheus et al. (1997) and shifting the focus to data sets that focus on *clinical* aspects of care, similar utility can be seen.

For example, if it is possible to predict a patient's health status movement away from the norm, the deviation can be translated into a risk analysis, and the information can be used to intervene at the most appropriate time to change the direction of the deviation to a more satisfactory level. The intervention could have an impact on the "bottom line," not only in quantitative cost savings, but in the qualitative measurements of human care. Such an approach may have particular utility in LTC, where prediction, notification, and timely intervention can be used to assist in the achievement of improved outcomes.

Data Sets in Long-Term Care

LTC centers have been slow to adopt information technology in any form other than claims-based systems. However, the health care reform movement and increased emphasis on evidence of quality care are driving the impetus for improved methods of information handling in long-term care centers. In 1990, federal mandates were enacted to require that all LTC centers perform periodic assessments of the functional capacity of residents. The outcome of these mandates was a resident assessment instrument (RAI) called the minimum data set (MDS). MDS was designed as a paper-based assessment tool that contains over 350 variables that are used to measure functional, interventional, demographic, and administrative elements for each resident. The RAI contains resident assessment protocols (RAPS), which are triggered by certain combinations of measurements obtained from the MDS. The RAPS are designed to offer a decision framework that stimulates additional assessments to positively impact an individualized care plan. Two studies of particular importance focused upon the use of the MDS in U.S. long-term care facilities (Hawes et al., 1997; Fries et al., 1997). The results of these two studies demonstrated a positive impact in three separate areas; resident outcomes, processes of care, and administrative perspectives. The MDS was shown to perform well as an outcome measurement tool in which data was collected, aggregated, and analyzed to examine processes and quality of care.

These assessments are performed quarterly in every nursing home in the United States that participates in the Health Care Financing Administration (HCFA) Medicare and Medicaid program. From the outset, HCFA anticipated that a national MDS data collection method would:

- Stimulate the growth of management information systems in LTC
- Improve the quality of care for LTC residents
- Improve the cost-effectiveness of LTC
- Encourage quality monitoring by focusing on targeted reviews
- Facilitate benchmarking and trending

Historically, the use of information technology to support these efforts in LTC has lagged. However, in the summer of 1998, HCFA began requiring all long-term care facilities to use automated and standardized methods of recording, collecting, storing, and transmitting MDS data (Department of Health and Human Services, 1997).

The required automation of MDS data brings challenges as well as benefits. The creation and proliferation of data warehouses that can be used for analysis are greatly anticipated. The conundrum arises when one examines the distribution, size, and complexity of the MDS dataset and the lack of integration with other separate but related data repositories. While the independent mining of the MDS warehouse has the potential to generate valuable information, the other factors that are suspected to contribute to patient outcomes (such as staffing ratios, ownership, reimbursement patterns, case-mix, etc.) will continue to be stored in separate and noninte-grated databases. Preliminary work aimed at incorporating separate but related data sets is warranted, as is the need to develop information systems solutions to facilitate the improvement of patient outcomes. Mechanisms for local retention and access to MDS and related data are needed. Management of outcomes and efforts to improve care will be less successful if assessment data are simply automated and shipped off to HCFA warehouses.

A critical component to adoption of systems that utilize the RAI is a loop of patient- and facility-specific information that is fed back automatically and quickly to clinicians. This goes beyond simply automating the RAPS and triggers component of the RAI, although that is a step in the right direction. While one may intuitively expect that the provision of patient/facility-specific information would positively impact clinical decision-making, further research is warranted. Measurement of impact on subjectively derived probability estimates, decision-making, and patient outcomes are areas of particular research value. Ultimately, work to leverage the value of the MDS for clinicians is critical.

Applying Discovery-Based Approaches to Long-Term Care Data

Many clinicians believe that the use of the federally mandated MDS is another example of governmental interference in the care of patients in long-term care facilities (Ouslander, 1997) and that improved utilization of this tool can do little to improve resident outcomes. It has been demonstrated (Abbott, 1999) that the MDS contains a wealth of untapped knowledge and, when examined in combination with certain factors specific to the facility and environment, has strong predictive abilities. Abbott (1999) demonstrated that via the use of KDD and connectionist machine learning techniques (using a conglomerate of a MDS warehouse, HCFA inpatient claims files, and OSCAR facility surveys), it was possible to predict admission from LTC to an acute care facility (a frequently negative outcome) with a sensitivity of 88%, a specificity of 99%, and an overall accuracy rate of 92%. This research also elicited the major predictors of admission. The potential exists for the incorporation of this machine learning algorithm into integrated decision support systems to assess levels of risk "on the fly" and then alarm clinicians of an impeding negative outcome. Although the intent of the system is the same, this research differs from other predictive systems such as APACHE due to use of the KDD process. No *a priori* hypotheses were generated; rather, the machine learning algorithm determined the major predictors while in the process of closely classifying the outcome. This discovery-driven approach can be used to predict and describe a variety of other phenomena whose data lie moldering in large LTC warehouses.

Summary

As health care moves into a highly automated future where massive data warehouses are the norm, innovative discovery-based approaches will become increasingly important. This will require adoption of techniques different from the familiar traditional statistical approaches so common to data analysis in health care today. Health care may find itself in a position similar to other industries, where the importance of prediction may begin to rival that of explanation.

Management of patient outcomes requires a linkage and analysis of cost data, resource data, and clinical data, creating massive data repositiories. Significant challenges present themselves due to the distribution, complexity, size, fragmentation, and frequently erroneous nature of health care data. However, when these components are merged, there is much to be discovered. What exists in the data that we do not know yet? How can we discover this knowledge and harness it to improve the quality of care? How can we handle huge sample sizes where the assumptions required of traditional approaches cannot be made? These questions will require that we begin to use new and innovative approaches to harness and analyze health care databases.

References

Abbott, P. (1999). *Predicting Long-Term Care Admissions: A Connectionist Approach to Knowledge Discovery in the Minimum Data Set.* (Doctoral dissertation, University of Maryland, Baltimore, Maryland). *Dissertation Abstracts International.*

Abbott, P. (2000). Knowledge discovery in large datasets: A primer for data mining applications in healthcare. In M. Ball, K. Hannah, S. Newbold, and J. Douglas (Eds.), *Nursing Informatics: Where Caring and Technology Meet* (3rd ed.). New York: Springer-Verlag.

Brachman R., and Anand, T. (1996). The process of knowledge discovery in databases. In U. Fayyad, G. Piatetesky-Shapiro, and P. Smyth (Eds.), *Advances in Knowledge Discovery and Data Mining* (pp. 37–57). Cambridge, MA: MIT Press.

Department of Health and Human Services. (1997). Medicare and Medicaid; Resident Assessment in Long Term Care Facilities. *Federal Register, 62*(246), 67174–67213.

Fayyad, U., Piatetesky-Shapiro, G., and Smyth, P. (1996). From data mining to knowledge discovery. In U. Fayyad, G. Piatetesky-Shapiro, and P. Smyth (Eds.), *Advances in Knowledge Discovery and Data Mining* (pp. 1–36). Cambridge, MA: MIT Press.

Fries, B., Hawes, C., Morris, J., et al. (1997). Effect of the national resident assessment instrument on selected health conditions and problems. *Journal of the American Geriatrics Society, 45,* 994–1001.

Goodwin, L., Schlitz, K., and Jasion, B. (1997). Data mining for improved patient outcomes. *Tarheel Nurse, 59*(4), 21–22.

Hawes, C., Mor, V., Phillips, C., et al. (1997). The OBRA-87 nursing home regulations and implementation of the resident assessment instrument: Effects on process quality. *Journal of the American Geriatrics Society, 45,* 977–985.

Keppel, G. (1991). *Design and Analysis: A Researchers Handbook* (3rd ed.). Upper Saddle River, NJ: Prentice Hall.

Matheus, C., Piatetsky-Shapiro, G., and McNeill, D. (1997). Selecting and reporting what is interesting. In U. Fayyad, G. Piatetsky-Shapiro, and P. Smyth (Eds.), *Advances in Knowledge Discovery and Data Mining* (pp. 496–515). Cambridge, MA: MIT Press.

McCormick, K. (1981). Nursing research using computerized data bases. In H. Heffernan (Ed.), *Proceedings of the 5th Annual Symposium on Computer Applications in Medical Care.* Silver Spring, MD: IEEE Computer Society Press.

Moriarty, T. (1998). Building the customer. *Intelligent Enterprise, 1*(4), 56–59.

Munhall, P. (1997). Out of the box. *Image: Journal of Nursing Scholarship, 29*(3), 203.

Ouslander, J. (1997). The resident assessment instrument (RAI): Promise and pitfalls. *Journal of the American Geriatrics Society, 45,* 975–976.

Pauker, S., Gorry, G., Kassier, J., and Schwartz, W. (1976). Towards the simulation of clinical cognition: Taking a present illness by computer. *The American Journal of Medicine, (60),* 981–996.

Peng, Y., and Reggia, J. (1990). *Abductive Inference Models for Diagnostic Problem Solving.* New York: Springer-Verlag.

Saarenvita, G. (1999). Data modeling for direct mail: A lesson in predictive modeling. *DB2, 4*(1), 40.

Shortliffe, E. (1991). Medical informatics and clinical decision making: The science and the pragmatics. *Medical Decision Making, 11*(4 Suppl), S2–14.

Stevens, J. (1996). *Applied Multivariate Statistics for the Social Sciences.* (3rd edition). Mahwah, NJ: Lawrence Erlbaum Associates.

Wreden, N. (1997). The mother lode: Data mining digs deep for business intelligence. *Communications Week,* Feb. 17, 1997, 43–47.

PART 7

Consumer Use of Informatics

21

Consumers in Health Care

Helga E. Rippen

OBJECTIVES

1. Review how computers are being used by consumers.
2. Identify issues relating to the use of health care applications by consumers.
3. Provide a general methodology to assess health care applications for consumers.

KEY WORDS

information systems
consumer
online systems
health education
internet
computer communication networks

O ver the last 10 years, there have been significant changes in the health care industry. The drive to control health care costs, coupled with decreasing costs of information technology, has resulted in our increasing reliance on information technology to support a variety of health care delivery needs, ranging from the medical record to disease management to education. In addition, less expensive computers, increased availability of local Internet service providers, and expanding Internet resources are drawing an ever increasing number of patients, caregivers, and health care providers to the computer and on-line. A 1999 study reported that 70% of health care providers have Internet access in their offices (Evans, 2000) and 90 million Americans are on-line (Panel News, 2000). Of these, 57% are accessing health information. As a result, consumers and health care providers are being exposed to information technology from a variety of sources and settings.

Given the time constraints and the increasing and expanding responsibilities of the nursing profession, the importance of consumer health care applications cannot be minimized. Since nursing has always played a central role in the delivery of health information to patients and their families, it can play a vital role in how health care applications are used by the consumer. In fact, the nursing profession can take the lead in being the conduit to

and development of health care applications. For these reasons, it is important to become familiar with the topics covered in this chapter.

This chapter will provide the necessary background to understand health care applications, the issues relating to their use, and the impact they will have on the health of the patient and general public. This chapter includes the following:

- Overview of consumer health care applications
- Delivery modalities
- Roles and responsibilities
- Issues

Overview of Consumer Health Care Applications

When discussing any topic, it is useful to define the terms used. In this chapter, a consumer will be defined as an individual who is the target of health information. A consumer health care application (CHA) is defined as an "intervention" that provides health information for the consumer through information technology. Information technology includes the hardware (e.g., computer, telephone), software (e.g., program), and conduit (e.g., Internet). The application can be static or interactive, algorithm-based or not, reactive or proactive. It can be provided through the consumer's health care provider or independently through a third party. CHA is a more restrictive term than interactive health communication (IHC) in that it focuses on the consumer. IHC is defined as "the interaction of an individual—consumer, patient, caregiver, or professional—with or through an electronic device or communication technology to access or transmit health information, or to receive or provide guidance and support on a health-related issue" (Eng and Gustafson, 1999).

The most basic CHA is static information. Static information does not change based on who is using it, requires no interaction, and is most similar to traditional print information. Static does NOT refer to the currency of the information. For example, text posted on an Internet Web page or a CD-ROM reference book provides information that is static. The consumer needs to find and decide what is relevant to him or her (i.e., process the information).

Interactive CHAs require consumer input and can be algorithm-based or not. Algorithm-based CHAs are applications whose responses are preprogrammed. Non-algorithm-based CHAs are primarily applications that support the communication of information between users. Examples include chat rooms (Web-based sites that allow real-time interaction with individuals and/or groups), newsgroups (Web-based sites that allow posting of comments by individuals on a topic), and listservs (a list of E-mail addresses that allows the exchange of E-mail to the entire group). Most often, in non-algorithm-based CHAs, the exchange of information is not between the health care consumer and the health care provider. Communication-focused CHAs are becoming increasingly important to patients and their families by providing a mechanism to obtain information and social support. These interactions are often described as an on-line community.

In algorithm-based CHAs, the input can be anything from demographic, preference, or health-related information. An example of an interactive-targeted CHA is a cardiovascular risk assessment. The consumer enters information relating to his or her age and other cardiovascular risk factors. Based on this information, the application "calculates" the consumer's relative risk for developing heart disease. This information is specific to the individual's characteristics.

Interactive risk management programs go one step further than risk assessments. Based on an initial risk assessment, the program helps consumers manage their risk. This could be as simple as providing exercise information to a consumer with a sedentary life style.

Decision support provides consumers and/or their health care provider with information to help consumers make a decision. A consumer enters specific health information and preferences, and the program recommends an approach, based on the algorithm and the entered information. For example, a patient with prostate cancer would like to determine the best treatment option. Based on the algorithm, his preference (e.g., treatment side effects, risks), age, and disease stage, the CHA provides a "recommended" course of action.

Consumers can use disease management CHAs to help them better manage their disease. This type of application can be illustrated by a diabetes management CHA. The CHA collects relevant health information, and the user enters all measured blood glucose levels and insulin dosages. As a result, the CHA can share this information with a health care provider, recommend an insulin dosage, recommend additional tests (e.g., ophthalmology consult), and provide the user relevant information (e.g., diet and nutrition, foot care).

Most CHAs are reactive. This means that they provide an output when the user selects the application and enters information. Proactive CHAs are applications that will provide users with information (e.g., a reminder) when they have not necessarily accessed the application. An example of proactive technologies is push technology. These applications "push" information, through an application, to a user. A screen saver that accesses Internet-based information and forwards the latest scientific information on breast cancer is an example of push technology.

Delivery Modalities and Provider

There are four ways to deliver CHAs, through a network (e.g., Internet, intranet), a nonnetworked computer (kiosk, laptop), CD-ROM (or diskette), or an automated phone application. A network can be very public, such as the Internet (described in more detail in Chap. 7) or private (e.g., intranet or a non-Web network). A benefit of using a network is that many people can access the CHA at the same time at many locations. The Internet provides the most flexibility and access but requires more attention to security.

Programs residing on a computer such as a kiosk or laptop are common. Kiosks are often found in health care settings or a public location (e.g., mall). Consumers often have access to computers at home where they can install CHAs and access them as needed. Applications that run through CD-ROM/diskettes are portable and allow consumers to use them on other computers (e.g., at school or a library). Unfortunately, computer and CD-ROM/diskette-based CHAs can only be accessed by one person at a time.

Automated phone health care applications (e.g., medication reminder systems or blood pressure checkups) provide a low technology interface on the consumer side. These applications allow many users to access the system simultaneously without requiring a computer in the home.

The mechanism by which the application is delivered is, in general, not as important as who provides it. It is the responsibility of the provider of the application to ensure the quality of the CHA. However, the quality of the CHA can vary dramatically. There are no regulating bodies that provide certification of CHAs. For this reason, it is important that CHAs provided in the health care setting be evaluated and tested prior to use.

Applications can be provided through the consumer's health care provider or a third party. Some health care settings provide CHAs at their offices, where it is tied to the patient's medical record. For example, a patient's answers to an electronic medical history survey are automatically incorporated into the patient's medical record. As a result, the patient will get a tailored patient information package, and the health care provider is alerted for intervention recommendations (e.g., mammography for a woman with known risk factors).

Some health care delivery organizations are providing their patients access on Internet-based CHAs as a member service, while others provide CHAs internally and allow access at specific sites. In general, the health care community has been slow to adopt the use of CHAs. For example, approximately 5% of physicians provide information for their patients on the Internet, though 77% of Internet health information retrievers would prefer health information from their physicians (Internet Source of Preferences, undated). This highlights the opportunity for health care providers to use the Internet as a delivery vehicle for CHAs and that the nursing profession can play a critical role.

Most applications are not provided through a consumer's health care provider. Many Internet-based CHAs are provided by other health care organizations, nonprofits, or government entities. Examples include Oncolink provided by the University of Pennsylvania's Cancer Center (*www.oncolink.org*), the American Heart Association (*www.amhrt.org*), and the National Cancer Institute's clinical trial information database (*cancertrials.nci.nih.gov*). They provide CHAs as a public service, a mechanism to increase their market share, or a revenue stream.

Most consumer-centered CHAs in CD-ROM/diskette format are developed by third parties that are not involved in the health care management of the consumer. Historically, many are CD-ROM versions of popular selling health books. But this is changing as more CHAs are being developed that provide consumers treatment decision support (e.g., when to call a health care provider), clinical preventive reminders, and a way to document their health record.

Roles and Responsibilities

Developer

The developer is responsible for the quality of the CHA it creates. This includes thorough evaluation and testing of the application and proper documentation. To help users assess the quality of the CHA, developers should provide the information summarized in Table 21.1. In addition to ensuring the quality of the content and algorithm, the developer should also ensure maximum usability and effectiveness (impact). Since there are no regulation or licensing/evaluation requirements for CHA developers, it is often up to the user to assess CHA quality.

Health Care Provider

The health care provider has a responsibility to ensure that patients are provided the best quality health care possible. This includes the availability of CHAs that have been shown to improve outcomes and quality of care. In a health care setting, it is important to ensure that the CHA can be successfully integrated into the practice. Table 21.2 summarizes major questions for health care providers to consider. Unfortunately, only a few CHAs have been evaluated in the health care setting. For this reason, health care providers should incorporate an evaluative component as part of their CHA implementation plan.

If CHAs are provided through their providers, consumers should be encouraged to provide feedback. Patients and families should be encouraged to discuss their experiences with CHAs. This is true even when the CHA is not provided through the health care provider. In this scenario, the role of the health care provider is to

Table 21.1   Information that should be provided by the developer

1) Credibility
    a) Source (developer)
       i)   Organization name and authors listed
       ii)   Credentials
       iii) Disclosure of any conflicts of interest

    b) Context clearly defined
       i)   Target of CHA
       ii)   Purpose of CHA

    c) Currency
       i)   Date
       ii)   "Expiration date" or date of expected update (if known)

    d) Relevance/utility

    e) Review process

    f) Contact mechanism

2) Content
    a) Scientific basis of the CHA
       i)   Scientific evidence
       ii)   The effectiveness of CHA

    b) References to original sources

    c) Disclaimer (limitations, purpose, scope, authority)

    d) Omissions noted (balanced information)

3) Disclosure
    a) Data collection disclosure
       i)   Who is collecting the information and why
       ii)   Who will have access
       iii) How privacy and confidentiality will be maintained

Reprinted, with permission, from Health Summit Working Group (1997).

put the externally acquired information into the appropriate context.

Consumer

Consumers are taking a greater role and responsibility in the management of their health or that of a loved one. This creates a dichotomy. They are seeking more information and increasing their independence from the health care community but are increasing their exposure to misinformation at a time they might be most vulnerable. It is important for consumers to discuss their use of CHAs with their health care provider. The nursing profession should facilitate this discussion.

Consumers have a responsibility for evaluating the quality of CHAs if obtained outside of the clinical setting.

Table 21.3 summarizes the criteria that consumers should use in evaluating a health site. There is a Web-based tool to help consumers evaluate Internet-based CHAs based on these criteria (*hitiweb.mitretek.org/iq*).

Government

The government is a major provider and funding source for the development and testing of CHAs. As a provider, the government is responsible for ensuring the quality of its work. When funding the development of CHAs, the government should require proper evaluation. In addition, the government may need to determine whether or not CHAs should be regulated or certified. This will become an ever-important issue as CHAs become a more integral part of the health care delivery system.

Issues

Approaches to Quality

As alluded to earlier, anyone can develop a CHA. This means that quality can range from poor to excellent. The previous section identified some of the criteria for assessing the "quality" of a CHA, but there are many strategies to ensure access to quality CHAs. These strategies include "trusted" sources, metalink sites, seals and awards, evaluation tools, education, and filtering.

Users of CHAs have their own preference for what they would identify as a "trusted source." For example, some individuals would trust information provided by the government, while others would not. Metalink sites provide a listing of sites (resources), often listed by disease topic, that users can use to obtain information. As with any site, there is no guarantee that any quality control mechanism was used to evaluate these links. Metalink sites that provide an appropriate quality review are a great resource.

There are several examples of organizations that provide seals or stamps of approval. What is their methodology of review? Most Internet seals of approval are based on characteristics that are not related to quality of content or health outcomes. In addition, seals are often forged. A unique example is one based on the honor system, HONCode. The HONCode logo can be displayed on a site that complies with a set of eight principles that cover everything from intent and disclosure to privacy issues. If a site displaying the logo is found not to adhere to the code, HONCode requires the site to remove its logo. This approach implies that intent assures quality.

There are many approaches to evaluating CHAs. One researcher, upon review of 47 rating instruments, concluded that there were many "incompletely developed instruments" and that none provided information on the validity and reliability of the measures (Jadad and Galiardi, 1998). The Health Summit Working Group (HSWG) is currently studying the validity and reliability of a quality-rating tool, known as the Information Quality Tool (IQ) (Health Summit Working Group, 1997). Preliminary results look promising. The IQ Tool is based on the criteria developed by the HSWG. This group represents a diverse set of views including the consumer, health care provider (physicians, nurses, pharmacists), government, academia, nonprofit organi-

---

Table 21.2 Health care provider's evaluation checklist of CHAs

1) Why was the CHA developed?
   a) What clinical problem does the application solve?

2) What does the CHA propose to do?
   a) What types of outcomes are expected?
   b) What are the findings from related literature? How did they guide the developer?
   c) Can the program be tailored to individual patients?
   d) How does it link with care delivery?
   e) What setting is most appropriate for the program?

3) What are the technical requirements of the application?
   a) How are the data collected and stored?
   b) What training do providers need to use the application?
   c) What personnel infrastructure is needed to implement the program?
   d) What technical infrastructure is needed?
   e) How often does the CHA need to be updated?

4) Does the program work as described?
   a) What are the limitations of the CHA?
   b) How has feasibility testing been done?
   c) How were the intended outcomes evaluated? What were the results?
   d) What is the user experience?

Adapted from Eng and Gustafson (1999).

Table 21.3   Criteria for the consumer to use to assess the quality of the CHA

1) Credibility
   a) Source (developer)
      i)   Organization name and authors listed
      ii) Credentials
      iii) Disclosure of any conflicts of interest
   b) Context clearly defined (e.g., advertisement or education)
      i)   Target of CHA
      ii) Purpose of CHA
   c) Currency
      i)   Date
      ii) Possibly an "expiration date" or date of expected update
   d) Relevance/utility
   e) Review process
   f) Contact mechanism

2) Content
   a) Scientific basis of the CHA
      i)   Scientific evidence
      ii) The effectiveness of CHA
   b) References to original sources
   c) Disclaimer (limitations, purpose, scope, authority)
   d) Omissions noted (balanced information)

3) Disclosure
   a) Data collection disclosure (e.g., who is collecting the information and why,
      who will have access, how privacy and confidentiality will be maintained)
   b) Does the content match the developers mission or purpose?

4) Links
   a) Is a selection process appropriate?
   b) Are the links appropriate?
   c) Can you navigate back and forth?
   d) Do the linked sites provide quality content?

5) Design
   a) Is the site readily accessible with your browser?
   b) Is the site easy to use and find things?
   c) Is there a search engine?

6) Interactivity
   a) Mechanism for feedback
   b) Interactive components (chat rooms, bulletin boards)
      i)   Moderator present?
   c) If information tailored, what is the clinical algorithm used?

7) Caveats
   a) Does a site sell products or provide services?
   b) Has this CHA been shown to be effective?

(Reproduced, with permission, from Health Summit Working Group (1997).

zations, professional health organizations, librarians, and developers. The purpose of including such a wide range of perspectives was to work towards establishing an unbiased consensus. The group started its effort in November 1996.

The IQ tool is Internet-based and is being continually refined to serve a variety of interests—to be used by consumers to rate sites, as an educational tool, and for helping developers provide a mechanism to make linking decisions. The focus of this tool is primarily on the quality of the content and not on the effectiveness of the CHA in achieving a defined outcome. The Science Panel on Interactive Health Communications' focus is on the evaluation of effectiveness (Eng and Gustafson, 1999).

Filtering technology could be applied to health information. The issues that arise with the use of this technology are similar to those with all approaches: what guidelines will be used to filter the information, how current will it be, and can it be "fooled"? In addition, filtering also brings up concerns of censorship and its implications.

Privacy, Confidentiality, and Security

To facilitate the discussion of privacy, confidentiality, and security, it is important to understand the defini-

tions of these terms (please refer to Chap. 9). In a health care setting, privacy and confidentiality are assumed. Make sure to find out what privacy, security, and confidentiality policies and procedures are in place in any setting that you use a CHA. When accessing CHAs provided by a third party, be especially wary of the information that is collected. There is no "protected" relationship, and many of the policies that are being developed (e.g., the Health Insurance Portability and Accountability Act [HIPAA]; see Chap. 10) do not cover health information collected by a third party outside of the health care setting. Review the data policy and the site's business model. If the data policy states that identifying information (e.g., name, social security number) is not distributed, realize that other information can be used to identify you indirectly. For example, zip code, birth date, and sex can identify 80% of individuals (Simmons, 1999).

The Consumer-Provider Relationship

The consumer interacts with numerous CHAs from a variety of sources (Fig. 21.1). Most CHAs are not provided through their health care provider. Therefore, it is not surprising that CHAs have not necessarily brought physicians and patients closer together. In fact,

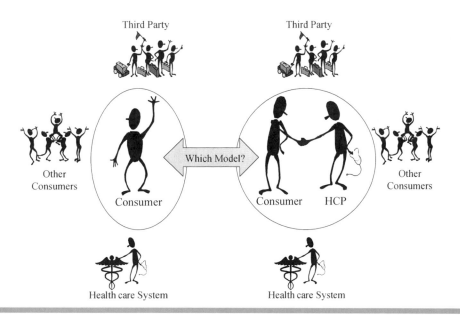

Figure 21.1
Interaction between consumers and CHAs. The health care provider (HCP) can be either another CHA source or a partner in the use of CHAs.

according to a study done on on-line patients, on-line health communities were rated superior to physicians in convenience, cost-effectiveness, emotional support, compassion/empathy, issues of death and dying, best source of medical referrals, best source of in-depth information about the conditions, best source of practical coping tips for the condition, and "most likely to be there for me in the long run" (Ferguson and Kelly, 1998). Specialist physicians rated best for diagnosing a condition correctly and helping in managing a condition after diagnosis, they did not rate as a superior source of technical medical knowledge about the condition (Ferguson and Kelly, 1998). This is despite the fact that 77% of the retrievers of health information on the Internet preferred their own physician as the source of accurate, timely, relevant, and objective health information on-line (Brown, 1998).

What does this mean? The "health information revolution" is changing the health care environment and the relationship between the patient and the health care provider. The nursing community has been a leader in patient education. This leadership role will become increasingly important in the information technology age. Where will we go? It will depend on which model you choose to pursue (see Fig. 21.1).

References

American Internet User Survey. (1998). http://www.cyberdialogue.com/press.html

Brown, M. S. (1998). Healthcare information seekers aren't typical Internet users. *Medicine on the Net*, 4(2), 17–18.

Eng, T., and Gustafson, D. (Eds.). (1999). *Science Panel on Interactive Communication and Health, Wired for Health and Well-Being, The Emergence of Interactive Health Communication*. Washington, D.C.: Department of Health and Human Services.

Evans, J. (2000). *The Bookend Channel @ e-Business World*. Boston: IDG News Service, Boston Bureau.

Ferguson, T., and Kelly, B. (1998). Online patients rate online health communities superior to physicians in ten of twelve aspects of health care. Austin, Texas: Ferguson Report.

Health Summit Working Group. (1997). White Paper: Criteria for Assessing the Quality of Health Information on the Internet. http://hitiweb.mitretek.or/docs/criteria.html

Internet Source of Preferences. SPV/Find.

Jadad, A., and Gagliardi, A. (1998). Rating health information on the Internet. *Journal of the American Medical Association*, 279, 611.

Panel News (1999). *Internet Access*.

Simmons, L. (1999). Personal communication.

22

Health-Related Decision-Making by Patients

Patricia Flatley Brennan
Shirley M. Moore

OBJECTIVES

1. Describe patient decision-making, and identify three reasons why it is complicated.
2. Explain the role of preferences in patient decision-making
3. Critically appraise two special-purpose and two general-purpose computer-based decision support tools.
4. Differentiate between decisions characterized by one-time, specific choices and those characterized by incremental behavior change.

KEY WORDS

consumer health
decision support
decision theory

Quality health care demands that patients assume increasingly central and active roles in personal health promotion and disease management. The kinds of decisions that patients face and that they must make range from the exotic, one-time treatment choices to the daily affirmations of actions and attitudes that give evidence to a commitment to a healthy lifestyle. Computer technologies, including telecommunications systems, the Internet and World Wide Web (WWW), and CD-ROM, hold great promise for supporting patients, their family caregivers, and concerned others.

The previous 10 years have witnessed an explosion of computer tools designed to help patients make better decisions about the health services they need and the health behaviors they must adopt. Some of these tools employ models from decision theory to guide patients in an analysis of the choices they face and the values they wish to employ as they make these choices. Other approaches employ an expert decision-making model, where the computer tool is used to provide advice and coaching based on the experiences of other patients who have had similar health problems or clinicians who diagnose and treat those problems. A third approach uses general-purpose computer tools, including the World

Wide Web, to help laypersons reflect on their behaviors and sense of self and incorporate incremental choices into a healthy lifestyle. Still other approaches to computer-based decision support work to provide patients with tools that let them view their clinical records and link these records with current literature databases.

This chapter will explore the many aspects of health-related patient decision-making, with particular emphasis on patient preferences, and examine experiences with computer tools designed to aid patients in the decision-making process.

Health-Related Decision-Making

Health-related decision-making is challenging for patients for several key reasons. First, decision-making itself is a complex perceptual, cognitive, and social process. The talents and limits of humans as decision-makers are well-known and well-described in the work of the human information processing theorists (Tversky and Kahneman, 1972). Essentially, information processing is a complex challenge, and humans employ mental mechanisms as coping strategies to help them sort significant from insignificant facts, to organize and interpret complex observations, and to facilitate recall and synthesis of known knowledge with new facts. Stressors, such as uncertainty, time pressures, and lack of knowledge, lead these efficient processes to deteriorate in such a way as to lead to suboptimal decision processes. Laypersons facing health crises experience many stressors; thus, their information processing skills are taxed repeatedly in a health crisis.

Second, health-related decision-making is complicated because the substance of the problems and choices is itself complex and exceeds the knowledge base of most laypersons. At the very point that patients face a threat to their integrity as persons, they must manage and understand large amounts of new and complex information. So, with diminished information processing skills the individual must attempt to comprehend and interpret new and unfamiliar facts. Even those persons who are not in a health crisis may have difficulty locating and evaluating the quality and relevance of health information. Facts mix with hearsay, providing an unsteady basis for health-related decisions such as following primary prevention recommendations or carrying out healthy lifestyle choices.

Finally, health-related decision-making is complex because it generally involves more than a single person. Two key groups must be considered: the family members of the person facing a health crisis or in need of health information, and the health care delivery team. Family members hold values, beliefs, and attitudes that implicitly or explicitly influence the health choices of an individual. The health care industry holds clinical care standards, values, and attitudes about the patient's responsibilities for her care and traditions that may interfere with the person's right to self-determination and self-care.

Health care decision-making is challenging because it taxes human information processing capabilities, it deals with subject matter that is unfamiliar to the involved person, and there are multiple constituents. A key determinant of choice and decision-making are the values held by an individual; therefore, in this discussion of health-related decision-making, we now turn attention to the concept of patient preferences.

Patient Preferences

Attention to patient preferences as an input into health care decision-making is rooted in the application of decision theory to understand personal choice. von Neumann and Morgenstern (1964) first proposed that the personal values and attitudes that drive individual

choice could be understood through mathematical formulations. Following on their work, Ledley and Lusted (1968) introduced the concepts of mathematical reasoning to medical decision-making, with particular attention to decision-making under uncertainty. Raiffa (1968) explicated decision analytical strategies that brought the treatment of personal preference and uncertainty into a form accessible in an interpersonal interview. Recently, work of Pauker and McNeil (1981), Sonnenberg and Pauker (1986), and Pauker et al. (1981) demonstrated the feasibility of using decision analysis to better understand treatment choices complicated by multiple uncertainties and personal values. These works offer a theoretical foundation for building health informatics tools that aid in the assessment of patient preferences.

The two main branches of decision theory, decision analysis and normative decision theory, both help make patient preferences accessible for clinical decision-making. Decision analysis helps in choosing one course of action from several when the most desired strategy depends, in part, on knowledge of the resolution of the outcomes of that strategy.

Multiattribute utility theory provided the mechanisms for quantifying the subjective value of health states and therefore can be very useful to patients who must make health care decisions (von Neumann and Morgenstern, 1964; Keeney and Raiffa, 1976). It defined preference as the ordering of entities over a value space (Keeney and Raiffa, 1976). The entities about which one develops preferences are discrete objects, such as cars or job candidates, or, in health care parlance, specific health outcomes. Entities were viewed as multidimensional. The value space described the n-dimensional intersection of a specific entity described simultaneously on all dimensions. The set of dimensions and their relative weights defined the preference structure. Multiattribute utility theory provided a way to establish a quantitative expression of an individual's values, with preference for a given health outcome being expressed as a score on the weighted sum of the dimensions and their relative weights.

The work of Pauker and colleagues provided the operational strategies to move decision analysis into the clinical arena. Pauker's group employed decision analysis to aid patients and clinicians in the challenges of selecting treatment courses when the choice of an intervention depended on two key unknowns: the extent to which a patient preferred the outcomes likely to follow the treatment and the probabilities that those outcomes would occur. Importantly, they devised the strategies to elicit from patients the quantitative estimates of the patient's assessment of the desirability of various outcome states. In a series of studies, this group explored preferences for cancer treatment (Sonnenberg and Pauker, 1986), prenatal testing (Pauker et al., 1981), and surgical intervention for cardiac disease (Pauker and McNeil, 1981). A utility function computed a score for each treatment alternative that explicitly incorporated the probability of each outcome of each treatment and a quantitative estimate of the desirability of the outcomes following each treatment. The treatment with the highest utility value became, by definition, the patient's preference. This use of preference as a synonym for the most desired action is consistent with but not identical to its use within normative decision theory, where an individual's preference for an entity is its utility, a composite of how well that entity performed on each important dimension.

Most informatics tools designed to elicit patient preferences are grounded in these decision theoretic conceptualizations (Lenert and Soetikno, 1997). In this context, the preference statement denotes the extent to which given health states are desirable according to some implicit or explicit valuing scheme. Other uses of the term patient preference also exist.

Alternative Meanings of the Term "Preferences"

The distinction between preferences as formalization of values, vis-à-vis a set of health care entities and preferences as the identified option chosen from the set of health care-related entities, becomes important when one examines how computers could be of assistance in patient preferences. Different kinds of computer programs and utilities support decision-making; some consider preference as an input to a decision or view preference as the final choice resulting from a decision. Clarifying the exact referent of preferences is a necessary precursor to the design of computer systems to support the use of patient preferences in health care. Donabedian's three-part quality model (Donabedian, 1968) provides a useful heuristic for sorting out the various referents about which individuals may develop preferences. Individuals may establish preferences about *structural* aspects of health care, such as belonging to a health maintenance organization (Sainfort and Booske, 1996) or their preferences for information or decision-making (Deber et al., 1996). Preferences for treatment options, such as surgical versus medical interventions, represent the individual's appraisal about *process* aspects

of health care. A third referent for preference is *outcomes* of health actions.

Some use the term "preference" to represent an individual's final choice of one option from many possible treatment options. For example, the man coping with an enlarged prostate may be said to have a "preference for surgery" if, after considering watchful waiting, medications, or surgical treatment, he finally decides on the surgical intervention as his final choice of treatment (Barry et al., 1995). However, this perspective introduces confusion in that the same term is used to refer to the general concept (valuing of a set of treatment) as well as a specific instance (most desired treatment).

Moore and Kramer (1998) used the term "preferences" to identify those features of cardiac rehabilitation programs deemed most desirable by patients. In this case, the preferences express the desirability to an individual of the features of a program, not the program (entity) itself. Henry and Holzemer (1995) identified preferences as "patient-specific inputs to the care process." Under this definition, preferences are atomic judgements that can be integrated with other components of the patient assessment and subsequently used to select treatment strategies.

Computers and Patient Health-Related Decision-Making

Computer technology can support health-related decision-making by patients through assistance with (1) preference clarification and elicitation, (2) effective data management and communication, and (3) ongoing support for health behavior change. Most of the existing applications demonstrate how computer technologies aid in preference clarification and elicitation (see Table 22.1 for a summary of the results of the effects of patient informatics tools and decision aids). Computerized versions of decision analytic algorithms follow the same normative decision-making principles that decision analysts do but allow patients the privacy and time flexibility sometimes not feasible in a one-to-one interaction. Prototype computer networks and computer-based patient records exist that could be modified and expanded to include patient preferences as data types, complementing the more familiar data types such as blood pressures and laboratory reports. In the areas of patient education, much work has been done capitalizing on the computer's ability to present multiple interfaces to the same information or to selectively present information that is relevant to the individual's concerns.

Table 22.1 Summary of the Effects of Patient Informatics Tools and Decision Aids on Treatment Selection

Study & health condition	Intervention & control conditions	Population	Design	Percentage using the informatics tool	Treatment choice	Findings Percentage among intervention group	Percentage among control group	Difference (Percentage points)
Adult Immunization:								
Carter et al., 1986[a] *Influenza vaccination*	Letter & brochure vs. Letter only	Veterans 65+	RCT 112/cell	Not reported	Flu shots vs. No shot	36%	23%	13%*
BPH and Prostate Cancer Screening:								
Wagner et al., 1995 *Benign prostatic hyperplasia*	Interactive videodisc vs. Nothing	Men 50+ in HMOs with BPH	Compare trends in other HMOs	CO HMO: > 50% WA HMO 1990: 41% 1991: 13%	Age-adj. rate of prostate surgery per 1000	Rate/1,000 1988: 6.0/1,000 1990: 3.6/1,000 1991: 2.5/1,000 1988: 4.8/1,000 1990: 2.3/1,000 1991: 3.3/1,000	Other HMOs: 1988: 4.7/1,000 1990: 4.0/1,000 1991: 3.7/1,000 1988: 5.3/1,000 1990: 4.6/1,000 1991: 3.3/1,000	1988–90: −25%* 1988–91: −29%* 1988–90: −39%* 1988–91: −11%*
Flood et al., 1996 *PSA screening*	Video decision aid vs. Nothing	Men 50+ in family practice clinic	Pre-/Post-cohort design (3 months per cohort): Intervn.: 103 Control: 93	85.5% recruited	PSA test by next visit	11.7%	22.6%	9.9%*
	Video decision aid vs. Basic video	Men 50+ in free prostate screening clinic	Randomized by day of week: Intervn.: 184 Control: 188	92.6% recruited	PSA test at visit	98.4%	100%	n.s.[b]
Wolf et al., 1996 *PSA Screening*	Script with risks & benefits vs. scripts with only benefits	Men 50+ with no history of prostate cancer	RCT: Intervn.: 103 Control: 102	Not reported	Preference for PSA test	28%	58%	−30%
Barry et al., 1997 *Benign prostatic hyperplasia*	Interactive videodisc vs. Brochure	Men with BPH in an HMO	RCT: Intervn.: 104 Control: 123	69% intervn., 85% control recruited	Prostatectomy surgery after 12 months	7.7%	13.0%	n.s.

Contraceptive Choice:

Study	Intervention	Population	Design		Outcome measure	Control	Intervention	Difference
Storey, 1991 *Vasectomy*	Video aid; Printed decison aid; vs. Nothing	Men planning to undergo vasectomy	RCT: ~100/cell	Not reported	Vasectomy	Not reported	Not reported	n.s.
Chewning, 1996[1]	Interactive computer vs. Nothing	Low-income minority women <20	RCT: Intervn.: 190 Control: 129	High	Use of oral contraceptives after 12 months	72.7%	56.9%	16.8%*
Oral contraceptives		Moderate-income women <20	RCT: Intervn.: 202 Control: 247	Not reported		72.5%	70.3%	n.s.

Ischemic Heart Disease:

Morgan et al., 1997 *Ischemic heart disease*	Interactive videodisc vs. Nothing	Patient with stable angina who completed coronary angiography	RCT: ~90/cell	Not reported	Coronary bypass surgery and/or angioplasty vs. Medical therapy	59% selected surgery	76% selected surgery	−17%*

Lower Back Pain:

Kamas, 1995 *Lower back pain*	Interactive videodisc vs. Nothing	HMO patients with back pain	Nonrandom: 53 users vs. 332 nonusers	14% of eligibles used tool	Surgery after 11 months	76.9/1,000	99.7/1,000	−22.8%*

Hormone Replacement Therapy:

O'Connor et al., 1995b *Hormone replacement therapy*	Audiotape with decision aid booklet vs. Nothing	Post-menopausal women	RCT: Intervn.: 81 Control: 84	Not reported	Use of HRT	Approx.: 25%	Approx.: 25%	n.s.
Rothert et al., in press *Hormone replacement therapy*	Brochure; Brochure and lectures; Brochure, lectures, and discussion group	Post-menopausal women	RCT: ~100/cell [no non-treatment control]	Not reported	Use of HRT	Approx.: 30%	Approx.: 30%	n.s.

Table 22.1 Summary of the Effects of Patient Informatics Tools and Decision Aids on Treatment Selection (continued)

Study & health condition	Intervention & control conditions	Population	Design	Percentage using the informatics tool	Treatment choice	Percentage among intervention group	Percentage among control group	Difference (Percentage points)
Study Descriptions				**Findings**				
Specialized Populations								
Decisions by Parents to Circumcise Infants:								
Herrera et al., 1982	Script with decision aid vs. Nothing	Women of lower SES	RCT: ~ 100/cell	Not reported	Circumcise male infants	98%	95%	n.s.
Herrera et al., 1983	Script with decision aid vs. Nothing	Women of higher SES	RCT: ~ 100/cell	Not reported	Circumcise male infants	84%	87%	n.s.
Maisels et al., 1983	Brochure vs. Nothing	Pregnant women	RCT: 51/cell	Not reported	Circumcise male infants	Not reported	Not reported	n.s.
Christensen-Szalanski et al., 1987	Counseling and fact sheet vs. Nothing	Middle-class women	RCT: ~ 100/cell	Not reported	Circumcise male infants	57%	56%	n.s.
Decisions by Medical Personnel to become Vaccinated for Hepatitis B								
Clancy et al., 1988	Decision aid and brochure; Brochure only; Letter only	Medical residents and faculty	RCT: Aid: 753 Info: 264 Control: 264	Medical residents: 11%	Hepatitis B shots vs. No shot	Aid users: 50% Aid group: 31% Info group: 24%	22%	28%* 9%* n.s.
Hepatitis B vaccination				Medical faculty: 16%		Aid users: 8% Aid group: 3% Info group: 3%	2%	6%* n.s. n.s.

*Difference statistically significant at a $p < 0.05$ level (two-tailed).

(a)To facilitate reading, this report references personal communications (e.g., Chewning, 1996) with the same convention used for publications. Details about the communications (i.e., person, affiliation, date of contact) and references are included in the reference list of Hersey et al. (1997).

(b)n.s. Not statistically significant at a $p < 0.05$ level (two-tailed).

Notes: This table summarizes the effects of informatics tools and decision aids on treatment choice. The left-hand columns of the table show intervention and control conditions, the study population, and the design of the study. For instance, a study by Carter et al. (1986) involved use of a personalized letter and a brochure about the risks and benefits of the influenza vaccine in the intervention condition (n = 112) compared to just a letter in the control condition (n = 112). This was an RCT among veterans 65 and older. The right-hand columns of the table summarize study findings. They report, if known, the percentage of the eligible patients who used the informatics tool and the percentage of patients in the intervention and comparison groups who selected the treatment described. The last column of the table shows the difference between the intervention and control groups. For instance, in the Carter et al. (1986) study, 36 percent of patients in the intervention group received the flu shots compared to 23 percent in the control group—an absolute difference of 13 percent. HMO, health maintenance organization; PSA, prostate-specific antigen; RCT, randomized central trial; BPH, benign prostatic hyperplasia. Reproduced with permission, from Hersey et al. (1997).

Agency for Health Care Policy and Research. (1997, September). *Consumer Health Informatics and Patient Decisionmaking: Summary.* (AHCRP Pub. 98-N001). Rockville, MD: AHCPR, DHHS.

Challenges to Using Patient Preferences for Health-Related Decision-Making

While the value of understanding and using patient preferences in health care is well-recognized (Earker et al., 1984), actually doing so presents a daunting challenge to patients (Gerteis et al., 1993). Imagining what a future health state could be like and determining the desirability of that future state is a complex cognitive task. Additionally, many patients lack experience with thinking about abstract concepts such as values and preferences. Attempting to do so under the stressful circumstance of the clinical encounter taxes the patient to an even greater degree. Skilled interpersonal interaction can lead to greater understanding of an individual's preferences (Raiffa, 1968; Pauker and McNeil, 1981). The fragmented, time-limited nature of contemporary health encounters leaves little opportunity to conduct the intense, interpersonal exploration needed to elicit and use patient preferences. Furthermore, under traditional models of care, patients and clinicians both presumed clinician preeminence in decision-making, and frequently patients prefer to defer to the judgement of the clinician. However, the scientific and clinical knowledge of clinicians does not always provide adequate direction for treatment of complex illnesses (Gerteis et al, 1993).

Preference assessment is an iterative, cognitive process designed to help a person understand and clarify personal values, health care situations, treatment options, and likely outcomes and elicits statements of preference. Benefiting from behavioral decision-making research, an interactive analysis process is used to help an individual focus on key components. Preference assessment can be conducted by a skilled interviewer using probes and reflection. Recently, Ruland demonstrated that staff nurses can be trained to effectively elicit patient priorities regarding the focus of care and that such elicitation leads to improved satisfaction with care (1998). Interactive computer systems can either supplement or supplant the human analyst.

Computer technology can assist in meeting the challenges inherent in employing patient preferences in health care practices. Computer packages that focus on elicitation and values clarification may serve to help patients think hard about complex, abstract issues, such as the desirability of future states (Barry et al., 1995). Multimedia displays use sound and full-motion video to help patients envision future states with greater clarity. When delivered via the World Wide Web (WWW), these programs facilitate patients' exploration of preferences in the privacy of their homes or away from an anxiety-producing health encounter (Lenert and Soetikno, 1997). Additionally, computer technology can store and communicate assessment data gleaned through a human- or computer-directed analysis. Such use of computer technology reduces the demand for repetition on the part of the patient and helps to ensure that data collected once are transmitted in a timely fashion to involved clinicians. Generally, the patient is the direct user in these applications of computer technology. Reviewed next are prototype, experimental systems that aid in the assessment of patient preferences and in using those preferences for making health-related decisions.

Computer Technology and Patient Decision-Making

Assessing Utilities of Health Outcomes

The Stanford Center for the Study of Patient Preference (the Center) has pioneered the use of computers and the Internet for low-cost elicitation of patient preferences for health states. Initially, computerized surveys and instructional programs walk the patient through classic decision analytic methods to help them clarify their preferences. Next, patients approach the rating task through programs that elicit preferences for specific health states (Lenert and Soetikno, 1997; Goldstein et al., 1994). These preference assessments use visual analog scales, pair-wise comparisons and standard gamble methods to measure patient utilities. Through tools developed by the Center, data can be collected on an appropriately equipped computer connected to the Internet. Patient preference data are then checked and stored rapidly and confidentially, ready for analysis.

Cognitive processes involved in the assessment can be quite demanding. For example, the standard gamble and the time trade-off methods deal with abstractions and expression of preferences for life and death and varying degrees of impairment and health conditions. Despite the complexity of the activity, the Center has shown that computer elicitation of preferences produces valid and reliable results and that this means of preference elicitation is well accepted by the patients. Investigators using the services of the Center can download their patients' responses over the WWW. In addition to the Internet-based assessments, a stand-alone multimedia preference elicitation software that incorporates health state descriptions (IMPACT) has been tested by the same group. Multimedia descriptions of health states the patients have not yet experienced have been shown to improve patients' understanding of these states' impact on quality of life (QOL) and to improve their abilities to rate preferences. Multimedia presentations have been used in some Center studies to describe the effects of anti-psychotic drugs and Gaucher Disease (Goldstein et al., 1994).

Choosing Treatment Options

The Comprehensive Health Enhancement Support System (CHESS) is a health promotion and support network application that operates as a module-based computer system for in-home or health care setting use (Gustafsen et al., 1994). People with major illnesses or health concerns can access information, decision support, social support, skill training, and a referral resource. Several of the CHESS services help the patients to clarify their values in preparation to make decisions that are consistent with their preferences.

Decision aid, based on an additive multiattribute utility model, can be used for condition-specific treatment decisions. The process involves the patient in understanding available options, in choosing possible decision criteria, in assigning weights to the criteria based on preference, and in assignment of a utility score to each criterion-option pair. Descriptions of suggested options and criteria or a personal story of someone who chose that option are offered. The program can also accommodate user-preferred options if the expert-generated lists do not contain the desired one. User-weighted decision criteria are shown in bar graph form, displaying the relative importance of all criteria. Likert-type utility scoring of criterion-option pairs are also graphically displayed in conjunction with summaries of how well each option satisfies its paired criterion. The system can also predict the decision the user will make. When used as a conflict analysis aid, CHESS will compare the different weights and utilities and identify areas in which compromise is possible (Boberg et al., 1997).

Network-Based Home Care Support: ComputerLink

Most of the computerized decision-making tools described so far in this chapter exist as free-standing programs. While this approach to decision support is valuable, it can also lead to artificial separation of the decision support tool from the patient's day-to-day health information management. In the ComputerLink project, an attempt was made to provide a range of inte-

grated electronic services. ComputerLink provided participants with access to an integrated set of computer utilities targeting the needs of home-bound patients and their family caregivers: coping with social isolation, managing novel and unexpected problems, and fulfilling unpredictable needs for health information (Brennan, 1994; Flatley-Brennan, 1998). Participants in the research projects used Wyse30 computer terminals based in their homes and linked via ordinary telephone systems to a computer network.

The ComputerLink project provided three services. The electronic encyclopediae consisted of information screens designed to enhance self-management, promote effective home-based treatment of patients, and promote patient/caregiver understanding of illness-specific issues. The communication service included several public/private options: (1) an unrestricted public bulletin board, which allowed users to post by name or anonymously anything that was on their minds for open, ongoing discussion; (2) a private electronic mail (E-mail) service, through which users could send and receive their own private E-mail, including messages from the nurse responding to their personal health care inquiries; (3) a question/answer area, in which answers to questions posed anonymously by users were posted by the nurse moderators. The third service, decision support, helped ComputerLink users make choices about which personal decisions were necessary, how they could best express these decisions, and how they could best generate insights for such decisions.

The effects of the ComputerLink interventions were evaluated in a field experiment. One study involved 60 persons living with AIDS (PLWAs). Sixty PLWAs participated in a 6-month field evaluation. Each group was randomly halved, with one group receiving typical home care and the other using ComputerLink. There were approximately 15,000 log-ons to each of the ComputerLink systems, averaging 10–13 minutes per log on. Participants' use of the decision support system provides some insight into how and why laypersons would use computer support tools.

Several approaches were used to measure the impact of the decision support system. Participants responded to a 15-item survey assessing decision-making confidence and related a recent decision situation, recounting the alternatives chosen and the rationale for their choice. This strategy to obtain information about decision-making skill followed that suggested by von Winterfeldt and Edwards (1986) and others, who recommended that appraisal of the effects of a decision support system target those dimensions of the decision problem likely to be amenable to ComputerLink influence. In MAU modeling, the perceived benefit arises from an increased ability to generate alternatives (Humphreys and McFadden, 1980) and an improved ability to understand their rationale (Fisher, 1979). Because decision situations familiar to the subject were used as a data source, this strategy avoided the biases engendered by posing hypothetical situations to the respondent. The strategy does, however, suffer from the bias of recency and saliency (Tversky and Kahneman, 1972); therefore, subjects were instructed to consider only decisions faced within the past 2 weeks. In addition, the effect of the substantive aspects of the decision problem on the number of alternatives generated could not be controlled.

A PLWA choosing to analyze a decision problem using ComputerLink would first make modem access to ComputerLink from the home-based computer terminal and then select the option "Make a Decision" from the opening menu. English-language prompts guide the analysis, sometimes incorporating words and phrases into subsequent questions typed by the PLWA in response to earlier items. First, the PLWA responds to a request to label the decision problem. This step is believed to help focus the user to the problem at hand. By permitting the PLWA to employ his/her own words for problem definition, the ComputerLink supported the analysis of problems as viewed by the individual. Next, the ComputerLink screens prompted the PLWA to list the alternatives under consideration, followed by the factors or characteristics deemed by the PLWA as important to the problem. By responding to a sequence of screens, one for each factor, the PLWA then designated on a visual-analog scale each of the options under consideration that met the factor or characteristic presented on the screen. The length of this line in millimeters became the single-attribute score. To assess the relative importance of each factor to solving the decision problem, subjects completed a weighting scheme suggested by von Winterfedt and Edwards (1986), in which they assigned 10 to the least important factor and then assigned a multiple of 10 to indicate how much more important than the index factor was each additional factor. To construct a recommendation, each alternative received a score computed as the weighted sum of each single attribute score times the weight of the attribute. The final screen presented a list, in rank order, of the alternatives under consideration. Interested subjects could call for detail screens that provided explanations of the computations.

The 29 PLWAs involved in the computer network experience used the decision support tool 195 times over the course of the experiment, each session lasting less than 10 minutes. Subjects used the ComputerLink for a wide range of decision problems. Labels provided by the PLWA of their decisions were classified by their manifest content as either relating to "day-to-day choices" or "health management."

It is impossible to separate out the effects of one part of the computer network intervention on global measures of impact. However, there is evidence of the effect of the overall ComputerLink use, which on some occasions involved use of the decision support system on decision-making-related outcomes.

No evidence was seen, however, to suggest that access to the ComputerLink improved decision-making skill (t − test of difference in the number of alternatives generated = .237, 46 df, $p>.05$). PLWAs with access to the decision support system generated a mean total of 4.5 alternatives solutions to two decision problems before the experiment and 5.4 following the experiment. Control subjects showed a mean gain of .7 in decision skill scores. Thus, the effect of using a computer network incorporating a decision support function appears to be an increase in decision-making confidence but no change in decision-making skill.

Many of the decision topics analyzed by PLWAs using the ComputerLink addressed issues faced by PLWAs in their day-to-day living. Twelve of the analyzed decisions were directly related to health issues; most of these dealt with choices about treatment or illness management. Topics included "Quit smoking," "decide whether or not to go to an analyst," and "bone marrow transplant." Only one decision suggested that the PLWA may have used the ComputerLink to help resolve an emergent health crisis; this person indicated that his decision was to "DECIDE TO CALL A DOCTOR" (upper case characters provided by PLWA). Other decisions analyzed using this system reflected daily living concerns. It is possible that the decision support tool provided in the ComputerLink was better suited to the one-time, exotic decisions and less well-suited to the day-to-day choice challenges faced by individuals. We now turn to other uses of computer tools for decision-making, including data management, future state visioning, and health behavior change support.

 ## Data Management and Health-Related Decision-Making

In addition to helping patients clarify preferences for health states, and select alternatives in accord with those preferences, computers can aid in the decision-making process by (1) facilitating data management related to information needed for health-related decisions, (2) helping patients envision the consequences of health decisions, and (3) supporting patients' access to personal and professional information that can lead to informed decision-making.

Facilitating Data Management

At Dana-Farber Cancer Institute, reports of health-related quality of life (HRQOL) are obtained from cancer patients each time they go to the breast cancer outpatient clinic. Patrick and Erikson define HRQOL as "the value assigned to the duration of life as modified by the social opportunities, perceptions, functional states, and impairments that are influenced by disease, injuries, treatments, or policy." The patient's assignment of a value to her current quality of life, vis-à-vis her preference for a health state, can be quantified on a continuum from 0 to 1. The longitudinal elicitation of the patient's perceptions of the effects of both the cancer and the treatment on her quality of life presents the clinician with multiple opportunities to improve patient care. The clinician receives self-reported information that can instigate further discussion with the patient about her preferences during the visit. These elicited data also act as feedback to the clinician about the outcomes of care since the last visit. At each point of contact, there is patient-reported information that can provide the basis for customizing patient care plans. In addition, the pen-based application utilized for the assessment has proven acceptable to patients, minimizes data entry, generates reports, is integrated with the institution's Oracle database, and works on a hand-held computer called the Newton MessagePad (Le, Kohane, and Weeks, 1995).

Envisioning Treatment Options

The technology-based Shared Decision-Making Program (SDP) was developed within a framework grounded in the idea that rational treatment decision-making considers both what the patient wants and what the clinician views as appropriate. The SDP was designed for use in the clinic setting to aid patients facing complex treatment choices (Kasper et al., 1992; Liao et al., 1996). The SDP for benign prostatic hyperplasia (BPH) has been clinically tested and evaluated since 1989, and the Foundation for Informed Medical Decision-Making has gone on to develop similar programs for other medical conditions, such as low back pain, mild hypertension,

breast cancer, and, lately, ischemic heart disease (Barry et al., 1997). In the SDP designed for BPH, following diagnosis and introduction to the program, patients receive an informational brochure and complete a questionnaire about demographics, current symptoms, feelings about symptoms, and health outcome preferences. Self-reported and other data are entered into the program, which then tailors estimates of risks and benefits to specific patient situations. In addition to verbal and graphic display of patient-specific probabilities, SDP presents videotaped interviews with individuals facing similar problems. For example, in the BPH program, a taped interview with two physicians-patients who chose either prostatectomy or watchful waiting is shown so that an understanding of the possible outcomes is made more real. This "core" segment lasts 22 minutes. In the "elective" segment that follows, the patient may view additional offerings on acute retention, sexual dysfunction, incontinence, and emerging treatments. The elective segments can add up to 25 minutes of material. Printed summaries for the patient and clinician are made available (Barry et al., 1995).

A prospective randomized trial to evaluate the impact of SDP for BPH on subsequent treatment decisions was recently carried out in Washington State. After a one-year follow-up, SDP subjects had significantly better scores than control subjects on BPH knowledge, satisfaction with the process of decision-making, general health perceptions, and physical functioning. The distribution of treatment decisions did not differ between groups. No difference was also found on satisfaction with the decisions themselves, BPH severity, social functioning, and preference for decision-making participation (Longo, 1993).

Linking Preferences with Treatment Decisions

The Department of Family Practice at the Medical College of Virginia, Virginia Commonwealth University, designed HealthTouch, a computerized health information system for health promotion and disease prevention for use in primary care. Evaluated in a randomized clinical trial involving 29 primary care practices, HealthTouch was intended to supplement clinician involvement in patient-focused preventive services. As factors that contribute to variation in health and prevention outcomes, patient preferences regarding diet management, exercise routines, weight control strategies, and other practices served as the basis for the customized computer recommendations for prevention (Williams, Boles, and Johnson, 1995). The preference assessment in HealthTouch is semantic in nature and does not rely on an explicit decision theoretic model.

Patients used a touch screen to answer 20 to 25 questions on personal and family history and patient preferences that affect lifestyle. The system then generated patient-specific intervention criteria and education materials as well as clinician chart reminders, reports, and order forms that facilitated both prescribing interventions and documenting the interaction with the patient. The clinicians were able to modify the recommendations, to further document patient preference to accept or decline implementation of the recommended activity, and to order the interventions or screenings if appropriate.

HealthTouch was incorporated into clinic practices in two ways: actively, by staff directing the patients to complete the survey, or passively, by placing the computers in the waiting area and allowing use based on patient choice. Regardless of the circumstances, follow-up surveys revealed that 77% of the patients who used HealthTouch received copies of their personalized health promotion recommendations, and of these patients, 93% read the reports. Patients who were actively asked to complete the questionnaire were more likely to have had their practitioner discuss the report with them and to have completed suggested interventions than were patients who completed the survey at their own initiative. Nearly 9 out of 10 patients reported being very satisfied with HealthTouch and saw it as a personally valuable tool for their health.

Decision-Making to Promote Health Behavior Change

Several models of health behavior change provide insight into individuals' decision-making and motivation about changing health and lifestyle habits. Effective behavior change is needed in diverse areas such as weight control, good nutrition, smoking cessation, or substance abuse treatment. In addition, behavior modification methods are important in increasing compliance with medication in conditions such as hypertension, asthma, diabetes, and HIV-AIDS. More than a dozen theoretical models have been proposed for how to bring about change in health behaviors and lifestyles. According to Glanz and colleagues (Glanz et al., 1997), these proposed changes fall into three broad categories: individual change, interpersonal change, and community change. Four theories for individual change are the health belief model (Rosenstock, 1960; Janz and Becker, 1984), stages of change model (Prochastka, 1984), reasoned action

(Fishbein, 1967), and stress and coping model of change (Lerman and Glanz, 1997). These theories focus on the individual and imply that change or the lack of it can be explained by individual characteristics. Three theories of interpersonal health behavior are social cognitive theory (Bandura, 1977), social support theory (Israel and Rounds, 1987; Cassel, 1976), and patient-provider communication (Roter and Hall, 1997). These focus on the interaction of two or a group of individuals and how these interactions can promote change. Four theories of community or group intervention models are community organization (Garvin and Cox, 1995), diffusion of innovations (Rogers, 1983), organizations change (Kaluzny and Hernandez, 1988), and communication theory (Bryant and Zillman, 1994; Gerbner, 1983). These models are helpful for leaders who want to make change in organizations. In addition, other scientists have combined several existing theories into broader sets of models for behavior change (Stokols, 1992; Petraitis et al., 1995; Ewart, 1989).

However, most behavior change models assume that individuals are aware of their alternatives, know their own values, and process information quickly and efficiently to choose what is in their best interest. Widespread data suggest that these models posit a degree of decision-making about everyday aspects of our lives that is just not that systematic (Nisbett and Ross, 1980). One conceptualization is that people attempting health behavior changes do not decide about single behaviors; they follow that which is implied by their habits from a web of prior decisions (Alemi et al., 2000). In this view, lasting change is a function of multiple decisions over a long time. During that time, a series of interrelated and dependent decisions are made. These decisions lead to actions that both are affected by and alter the state of the world and the rewards the decision-maker receives. When actions are repeated frequently over time, habits are formed. Decisions are linked to many prior large and small choices and affect future options. It is necessary to go beyond the immediate decision about a single act to see how prior choices concerning a number of related behaviors affect current events. In this conceptualization, habits emerge from a series of linked decisions as opposed to a single decision. There is a shift away from a focus on will power and self-discipline to a focus on problem-solving.

To change habits, it is not enough to change a single act. All related decisions and reinforcements also must be examined and modified. Successful change requires careful study of reinforcements and an understanding of linkages among decisions so that all decisions support the same action. For example, the decision to reduce fat intake does not make sense when people continue shopping the same way as before. To maintain new habits, behaviors and decisions that promote the needed change should be coupled with or incorporated into existing routines so that they occur without thought and effort. An avalanche of related small and large decisions is made to make one habit change. This could be seen as analogous to a personal pyramid scheme in which the choice of continuing with an unwanted habit is no longer possible.

It is proposed that to change the system that maintains a habit one must (1) identify and examine the linkages among decisions, (2) measure and receive feedback about behaviors, (3) propose and try out new activities to improve these habits, and (4) build these decisions and behaviors into everyday routines that continue over a long period of time (Alemi et al., 2000). In this context, will power and discipline are organized and enhanced by changing the system of linked decisions. The conscious decision is not in changing the behavior but in changing the system that produces the behavior.

Initiatives in the design of computers to aid the decision-making process to date primarily have focused on the construction of tools with a discrete application, such as breast cancer treatment or hormone replacement therapy, for special purpose. The use of computers to assist decision-making for more general purposes, such as making health behavior and lifestyle changes, may require computer tools that focus on the process of decision-making more than the specific content of any one decision. Under the directed access of a clinician, a client could learn to examine a series of decisions about his or her health behaviors and the linkages among them. This approach to making health behavior change is being refined in a project in which interdisciplinary clinical teams work with an electronic community of individuals to change cardiac risk factors (Moore, in press). As part of an interdisciplinary course in quality improvement, clinical teams (1) develop a therapeutic relationship with clients over a computer network, (2) assess clients' current health patterns regarding diet and exercise compliance with heart-healthy lifestyle guidelines, (3) coach clients to make self-improvements in health behaviors, and (4) track and trend data related to diet and exercise behavior over the project period. Using a self-improvement Web site created by the authors (*www.csuohio.edu/hca/hca615/improve.htm*), interdisciplinary clinical teams apply several theories of health behavior change, including the health belief model, reasoned action, self-efficacy enhancement, stage of change,

and relapse prevention. Clients are electronically "coached" using strategies of goal-setting, benefits/barriers assessment, problem-solving skills, diary keeping, social support, buddy system, contracting, tailored messages, relapse analysis, and feedback. Clinicians successfully conduct learning needs assessments with clients, implement strategies to change behaviors, and evaluate client outcomes using on-line methods. In this project, 95% of the 15 clients using this approach have made their desired health behavior changes. They reported feelings of connectedness to their care provider (electronic coach) and stated that the emphasis on making small changes and receiving frequent data and feedback about the changing trends in their behavior were particularly important to making the behavior change.

Although computer interactions between clinicians and clients are not required to apply this approach to health behavior change, computers offer the ability to efficiently provide information to increase understanding, provide timely feedback, and track and display behavior data in ways that are easily understood by clients, and they offer an ongoing (almost daily) presence in someone's life. Although the role of computers to provide social support to users is controversial, it appears that directed support or coaching from a clinician may work because it brings new information and feedback to the problem (Cobb, 1976; Cassel, 1976). Kessler and McLeod (1985) suggest that support works because it reduces stress and provides a sense of belonging and happiness. Sarason et al. (1990) argue that support works because individuals worry less about where help might come from and spend more time facing their problems. In addition to professional support, this approach encourages (demands) that clients participate in understanding and changing the web of decisions that comprise their behavior pattern. Data show that participation in decision-making enhances implementation chances (Roter and Hall, 1997). Also, early and frequent feedback may be an important reinforcement for maintaining a behavior or abandoning a behavior. Data about behaviors help an individual to understand. Data are needed to discipline our intuitions and prevent us from making false claims and attributions. Lasting change requires changes in understanding, not changes in attitude.

Some challenges to using an electronic care delivery system to support decision-making for health behavior change include obtaining patient hardware for electronic communications needed for Internet access and obtaining sufficient software to graphically display patient data to support behavior change. Clinicians also must increase their learning about combining and applying knowledge from the disciplines of health behavior change and computer science. For example, what is the ideal "client load" that can be reasonably managed electronically by a clinician or team, how much electronic client contact should be done individually or in groups, to what extent should clients' families be involved, and what is the correct balance between the amount of work done with clients on-line and using other forms of communication (i.e., telephone, written, or face-to-face)? Importantly, experience also has shown that electronic delivery of care to clients is a good way to foster interdisciplinary approaches to care. This approach broadens clinician exposure to different views of patient problems and interventions from multiple disciplines.

Summary

Decision-making and choice in health care are shaped by three important trends: a recognition of both the value and limits of science as a guide for care, a philosophy of care management that emphasizes standards and coordination, and a growing importance of the patient as a key participant in selecting and implementing clinical treatment. Each of these trends supports the need for explicit consideration of patient preferences as a guide to choosing health care practices, yet each poses specific barriers to the use of patient preferences. Scientific advances that can be made explicit and stated in a logical fashion may overshadow the more elusive, difficult to characterize, patient values. Managed care models may establish clinical care practices that leave little time for the intense, interpersonal process necessary to elicit a coherent understanding of patients' values and preferences. Patients themselves may hold personal attitudes that interfere with their ability or desire to explore these intimate parts of the self, to uncover and make explicit personal preferences, and choose care in accord with those preferences.

Computer technology can solve some, but not all, of the challenges inherent in employing patient preferences in health care practices. As new computer tools are developed to support health-related decisions, clarity about the models of decision-making being employed and their match to the type of decisions being addressed are crucial. Given the wide range and vastly different characteristics of various types of health decisions, computer tools of both general purpose and specific purpose and requiring both directed and nondirected access are most likely needed. Computer packages that focus on elicitation and values clarification may serve to help patients think hard about complex, abstract issues such

as preferences for life support or health outcomes. Computer networks can ensure the rapid, efficient transmission of patient preferences from the point of elicitation to the point of care and may facilitate patients' exploration of preferences in the privacy of their homes or away from an anxiety-producing health encounter. Computer algorithms, built and integrated into a computer-based patient record, have the ability to ensure that care is in accord with patient preferences by producing alerts when care deviates from explicit patient preferences. The WWW, CD-ROMs, and other computer tools can deliver informational interventions tailored to the needs, interests, and display requirements of individuals.

References

Agency for Health Care Policy and Research. (1997, September). *Consumer Health Informatics and Patient Decisionmaking: Summary.* (AHCPR Pub. 98-N001). Rockville, MD: AHCPR, DHHS.

Alemi, F., Neuhauser, D., Ardito, S., Headrick, L., Moore, S., Hekelman, F., and Norman, L. (2000, Feb). Continuous self-improvement: Systems thinking in a personal context. *Joint Commission Journal on Quality Improvement,* 26(2), 74–86.

Bandura, A. (1997). *Social Learning Theory.* Englewood Cliffs, NJ: Prentice Hall.

Barry, M. J., Cherkin, D.C., Chang, Y., et al. (1997). A randomized trial of a multimedia shared decision-making program for men facing a treatment decision for benign prostatic hyperplasia. *Disease Management and Clinical Outcomes,* 1(1), 7.

Barry, M. J., Fowler, F.J., Mulley, A. G., et al. (1995). Patient reactions to a program designed to facilitate patient participation in treatment decisions for benign prostatic hyperplasia. *Medical Care,* 33(8), 772–773.

Boberg, E. W., Gustafson, D. H., Hawkins, R. P., et al. (1997). CHESS: The comprehensive health enhancement support system. In P. F. Brennan, S. J. Schneider, and E. Tornquist (Eds.), *Information Networks for Community Health* 1997. New York: Springer-Verlag Publishers.

Brennan, P. F. (1994). Use of a computer network by persons living with AIDS. *International Journal of Technology Assessment in Health Care,* 10, 253.

Bryant, J., and Zillman, D. (Eds.). (1994). *Media effects: Advances in theory and research.* Hillsdale, NJ: Erlbaum.

Cassel, J. (1976). The contribution of the social environment to host resistence. *American Journal of Epidemiology,* 104, 107–123.

Cobb, S. (1976). Social support as a moderator of life stress. *Psychosomatic Medicine* 38, 300–314.

Deber, R.B., Kraetschmer, N., and Irvine, J. (1996). What role do patients wish to play in treatment decision-making? *Archives of Internal Medicine, 156*(13), 1414–1420.

Donabedian, A. (1968). Promoting quality through the evaluation of patient care. *Medical Care,6*, 181–202.

Earker, S. A., Kirschtk, J. P., and Becker, M. H. (1984). Understanding and improving patient compliance. *Annals of Internal Medicine, 100*, 258–268.

Ewart, C. K. (1989). A social problem-solving approach to behavior change in coronary heart disease. In S. A. Shumaker, E. B. Schron, and J. K Ockene (Eds.), *The Handbook of Health Behavior Change* (pp.153–190). New York: Springer Publishing Co.

Fishbein, M. (Ed.). (1967) *Readings in Attitude Theory and Measurement*. New York: Wiley.

Fisher, G. (1979). Utility models for multiple objective decision making: Do they really represent human judgment? *Decision Science, 10*, 451.

Flatley-Brennan P. (1998). Computer network home care demonstration: A randomized trial in persons living with AIDS. *Computers in Biology & Medicine, 28*(5), 489–508.

Garvin, C. D., and Cox, F. M. (1995). A history of community organization since civil war with special reference to oppressed communities. In J. L. Erlich and J.E. Tropman (Eds.), *Strategies of Community Organization* (5th ed.). Itasca, IL: Peacock.

Gerbner, G. (1983). Field definitions: Communication theory. In *1984–85 US Directory of Graduate Programs* (9th ed.). Princeton, NJ: Educational Testing Services.

Gerteis, M., Edgman-Levitan, S., Daley, J. and Delbanco, T. L. (1993). *Through the Patient's Eyes*. San Francisco, CA: Jossey-Bass Publishers.

Glanz, K., Lewis, F. M., and Rimer, B. K. (Eds.). (1997). *Health Behavior and Health Education: Theory, Research and Practice*. San Francisco: Jossey-Bass, Inc.

Goldstein, M.K., Clarke, A. E., Michelson, D., et al. (1994). Developing and testing a multimedia presentation of a health-state description. *Medical Decision-Making, 14*, 337.

Gustafson, D.H., Hawkins, R., Boberg, E. W., et al. (1994). The use and impact of a computer-based support system for people living with AIDS and HIV infection. *Journal of the American Medical Informatics Association* Suppl, 599–605.

Henry, S.B., and Holzemer, W.L. (1995). A comparison of problem lists generated by physicians, nurses, and patients: Implications for CPR systems. *Proceedings of the Annual Symposium on Computer Applications in Medical Care, 382*–386.

Hersey, J. C., Matheson, J., and Lohr, K. N. (1997). *Consumer Health Informatics and Patient-Decision-Making*. Final Report. Rockville, MD: AHCPR Publication No. 98–N001.

Humphreys, P., and McFadden, W. (1980). Experiences with MAUD: Aiding decision structuring vs. bootstrapping the decision maker. *Acta Psychological, 45*, 51.

Israel, B. A., and Rounds, K. A. (1987). Social networks and social support: A synthesis for health educators. *Advances in Health Education and Promotion, 2*, 311–351.

Janz, N. K., and Becker, M. H. (1984). The health belief model: A decade later. *Health Education Quarterly, 11*, 1–47.

Kaluzny, A. D., and Hernandez, S. R. (1988). Organizational change and innovation. In S. M. Shortell, and A. D. Kaluzny (Eds.), *Health Care Management: A Text in Organization Theory and Behavior* (2nd ed.). New York: Wiley.

Kasper, J.F., Mulley, A. G., Wennberg, J.E. (1992). Developing shared decision-making programs to improve the quality of health care. *Quarterly Review Bulletin, 18*(6), 183–190.

Keeney, R. and Raiffa, H. (1976) *Decisions with Multiple Objectives*. New York: Wiley Publishers.

Kessler, R. C., and McLeod, J. D. (1985). Social support and mental health in community samples. In S. Cohen and S. L. Syme (Eds.), *Social Support and Health*. Orlando, FL: Academic Press.

Le, P.P., Kohane, I.S., and Weeks, J.C. (1995). Using a pen-based computer to collect health-related quality of life and utilities information. In R. M. Gardner (Ed.), *Proceedings of the Nineteenth Annual Symposium on Computer Applications in Medical Care* (pp.839–843). Philadelphia: Hanley and Belfus, Inc.

Ledley, R. S., and Lusted L. B. (1968). Reasoning foundations of medical diagnosis. *Science 1959*(130), 9–21.

Lenert, L. A., Soetikno, R. M. (1997). Automated computer interviews to elicit utilities: Potential applications in the treatment of deep venous thrombosis. *Journal of the American Medical Informatics Association, 4*(1), 49–56.

Lerman, C., Glanz, K. (1997). Stress, coping and health behavior. In K. Glanz, F. M. Lewis, and B.K. Rimer, (Eds.), *Health Behavior and Health Education: Theory, Research and Practice*. San Fransisco CA: Jossey-Bass, Inc.

Liao, L., Jollis, J. G., DeLong, E. R., et al. (1996). Impact of an interactive video on decision-making of patients with ischemic heart disease. *Journal of General Internal Medicine, 11*, 373.

Longo, D. R., (1993). Patient practice variation: A call for research. *Medical Care, 31*(5), YS82–83.

Moore, S. M., and Kramer, F. M. (1998). Women's and men's preferences for cardiac rehabilitation program features. *Journal of Cardiopulmonary Rehabilitation, 16*(3), 163–168.

Moore, S. M. (In press). Expanding information for clients: Using continuous improvement techniques to achieve health behavior change. *Quality Mangement in Health Care.*

Nisbett, R., and Ross, L. (1980). *Human Inference: Strategies and Shortcomings of Social Judgement.* Englewood Cliffs, NJ: Prentice Hall, Inc.

Patrick, D.L., and Erickson, P. (1988, August). What constitutes quality of life? Concepts and dimensions. *Qual Life Cardiovascular Care,* 104.

Pauker, S. G., and McNeil, B. J. (1981). Impact of patient preferences on the selection of therapy. *Journal of Chronic Diseases, 34*(2–3):77–86.

Pauker, S. G., Pauker, S.P., and McNeil, B.J. (1981). The effect of private attitudes on public policy: Prenatal screening for neural tube defects as a prototype. *Medical Decision Making 1*(2), 103–114.

Petraitis, J., Flay, B., and Miller, T. (1995). Reviewing theories of adolescent substance use: Organizing pieces in the puzzle. *Psychological Bulletin, 117*(1), 67–86.

Prochaska, J. O. (1984). *Systems of psychotherapy: A transactional analysis* (2nd ed.). (Originally published 1979). Pacific Grove, CA: Brooks-Cole.

Raiffa, H. (1968). *Decision Analysis:Introductory Lectures on Choice Under Uncertainty.* Reading, MA: Addison-Wesley Publishing Co.

Rogers, E. M. (1983). *Diffusion of Innovations* (3rd ed.). New York: Free Press.

Rosenstock, I. M. (1960). What research on motivation suggests for public health? *American Journal of Public Health, 50,* 295–301.

Roter, D. L., and Hall, J. A. (1997). Patient provider communication. In K. Glanz, F. M. Lewis, and B. K. Rimer (Eds.), *Health Behavior and Health Education: Theory, Research and Practice.* San Francisco, CA: Jossey-Bass, Inc.

Ruland, C. M. (1998). Improving patient outcomes by including patient preferences in nursing care. *Proceedings / AMIA Annual Symposium,* 448–452.

Sainfort, F. and Booske, B. C. (1996). Role of information in consumer selection of health plans. *Health Care Financing Review, 18*(1), 31–54.

Sarason, B. R., Pierce, G.R., and Sarason, I. G. (1990). Social support: The sense of acceptance and the role of relationships. In B.R. Sarason, I. G. Sarason, and G. R. Pierce (Eds.), *Social Support: An Interactional View.* New York: John Wiley & Sons.

Saunders, G., and Courtney, J. (1985). A field study of the organizational factors influencing DDS success. *MIS Quarterly, 9*(1), 7.

Sonnenberg, F. A., and Pauker, S. G. (1986). Elective pericardiectomy for tuberculous pericarditis: Should the snappers be snipped? *Medical Decision Making, 6*(2), 110–123.

Stokols, D. (1992). Establishing and maintaining healthy environments: Towards a social ecology of health promotion. *American Psychologist, 47*(1), 6–22.

Tversky, A., and Kahneman, D. (1972). Judgment under uncertainty: Heuristics and biases. *Science, 185,* 124–131.

Von Neumann, J., and Morgenstern, O. (1964). *Theory of Games and Economic Behavior.* New York: Wiley Publishers.

von Winterfeldt, D., and Edwards, W. (1986). *Decision Analysis and Behavioral Research.* Cambridge: Cambridge University Press.

Williams, R.B., Boles, H.M., and Johnson, R.E. (1995). Patient use of a computer for prevention in primary care practice. *Patient Education and Counseling, 25*(3), 283–292.

PART **8**

Educational
Applications

23

The Nursing Curriculum in the Information Age

Barbara Carty
Elizabeth Phillip

OBJECTIVES

1. Understand the paradigm shift from computer applications to information management in nursing education.
2. Describe strategies to integrate information and computer technology into the nursing curriculum.
3. Describe the nursing informatics curriculum.

KEY WORDS

curriculum
informatics
faculty development
cognition
information technology
information systems
computer literacy
computing methodologies

This chapter presents nursing education within the context of information management and technology applications in society today. Curriculum implications including faculty development, interactive learning, cognition, electronic communications, and informatics are summarized. Models are presented and strategies suggested for meeting the educational challenges of the information age.

Nursing is an information-intensive profession, and nursing education relies heavily on the acquisition of information to educate students in their professional programs. Thus, the acceleration of technological development and availability of information will have profound effects on how students learn, how nursing is taught, and how care is delivered. Hairston (1996) states that the streamlining of businesses in the information age has set a precedent for education. No longer should education be constrained by department and discipline boundaries, but rather information technology should facilitate interactions and connectivity should promote the flow of information, the "lifeblood" of educational institutions.

In a very short period of time, higher education in general, and nursing education in particular, has moved from the delivery of educational content via isolated networked computer-assisted instruction (CAI) to the development of dynamic Web-based sites with interactive voice, video, and text. The acquisition of educational materials and information now involves sophisticated graphic communication and information systems that students can access from home, classroom, and clinical settings. Additionally, informatics, a discipline in its embryonic stage, has become intricately related with the delivery of information in education and practice, and research indicates that the concept of informatics needs to be articulated in curricula in the context of cognition and information processing, including information science as well as the technology that supports these functions (Patel and Kaufman, 1998; Ribbons, 1998a; Carty and Rosenfeld, 1998). In short, when curriculum and nursing education are examined, it needs to be done through the lens of information technology and information science. This is the future vision of education.

Informatics as applied to health care and education has changed dramatically in the past decade. Propelled by the advances in information and computer technology, we are now poised for yet another paradigm shift in the information era of the new millennium. The experience we have had with computers and information technology over the past decade allows us to incorporate new information, develop innovative models, and apply research findings to the field of informatics as it relates to nursing education and practice.

In the past, literature on educational applications related to the use of computers to enhance and promote education. There is currently a paradigm shift in society, generally, and informatics specifically that emphasizes the communication and collaborative components of information technology rather than the computing aspects (Carty and Rosenfeld, 1998). Nursing literature supports that the teaching of computer literacy or skills alone will not prepare nurses for the knowledge and integrative competencies they will need for the adequate managing of information in their profession (Travis and Brennan, 1998).

This chapter will present the rapidly evolving changes taking place in the development and delivery of education material in nursing education and will focus on the processes of information management and technology as they apply to the nursing curriculum. Education will be discussed within the context of information technology and information science and specifically related to:

1. Information management and the educational environment

2. Faculty development

3. Cognition and interactive learning

4. Nursing informatics and the curriculum

Information Management

The management of information is and will continue to become one of the most daunting challenges for faculty, students, and nurses. Simply being a citizen in the information technology era predisposes one to this challenge. In 1993, the National Information Infrastructure: Agenda for Action resulted in the formation of the National Information Infrastructure (NII). Among the many purposes of the NII is the promotion of access to health care and health care information through a global and national electronic infrastructure. A number of other efforts both within and outside of nursing support the necessity for

nurses to be able to process, manage, and access information in education and nursing practice (Ribbons, 1998b; Porritt, 1997; Arnold, 1996). These demands will only increase as our society becomes more dependent on information and technology continues to move to seamless interactive systems that incorporate cognition and decision support into the ebb and flow of education and practice.

Studies indicate that in many ways nursing education programs have neither incorporated information technology nor developed strategic plans that promote faculty development, financing, and support for information management in a comprehensive and measurable way (Carty and Rosenfeld, 1998; Arnold, 1996). Of primary importance for the successful integration of information management in education is an organizational infrastructure that supports resources both human and technical, promotes faculty development, and incorporates information science (informatics) into the curriculum.

Educational Environment

A discussion of the process of education in the context of information technology and information management necessitates inclusion of the educational environment to promote the delivery of curriculum content. A recent survey by Carty and Rosenfeld (1998) demonstrates that the majority of nursing schools have technology in place to deliver basic CAI and interactive video (IAV) material, but few schools have the capability to support more sophisticated delivery of CD-ROM and interactive Web-based technology.

The use of traditional methods of computer instruction has limited applications in the fast moving world of interactive, multimedia Web-based information. Students as well as faculty need to learn how to access information, integrate it, and apply it in the learning environment as well as the practice environment. The use of appropriate technology for course delivery and assessment and management of health care information must be fostered in an environment of collaboration among departments and institutions to assure adequate distribution of resources, quality assurance, and professional recognition (Porritt, 1997; Carty and Rosenfeld, 1998).

A successful plan for the integration of information technology into the education process requires the presence of an environment that supports and sustains (1) a supportive infrastructure, (2) the availability of centralized technology resources, and (3) collaborative, interdisciplinary courses supporting information management. Such a model, which crosses department lines and assures adequate resources to all members of the educational community, can effectively and efficiently prepare faculty and students to manage information for education and practice (Green, 1996; Lewis et al., 1997; Narsavage and Beidler, 1997).

Supportive Infrastructure

The educational and curriculum goals of nursing education are forced by the nature of information technology to operate within an infrastructure that shares and supports access to available technology and technological innovations. Such an environment includes (1) adequate technical support, including personnel, (2) an educational resource/technology planning committee, and (3) allocation of financial resources. Administrators and faculty in nursing education should assure their consumers that planning and resources in information technology will be integral to the governance and delivery structure of the institution. Nelson and Anton (1997) suggest that one of the first steps in assuring organizational recognition for information technology is a study of the computer and information learning needs within the organizational structure. An assessment of resources as well as learning needs of both faculty and students will provide data to support informed decision-making for both computer technology and information management planning.

Financial resources and budget allocations have been one of the most difficult challenges for educators to reconcile in planning for technological resources. Schools of nursing throughout the country have reported financial resources for technology ranging from no monies to as high as $156,000 annually, but the mean was only $7,000, and the most frequently allocated amount was $1,000. Likewise, only one-third of schools have reported monies allocated for personnel, with the mean reported as $8,000 (Carty and Rosenfeld, 1998). Clearly then, schools of nursing need to examine their strategies and formulate innovative methods to assure that resources are made available to both faculty and students.

Centralized Resources

With the availability of interconnectivity and both Internet and intranet capability, schools are in a position to develop and share resources with other departments and divisions in an academic setting. Centralized resources are a natural extension of the information superhighway and the Internet II initiative of the government. The evolution of the Web-based platform not only allows for the transfer of information, but also the sharing of data, group discussions, access to educational programs, and the facilitation of research. Local area networks (LANs) within schools of nursing promote immediate access to large shared databases and the pooling of resources. Current findings indicate that only a small minority of nursing programs have a plan for the implementation of technology into their programs (Carty and Rosenfeld, 1998). As academic settings expand their connectivity and Internet capability, nursing programs should have a seat at the table and contribute to the planning and allocation of resources. Representation on interdisciplinary strategic planning committees for technology implementation is essential as universities restructure and chief information officers (CIOs) form teams to develop long-range plans and goals. Similarly, technical support can be jointly supported by a number of departments, and nursing students can be encouraged to collaborate with students from other disciplines, including business and computer science. Such collaborative methods can decrease operational costs and provide for access to a large array of digital information including library databases, educational software, and research resources.

Collaboration

Rogers (1996, p. 29) maintains that the rapid advances in technology will continue to "create financial and infrastructure needs that university campuses will be forced to address: new equipment, more user training and new courses." The development of collaborative models in which faculty formulate interdisciplinary courses, share resources, and promote student interaction can be an exciting paradigm of the future. Hairston (1996) states that "for tomorrow's successful college and university, it will matter much less that departments exist, but far more that faculty, students, and all others interrelate."

The development of interdisciplinary courses and the cross-fertilization of experiences can benefit both faculty and students as they acquire skills in computer literacy and knowledge of information management. Various course models (Narsavage and Beidler, 1997) have recently been proposed by educators as successful strategies to enhance education, maximize resources, and promote innovative learning. Hodson describes a collaborative model for preparing health care practitioners for the future (Fig. 23.1). This model emphasizes the concept of information and communication technology as essential to education and practice. Indeed, both faculty development and student learning are dependent on interdisciplinary

Proposed Collaborative Operational Model for Preparing Health Care Practitioners for the Future

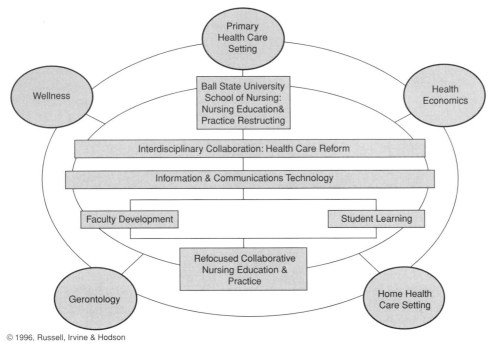

© 1996, Russell, Irvine & Hodson

Figure 23.1
Proposed collaborative model for preparing health care practitioners for the future.
(Courtesy of Kay Hodson, University of Indiana.)

collaboration and the use of information and communications technology.

Clearly, in a number of college settings, a subtle transformation is taking place in which technological innovations are being incorporated into the infrastructure and instructional operations of colleges. The collaborative paradigm in health care practice in which nurses work with information specialists, system designers, and technical experts should be emulated in the education setting.

Faculty Development

In order for faculty development programs to be successful at integrating information technology into the curriculum, they must be sensitive to both faculty interests and time limitations. Faculty value can be used to improve student learning, research projects, or service, so it is important that these benefits are emphasized. Harris (1995) indicates that faculty move through several phases as they integrate the use of computers and instructional technology. This suggests that technical aspects should be taught before moving on to instructional applications of information technology. Table 23.1 lists categories and examples of content for faculty development programs designed to integrate information technology into the curriculum.

Barriers to Faculty Development

Integration of information technology into the curriculum creates major change within an organization. As with any change, driving and restraining forces exist that impact on the integration of this innovation. Attention to the change process is crucial if information

Table 23.1   Content for Faculty Development Programs to Integrate Information Technology into the Curriculum

Computer Literacy Skills	Information Literacy Skills	Technical Skills	Skills for Teaching Information Technology Strategies
Computer systems for delivering health care	Electronic mail and Internet/WWW access	Campus and distance course delivery skills such as Internet skills, video-conferencing, and multimedia	Cognitive theories and information technologies
Software packages such as word processing, spreadsheet applications, database, and computer-based testing systems	Library database access Understanding the impact of automation on health care delivery		Evaluating the quality of information on the Internet

technology is to be successfully integrated into nursing curricula. Cravener (1998) developed a faculty development paradigm for integrating information technology into nursing education. Underlying this paradigm is the principle that adoption of information technology for teaching and scholarship is an innovation issue requiring application of change theory so that faculty's affective responses to change are understood and the desired outcome of change in faculty teaching behaviors are achieved (Fig. 23.2).

The model illustrates a paradoxical disjunction between the information technology approach to faculty development and the psychosocial concerns that tend to inhibit faculty participation. A psychosocial systems checklist serves as a guide for identifying critical areas to be addressed during faculty development programs.

Faculty development programs that focus on enhancing faculty skills with the use of information technologies will be most successful if known areas of resistance to change are specifically addressed during the planning and implementation phases of program development. Resistance to the integration of technology comes from the feelings, anxieties, and fears that people have when faced with major personal and institutional changes. From a faculty perspective, issues commonly associated with resistance to change and some strategies to overcome these barriers include institutional cultures, affective responses to the challenge of learning new instructional strategies, competing demands on faculty time, and perceived validity of computer-mediated teaching and learning.

Institutional Cultures   Traditionally, institutions of higher learning have been authority- and knowledge-centered. The provision of distance education creates a shift to a more lateral structure and a perceived threat to traditional faculty roles along with a perceived inability to control the teaching process. Integration of information technology can also create fear of loss of employment.

Affective Responses   Integrating information technology can create a potential threat to faculty self-concept in a variety of ways. Proposing that an educator needs to learn new media for teaching implies that the old way is not optimal. Faculty development programs should emphasize that new technologies are neither good nor bad, but merely a means for solving new problems. An educator's beginner role with instructional technology and/or Internet communications contrasts with his or her normal view of the self as a scholar and discipline expert. Development of technical skills needs to be taught in a nonthreatening manner.

Competing Demands   Integration of information technology into the curriculum is a time-intensive process. A realistic assessment of this time variable and the impact of information technology on faculty workload needs to be addressed to prevent faculty disillusionment with the process. Faculty participation in information technology training sessions should be recognized as valid continuing professional education programs by their department chair, and integration of information technology into the curriculum should be part of the tenure and post-tenure review criteria.

Nursing faculty in particular may feel that computers disrupt interpersonal relationships with students and patients that are central to building caring, therapeutic relationships. Forces promoting the integration of information technology that can be used to encourage its adoption include new social and economic con-

ditions, technology supports of excellence, risk-taking faculty, and change agents.

As the need for adult lifelong learning gradually spreads through educational systems, the introduction of Web-based instruction provides opportunities to enroll new populations of adult students. Uses of technology to support high-quality teaching and learning can serve as strong selling points during faculty development

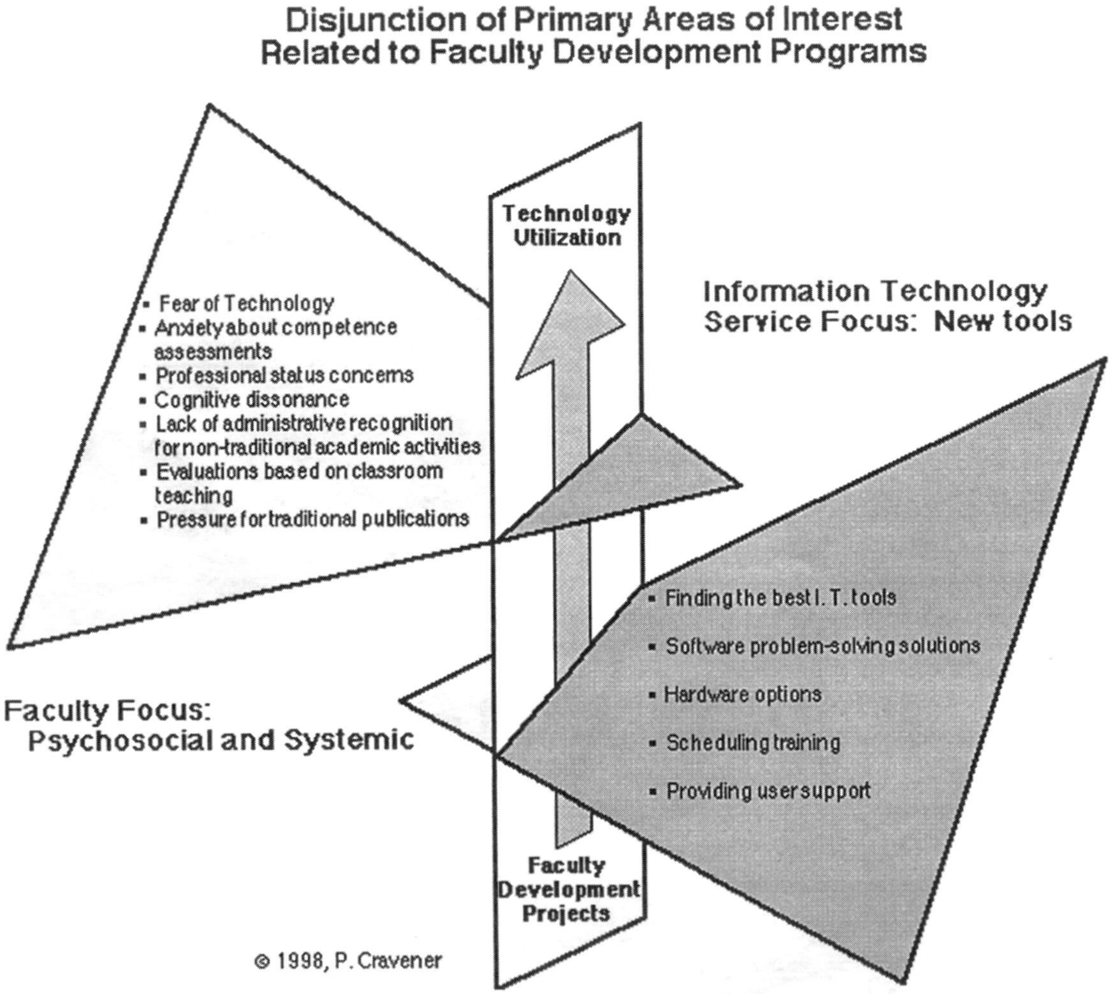

Disjunction of Primary Areas of Interest Related to Faculty Development Programs

Technology Utilization

Information Technology Service Focus: New tools

- Fear of Technology
- Anxiety about competence assessments
- Professional status concerns
- Cognitive dissonance
- Lack of administrative recognition for non-traditional academic activities
- Evaluations based on classroom teaching
- Pressure for traditional publications

Faculty Focus: Psychosocial and Systemic

- Finding the best I.T. tools
- Software problem-solving solutions
- Hardware options
- Scheduling training
- Providing user support

Faculty Development Projects

© 1998, P. Cravener

Figure 23.2
The paradoxical disjunction model.
(Courtesy of P. Cravener.)

programs. Reinforcing the fundamental rationale for academic use of Web-based resources, potential advantage for individual faculty, the institution, and students, is crucial to the success of any faculty development program.

Rogers (1983) divides various individual responses to technology into ideal adopter categories. These categories are useful in planning faculty development programs, anticipating possible reactions to a change, and implementing it. In order to keep pace with rapidly changing technological innovations, ongoing faculty development programs for the integration of information technology should be provided. Additionally, adequate resources in the form of hardware, software, and technical support need to be available immediately and on an ongoing basis in order to decrease faculty frustration while they integrate technology. Faculty development programs need to occur not only on an institutional level but also on the national level. Recently, the Division of Nursing, U.S. Department of Health and Human Services, funded continuing education courses in nursing informatics for nursing faculty that were offered across the nation in conjunction with regional nursing organizations. The anticipated outcomes of these sessions include increased knowledge and skills of nursing informatics, diffusion of informatics in nursing education, development of mentorships in nursing informatics to help nursing faculty to expand their use of computer based systems, and replication of models of continuing education in nursing informatics.

Cognition and Interactive Learning

With the complex clinical practice environment of the next millennium, it is anticipated that nurses will face escalating information management challenges as well as require psychomotor skills to use ever-changing technology in their nursing practice. As the American Association of Colleges of Nursing (AACN) has stated in *Position Statement: Nursing Education Agenda for the 21st Century* (1993), nursing education must encompass the requirements for entry into practice and, to the greatest extent possible, anticipate the requirements for nursing practice in the future. This challenges nursing education to prepare practitioners who have not only appropriate computer literacy skills but also cognitive skills for the effective use of information technologies. Skills and methods for integrating these skills into nursing curricula have been addressed by various authors (Nelson and Anton, 1997; Ribbons, 1998a).

Nelson and Anton describe the need for both computer literacy and information literacy in nursing curricula. Computer literacy is the ability to perform computer operations at a skill level high enough to meet the demands of society (Joos et al., 1996). In health care environments, it involves the computer systems that are used to deliver health care and the common microcomputer software packages. Information literacy is the ability to use the tools of automation in the process of accessing, evaluating, and utilizing information. This includes understanding the impact of automation on health care.

Ribbons (1998a) discusses the potential that information technologies hold as tools for the development of cognitive skills. The foundational cognitive skills of information acquisition, assessment, management, and use are necessary for effective problem-solving and clinical decision-making. Cognitive tools are any innovative use of information technologies to facilitate the development of metacognitive skills (Jonassen, 1995). This is in contrast to using knowledge domain software, as seen in computer-assisted instruction, that supports context-specific knowledge reproduction. Ribbons (1998a) and Nelson and Anton (1997) suggest using cognitive tools such as word processing, spreadsheets, hypertext applications, and E-mail to promote knowledge construction or learning outcomes to apply knowledge across a wide variety of content and context domains. These broader based learning outcomes occur as a result of cognitive residue. Cognitive residue is the skills, understanding, and attitudes that remain with the individual as a result of human-computer interaction. Ribbons (1998a) suggests that when using technology as a cognitive tool, educators develop educational experiences that foster the development of higher order thinking skills required for the effective acquisition, management, and use of health care information. There is very little research related to cognitive tools and metacognition in relation to computers and information technology in the nursing literature. Future research directions for the application of computers as cognitive tools in education and health care settings are promising areas of research.

Cognition and Hypertext

Hypertext is a "nonlinear, multidimensional, semantic structure in which words are linked by associations" (Tripp and Roby, 1990). Cognitive learning theories can be used to inform decisions about placement of hypertext links and customize the production of hypertext-based materials for nurse education.

Two theoretical approaches differ in the need for structural guidance for hypertext links. Schema theorists advocate hierarchical hypertext materials to provide high levels of guidance for novice users (Shin et al., 1994). Schema theory emphasizes the need for newly acquired knowledge to be linked to existing foundational knowledge (Driscoll, 1994). Applying this theory suggests that hypertext materials should be presented in a consistent format so that students can locate their new learning in an overall scheme or structure (Gillham, 1998). Cognitive flexibility theory offers a contrasting view of knowledge acquisition through hypertext. Cognitive flexibility theory is based on the assertion that advanced learning involves the development of flexible representations of knowledge that will help promote deep conceptual understanding and the ability to adaptively use knowledge in new situations. Application of cognitive flexibility theory should incorporate use of rich cases and examples, facilitate multiple forms of knowledge representation, and identify links between abstract concepts and case examples (Jacobsen, 1994). These representations link favorably to holistic care and problem-based learning that are both favorably applied to nursing education. There are numerous potential uses of hypertext in nursing education including linking nursing care data found on hospital information databases to theoretical information. This application can provide on-line clinical information to practicing nurses as well as provide students with detailed explanations of terminology within the same hypermedia resource.

Table 23.2 provides a summary of information required for hypertext materials by various user groups, specific design recommendations, and the theoretical basis for these recommendations.

Multimedia

Multimedia, with its ability to deliver text, full color graphics, sound, video, and animation, provides an excellent example of how cognition can be enhanced by computer-based systems. The most important characteristic of multimedia is its ability to offer an enjoyable, effective, and flexible method of instructional delivery that attracts the learner's interest, maintains attention, and accommodates a diversity of learning styles (Hazari, 1992). Ribbons (1998c) offers a variety of practical guidelines for the development of interactive multimedia applications in nursing education. In order for multimedia to be an effective teaching tool, it is essential that the application be based on firm pedagogical principles.

World Wide Web

The Web represents the graphical part of the Internet, incorporating text, full-color graphics, sound, and video. Intranets work in the same way as the Internet, but the information is only available to users within a LAN for in-house consumption. Course outlines and material, school information, evaluations, application forms, and the like can be carried on it. Students and faculty can also publish their work on the Internet using software applications such as Microsoft FrontPage. Publishing quality work on the Internet can make more nursing resources available. The volume of information

Table 23.2   Hypertext: Suggested Design Characteristics for Nurse Education

User	Information Required	Design	Theoretical Basis
Low computer literacy	Details on actual use of hypertext	User-friendly Consistent screen structure	Schema theory
Good computer literacy	Storyboard detailing content	Well indexed Design to facilitate navigation	Schema theory Cognitive flexibility theory
Undergraduate students	Detailed nursing care instructions	Hierarchical structure Detailed within linear structure	Schema theory
Practicing nurses	Evidence-based research Information directly relevant to clinical practice	Rapid navigation Networked web structure Well indexed	Schema theory Cognitive flexibility theory

Reproduced, with permission, from Gilham (1998).

on the World Wide Web (WWW) serves to remind students of the need to develop effective search skills and critical analysis of information.

A recent consumer survey (FIND/SVP, 1997) indicates that more and more consumers are obtaining a greater proportion of their health information from the World Wide Web. In order for nurses to fulfill their role as patient advocates and educate consumers on how to critically analyze health information, students need to gain experience in evaluating the quality of health education information on the Internet. Figure 23.3 illustrates a valid and reliable tool to evaluate the quality of health-related WWW sites. There are many such tools available on the Internet and in the literature. The benefit of this tool is that content validity is assessed by a group of library and information science professionals.

CD-ROM

The benefit of CD-ROMs as teaching-learning tools for clinical nursing education include multimedia capabilities, portability, and large storage capacity. The multimedia capability of CD-ROM technology allows for an interactive on-screen situation that mimics reality with graphics, sound, and movement. The technology and materials needed to record CD-ROMs are now available for personal computer production (Schroader, 1994). CD-ROMs can store 650 megabytes of data or the equivalent of 1,500 high density floppy disks, 12,000 scanned images, or over 250,000 pages of printed text (Nicoll, 1994; Gleydura et al., 1995). A CD-ROM drive is necessary to use the material found on a CD-ROM. These drives, which are located either internally or externally, can currently be purchased for less than $100 (Sengstack, 1998). CD-ROM technology has become less expensive and faster (currently, $32\times$ speed is available), making it popular.

Computer-Assisted Instruction

CAI is a software program designed to achieve greater mastery of content and learning than is possible with didactic instruction. This is achieved by allowing the learner to interact with the computer at his or her own pace and as many times as needed to master content. Most CAIs are text-based, but some include illustrations and minimal visual graphics of a procedure. The sound and motion characteristics of CD-ROM or Web-based applications are not present in CAI. There are several types of CAI software available including drill and practice, tutorials, and simulations. Drill and practice routines allow the student to practice previously learned material through answering multiple choice questions. The CAI scores and tracks the student's progress and provides feedback to the student. Tutorials or remedial instructions are CAI software that provides didactic information and includes drill exercises to provide the learner with feedback about his or her mastery level of content. Simulations are case studies and/or models designed to provide opportunities to deal with realistic clinical or administrative problems. Clinical simulations provide the learner with opportunities to develop clinical decision-making skills in a nonthreatening environment.

CAI programs are frequently used because they are cost effective and can be user-friendly, and the content can be easily changed by adding another database. The downfall is that they can foster a surface approach to the learning task (Conrick and Foster, 1992). In order for CAI to be an effective educational tool, it must be designed in a stimulating and motivating way. It is essential that the educational strategy be clear and the program be appropriate to course objectives and the level of the student. There are several evaluation tools that can be used to review, score, and determine the usefulness of the CAI programs.

Testing System

Since April 1994, the National Council Licensure Examination for Registered Nurses (NCLEX-RN) has been an on-line, computer-based test administered in selected locations in every state and United States territory. Although computer literacy is not essential for taking the test, student familiarity and comfort with computer adaptive testing prior to taking the licensure examination are helpful to decrease anxiety levels and improve computer literacy. In response to this need, testing systems or software programs designed by developers or teachers as computerized evaluations or programmed tests have been developed. The first published report of computerized testing in nursing education found that students taking examinations on computer performed "as least as well as, and in some cases better than" those given paper and pencil tests. The study further concluded that computerized testing was not detrimental to grades or to learning for the limited number of students who participated in the study (Bloom and Trice, 1997). Concerns related to this type of testing include test security, use of honor codes, and positive student reactions to the choices accompanying computer testing.

Reported benefits of computerized testing for faculty include a reduced amount of time invested in the

Title: _____ **URL: http://** _____

Date: _____ **Evaluator:** _____

Information

Step 1: Check 'Y' (Yes) if statement applies 'N' (No/Not Sure) if statement does not apply.

Criteria 1: Scope	Y	N
A. Many different aspects of the topic are presented.		
B. Each aspect is presented in depth.		
Tally		

Criteria 4: Currency	Y	N
A. The information presented is up-to-date.		
B. The information builds on previous knowlege.		
Tally		

Criteria 2: Accuracy	Y	N
A. The information is consistent with other resources on the topic.		
B. The information presented is properly referenced.		
C. The information is based on scientific data.		
D. The site includes a disclaimer.		
Tally		

Criteria 5: Purpose	Y	N
A. The purpose of the site is identified.		
B. The information is appropriate for the intended purpose.		
C. The intended audience is specified.		
D. The source funding the site is identified.		
Tally		

Criteria 3: Authority	Y	N
A. The author(s)/organization(s) supplying the information are identified.		
B. The author(s)/organization(s) are recognized in the field.		
C. The credentials of the author(s) are identified.		
D. The author(s) are writing in their discipline.		
Tally		

Step 2: Sum the Y's from each criteria.

C1 ☐ + C2 ☐ + C3 ☐ + C4 ☐ + C5 ☐ = ☐

Step 3: Rate the site by comprehensiveness of information.

☐ 13 - 16 = Credible site: Convincing evidence exists

☐ 7 - 12 = Ambivalent site: inconclusive evidence exists

☐ 0 - 6 = Red Flag Site: Insufficient evidence exists

Design

Step 4: Check 'Y' (Yes) if statement applies 'N' (No/Not Sure) if statement does not apply.

Criteria 6: Organization, Structure & Design	Y	N
A. The information presented in the site is well-organized.		
B. The terminology used is meaningful to the subject area.		
C. The site contains a table of contents or provides an organizational structure to easily access content.		
D. The site contains specific links to data referenced.		
E. The site contains internal search engines.		
F. The document has a distinguishable header and footer.		
G. The major headings and subheadings are identifiable.		
H. The loading time for the site is reasonable.		

Organization, Structure & Design	Y	N
I. The site's creation date is clearly displayed.		
J. The date of the last revision is clearly displayed.		
K. The reading level and material presented is appropriate for intended audience.		
Tally		

Step 5: Rate the site by "net appeal."

☐ 6 - 11 = Accommodating site

☐ 0 - 5 = Hindering site

Step 6: Personal Comments: Now compare this source to other sources you have on this topic.

Figure 23.3
Health-related WWW site evaluation tool.
(Reproduced, with permission, from Kotecki and Chamness (1999).)

development, administration, and scoring of tests; the ability to generate a variety of question types; establishment of test banks with varying degrees of psychometric properties; the ability to import questions from textbook computerized test banks; and prompt processing of grades and analysis of questions through access to students' answer files. Students report that feedback on questions during or immediately after the test promotes their learning. Other student benefits reported include immediate reports on their grades and scheduling of testing dates and times spread over several days to fit their academic and personal needs. Students feel that exposure to computers for evaluative purposes prepares them for taking the licensing exam on the computer. The one drawback reported by students is the restriction from moving freely about the exam and from reviewing previously answered questions. However, since this is how NCLEX-RN is structured, this restriction does prepare them for the licensing examination (Anna, 1998). The selection of a computerized testing system for institutional adoption can be made easier through the work of Kirkpatrick et al. (1996), who conducted a comparative review of seven computerized test development programs. The features of each of the systems are reviewed along with suggestions on foundational aspects of implementation.

The next generation of testing methodology currently being researched by the National Council of State Boards of Nursing for potential use in the NCLEX-RN is computerized clinical simulation testing (CST). CST is designed to measure application of the registered nurses' independent clinical decision-making related to the management of client care through a series of interactive client care scenarios. Underlying the CST is the Nursing Information Retrieval System (NIRS), a relational database of tables of nursing and medical terms that is used to facilitate the retrieval of related medical and nursing information for developing, delivering, and cataloging CST cases and case materials. Terms in the NIRS tables are linked through a simple coding system that contributes to standardization across the varied vocabulary and classification systems used in medicine and nursing. The NIRS includes medical subject heading and North American Nursing Diagnosis terms and codes from the National Library of Medicine's unified medical language system metathesaurus. Also included in the NIRS is a nursing activity database that is linked to the patient problem/nursing diagnosis table, the NCLEX-RN test plan table, and a time and cost of care table.

CST permits evaluation of clinical decision-making competence, which is defined as the appropriate and timely sequencing of nursing actions taken with, or on behalf of, the client. Evidence of competence in clinical decision-making is demonstrated by specifying assessment, diagnosis, intervention, and evaluation actions on behalf of a client during an unprompted, time-sensitive, dynamic scenario.

A pilot study of CST's usefulness, psychometric soundness, and legal defensibility as a potential component of the NCLEX-RN examination was undertaken from April through July 1998. In August 1999, based on a report of the study findings, the National Council's Delegate Assembly will make a decision regarding the use of CST as a component of the NCLEX-RN examination. If the decision is to incorporate CST as a component of the NCLEX-RN examination, an implementation plan will be initiated, and CST will become part of the NCLEX-RN examination sometime after the year 2001. This movement toward a more realistic measure of clinical decision-making will require further integration of information technology into nursing curricula (Bersky et al., 1998).

Electronic Communications

The Internet with the World Wide Web as a platform offers access to a host of information and communication resources for students and educators. Multiple benefits include the ability to exchange E-mail messages, transfer computer files, connect to and use distant information services/databases, participate in and obtain information from special interest group mailing lists, and obtain electronic journals. The literature includes many examples of the benefits of Internet applications in nursing practice (Sparks, 1993; Dubois and Rizzolo, 1994; Wright, 1996). In order to prepare students for the practice environment in which they will be working, experience in using these applications during their educational program is essential.

There is little research reported in the literature about the use of these applications in nursing education. A number of articles have addressed methods for integrating technology into the nursing curriculum (Mastrian and McGonigle, 1999; Shellenberger, 1999; Clark D., 1998; McGonigle and Mastrian, 1998). It has been found that classes using the Internet as a teaching medium differ from traditional classes in that the active participation of each student is required, there is a greater level of personal interaction and sharing of information among students, the learner's independence is fostered, and scheduling is flexible. These differences promote a shift in emphasis on the part of the educator from lecturing to guidance and facilitation (Connors et al., 1996; Bachman and Panzarine, 1998). Bachman and Panzarine (1998) studied the impact of using a variety of information technologies on a group of RN to MSN students. Although the study had a small sample size, the findings suggest that these students used computer and information technologies more effectively for the acquisition, management, and use of health care information than 23 students at a similar stage of their nursing program. This report also recommends that Internet activities be functionally relevant for nurses and their work.

E-mail

The fastest growing domain of computer use at colleges has been E-mail; the percentage of college courses using E-mail jumped from 8 percent in 1994 to approximately 20 percent in 1995 and 25 percent in 1996 (Green, 1996). E-mail can be used for computer-mediated communication (CMC) between faculty and students, to facilitate group work, and to distribute lecture notes and tutorial information. Rohfeld and Hiemstra (1995) reported benefits of CMC as perceived by distance learning students. These benefits included increased control over learning environment, satisfaction in having mastered technical skills, the timeliness and convenience of personal communication with their instructor, and student belief that their responses were more thoughtful/reflective because of the delay imposed by writing. Students who described themselves as timid or unable to think quickly in face-to-face situations stated that CMC gave them time to reflect and compose their contributions to class discussion. Cravener and Michael (1998) conducted a study designed to investigate the extent to which campus-based students who were not inclined to participate in classroom discussions would use CMC for that purpose and to determine which individual differences among students appeared to be associated with student selection of class discussion or CMC. The study findings support the belief that students who used class and office time to talk about education-related concerns were the same individuals who used computer-mediated communications. For campus-based students who communicated frequently with faculty, the educational advantage of CMC was related to expansion of time for access to faculty. Todd (1998) used E-mail in an undergraduate child health nursing course to promote critical thinking by requiring students to respond to 10 critical thinking questions posted by the faculty. As a result of the electronic dialogue, misconceptions were clarified and students with learning disabilities participated more readily than in a traditional classroom discussion.

Internet communication can be enhanced by the addition of internet video and sound. Video software such as CU-See Me can be used to transfer audio and video for video-conferencing through the Internet. Both parties need this technology for the sound and picture to be transmitted.

Listservs and Forums

Enormous numbers of listservs covering a wide range of nursing interests including research and clinical practice are available. A user subscribes to the group by sending an E-mail to a listserv. These mailing lists give the user direct access to hundreds of like-minded clinicians and academics throughout the world. Listservs can be used in nursing courses to facilitate faculty and student communication and interaction. They provide a forum for class content and related topics of discussion.

Newsgroups

Newsgroups work by posting messages, much like putting a message on a bulletin board. The most common newsgroup network is Usenet. Newsgroups can be set up to run on a LAN, acting very much like an electronic bulletin board to be used for facilitating an electronic tutorial or a virtual classroom. Electronic tutorials can be used for sharing information and may facilitate critical thinking and questioning. Specific nursing-related newsgroups can be found at *sci.med.nursing*, a general forum for all nursing issues (Ribbons, 1998b).

Electronic Meeting Software

Electronic meeting software is a collection of software tools to automate and improve the quality of group process and team building. It can be used to support a variety of processes in higher education including strategic planning, research collaboration, student program evaluation, and classroom instruction. A meeting support software system consists of a suite of decision support tools. Several advantages of electronic meetings over traditional meetings have been identified. The ability to work in the same area or at remote sites allows for greater control of personal time. The expression of ideas is promoted through maintaining anonymity. The ability of all members to express ideas at the same time, speaking in parallel, increases participation and idea building. An increased awareness of and value for different perspectives is promoted through expression of ideas in a nonjudgemental environment (O'Brien and Renner, 1998; O'Brien and

Renner, 1999). A study of the effectiveness of group system software for teaching a nursing management course indicated that examination scores and frequency of class participation were higher for the study group than the control group of students who experienced the same course using lecture. Student evaluations revealed that they believed the process enhanced application and understanding. Negative aspects of this methodology were increased preparation time for faculty and students' lack of tolerance when technical difficulties were encountered (Ayoub et al., 1998)

 ## Nursing Informatics and the Curriculum

In 1994, the American Nurses Association (ANA) defined the scope of informatics practice as "the specialty that integrates nursing science, computer science, and information science in identifying, collecting, processing, and managing data and information to support nursing practice, administration, education, research, and the expansion of nursing knowledge." The position of the ANA was a direct outcome of the national endorsement of automating health care information, the establishment of the computer-based patient record, and the development of standards to facilitate the transmission of health care information across settings.

Prior to the ANA recognition, Corcoran-Perry and Graves (1989) defined nursing informatics as the "combination of computer science, information science, and nursing science, designed to assist in the management and processing of nursing data, information, and knowledge to support the practice of nursing and the delivery of nursing care."

Further clarification of the scope of nursing informatics was provided by the expanded definition of nursing informatics practice to include "the full range of activities that focus on the methods and technologies of information handling in nursing. Informatics nursing practice includes the development, support and evaluation of applications, tools, processes and structures which assist the practice of nurses with the management of data in direct care of patients" (American Nurses Association, 1995).

The emphasis on automated health care systems has created within the professions an imperative to identify, develop, and design data and information that reflects discipline specific as well as interdisciplinary domains. Nursing informatics is an area of practice that is being propelled by the advances of information technology in health care and the rapid

evolution of the automated patient care record. Professional opportunities and roles are evolving at a rapid rate, and nurses are searching for educational programs to meet their needs. In a national study of undergraduate and graduate nursing programs, fewer than one-third of the schools reported that informatics was incorporated in their programs, and only 10 percent reported that nursing informatics was presented as a separate course (Carty and Rosenfeld, 1998). In a study conducted on a nationwide sample of informatics specialists, the majority of nurses sampled attributed their learning of informatics to "on the job training" (Carty, 1994). A study by Arnold (1996) supported the need for educational programs for nurses in informatics, the majority of nurses in the study sample identified the need for education in informatics; even though 71 percent had higher degrees. In 1997, the National Advisory Council on Nurse Education and Practice issued a report to the Secretary of the Department of Health and Human Services on "A National Informatics Agenda for Education and Practice." Among the many issues addressed in the report was the call for nursing informatics education including:

- Identification of core informatics content for students and practicing nurses
- Advanced informatics preparation for nurses
- Faculty preparation in informatics

It is imperative, therefore, that nursing education address the learning needs of students and prepare them to practice in the next millennium of health care. Mastery of information technology and managing health information are essential areas of curriculum content for all undergraduate and graduate nursing programs.

Nursing Education Informatics Models

In the past, emphasis has been on acquiring basic computer skills and knowledge of generic applications such as word processing and spread sheets. The focus now is on mastering information technology and information management as it applies to nursing information and knowledge. The rapid advances in information technology; the availability of information in flexible, retrievable formats; and the need for faculty, students, and nurses to manage large amounts of data and information have driven this shift. The change in education and informatics has been from computer literacy to information literacy and management (Nelson and Anton, 1997).

A number of models have been presented for educators to emulate in designing curriculum for the inclusion of nursing informatics. Travis and Brennan (1998) propose a model that emphasizes the inclusion of information science as essential in the undergraduate curriculum (Fig. 23.4).

Focusing on the three concepts of information, technology, and clinical care processes, the authors support the incremental progression of informatics in the undergraduate curriculum. Such a model provides for both the theoretical and practical components of informatics and emphasizes the smooth integration into course sequencing. Mastering the basics of information technology in the first and second year, students progress to the actual application of information technology to the science of nursing in the third year. The correlation between information tech-

nology and patient care is reinforced in the clinical environment. A final project concludes the students' understanding of the information of nursing by requiring the completion of a project in a selected area of nursing informatics that has practice implications (Travis and Brennan, 1998).

Another approach to integrating nursing informatics into the curriculum has been proposed by Riley and Saba (1996). In the Nursing Informatics Education Model (NIEM) (Fig. 23.5), the domains of computer science, information science, and nursing science are integrated throughout the curriculum in a progressive leveling to ensure the development of nursing informatics competencies. In the Riley and Saba model, undergraduate students master computer literacy and progress to information management and its application to the clinical setting.

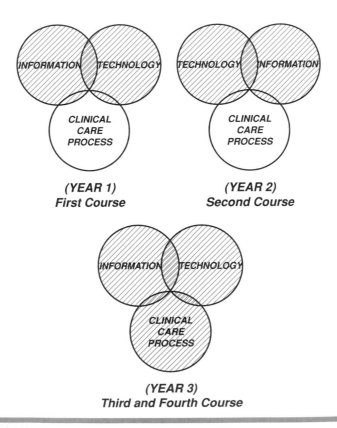

Figure 23.4
Travis and Brennan model.
(Reproduced, with permission, from Travis and Brennan (1998).)

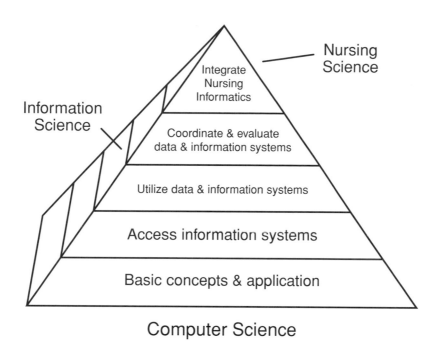

Figure 23.5
Nursing Informatics Education Model (NIEM).
(Reproduced, with permission, from Riley and Saba.)

The challenge remains to determine and develop strategies for integration into the undergraduate curriculum. Current efforts are under way to identify competencies in nursing informatics across the spectrum from beginner to expert (Staggers and Gassert, 2000). This effort also requires the recognition to develop and implement faculty education programs in nursing informatics.

Nursing informatics on the graduate level has a vital role in both education and practice, but currently there is a dearth of programs available. Several schools offer graduate nursing informatics specialization, and several more offer graduate courses in the area. As nursing informatics attempts to define its role in the education and health care arena, there is discussion on the nature of the discipline. Some proponents see it as more of an interdisciplinary focus, while others propose a nursing focus. Current research efforts to support the domain of nursing, by developing nursing taxonomies, language, and classification systems, and designing clinical systems that reflect patient outcomes and effective nursing interventions,

champion the recognition of an area of informatics specific to nursing (National Center for Nursing Research, 1993; McCormick, 1994; Zielstorff, 1995; Maas et al, 1996; Brennan et al., 1997; Clark, 1997; Henry and Mead, 1997).

Nursing Informatics Education: Domain-Specific and Interdisciplinary

It has been suggested that nursing informatics has a specific nursing focus, but there are acknowledged areas of interdisciplinary and collaborative foci that need to be explored and studied. Turley (1996) proposes a model for nursing informatics that incorporates other disciplines including cognitive science that has implications for education. This model supports a multidisciplinary approach and encompasses computer science, information science, and, cognitive science within the domain of nursing science. The intersection of the information, cognitive, and computer sciences underpins informatics (Fig. 23.6). The Turley model gives credence to the importance of cognition in the application of information technology and management in nursing education.

In addition to Turley, several others have supported the inclusion of the science of cognition within a model of informatics (Patel and Kaufman, 1998; Ribbons, 1998; Gillham, 1998). The paradigm shift from emphasis on technology to the cognitive or human computer interaction has important implications for nursing education. How do students learn with technology, and how does technology affect the learner? These are fertile areas for the emerging field of informatics and pose exciting research initiatives for educators.

Another interdisciplinary focus of informatics specifically relates to the collaborative nature of the discipline (National Advisory Council on Nurse Education and Practice, 1997; Gassert, 1998), nurse informatics specialists work with programmers, information management teams, and system designers. Many nurse educators collaborate with other departments including computer sci-

entists, education design specialists, and system analysts. This trend will continue as the need to manage and deliver information becomes the essential component of education and health care.

As computer hardware and software become more powerful and sophisticated, the ability to manage data and information and represent knowledge will affect how students learn in an educational environment and clinicians practice in a health care environment. The incorporation of decision support systems into clinical systems and the ability to access knowledge sources and research repositories will provide users with sophisticated knowledge systems that will have the potential to improve care. The communication and collaborative capability of information technology will have the effect of producing seamless, interactive systems that will support knowledge representation, facilitate human interaction, and provide new avenues for research in both practice and education.

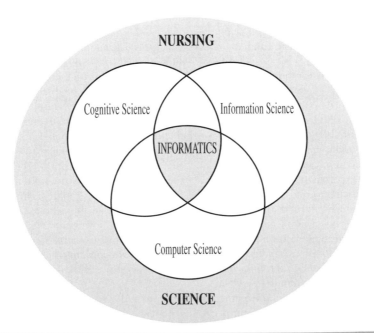

Figure 23.6
Turley model.
(Reproduced, with permission, from Turley (1996).)

Current and past literature reveal enormous efforts by nurse informaticians to develop, design, and research nursing-specific as well as interdisciplinary areas of patient care data. Specialists in nursing informatics will continue to expand their work with interdisciplinary teams to develop sophisticated programs for decision support, interactive multimedia health care, and tele-health delivery systems (Brennan, 1995; Lindberg, 1997; Schiffman, 1997; Campbell, 1997; Zielstorff, 1997; Zielstorff, 1998; Henry and Mead, 1997; Henry et al., 1998). At the same time, there will remain the necessity to educate nursing informatics specialists to contribute to the ever-expanding field of health care informatics. It will be these specialists who will be able to cross the interdisciplinary boundaries and advance nursing knowledge and promote the domain of nursing within systems. This new area in nursing will grow as our society essentially relies on information systems to deliver, research, and teach health care.

References

American Association of Colleges of Nursing. (1993). *Position Statement: Nursing Education's Agenda for the 21st Century*. Washington, D.C.: American Nurses Publishing.

American Nurses Association. (1994). *Scope of Practice for Nursing Informatics*. Washington, D.C.: American Nurses Publishing.

American Nurses Association. (1995). *Nursing Informatics Standards of Practice*. Washington, D.C.: American Nurses Publishing.

Anna, D. (1998). Computerized testing in a nursing curriculum. *Computers in Nursing, 23*, 22–26.

Arnold, J. (1996). Nursing informatics educational needs. *Computers in Nursing, 14*, 333–339.

Ayoub, J., Vanderboom, C., Knight, M., et al. (1998). A study of the effectiveness of an interactive computer classroom. *Computers in Nursing, 16*, 333–338.

Bachman, J., and Panzarine, S. (1998). Enabling students to use the information superhighway. *Journal of Nursing Education, 37*, 155–161.

Bersky, A., Krawczak, J., and Kumar, T. (1998). Computerized clinical simulation testing: A new look for the NCLEX-RN® examination? *Nurse Educator, 23*, 20–25.

Bloom, K.C., and Trice, L.B. (1997). The efficacy of individualized computerized testing in nursing education. *Computers in Nursing, 2*, 82–84.

Brennan, P. (1995). Patient satisfaction and normative decision theory. *Journal of the Medical Informatics Association, 2*, 250–259.

Brennan, P., Lorenson, P., and Rutland, C. (1997). Decision support for assessing patient preferences for geriatric care. In U. Gerdin, M. Tallberg, and P. Wainright (Eds.). *Nursing Informatics: The Impact of Nursing Knowledge on Health Care Informatics*. Amsterdam: IOM Press.

Campbell, J. (1997). Phase II evaluation of clinical coding schemes: Completeness, taxonomy, mapping, definitions and clarity. *Journal of the Medical Informatics Association, 4*, 238–251.

Carty, B. (1994). The protean nature of the nurse informaticist. *Nursing and Health Care, 15*, 174–177.

Carty, B., and Rosenfeld, P. (1998). From computer technology to information technology: Findings from a national study of nursing education. *Computers in Nursing, 16*, 259–265.

Clark, D. (1998). The international classification for nursing practice: A progress report. In U. Gerdin, M. Tallberg, and P. Wainright (Eds.), *Nursing Informatics: The Impact of Nursing Knowledge on Health Care Informatics* (pp. 62–68). Amsterdam: IOM Press.

Clark, D. (1998). Course redesign: Incorporating an Internet web site into an existing nursing class. *Computers in Nursing, 16*, 219–222.

Connors, H. R., Smith, C., and DeCock, T. (1996). Kansas nurses surf the Web for master's degrees. *Reflections, 22*, 16–17.

Conrick, M., and Foster, J. (1992). Clinical decision making in nursing using computer based education. In P. Weeks and D. Scott, Eds., *Exploring Tertiary Teaching Armidale, UNE*.

Corcoran-Perry, S., and Graves, J. (1989). The study of nursing informatics. *Image Journal of Nursing Scholarship, 21*.

Cravener, P., (1998). A psychosocial systems approach to faculty development programs. *http://horizon.unc.edu/TS/development/1998-11.asp*

Cravener, P., and Michael, W. (1998). Students use of adjunctive CMC. 5th Annual National Distance Education Conference. *http://www.cravener.net/articles/austin1.html*

Driscoll, M. (1994). *Psychology of Learning for Instruction*. Boston: Allyn and Bacon.

Dubois, K., and Rizzolo, M. A. (1994). Cruising the information superhighway. *American Journal of Nursing, 94*, 58–60.

FIND/SVP, Inc. (1997). The 1997 American Internet user survey. *http://etrg.findsvp.com/internet/top.html*

Gassert, C. (1998). The challenge of meeting patients' needs with a national nursing agenda. *Journal of Medical Informatics Association, 5*, 263–268.

Gilham, D. (1998). Using hypertext to facilitate nurse education. *Computers in Nursing, 16*, 95–98.

Gleydura, A. J., Michelman, J. E., and Wilson, C. N. (1995). Multimedia training in nursing education. *Computers in Nursing, 13*, 169–175.

Green, K. C. (1996). The coming ubiquity of information technology. *Change, 28,* 24–27.

Hairston E. (1996). A picaresque journey. *Change,* March/April: 32–37.

Harris, J. (1995). Curricularly infused telecomputing: A structured approach to activity design. *Computers in the Schools, 11,* 49–59.

Hazari, S. (1992). Multimedia: Is it the right tool for your instructional application? *The Journal of Educational Multimedia and Hypermedia, 1,* 143–146.

Henry, S., and Mead, C. (1997). Nursing classification systems: necessary but not sufficient for representing "What Nurses Do." For inclusion in computer-based patient record systems. *Journal of Medical Informatics Association, 4,* 222–232.

Henry, S., Warren, J., Lange, L., and Button, P. (1998). A review of major nursing vocabularies and the extent to which they have the characteristics required for implementation in computer-based systems. *Journal of the Medical Informatics Association, 5*(4), 321–328.

Jacobsen, M. (1994). Issues in hypertext and hypermedia research: Toward a framework for linking theory to design. *Journal of Educational Multimedia and Hypermedia, 3,* 141–154.

Jonassen, D. H. (1995). Computers as cognitive tools: Learning with technology, not for technology. *Journal of Computing in Higher Education, 6,* 40–73.

Joos, I., Whitman, N., Smith, M. J., et al. (1996). *Computer in Small Bytes* (2nd ed.). New York: NLN.

Kirkpatrick, J. M., Billings, D. M., Hodson-Carlton, K. H., et al. (1996). Computerized test development software: A comparative review. *Computers in Nursing, 2,* 113–125.

Kotecki, J., and Chamness, B. (1999). A valid tool for evaluating health-related WWW sites. *Journal of Health Education, 30,* 56–59.

Lewis, D., Watson, J., and Newfield, S. (1997). Implementing instructional technology: Strategies for success. *Computers in Nursing, 15,* 187–190.

Lindberg, C. (1997). Implementation of in-home telemedicine in rural Kansas: Answering an elderly patient's needs. *Journal of Medical Informatics Association, 4,* 14–17.

Maas, M., Johnson, M., and Mooched, S. (1996). Classifying nursing-sensitive patient outcomes. *Image: Journal of Nursing Scholarship, 28,* 295–301.

Mastrian, K., and McGonigle, D. (1999). Using technology based assignments to promote critical thinking. *Nurse Educator, 24,* 45–47.

McCormick, K. (1994). Toward standard classification schemes for nursing language: Recommendations of the American Nurses Association Steering Committee on databases to support clinical practice. *Journal of Medical Informatics Association, 1,* 421–427.

McGonigle, D., and Mastrian, K. (1998). Learning along the way: Cyberspacial quests. *Nursing Outlook, 46,* 81–86.

National Center for Nursing Research. (1993). *Nursing Informatics: Enhancing Patient Care.* (NIH Publication No. 93-2419). Bethesda, MD: National Center Nursing Research.

National Advisory Council on Nurse Education and Practice. (1997). *A National Informatics Agenda for Nursing Education.* Rockville, MD: Department of Health and Human Services.

Narsavage, G., and Beidler, J. (1997). Technology in nursing education: An interdisciplinary course. *Fifteenth Annual International Nursing Informatics Conference.* Atlantic City, NJ: Rutgers University.

Nelson, R., and Anton, B. (1997). Organizational diagnosis of computer and information learning needs: The process and product. *Sixth International Congress on Nursing Informatics.* Stockholm, Sweden.

Nicoll, L. (1994). Essential resources: Compact disks for computers. *Journal of Nursing Administration, 24,* 7–8, 27.

O'Brien, B., and Renner, A. (1998). Opening minds: Values clarification via electronic meetings. *Computers in Nursing, 16,* 266–271.

O'Brien, B., and Renner, A. (1999). Wired for thought: Electronic meetings in nursing education. *Computers in Nursing, 17,* 27–31.

Patel, V., and Kaufman, D. (1998). Medical informatics and the science of cognition. *Journal of American Medical Informatics Association, 5,* 493–501.

Porritt, N. (1997). Managing to learn with technology. *Active Learning, 12,* 7.

Ribbons, R. (1998a). The use of computers as cognitive tools to facilitate higher order thinking skills in nurse education. *Computers in Nursing, 16,* 223–228.

Ribbons, R. (1998b). Practical applications in nurse education. *Nurse Education Today, 18,* 413–418.

Ribbons, R. (1998c). Guidelines for developing interactive multimedia applications in nurse education. *Computers in Nursing, 16,* 109–114.

Rogers, E., and Green, K. (1996). The coming ubiquity of information technology. *Change, March-April,* 2, 24–31.

Rogers, E. M. (1983). *Diffusions of Innovations* (3rd ed.). New York: The Free Press.

Saba, V., and McCormick, K. (1996). *Essentials of Computers for Nurses.* New York: McGraw-Hill.

Schiffman, R. (1997). Representation of clinical practice guidelines in conventional and augmented decision tables. *Journal of the Medical Informatics Association, 4,* 382–393.

Schroader, E. (1994). CD-R is becoming a storage option; falling prices, increasing CD-ROM use spur popularity of recording technology. *PC Week, 11,* 33.

Sengstack, J. (1998). 32X CD-ROMs up ante- but add little value. *PC World, 16*, 78.

Shellenberger, T. (1999). Using CD-ROM technology to enhance clinical nursing education. *Nurse Educator, 24*, 20–22.

Shin E., Schallert D., and Savenye, W. (1994). Effects of learner control, advisement, and prior knowledge on young students' learning in a Hypertext environment. *Educational Technology Research and Development, 42*, 33–46.

Sparks, S. (1993). Electronic networking for nurses. *Image; Journal of Nursing Scholarships, 25*, 245–248.

Staggers, N., and Gassert, N. (2000). Nursing informatics competencies. In B. Carty (Ed.), *Nursing Informatics: Education for Practice*. New York: Springer.

Stead, W. (1998). It's the information that's important, not the technology. *Journal of American Medical Informatics Association, 8*, 131.

Todd, N. (1998). Using e-mail in an undergraduate nursing course to increase critical thinking skills. *Computers in Nursing, 16*, 115–118.

Travis, L., and Brennan, P. (1998). Information science for the future: An innovative nursing informatics curriculum. *Journal of Nursing Education, 37*, 162–168.

Tripp, S., and Roby, W. (1990). Orientation and disorientation in a hypertext lexicon. *Journal of Computer-based Instruction, 17*, 120–124.

Turley, J. (1996). Toward a model of nursing informatics. *Image: Journal of Nursing Scholarship, 28*(4), 309–313.

Wright, K. B. (1996). The internet and nursing: A vital link. *MEDSURG Nursing, 5*, 209–211.

Zielstorff, R. (1995). Capturing and using clinical outcome data: Implications for information systems design. *Journal of the Medical Informatics Association, 2*, 191–196.

Zielstorff, R. (1997). A knowledge-based decision support system for the prevention and treatment of pressure ulcers. In U. Gerdin, M. Tallberg, and P. Wainright, (Eds.), *Nursing Informatics: The Impact of Nursing Knowledge on Health Care Informatics*. Amsterdam: IOM Press.

Zielstorff, R., et al. (1998). Mapping nursing diagnosis nomenclatures for coordinated care. *Image: The Journal of Nursing Scholarship, 30*, 369–373.

Recommended Reading

American Nurses Association. (1996). *Nursing Data Systems: The Emerging Framework*. Washington, D.C.: American Nurses Publishing.

Anderson, B. (1992). Nursing informatics: Career opportunities inside and out. *Computers in Nursing, July/August*, 165–169.

Bruner, J. (1962). *On Knowing*. Cambridge, MA: Harvard University Press.

Carty, B., and Rosenfeld, P. (1997). The information age: The status of technology in nursing education programs in the United States. In U. Gerdin, M. Tallberg and P. Wainright (Eds.), *Nursing Informatics: The Impact of Nursing Knowledge on Health Care Informatics* (pp. 125–131). Amsterdam: IOM Press.

Cohen, P., and Dacanay, L. (1994). A meta-analysis of computer-based instruction in nursing education. *Computers in Nursing, 12*(2), 89–97.

Daly, J., Button, P., Prophit, C., et al. (1997). Nursing interventions classification implementation issues in five sites. *Computers in Nursing, 15*, 23–29.

Dolence, M., and Norris, D. (1995). *Transforming Higher Education: A Vision for Learning in the 21st Century*. Ann Arbor, MI: Society for College and University Planning.

Dorenfast, S. (1997). Health care informatics editorial. *http//www.healthcare.com*

Edmonds, G. (1999). Making change happen: Planning for success. *http://horizon.unc.edu/TS/development/1999-03.asp*

Fullerton, J., and Graveley, E. (1998). Enhancement of basic computer skills: Evaluation of an intervention. *Computers in Nursing, 16*(2), 91–94.

Federal Coordinating Council for Science, Engineering, and Technology. (1994). *High performance computing and communications: Toward a national information infrastructure*. Washington, D.C.: Office of Science and Technology.

Gassert, C. (1995). Academic preparation in nursing informatics. In M. Ball et al. (Eds.), *Nursing Informatics: Where Caring and Technology Meet* (pp. 333–349). New York: Springer-Verlag.

Goodman, J., and Blake, J. (1996). Multimedia courseware. Transforming the classroom. *Computers in Nursing, 14*(5), 287–296.

Hardin, P. C. (1997). Interactive multimedia software design: Concepts, process, and evaluation. *Health Education & Behavior, 24*(1), 35–53.

Hardy, J., Conrick, M., Foster, J., et al. (1996). Computerised education for health professions. In E. Hovenga, M. Kidd, and B. Cesnik (Eds.), *Health Informatics: an Overview*. Melbourne, Australia: Churchill Livingstone.

Kannery, J. (1996). Portability issues for a structured clinical vocabulary: Mapping from Yale to the Columbia medical entities dictionary. *Journal of the Medical Informatics Association, 3*, 66–78.

Kirkpatrick, M. K., Brown, S., and Atkins, B. A. (1998). Using the Internet to integrate cultural diversity and global awareness. *Nurse Educator, 23*, 15–17.

Miller, J. G., and Wolf, F. M. (1996). Strategies for integrating computer-based activities into your educational environment: A practical guide. *Journal of the American Medical Informatics Association, 3*(2), 112–117.

Petryshen, P., Pallas, L.L.O., and Shamian, J. (1995).
      Outcomes monitoring: Adjusting for risk factors,
      severity of illness, and complexity of care. *Journal of
      the Medical Informatics Association, 2,* 243–249.
Poirrier, G. P., Wills, E. M., and Payne, R. L. (1996).
      Nursing information systems: Applications in nursing
      curricula. *Nurse Educator, 21*(1), 18–22.
Richards, P. L. (1997). Conquering technophobia:
      Preparing faculty for today. *Sixth International
      Congress on Nursing Informatics.* Stockholm, Sweden.
Rohfeld, R. W., and Hiemstra, R. (1995). Moderating
      discussions in the electronic classroom. In Z. L. Berge
      and M. P. Collins (Eds.), *Computer Mediated Com-*

munication and the Online Classroom, vol. II, *Higher
      Education* (pp. 22–24). Cresskill, NJ: Hampton Press.
Saranto, K., Leino-Kilpi, H., and Isoaho, H. (1997). Learn-
      ing environment in information technology: The views of
      student nurses. *Computers in Nursing, 15,* 324–332.
Witucki, J. M., Hodson, K. E., and Malm, L. D. (1996).
      Electronic education: Integrating electronic
      conferencing to enhance problem solving in nursing.
      Nurse Educator, 21(4), 8–12.
Wong, J., Wong, S., and Richards, J. (1992).
      Implementing computer simulations as a strategy for
      evaluating decision-making skills of nursing students.
      Computers in Nursing, 16, 264–269.

24

Distance Education: Using Technology to Learn

Myrna L. Armstrong

OBJECTIVES

1. Define distance education.
2. Describe the historical approaches and current development.
3. Discuss important interactive strategies and support needed for learning at a distance.
4. Identify essential support required for course development.
5. Explore the associated research needed to assist future trends in nursing education.

KEY WORDS

distance education
distance learning
telecommunications
consumer-driven education
research
learning interactively
Internet courses

Programs for distance learning are flourishing, especially Internet courses. The advertisement "new distance learning programs for working professionals" certainly has appeal, capturing the attention of many people seeking to fit further education into their busy schedules. Yet, many questions are frequently asked: are these courses for "real"; can I actually acquire a degree in my home or workplace without driving long distances and sitting in tedious lecture classes, and do they really have application to nursing, especially for the clinical work I want to do? This progressive movement toward another way of providing both academic and continuing nursing education is not only due to the development and use of technologies (video, audio, and computer equipment) that can be used for distance education, but also the market-driven demands of educational reform. The result of this education will be the empowerment of the nursing student and working professional to make important educational choices. Often these decisions will be based on accessibility and the amount of time needed to complete the course or program.

While distance education has been available in this country since before the turn of the nineteenth century, many methodology changes, especially in synchronous and asynchronous technologies, have occurred. Consumers who have needed access to education have always been willing to participate in this type of education. On completion, the learners are frequently pleasantly surprised with the educational quality.

Following a review of the historical approaches to distance education and the present-day movement, this chapter will examine today's high-quality, cost-effective, learner-centered approach to distance education, from both the student and faculty perspectives. This will include the importance of applicable educational principles needed to promote interactivity, active learning, and effective learner support, as well as some of the major academic and pedagogical issues impacting faculty developing creative courses. Last, in order to enhance the quality, effectiveness, and efficiency of nursing education at a distance, ideas for research associated with distance education need to be explored. These suggestions for research-based assessments and evaluations of distance education can assist future educational decision-making in the design, development, and dissemination of information to nursing professionals. This chapter will include the following:

■ A definition of distance education

■ Strategies and support for the learner

■ Faculty support for course development

■ Legal, ethical, and public policy issues

■ Future trends and associated research

Distance Education: Historical and Current Perspectives

What Is Distance?

In the past, schools and educators needed an excuse to develop and conduct distance education. Off-campus or extension sites could be approved by regulatory agencies when the sites were great distances away from the originating school or when geographical barriers existed. Some states even defined the number of miles for approval. Documentation of need frequently had to be substantiated (Clark, 1993a). Distance education, depending on the school's technological resources, could also mean that the faculty drove "the distance" to the off-campus site. Today, the term "distance" education has to do more with learner accessibility. Mileage is not counted or traveled; rather, learning is experienced locally or globally, at home or in the workplace, regardless of a rural or urban setting, across state lines and even internationally.

What Is Distance Education?

Distance education differs from the traditional classroom in two essential elements. The majority of a course or program of study, whether with teachers and students or with students and students, is separated by (1) physical distance and often (2) time. A motto of distance education could be "education—anytime, anywhere, at reasonable rates" (Neal, 1999). This education is not bound by time; it can occur in "real time," a synchronous mode where the teacher and students (or student and students) have active dialogue simultaneously (Milsead and Nelson, 1998). To accomplish this, an on-line computer "chat" could be used, while the participants are still separated by distance. In an asynchronous mode, or "delayed" time, students and

faculty can interact with each other, but not at the same time. For example, the student may send electronic mail (E-mail) or use an electronic bulletin board. The message is received immediately, but the faculty may not see the message until they check their E-mail, which may be in an hour or the next day (Billings, 1996a; Massoud, 1999).

The Evolution of Distance Education

Distance education has experienced bumps and surges of acceptance with the evolving use of print, audio, television, and the various computer interactive technologies. Distance education courses started out focusing on vocational training, but as people have become comfortable with them, many different topics have been presented and many disciplines have used distance education as an option of instruction (Neal, 1999). Over the years, learners in underserved and unserved areas have always identified with the concept of education at a distance because it provided access to education previously not available (Pym, 1992). Currently, the twenty-five-year-old and older age group is the major group participating in distance education courses (Neal, 1999). The traditional student did not pay much attention to distance education because the educational opportunities and the typical classroom setting were nearby. Many faculty avoided the concept by raising questions of quality rather than exploring the educational principles used in distance education (Shomaker and Fairbanks, 1997). While some of those feelings still exist, distance education has moved on, capturing new types of educational experiences and innovative kinds of pedagogy and transforming education for both the students and faculty. In essence, what has been learned is that good distance education theory and good education theory are actually the same; the education just transcends the barriers of time and space (Armstrong and Mahan, 1998; Dede, 1990; Schlosser and Anderson, 1994).

Correspondence and Radio Courses

While it can be said that today's distance education is new, the earliest form began in the 19th century as correspondence courses in Sweden. In the United States, support for this educational movement was taken by the Boston-based Society to Encourage Studies at Home in 1873. By 1891, a commercial school for correspondence studies had developed in Pennsylvania. The 1900 enrollment figure was 224,000, and by 1920, enrollments had risen to more than 2,000,000 (Schlosser and Anderson; 1994). Unfortunately, dropout rates averaged around 65%. In 1885, the University of Wisconsin developed "short courses" and farmer's institutes. In 1919, they added radio, the first technology used for distance education, and it provided one-way communication from the faculty to the students. By the early 1920s, at least 176 radio stations were constructed at land grant colleges to promote this type of education.

Telephone, Television, and Satellite Courses

The ongoing changes in distance education have been termed as moving from plain old telephone service (POTS) to pretty amazing new stuff (PANS) (Zetzman, 1995). The inclusion of audio conferencing in the early 1950s used telephone handsets, speaker phones, and an audio bridge to connect multiple phone lines. This provided the first two-way interaction within distance education for physicians and nurses in Wisconsin. Early experimental television in 1935 added another idea for motion and visuals so that complex and abstract concepts could be illustrated through visual simulation. The first educational television license was issued in 1945, yet this additional technological idea for distance education did not become practical, feasible, and finally a reality until the 1950s (Neal, 1999; Armstrong and Mahan, 1998; Schlosser and Anderson, 1994).

In 1971, the Open University of the United Kingdom began offering full degree programs through the innovative use of media. The popularity of this concept was astounding. By 1984, over 69,000 students had completed requirements for their Bachelor of Arts degree (Schlosser and Anderson, 1994). A United States campus of the Open University has now opened. Many more universities whose mandate is exclusively distance education with technology have opened since that time including the British Open University, the German FernUniversitat, and, in Canada, the Open Learning Agency and Athabasca University (Pym, 1992).

Satellite technology for distance education in the United States was implemented in the early 1980s. Since that time, further refinement and inclusion of interactive technologies such as cable, compressed video, and video teleconferencing have continued to pave the way for more simulated face-to-face contact and two-way interaction. This offered distance students greater transparency of technology and provided an expansion of the traditional classroom setting experiences.

Computer Technology and the Internet

Computer technology came slowly to the forefront of distance education, and then it exploded. In the late 1970s computer technology arrived in the traditional university classroom. Computer-based education (CBE), which encompasses computer-assisted instruction (CAI) and computer-managed instruction, was implemented cautiously. In nursing education, CAI first supported teaching and learning by supplementing traditional classroom courses. Now, according to a recent National League for Nursing survey, CAI is the "most prevalent educational application" used in 135 undergraduate nursing schools (Carty and Rosenfeld, 1998). CAI continues to evolve into stand-alone education with such multi-hour continuing education programs as the *Pharmacokinetics Primer* for advanced practice nurses (Neafsey, 1997). With the continual refinement of computers and computer networks of today, the delivery of faculty and student education is moving to use of the Internet, a powerful worldwide "network of networks" connecting people globally using specific software protocols (Billings, 1996b). Additionally, the Internet provides several major services for communication, file transfer protocols, and worldwide access to vast sources of information (Plank, 1998; Sparks and Rizzolo, 1998). Moving forward, distance education continues to add and incorporate multimedia, including animations, graphics, print, audio, and video to the Internet technology (Ribbons, 1998).

As information continues to become an important resource, moving and accessing that information is becoming a fast-growing industry. Several university systems and state networks for distance education are now available in Colorado, Oregon, Iowa, Kentucky, and Wisconsin (National Center for Education Statistics, 1997). The Western Governors University is a "virtual university" sponsored by 15 states and one U.S. territory as well as consortia such as the Committee on Institutional Cooperation made up of 12 large universities. The Southern Regional Electronic Campus spans 15 states and includes 200 educational institutions (Neal, 1999). About a third of higher education institutions have distance education programs with another 25% planning to implement them. Internet courses can be presented in textbook-based formats to complex learning situation experiences. Use of the Internet for academic courses has exceeded more than 4 million users in a short period of time (Dawes, 1998).

Nursing Education at a Distance

Nursing education, especially for the Registered Nurse (RN), has a long history of using various modalities to deliver RN-BSN and graduate programs, as well as continuing nursing education (CNE). The use of distance education has been an effective way to increase RN retention at health care facilities, build professional commitment, and promote quality care, while the nurse stays in her community (Sherwood et al., 1994). Additionally, there tends to be a higher enrollment and completion rate of minority students in distance education programs, because after they have their basic nursing education, they do not leave the community to take further courses due to family and work demands (Shomaker and Fairbanks, 1997). A variety of instructional technologies including satellite, microwave, compressed video, videotapes, audiographics, video-teleconferencing, and now Internet technologies (Table 24.1) have all been used to deliver that education (Armstrong, 1984; Boyd and Baker, 1987;

Table 24.1   Types of Technologies That Can Be Used with Distance Education in the 21st Century

Audio conferencing: provides the two-way interaction support needed when one-way communication technology like videotapes or live satellite are used.

Audiographics: a computerized slow scan or compressed video system (Fig. 24.1) that provides real-time simultaneous voice and graphic interaction via phone lines (Frazier et al., 1998).

Bulletin board system (BBS): a multiaccessed communication system shared by all the users of a group. It often is used to post messages and provide information or for discussions about various topics.

CD-ROM: a round, metal-coated plastic disk used to store large volumes of digital data. Multimedia for distance education purposes is also being added.

Chat conferences: on-line discussions conducted in real time so that students can receive immediate feedback. Chats may be between faculty and students or between students and students (Milstead and Nelson, 1998).

E-mail: an effective computer-based method to store and forward messages, present stimulating questions to students, and attach files for interchange.

Fax: a low-cost approach using a telefacsimile machine to electronically reproduce visuals and text. The information is quickly transmitted or "faxed" over telephone lines.

Interactive television: faculty use an electronic podium to access sites via telephone, closed circuit, cable, satellite, fiber-optics, or microwave. It may be one- or two-way video and audio. Monitors display projected images to students at designated sites.

Internet: computer-based classes/courses/degree programs on-line, simultaneous conferences with faculty and students, and links to informative Web sites.

Microwave: a terrestrial point-to-point telecommunications system that requires line-of-sight transmission between sending and receiving antennas. It is capable of carrying various types of audio, video, and data signals and can be used in conjunction with copper, fiber-optics, and satellite to carry information.

Print material: a relatively inexpensive way to disseminate information that still yields effective learning outcomes. Additionally, hard copies from World Wide Web (WWW) sites are read.

Satellite: an orbiting communication system (22,000 miles in space) capable of transmitting and receiving a variety of video and audio signals from a single source. The signals are then retransmitted over a wide geographic area known as the satellite's footprint. It also may be used with other telecommunication technologies such as copper, fiber-optics, and microwave systems to carry the signals.

T1 line: leased terrestrial communication system commonly used to carry voice-grade digital or compressed video signals. TI circuits can consist of copper wire, fiber-optics, microwave, and/or satellite circuit segments to carry the signals.

Video, compressed: a digital compression technique used to remove redundant information from the video images, thus creating signals that require less bandwidth and also reduce transmission costs.

Video, desktop: through telephone lines, signals are transmitted by use of a small camera on top of the computer and a computer card. This enables people to capture and transmit a small, live image to a computer screen at another location, thus seeing each other while conducting classes. While the image currently is jerky, improvements are being made (Billings, 1996).

Video, live streaming: "moving" images sent in compressed form over the Internet. The video is usually sent from prerecorded video clips and then is transmitted as a continuous stream of images to the learners (Green, 1999).

Reproduced with permission, from *Journal of Continuing Education in Nursing*, vol 31, issue 2, p. 67. Slack, Incorporated.

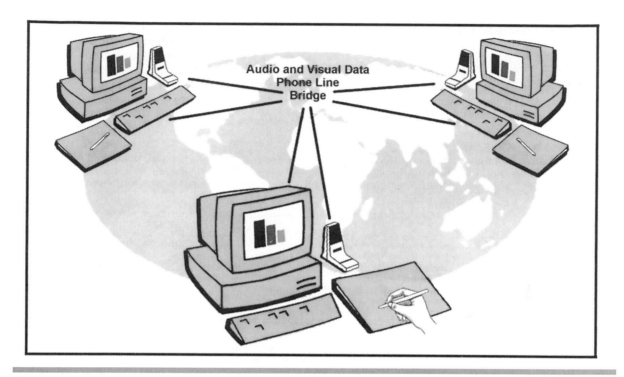

Figure 24.1
Audiographics interaction.
[Illustration by Anna Wittman-Meise, University of Wisconsin-Extension. (Used by permission from Armstrong, M.L. *Telecommunications of Health Professionals*, 1998. Springer-Verlag Publishing Company, Inc., New York 10012.)]

Carlton et al., 1998; Clark, 1993b; Cravener, 1999; Douglas and Fotos, 1989; Frazier et al, 1998; Hegge, 1993; Major and Shane, 1991; McGonigle and Mastrian, 1998; Reinert and Fryback, 1997; Shomaker and Fairbanks, 1997; Sherwood et al., 1994). A recent survey of nursing schools ($n = 358$) documents 38% with distance education programs; 41 more schools are planning for future extension programs (Reinert and Fryback, 1997).

Effectiveness of Distance Education

The effectiveness of distance education has been documented in numerous studies over the years both for general secondary and academic distance education and for nursing education (Armstrong, 1984; Armstrong et al., 1999, Boyd and Baker, 1987; Carlton et al., 1998; Clark, 1993b; Douglas and Fotos, 1989; Hegge, 1993; McGonigle and Mastrian, 1998; Reinert and Fryback, 1997; Sherwood et al., 1994; Shomaker and Fairbanks, 1997). Educational outcomes are similar for both the on and off campus students. Students usually drop out for personal and family

crises rather than the educational modality (Pym, 1992). Off-campus students, regardless of the delivery methods, receive the same grades or do better than those students receiving traditional instruction. Overall, student evaluations are good to very good following distance education activities. One factor commonly identified by students as a tremendous value in distance education is a collection of learners at a location that promotes the sharing of ideas, partners to debate the issues, and educational camaraderie (Shomaker and Fairbanks, 1997).

Nurses know that knowledge is power. Power to control their nursing practice and access to educational opportunities is a vital way to maintain their professional practice, to meet the challenges of health care changes, and to effectively participate in the health team (McGonigle and Mastrian, 1998; Bachman and Panzarine, 1998). Yet, the ability to "keep up" will be intensified as dollars for travel and conferences continue to disappear, while the demands of rotating shifts, marketing for future opportunities, and family commitments continue (Dawes, 1998; Carlton, 1997).

The Distance Education University of the 21st Century

Augmenting existing technological skills while pursuing new informational skills will help nurses remain competitive in the health care market. Thus, when nurses take on this life-long learning commitment, distance education should become a tremendous mechanism for nurses to become "adept users and information connoisseurs…discriminating users of the cyberspacial arena that spans the informational gambit from junkyard to gold mine" (McGonigle and Mastrian, 1998). The distance education university of the 21st century will incorporate some or all of the following multimedia (see Table 24.1) to offset the disadvantages and enhance the advantages of each medium (Billings, 1996a; Ribbons, 1998; Carlton et al., 1998).

Strategies and Support for the Learner at a Distance

Principles and Evaluation Criteria

Any quality education should be based on learning objectives and educational outcomes. Distance education courses and programs are no different (Massond, 1999). They need to adhere to the same national accreditation and educational standards of the originating school (Hanna et al., 1998; Milstead and Nelson, 1998). Students should seek information about the course design, expectations, and method of interaction between faculty and student and between students. A self-assessment quiz for aspiring distance education learners can be found *(http://www.wgu.edu/)* with accompanying rationale for the potential student's responses. It is important to determine if course credits can be transferred to other universities. Additionally, students should determine what arrangements are needed for technology trouble-shooting, registration, student services, literary sources, and textbook acquisition (Milstead and Nelson, 1998). Samples of criteria that the student (and faculty) can use for evaluating effective distance education programs are available from the Western Cooperative for Educational Telecommunications *(http://www.wiche.edu)*. To foster and support quality higher education programs, they have developed "Principles of Good Practice for Electronically Offered Academic Degree and Certificate Programs." The Southern Association of Colleges and Schools *(http://www.sacs.org/)* also has evaluation

criteria. Overall, these two organizations advocate the major components of instruction, institutional commitment, and evaluation as they relate to:

Instruction: Pacing and progression of content, effectiveness of materials, and development of methods to provide feedback, counseling, and evaluation. Formation of support and discussion groups.

Management: Organizational structure and support from the originating departments and the educational institution. Includes the telecommunications infrastructure, creation of internal policies, and any linkages with other educational institutions.

Logistics: Quality of programming, moving the course along with tests and readings. Overall helpfulness and instructional support including student services and literary sources (Armstrong and Mahan, 1998).

The Role of Faculty Will Change

While the course content will most likely remain the same as in the traditional classroom, providing education via distance will mean some methodological changes from the traditional classroom when delivering the educational materials. The Internet has been described as the "library card to the world" (Smith, 1997). Thus, the faculty role will change to more of a facilitator of learning rather than an imparter of all the information (Bachman and Panzarine, 1998; Billings, 1997; Scott and Armstrong, 1998). With information so accessible, the emphasis will go beyond just locating the information to a role of filtering the information. In order to help the student, "the faculty's role will be to teach the student how to swim because they will be drowning in data" (Dede, 1990; Scott and Armstrong, 1998). This major change in faculty role will also impact the student-faculty and student-student interaction. Additionally, not only will the virtual classrooms incorporate faculty, but the student will interact with many other sources including the local site coordinator(s), community experts, colleagues, course instructional materials, and national and international information from the World Wide Web (WWW) (Scott and Armstrong, 1998). Other student adaptation will involve clinical coordination, technological flexibility, and the development of self-directed learning skills.

Importance of Communication and Flexibility

Internet education may be partially or fully text-based, so the ability to carry on a dialogue/discussion/interchange, whether in a synchronous or asynchronous mode, is vital to the connectivity of the student's experiences with the faculty and fellow students. Strategically placed questions in the text will be helpful in extracting major concepts; computer-based conferencing tools such as chat sessions and/or bulletin boards can provide further opportunity to explore important concepts with synchronous or asynchronous feedback (Milstead and Nelson, 1998; Carlton et al., 1998). The knowledge and the willingness to learn how to use the equipment for communication, the accessibility of the equipment, and the required computer capabilities as well as the commitment to be an active participate in the interchange format will be valuable tools for student success (Plank, 1998; Sparks and Rizzolo, 1998). Otherwise, the education experience reverts to passive learning, similar to the old correspondence course model (Sherry, 1996).

An additional word here about too much text within Internet courses. Reading off the computer screen is difficult, takes more time than reading hard copy, and can be expensive if the student has to use long distance services to access the Internet. Additionally, the student in general spends a great deal of time printing hard copies of the information. This is another reason why synchronous chat and bulletin board exchanges are important. To avoid another form of a correspondence course with a bit of electronic sophistication, mixing mediums takes advantage of the visual, interactive, and electronic components of distance education, as proposed by one leader in this field, Ball State University (Carlton et al., 1998).

Both faculty and students will spend more time writing, actively promoting learning, and building knowledge by interaction (Cravener, 1999). Interestingly, developers of computer-based courses describe the increased amount of communication as richer in depth and content as well as exciting because it seems to better meet the needs of all the learners on-line (Carlton et al., 1998; Achterberg, 1996). This results from using computerized communication tools; they become "an equalizer because the message is sent with no signs of race, gender, physical appearance, shyness, or external socioeconomic and status cues, which may be especially attractive to students not comfortable in the traditional classroom" (Achterberg, 1996; Craig, 1994). Messages are also documented, so a running tabulation of responses can be recorded. Since writing is often improved with further writing, the interaction becomes an excellent method to encourage "an organized and fluent thought pattern, an application of learning, and an analysis of relationships" (Larson and Dunkin, 1997). This in turn assists both the faculty and student's evaluation of the learning process. Peer critique may also be part of the course interaction, leading to further

collegiality, networking, and perhaps even mentoring (Billings, 1996b; Larson and Dunkin, 1997).

Expected but frustrating obstacles will develop when working with any type of technology, especially at the initiation of the course (Milstead and Nelson, 1998; Todd, 1998). Flexibility is the watchword as both faculty and students experience problems with the lack of reliable access to Internet-connected hardware, difficult interfaces, and unresponsive technical support during the course (Achterberg, 1996; Bachman and Panzarine, 1998; Billings, 1996b; Craig, 1994; Cravener, 1999).

Incorporating Clinical Experiences

Clinical work can be supported by the use of faculty-appointable nurses (perhaps called site coordinators), who can facilitate learning in the local area or region (Major and Shane, 1991; Armstrong and Sherwood, 1994). These coordinators are an extension of the faculty. With regularly scheduled face-to-face contacts and discussion about clinical facilities with the site coordinator, RN students can design and implement their own learning activities based on the educational objectives of the course. These coordinators often act as the "eyes and ears" of the faculty, stimulating interaction when students are hesitant to ask or participate in discussion. They also are motivators to assist students as they progress through their educational program (Armstrong and Sherwood, 1994).

Student Development of Self-Directed Learning Skills

Computer-based course authors agree that successful distance education students become "more assertive, independent, and organized than in a traditional classroom setting" (Milstead and Nelson, 1998; Cravener, 1999; Achterberg, 1996; Craig, 1994). RN students in Craig's study (1994) cite the ability to "time-shift," or study when able to, as an important advantage to developing this independence as well as an increasing proficiency with computers. Thus, support is provided for the development of self-directed learning skills such as active listening, working independently in the absence of a live instructor, and time skill management. Students inquiring about new learning experiences and possessing diligence and a positive attitude will be supported (Billings, 1997).

Faculty Support for Course Development

When designing and implementing Internet courses, faculty commitment to change is also important, since there is a redistribution of responsibilities. Educational changes for faculty will evolve around course instruction delivery, on-line course management and logistics, and faculty workload, especially as faculty rethink their classroom habits and practices that have been taken for granted (Billings, 1996a; Cravener, 1999; Achterberg, 1996). For example, what kind of interaction can be planned with students when there are no face-to-face classroom entry and exit rituals nor the usual verbal or nonverbal clues such as intonation of audio presentation when teaching (Clark, 1993a)? Considerable thought must be given to the communication process in distance education as the "communication is judged by the words on the computer screen and the ideas expressed" (Milstead and Nelson, 1998). Recommendations to liven up the discussions and reduce the stiffness of entirely word-based material include using words (chuckle, chuckle), "emoticons" or Internet shorthand that helps the user express feelings (such as smiley faces [☺] or [:-)), and colloquialisms ("Go for it, keep cooking") (Bachman and Panzarine, 1998).

Effective Course Planning

Educational support personnel are essential to help faculty pull together courses for distance education. These experts include instructional designers and technical partners associated with the computing telecommunications systems. They will provide great assistance to altering teaching methods and modifying instructional materials (Billings, 1997). Their expert services are vital, so that nursing faculty have the time for additional preparation as the content specialist and planners of creative, interactive student experiences (Carlton et al., 1998; Scott and Armstrong, 1998).

Distance education courses need to be tightly organized (Massoud, 1999; Reinert and Fryback, 1997). "Last-minute" preparations are not easily accomplished and improvisation can be difficult (Cravener, 1999). Faculty should consider definite timetables, so that there is adequate time to grade and give feedback for improvement of writing assignments (Billings, 1996b). To cope with possible problems with the technology, faculty should plan how additional time will be allowed or should have a practice of accepting "late" papers and written work. The creation of either video or written user tutorials or specific Web pages dedicated to quick reference topics might overcome initial student unfamiliarity with such topics as the use of E-mail, network software, and file transfer (Milstead and Nelson, 1998; Ribbons, 1998; Cravener, 1999; Carl-

ton, 1995; Gravely and Fullerton, 1998). Depending on the number of students, designated coaching time from the technology team for individual learners on the system might be extremely valuable and proactive (Craig, 1994).

Teaching strategies that encourage active involvement and critical thinking with the course content are very important (Billings, 1996b; Carlton et al., 1998; Todd, 1998). The design and format of the education must foster relationships among the distance learners, providing the support and direction to enable them to make the transition from the traditional classroom to self-directed learning. Students seem to pass through a series of steps toward self-directed learning, almost like experiencing a sense of loss. Using Kubler-Ross's patterns of grieving (denial, anger, bargaining, depression, and acceptance), Cravener (1997) cites examples of students' grief as they move toward the resolution of a new learning role.

Milstead and Nelson (1998) describe student concerns when quick responses are needed during real-time chat conferences and faculty want to review student spelling and grammatical errors. These authors agreed that chats were for content and feelings and not for monitoring English, especially during the initial courses. Using bulletin boards can allow the student time to formulate thoughtful responses with the ability to check spelling, and the student will not feel so rushed to "chat." This may be a more comfortable way to start students out with discussion groups then moving them rapidly to chat conferences. Additionally, chat conferences may be student-led or only between students to bolster collegial interaction (Craig, 1994). Students can also be broken into groups within the chat room format and have a small group discussion before reassembling as a larger group and having a "spokesperson" report. Such formats for chat sessions will also help students overcome the "obstacles of isolation, intimidation, and insecurity, factors which in the past have been associated with distance education" (Larson and Dunkin, 1997). Use of case studies and clinical examples relevant to the target audience and personalizing the instruction are helpful. Effective distance education faculty need to be "enthusiastic about networking with and among the distance students to build a feeling of connectedness, safeness, respect, and community" (Billings, 1996b). Collegial student interaction can be encouraged by class rosters, student pictures, simple Web page development, and group assignments or dialogue. Interaction can be promoted by forming group activities in the same region of the course delivery. Evaluation of coursework will require the discussion and development of steps for test security and timely feedback.

An increase in faculty workload can be expected. At least one year of preliminary course planning is important to alter teaching methods and modify instructional materials (Milstead and Nelson, 1998). Proactive faculty development and ongoing institutional support can smooth out some of the frustrations. The Apple Classrooms of Tomorrow (Sherry, 1996) describe their perceptions of faculty response to distance education:

It may take at least two years to change [the] focus from being anxious about themselves and equipment malfunctions, ... to anticipating problems and developing alternate strategies, exploring software more aggressively, sharing ideas more freely, increasing student motivation and interest, and using technology to their advantage. Educational change takes time, a great deal of support, peer networking, and guidance. In general, teachers tend to focus on the increased workload and drawbacks associated with an innovation before the benefits of change emerge and the innovation takes hold.

Trying to get the on-line course to the desired level of efficacy will also take a good portion of time (Billings, 1996a; Achterberg, 1996; Clark, 1998). Boston (1992) believes at least three semesters are needed. Achterberg (1996) describes tripling the time (when comparing a traditional classroom setting) to implement an E-mail course, yet upon completing the course, she was ready to design more distance education because of the satisfaction of reaching so many students and stimulating a more "learner-centered system". Billings (1997) and Carlton et al. (1998) describe similar responses. Regardless of the time commitment, "adequate operational and administrative infrastructure to support the distance education teaching endeavors" is vital (Clark, 1993a; Bachman and Panzarine, 1998).

 ## Legal, Ethical, and Public Policy Issues

Legal, Ethical, and Copyright Concerns

The faculty are accountable for any kind of educational endeavor, including that for distance learning (Menix, 1998). Legal concerns relate to established laws associated with telecommunication technologies, whereas the ethical concerns relate to the rights and wrongs stemming from the values and beliefs of the various users of the distance education systems. Three major areas that are of concern regarding legal issues include copyright protection, interstate commerce, and intellectual property. Additionally, there are cyberethical issues such as "privacy, confidentiality, censorship, freedom of speech, and an ever-increasing concern for control of personal information" (Bachman and Panzarine, 1998).

The ongoing dilemma with copyright issues is the assurance of publisher protection if books and journals are used, the media interests, and the access of information. The media interests include the use of various information media (whether as images, text, or audio). "Any change of existing media may require appropriate copyright clearance or licensing arrangements" (Ribbons, 1998). While no new federal mandates except the Copyright Act of 1976 exist to address multimedia educational concerns, the Consortium of College and University Media Centers has published the *Fair Use Guidelines for Educational Multimedia* (Dalziel, 1996). Educational institution guidelines for distance education programs regarding copyright protection should also be written; currently, most of these educational perspectives seem to align with the traditional classroom setting (Menix, 1998).

With more Web-based courses, students need to examine their state's regulation for recognition of out-of-state academic and certificate programs. The lack of "established laws and legal precedence compel educational entities to collaborate and negotiate programs and courses" (Menix, 1998). Perhaps, with the further development of university consortia and multi-institutional agreements, this concern will be resolved.

Intellectual property should be explored from two perspectives: faculty ownership of distance education products and the need to obtain permission for the various pieces of intellectual property of others (Billings, 1996b). Faculty own the materials they have developed for use in their distance education programs, but it is always good to have a memo of understanding documenting the specific use of the materials as well as the accrued benefits (Billings, 1996b). For any type of written and nonprint materials, permission should always be obtained from the copyright holders, followed by the appropriate recognition of their work (Menix, 1998). The Copyright Management Center at Indiana University Purdue University at Indianapolis *(http://www.iupui.edu/it/copyinfo/home.html)* is a good source of further information (Billings, 1996b).

As course designers become more creative and flexible with distance education, the ethical and legal issues will continue. Specific regulatory boards of nursing are trying to adapt quickly to the changing environment of nursing education. The key is to write understandings of mutual agreement to avoid potential conflicts. For example, student privacy and confidentiality are vital. Universities with distance education programs should have students sign releases for the recording of their images. If student assignments are used for anything other than faculty-student interaction, permission should also be obtained. Also, links to Web-based sites to purchase books should be reviewed by the university because it can detract business away from locally owned bookstores.

Proactively, the distance educator should stay current with the law, seek guidance from knowledgeable resources when no legal precedence exists, assist with the development of institutional policies, document appropriately, and prevent problems by providing consistent student feedback with respect and dignity. The essence seems to be effective planning, coordination, and evaluation of established policies and then proper adherence to those policies.

Public Policy Concerns

The examination and viability of public policy with distance education lie primarily in the infrastructure problems of accessibility. According to Cotton (1998), "the most frustrating obstacle to the rapid deployment of new technology has been the lack of sophisticated telecommunications network infrastructure in most of rural American and in some urban areas," primarily in the cost-effectiveness of distance education and telephone networks. The person who often needs the distance education the most does not have access to the necessary sophisticated equipment to obtain the education and services. While the heightened competitive environment usually produces some legislative and regulatory changes, the push is often in the large urban markets, not necessarily for the good of universal accessibility. The other public policy issue is helping the public and the nursing profession to understand technology options are available as tools, to teach, to cure, and to communicate. "The public's [and the profession's] understanding of those emerging options lags far behind the technology itself" (Cotton, 1998).

 Associated Research for Distance Education

Most of the research associated with distance education in the past has focused on effectiveness of the instruction. Now, a more holistic evaluation of student issues is being sought. Issues include professional socialization, faculty and student interaction, and gender and environment issues.

Professional Socialization

As nursing students advance to higher levels of academic education, professional socialization or the identity of those expectations is part of role development. Students comment that after completion of their academic program they think differently. Yet, can that be accomplished when there is no face-to-face contact with faculty for role modeling and mentoring (Milstead and Nelson, 1998)? Reinert and Fryback, (1997) suggest that "sensitive indicators must be developed to determine when, how, and what socialization has occurred."

Faculty and Student Interaction

How much interaction is important during distance education, both between student and faculty and between student and student (Abrahamson, 1998)? With interactive video, Threlkeld and Brzoska (1994) report differing needs for interaction, depending on the age of students. They have found that adults tend to value the logistical elements of learning (rapid test return, feedback on writing assignments, etc.) more importantly than discussing the issues, whereas high school students report greater emphasis on course design and interaction. Further research is needed, since data from interactive video instruction may provide different findings than Internet courses. Additionally, as interaction is planned for distance education, what types of questions enhance critical thinking, what type of feedback is most beneficial, and at what time in the instruction is questioning most important (Gravely and Fullerton, 1998)?

Gender and Environment Issues

Even further, with the large numbers of women in nursing using distance education for academic and continuing education, is gender a variable (Craig, 1994; Green, 1987; Koch, 1998; Pym, 1992)? Nurses expect support from family, friends, employers, and co-workers when they return to school, yet this may or may not be the case. According to Koch (1998), "some faculty claim that women and men behave and learn differently with distance education, in course satisfaction, academic performance, and retention." Few studies have examined this notion, and further research is warranted, especially with the technology-filled Internet courses, where there is very limited or no campus or face-to-face contact with faculty and fellow students. Also, are there differences between RN students from rural areas and RN students from urban areas? Any gender differences should also be explored (Barker, 1985).

Can Everyone Be a Distance Learner?

Lastly, distance education is not for everyone (Pym, 1992; Billings, 1996b). Not all learners will be comfortable receiving education at a distance due to feelings of isolation or alienation as well as a reluctance to assume self-directed learning skills (Dawes, 1998; Craig, 1994). The creation and analysis of an assessment instrument to "screen out" high-risk students considering distance education is vital (Neal, 1999; Achterberg, 1996). While the retention rates associated with distance education are low (Pym, 1992), an ability to counsel students with multiple role demands seeking computer-based education opportunities would be extremely helpful in supporting academically successful students. Additionally, some faculty issues for research in this area include the identification of essential ingredients for successful distance education, methods to assist faculty in overcoming resistance to the various technologies, and determination of what types of specific course can or cannot be delivered via distance education (Scott and Armstrong, 1998). Further examination of those concerns will be beneficial for better implementation of distance education.

 ## Summary

Life-long learning to enhance professional competence is important for every nurse. Distance education has great potential to provide a wider variety of academic programs and continuing education courses by maximizing access to information and qualified instructors, freeing the learner from the structure of traditional classroom hours, offering the convenience of being able to learn when and where the student wants to learn, and offering the tremendous opportunity to develop self-directed learning skills. This certainly is a rich resource for progressive use of available and future computer technologies.

 ## References

Abrahamson, C. E. (1998). Issues in interactive communication in distance education. *College Student Journal, 32*(1), 33–42.

Achterberg, C. (1996). Tips for teaching a course by e-mail. *Journal of Nutrition Education, 28*(6), 303–307.

Armstrong, M. L. (1984). Video in the classroom: Use it like a telephone rather than television. *Journal of Continuing Education in Nursing, 15*(1), 13–15.

Armstrong, M. L., Gessner, B. A., and Kane, J. (1999). Does RN-BSN education foster professional reading? *Journal of Professional Nursing, 15*(4), 238–244.

Armstrong, M. L., and Mahan, K. (1998). Distance education: What was, what's here, and preparation for the future. In M. L. Armstrong (Ed.), *Telecommunications for Health Professionals: Providing Successful Distance Education and Telehealth* (pp. 23–41). New York: Springer.

Armstrong, M. L., and Sherwood, G. D. (1994). Site coordinators: A critical component in providing quality nursing education at distance sites. *Journal of Nursing Education, 33*, 175–177.

Bachman, J. A., and Panzarine, S. (1998). Enabling student nurses to use the information superhighway. *Journal of Nursing Education, 37*(4), 155–161.

Barker, B. O. (1985). Understanding rural adult learners: Characteristics and challenges. *Lifelong Learning, 9*(2), 4–7.

Billings, D. M. (1996a). Distance education in nursing. *Computers in Nursing, 14*(4), 211–212.

Billings, D. M. (1996b). Distance education in nursing: Adapting courses for distance education. *Computers in Nursing, 14*(5), 262, 263, 266.

Billings, D. M. (1997). Issues in teaching and learning at a distance: Changing roles and responsibilities of administrators, faculty, and students. *Computers in Nursing, 15*(2), 69–70.

Boston, R. L. (1992). Remote delivery of instruction via the PC and modem: What have we learned? *American Journal of Distance Education, 6*(3), 45–47.

Boyd, N. J., and Baker, C. M. (1987). Using television to teach. *Nursing & Health Care, 8*, 523–527.

Carlton, K. H. (1995). Establishing technological health care resources links with the distant learner. *Computers in Nursing, 13*(5), 206, 209–211.

Carlton, K. H. (1997). Refining continuing education delivery. *Computers in Nursing, 15*(1), 17–18, 22.

Carlton, K. H., Ryan, M. E., and Siktberg, L. L. (1998). Designing courses for the Internet: A conceptual approach. *Nurse Educator, 23*(3), 45–50.

Carty, B., and Rosenfeld, P. (1998). From computer technology to information technology: Findings from a national study on nursing education. *Computers in Nursing, 16*(5), 259–265.

Clark, C. (1993a). Teaching and learning at a distance. In D. M. Billings and J. A. Halstead, (Eds.). *Teaching in Nursing: A Guide for Faculty* (pp 331–346). Philadelphia: W. B. Saunders.

Clark, C. (1993b). Beam me up, nurse! Educational technology supports distance education. *Nurse Educator, 18*(2), 18–22.

Clark, D. (1998). Course redesign: Incorporating an Internet web site into an existing nursing class. *Computers in Nursing, 16*(4), 219–222

Cotton, S. (1998). Public Policy Issues: Achieving Public Access to Technology at Reasonable Cost. In M. L. Armstrong (Ed.), *Telecommunications for Health Professionals: Providing Successful Distance Education and Telehealth* (pp 264–282). New York: Springer.

Craig, C. E. (1994). Distance learning through computer conferences. *Nurse Educator, 19*(2), 10–14.

Cravener, P. A. (1997). Promoting active learning in large lecture classes. *Nurse Educator, 22*(3), 21–26.

Cravener, P. A. (1999). Faculty experiences with providing online courses. *Computers in Nursing, 17*(1), 42–47.

Dalziel, C. (1996). Fair Use Guidelines for Educational Multimedia. *http://www. libraries, psu.edu/mtss.fairuse/dalziel.html*

Dawes, B. S. (1998). Can distance learning provide a twenty-first century hallmark? *AORN Journal, 68*(2), 170, 172, 174.

Dede, C. J. (1990). The evolution of distance learning: Technology-mediated interactive learning. *Journal of Research in Computing in Education, 22*(3), 247–264.

Douglas, B. H., and Fotos, J. C. (1989). BSN courses for students via satellite. *Journal of Nursing Education, 28*, 428–430.

Frazier, S., Gessner, B. A., and Monson, M. (1998). Working with audiographics. In M. L. Armstrong (Ed.), *Telecommunications for Health Professionals: Providing Successful Distance Education and Telehealth* (pp. 107–125). New York: Springer.

Graveley, E., and Fullerton, J. T. (1998). Incorporating electronic-based and computer-based strategies: Graduate nursing courses in administration. *Journal of Nursing Education, 37*(4), 186–188.

Green, C. P. (1987). Multiple role women: The real world of the mature RN learners. *The Journal of Nursing Education, 26*(7), 266–271.

Green, M. (1999). Streaming Video and Streaming Media. *http://www.whatis.com/streamvd.html.*

Hanna, K. P., Wolford, N. R., and James S. G. (1998). Distance education and accreditation. *AANA, 66*(2), 113–116.

Hegge, M. (1993). Interactive television, presentation style, and teaching materials. *Journal of Continuing Education in Nursing, 24*, 39–42.

Koch, J. V. (1998). How women actually perform in distance education. *Chronical of Higher Education*, A60.

Larson, O. M., and Dunkin, J. W. (1997). Writing in the interactive classroom. *Journal of Nursing Education, 36*(6), 298–301.

Major, M. B., and Shane, D. L. (1991). Use of interactive television for outreach nursing. *The American Journal of Distance Education, 5*(1), 57–66.

Massoud, L. (1999). *So You Want to Be a Distance Learning Instructor.* Flint, MI: Mott Community College.

McGonigle, D., and Mastrian, K. (1998). Learning along the way: Cyberspacial quests. *Nursing Outlook, 46*, 81–86.

Menix, K. D. (1998). Ethics and legal perspectives in distance education and telehealth. In M. L. Armstrong (Ed.), *Telecommunications for Health Professionals: Providing Successful Distance Education and Telehealth* (pp. 245–263). New York: Springer.

Milstead, J. A., and Nelson, R. (1998). Preparation for an online asynchronous university doctoral course: Lessons learned. *Computers in Nursing, 16*(5), 247–258.

National Center for Education Statistics. (1997). Distance Education in Higher Education Institutions: Incidence, Audiences, and plans to Expand. *http://nces.ed.glv/pubs98132.html*

Neafsey, P. J. (1997). Computer-assisted instruction for home study: A new venture for continuing education programs in nursing. *Journal of Continuing Education in Nursing, 28*(4), 164–172.

Neal, E. (1999). Distance education: Prospects and problems. *Phi Kappa Phi Journal, 79*(1), 40–43.

Plank, R. K. (1998). Nursing on-line for continuing education credit. *Journal of Continuing Education in Nursing, 29*(4), 165–172.

Pym, F. R. (1992). Women and distance education: A nursing perspective. *Journal of Advanced Nursing, 17*, 383–389.

Reinert, B. R., and Fryback, P.B. (1997). Distance learning and nursing education. *Journal of Nursing Education, 36*(9), 421–427.

Ribbons, R. M. (1998). Guidelines for developing interactive multimedia: Applications in nurse education. *Computers in Nursing, 16*(2), 109–114.

Schlosser, C. A., and Anderson, M. L. (1994). *Distance Education: Review of the Literature.* Washington D.C.: Association for Educational Communications & Technology.

Scott, D., and Armstrong, M. L. (1998). Faculty development: A cornerstone of distance education. In M. L. Armstrong (Ed.), *Telecommunications for Health Professionals: Providing Successful Distance Education and Telehealth* (pp. 142–159). New York: Springer.

Sherry, L. (1996). Issues in Distance Learning. *http//:www.cudenver.edu/~lsherry/pubs/issues.html.*

Sherwood, G. D., Armstrong, M. L., and Bond, M. L. (1994). Distance education programs: Defining issues of assessment, accessibility, and accommodation. *Journal of Continuing Education in Nursing, 25*(6), 251–257.

Shomaker, D., and Fairbanks, J. (1997). Evaluation of a RN-to-BSN distance education program via satellite for nurses in rural health care. *Journal of Nursing Education, 36*(7), 328–330.

Smith, R. P. (1997). The Internet for continuing education. *MD Computing, 14* 414–416.

Sparks, S. M., and Rizzolo, M. A. (1998). World Wide Web search tools. *Image: Journal of Nursing Scholarship, 30*(2), 167–171.

Threlkeld, R., and Brzoska, K. (1994). Research in distance education. In B. Willis (Ed.). *Distance Education: Strategies and Tools* (pp 41–66). Englewood Cliffs, NJ: Educational Technology Publications.

Todd, N. A. (1998). Using E-mail in an undergraduate nursing course to increase critical thinking skills. *Computers in Nursing, 16*(2), 115–118.

Zetzman, M. R. (1995). Telemedicine, POTS, and PANS technology, and rural health care in Texas. *Texas Journal of Rural Health, XIV*, 1–4.

25 Innovations in Telehealth

Diane J. Skiba
Amy J. Barton

OBJECTIVES

1. Explore how telehealth innovations will transform health care, education, and research.
2. Examine the challenges and issues of these transformations.

KEY WORDS

information systems
telemedicine
telehealth
telephone consultation
Internet

"As we approach the new millennium, it is clear that that "information infrastructure"—the interconnected networks of computers, devices and software—may have a greater impact on worldwide social and economic structures than all networks that have preceded them" (President's Information Technology Advisory Committee, 1999).

Scientific advances in computing and communications technologies are transforming the way we live, work, and interact with each other. These technologies have transformed and will continue to transform the delivery of health care and learning in our society. These transformations will affect the practice of both health care and education. Telehealth applications will become commonplace and individuals will be able to participate in learning opportunities regardless of geographic location, age, physical limitation or personal schedule (President's Information Technology Advisory Committee, 1999). In the mid-1990s, Kassirer (1995) predicted that the rapid growth of computer-based electronic communication coupled with patient empowerment and patient comfort with the electronic retrieval of information would have a profound influence on the delivery of health care. He believed that the extension of telecommunications, particularly to rural areas in various forms would make "telemedicine" accessible to almost everyone. He stated that technology has already triggered widespread social transformations and would ultimately transform the delivery of health care.

This chapter explores the transformations in health care and education within the context of advances in computing and communications technologies. The goals of this chapter are twofold: to explore how telehealth innovations will transform health care, education, and research and to present the challenges and issues as a result of these potential transformations. The chapter covers such topics as the concept of telehealth; the progression of telehealth applications; future innovations in advanced practice, education, and research; and the challenges and issues as a consequence of these transformations.

The Concept of Telehealth

Providing health care and education at a distance is not a new phenomenon. Distance education, the provision of learning opportunities at a distance, can be traced to the 19th century soon after the introduction of the postal service (Phipps and Merisotis, 1999) Correspondence courses were commonplace. This trend continued into the 20th century with the arrival of new media such as radio and television. Similarly, telemedicine efforts can be traced to the late 1950s (Grisby and Sanders, 1998) with initial efforts focused on providing health care consultation to rural or remote environments (Bloch, 1999).

In order to understand the concept of telehealth, it is important to first define the term "telecommunications." According to the Institute of Medicine (IOM)

(1996), "it is the use of wire, radio, optical or other electromagnetic channels to transmit and receive signals for voice, data and video communications." In the world of telecommunications, the media are telephone, video, and computer systems, and the methods of transmissions are phone lines, fiber-optics, satellites, and microwave systems (Witherspoon et al., 1994).

The Institute of Medicine (1996) broadly defined telemedicine "as the use of electronic information and communication technologies to provide and support health care when distance separates the participants." Telemedicine has a variety of applications, some of which are often not thought of as telemedicine, since they are so commonplace. One such example is emergency calls to 911 that make use of "plain old telephone" technology (Institute of Medicine, 1996). Telephone triage, such as services like Ask a Nurse™, are also another example that is often overlooked. More recent applications include remote telesurgery. Almost every specialty in medicine has some form of a telemedicine application (Grisby and Sanders, 1998).

In nursing, the American Nurses Association (ANA) (1997) wanted a more inclusive term and proceeded to define telehealth as "delivery of health care services or activities with time and distance barriers removed and using technologies such as telephones, computers, or interactive video transmissions." This organization considers telehealth as an umbrella term that encompasses telemedicine, telenursing, teleradiology, and telepsychiatry. Accordingly, telenursing is considered a form of telehealth where nursing practice is delivered via telecommunications. Perhaps the broadest definition is provided in *Mosby's Medical and Nursing Dictionary* (1998). Telehealth is defined as:

> "use of telecommunication technologies to provide health care services and access to medical and surgical information for training and educating health care professionals and consumers, to increase awareness and educate the public about health related issues and to facilitate medical research across distances" (Mosby, 1998).

A similar definition is provided by Bloch (1999), "telehealth is a broad term that can refer to educating health professionals and consumers, disseminating information on public health, performing research, and administering health services." Thus, using the broadest definition of telehealth as a foundation, this chapter will explore the past, present, and future innovations as they apply to health care delivery, education, and research.

Progression of Telehealth Applications

For the last century, telehealth applications have evolved from simple communications to sophisticated two-way video transmissions. Trends in telehealth applications can be grouped according to the various media: voice, data, and video. Voice applications remain a mainstay of telehealth applications, since the telephone offers many advantages. According to Witherspoon et al. (1994), the telephone has the following advantages: relatively low cost for installation, low cost per use, minimal training for use, and ubiquity. Universal phone service was established as a public policy goal in the 1930s. Telephone service can be enhanced to provide the following: conferencing, voice mail, facsimiles, computer communications, and videophones.

Voice communications applications will continue to have a major impact on telehealth applications. Many are projecting that telephone-based health management will flourish in the age of managed care (Malloy, 1998). According to Bleich (1998), care delivery networks view telephone-based health management as a pivotal service strategy. Any health care plan interested in demand or disease management quickly realizes the potential of telephonic care.

Kinsella (1998) classifies telephone care in the following categories: "keeping in touch" calls, initiated calls, by either the patient or the nurse, computer-generated single purpose calls, or computer generated interactive calls. Her report claims that telephone care will be a mainstay in the next century. Her continuum of care ranges from simple telephone calls to talk with patients to computer-generated interactions using sophisticated decision support tools. An example of keeping in touch applications is the work by Shu et al. (1996), who initiated a "telephone reassurance program" with their Visiting Nurse Association (VNA) clients in Connecticut. Another example is the ParentLine Program (Moore and Krowchuk, 1997), where nurses initiated weekly telephone calls and provided a telephone hotline for new parents.

Two examples of interactive systems include Home Talk and the REACH project in Massachusetts. The first, HomeTalk, is an example of a demand management project in which clients in the community can complete preventive assessment screening provided by the Cleveland VNA through the telephone. Telephone screenings are available for elderly clients and families with children. The technology enabled the nurses to assess an additional 341 clients and to provide additional services to 1,000 clients in six different centers (Niles et al., 1997). The work by Mahoney et al. (1998) exemplifies the computer-generated interactions. This project, called REACH (Resources for Enhancing Alzheimer's Caregiver Health) for TLC (telephone-linked care), uses a telephone network system coupled with an interactive voice response computer network to support the caregiver. The caregiver can enter the password-protected system and interact with various modules, each designed to alleviate stress and provide support. One module engages the caregiver in a simple nondemanding conversation to distract him or her from the current situation. This module provides a respite conversation from the stresses of caring for an Alzheimer's patient. Without a doubt, the sophistication of the computer-generated interactions will increase as telecommunications technologies improve.

Data communications is the area where there is the largest projected growth in the next century. Numerous statistics are available to document the rapid and continuing growth of the Internet and usage of the World Wide Web by various users to access health care information. Here are just some examples of various statistics being reported on Web usage. Recent surveys indicate that 40–45 million Americans use the Internet, with 51 percent of those users earning an income under $50,000 (Baruch College-Harris Poll, 1998). Ferguson (1998) reported that 43 percent of the estimated 40.6 American users in 1997 accessed the Web to obtain health care information. Osheroff (1997) reported that the federal government-sponsored health care Web site had 4.8 million hits during its first month of operation. Additional information documents that the fastest growing segment of the population to use the Internet is adults aged 55 to 70. Another staggering statistic reported by Lindberg and Humphreys (1998) is that the number of on-line MEDLINE searches of medical literature has grown 10-fold (75 million searches annually) since this became freely accessible on the Web. Without a doubt, the Internet and its accompanying data communications applications will transform the way health care is delivered in the new millennium.

Data communications applications can be classified according to whether the application was developed by the consumer or by health care professionals. These applications have evolved from simple electronic bulletin board systems running on the FidoNet network (Sparks, 1992) to more elaborate multimedia systems designed to provide patient care in the home. Applications designed by clients are continually growing on the Internet. Historically, the first applications designed by consumers were the early electronic support groups developed for electronic bulletin board systems. For almost any diagnosis, there was an electronic support group that consumers could access. As an outgrowth of these electronic support groups, community computing systems were established in many communities across the United States. These networks allowed communities to design computer networks to support their needs, including health care information. The first community network was the Cleveland Free Net that was used as a basis for the pioneering work done by Brennan et al. (1991a). Again electronic support groups and health information dissemination were integral components of the health care sections of community networks (Skiba and Mirque, 1994). Both consumers and health care professionals designed many community networks. With the introduction of the World Wide Web (WWW), electronic support groups have expanded to another level as an information resource about a particular diagnosis. For example, the Colorado HealthNet (CHN) was founded by a consumer who wanted to share health care information about chronic diseases with consumers. Accordingly, CHN is a Colorado nonprofit corporation formed in 1995 to provide electronic access to factual and statistical information, support services, medical resources, and related health care information for persons with chronic medical conditions and for other users (*http://www.coloradohealthnet.org/*).

In addition, consumers were given access to electronic mail (E-mail), and there is a demand for increased use of E-mail as a means of communication between patients and providers. Consumers have increased the demand for E-mail access to their health care providers (Fridsma et al. 1994; Kane and Sands, 1998; Spielberg, 1998). Healtheon (1999) in their annual surveys of physicians found a 300 percent increase in the use of E-mail over the last 2 years. There have been several studies about the usage of E-mail with patients (Widman and Tong, 1997; Borowitz and Wyatt, 1998; Diepgen and Eysenbach, 1998). There are also excellent articles on the legal and ethical issues related to E-mail (Spielberg, 1998) and guidelines for the use of electronic mail with patients published by the American Association of Medical Informatics (Kane and Sands, 1998). Recent articles also focus on a research agenda for patient-provider communication (Mandl et al., 1998) and the evaluation of the efficacy of electronic communication with patients (Balas et al., 1997).

Health care professionals and health care institutions have been actively creating applications for the Internet. These applications have been focused on either information dissemination for patients or the direct delivery of health care for patients using Web-based applications. Perhaps one of the first sites to establish a patient care focus with extensive information dissemination was the University of Iowa Virtual Hospital. This Web site set the stage for patient education materials with the development of the Iowa Health Book and all the various on-line resources available to their patients *(http://www.vh.org/)*. This Web site served as a catalyst for the numerous institutions to create Web-based information sites for patients. The federal government has been active in creating a Web site called HealthFinder specifically targeted to consumers *(http://www.healthfinder.org/default.htm)*. This Web site contains numerous links to information across the entire spectrum of health care. Another site that is directed towards both consumers and professionals is Oncolink. This peer-reviewed site contains oncology information resources *(http://oncolink.upenn.edu/)*.

Health care professionals have also designed applications to deliver patient care. Brennan et al. (1991a, 1991b) conducted pioneering work on the use of computer-mediated systems to provide health care for persons living with AIDS and caretakers of Alzheimer's disease patients. In both instances, Brennan and colleagues used a community computing network, ComputerLink, to provide support services (contact with a nurse, informational resources, electronic support groups, and access to a decision-making tool) into the homes of patients and their caretakers. Results of these experiments (Brennan and Ripich, 1994; Brennan et al., 1995) demonstrated the value and effectiveness of computer-mediated support systems. As a continuation of this work, Brennan et al. (1998) have designed a project, HeartCare, that will design individual Web pages for cardiac artery bypass graft patients upon discharge. The delivery of this health care recovery series will use WebTV™ and provide direct communication via E-mail with the patient's health care provider. The Web-based group will be compared with a control group that receives an audiotape coaching program.

Other examples of provider-designed data communications applications include NetWellness, an electronic consumer health information service operated by the University of Cincinnati Medical Center (Morris et al., 1997). There are several computer-mediated support services for patients with cancer (Weinberg et al., 1996; Gustafson et al., 1993; Sharf, 1997; Klemm et al., 1998). It is clear that the Internet is a powerful channel for interactive health communication (Robinson et al., 1998). Interactive health communication (IHC) is defined as the "interaction of an individual—consumer, patient, caregiver or professional—with or through an electronic device or communication technology to assess or transmit health information or to receive guidance and support on a health related issue" (Robinson et al., 1998). The increased use of IHC has precipitated the creation of recommendations to serve as a basis for an evidence-based approach to the development and evaluation of IHC applications. These recommendations developed by the Science Panel on Interactive Communication and Health can be found at the following Web site: *http://www.scipich.org.*

The last type of telehealth applications uses video as its medium. Video applications are only beginning to evolve in nursing. Video communications can be broken into four basic types of transmissions: full-motion broadcast (TV quality), compressed video, slow-scan, and two-way video-audio (Witherspoon et al., 1994). For the past 30 years, medicine and psychiatry were the primary users of video applications. Store and forward radiology, dermatology, and pathology images were primary transmissions in medicine. There were also real-time patient visits for medical consults and telepsychiatry. There are numerous medical centers using teleconsultations, with the University of Texas Medical Center having the largest number of visits (2,000 to 3,000 consults per year) for the prison system (Crump et al., 1996). The Institute of Medicine (1996) reported that despite the many applications, there is limited evidence to support the cost-effectiveness of telemedicine.

In more recent years, video applications have moved from the hospital to the home environment. The growth in managed care and demand management strategies has increased the interest in using video technologies with chronically ill patients. Videophones, desktop video systems, and televisions are common methods used in the home care market. In addition, Kinsella (1998) reports that video visits are augmented with vital sign devices with telecommunication capabilities such as blood pressure cuffs and glucometers. As video applications move to the home market, there is more potential for use by the nursing profession.

There have been several projects in nursing demonstrating the use of video applications in the home. Schlachta and Pursley-Crotteau (1997) described an experimental program, Electronic Housecall, where chronically ill patients received health care through a personalized two-way interactive video system using a cable television network. In Kansas, nurses used a television screen equipped with a phone and camera to provide care to patients at home (Japsen, 1998; Miller, 1998). Kaiser Permanente in Sacramento established a program, Tele-Home Health, to deliver care to a group of patients with advanced medical problems. This project used a videophone augmented with an electronic stethoscope. Another example is the Home Assisted Nursing Care (HANC) device that is used in the home setting. This system collects and transmits data on heart rhythm, blood pressure, pulse, and temperature over telephone lines to a central nursing station (Crump et al., 1997). The device allows for patient-provider communication and can be programmed to provide self-care activities, dispensing of drugs, and health care instruction. To date, evaluations of these programs have demonstrated significant cost savings and patient satisfaction (Barrell, 1997; Council on Competitiveness, 1996; Schlachta and Pursley-Crotteau, 1997).

In summary, there has been a tremendous growth in the use of telehealth applications in nursing. Nursing applications have evolved over time and will continue to increase as we enter the next decade of health care. The rapid growth in home health care and managed care strategies will serve as a catalyst for continued explorations in telehealth applications. Growth in the next decade will occur across the spectrum of voice, data, and video applications. These applications are transforming the way nursing care is delivered to patients. In the next century, technological innovations will serve as a catalyst for many telehealth applications and continue to transform the way we live, work, learn, and conduct research.

Technological Innovations

Technological advances are providing health care with many opportunities to transform the business. This is particularly true in the area of telehealth. In the 20th century, health care was in the infancy stage of telehealth. As the 21st century unfolds, technological innovations will advance the ability of nurses to participate in telehealth applications. What follows is a brief overview of technological advances for the next decade.

In writing about the next 50 years of computing, Denning and Metcalfe (1997) project ways in which information technology will evolve and affect society. Fundamental forces, such as software engineering, microprocessor speeds, sensor technologies, and new dimensions in telecommunications and interfacing will greatly alter how information technologies will impact the global society (Crawford, 1997). Recent reports from both the

President's Information Technology Advisory Committee (1999) and the Working Group on Biomedical Computing Advisory Committee to the Director of the National Institutes of Health (1999) emphasize the potential advances in the new millennium.

According to Bell (1997), if hardware (such as semiconductors, magnetic memories, and fiber-optics) continues to evolve at the annual factor of 1.60, which we know as Moore's Law, then future computers will be 10 billion times more powerful by the year 2047. In 1996, an important milestone in supercomputing was reached. The "teraflop barrier" was broken; in other words, computers could process over a trillion floating-point operations per second (Clark, 1997). The computer, with 500 gigabytes of memory, could perform 1.8 teraflops. The Department of Energy's Accelerated Strategic Computing Initiative predicted that computing performance would triple every 18 months over the next 10 years. It is projected that in 10 years, we will see petaflops (quadrillion flops) as the supercomputing norm (Clark, 1997). A National Science and Technology Council report (1996) concurs and is encouraging the development of testbeds that support teraflop-class wide area computing. The placement of more transistors on a chip will allow for faster and cheaper technologies. The need to squeeze more transistors into a smaller space has led to research in the area of nanotechnology. Nanotechnolgy promises to determine how to place billions of transistors onto each chip. But the real payoff is that working at this molecular level could lead to advances in optical communications and photonics as well as ways to probe individual cells (Rothman, 1999).

Schneiderman (1997) extrapolates this concept even further and predicts that there will be a need for terabyte hard disks and Web spaces with petabytes (one million gigabytes) of information at our fingertips. Given the enormous digital repositories of information from the Human Genome Project, clinical trials, statistics, population genetics, information visualization, and imaging, a terabyte hard disk is needed (Working Group on Biomedical Computing Advisory Committee to the Director of National Institutes of Health 1999). As a matter of fact, the Working Group on Biomedical Computing Advisory Committee to the Director of National Institutes of Health (1999) predicts that a single biomedical laboratory will produce up to a terabyte of information a year. To place this in perspective, a terabyte is roughly equivalent to one million encyclopedias.

Bandwidth is also going to geometrically increase in the new millennium. According to Gilder (1997), over the next 30 years, bandwidth is going to be the fastest growing resource. Bandwidth is important, since it supports telecosm development (Gilder, 1991). "Telecosm" is a term used to describe broadband communications infrastructure that makes all knowledge accessible to anyone, anywhere and anytime. Cable modems, digital subscriber line technologies, satellites, and digital wireless technologies (personal digital assistants [PDAs] and wireless PCs) will influence bandwidth. Gilder (1997) predicts the following technologies in the near future: broadband digital radios, java teleputers (Internet access devices), household ethernets running on telephone wiring, smart cards so your PDA can become an internet transaction processor, direct broadcast and low earth orbit satellites, and media processors on DRAM that allow one-chip teleputers for Internet access. Farber's (1997) projections of direct broadcast satellites and mobile communications and the National Science and Technology Council report (1996) projections of large-scale wireline, optical, wireless, and mobile network technologies both coincide with Gilder's predictions. Chatterjee and Pawlowski (1999) project "that the future communications world will be two-layered—in that all communications between fixed points will take place by fiber-optics, while working from this backbone infrastructure will be a second world of untethered radio and infrared communication involving portable devices." Radio and infrared communications allow mobility but have limited bandwidth, whereas fiber has enormous bandwidth but limited distribution. In addition, fiber does not suffer from the bit-error rate that is inherent in copper and co-axial wires. Fiber allows for bandwidth in excess of 50 Tbps with a near zero bit-error.

Sensors and wearable computers are also on the horizon. According to Saffo (1997), cheap, ubiquitous, high-performance sensors will become available in the next decade. These sensors, embedded in objects such as phones, light switches, cars, buildings, and highways, will not only observe things, but they will manipulate things (Saffo, 1997). Billinghurst and Starner (1999) provide a good synopsis of where we are heading with wearable devices in the next century.

As the computer moves from the desktop to coat pocket to the human body, its ability to help manage, sort and filter information will become more intimately connected to our daily lives. In the next five years, we can expect to see wearable computer technology embedded in application-specific portable devices...such as personal organizers. A few years after that, we should see more general wearable computers in common use in the mobile workforce. These wearables will combine communication, computation and context sensitivity to enhance personal

productivity. By the next decade, you will have a device that gives continuous access to computing and communications resources on a machine intelligent enough to know who you are...(Billinghurst and Starner, 1999)

Information appliances are projected for the future (Birnbaum, 1997b; *Business Week*, 1996; *Business Week*, 1999). Users will think of information appliances in terms of what they do rather than how they do it. Information appliances will have essentially no learning curve, be specific to a particular task, and hide their own complexity (Birnbaum,1997b). Appliance names relate to function rather than to how the internal components work (Birnbaum, 1997a). The ultimate goal is to bring the unwired masses into the information age with appliances that in the next century will be as commonplace as telephones and automobiles (*Business Week*, 1996). Examples in *Business Week* (1999) show post-personal computer products such as the E-Book, Webtouch phone, wristwatch cell phone, and a cell phone that sends E-mail. Data International Data Corp. (*Business Week*, 1999) projects that in the year 2001, information appliances will outnumber personal computers. If we begin to think of these devices of the future as information appliances, will people expect an information utility, like phone service, to be universally accessible? According to Birnbaum (1997a, 1997b), client-utility computing will replace client-server computing. Client-utility will allow clients to connect to the utility (high-bandwidth digital multimedia networks) and pay for their computing by usage as we pay for our other utility bills (water, electricity, telephone, cable).

These are just some of the highlights of technology in the future. This chapter has only begun to scratch the surface. In the next section, we will explore how these advances in technology will impact applications and transform the way we practice, learn, and conduct research. Each transformation area (advanced practice, education, and research) begins with the vision from the *Information Technology Research: Investing in Our Future* report (President's Information Technology Advisory Committee, 1999). Telehealth examples for each vision are projected.

 ## Applications for Advanced Practice: Transforming the Practice of Health Care

Vision: Telemedicine applications are commonplace. Specialists use videoconferencing and telesensing methods to interview and even to examine patients who may be hundreds of miles away. Computer-aided surgery with Internet-based video is used to demonstrate surgical procedures to others. Powerful high-end systems provide expert advice based on sophisticated analysis of huge amounts of medical information. Patients are empowered in making decisions about their own care through new models of interaction with their physicians and ever-increasing access to biomedical information via digital medical libraries and the Internet. New communications and monitoring technologies support treatment of patients comfortably from their own homes. (President's Information Technology Advisory Committee, 1999)

Think about what this vision will mean to nursing and its involvement in telehealth applications in patient care. Increasing bandwidth will allow multimedia images to be transferred between providers and consumers. These multimedia images can be patient educational materials, vital signs, or video holograms of one's social support group. Wearable computer sensors will track valuable patient information and allow direct transmission to health care providers regardless of geographic and time boundaries. Here are two telehealth projections based upon these advanced technologies.

Cochrane et al. (1996) described remote monitoring devices for the aged that can be used in home health care. Wrist-sized computing can provide diagnostic information to providers, and patients can benefit from round-the-clock monitoring. Whenever vital signs or other diagnostic measures indicate an abnormality, the health care provider can be notified. Mann (1997) also projects that wearable computer or computer clothing will become a "visual memory prosthetic" and a perception enhancer. Full mediated realities and personal visual assistants for the visually challenged are one of Mann's applications of wearable computers. According to Mann (1997), a computer that is constantly attentive to our environment may develop situational awareness, perceptual intelligence, and an ability to see from the wearer's perspective and thereby assist in day-to-day activities. Imagine the possibilities for health care and for nursing practice.

Kinsella (1998) projects that more opportunities will arise to provide extended needed care services to patients using telecommunications-ready tools. According to Kinsella (1998), integrating telehealth will be a new way of doing business in the home care market. Here are some of her predictions.

■ Integrating telehealth tools into a care plan.

■ Adapting the focus to accommodate the 21st century patient who is more knowledgeable, empowered, and demanding.

■ Adapting the focus to changing definitions of home. Home may be the school, the work center, or the senior day care center.

■ New services and new techniques, such as videotherapy, will be available.

Remote telesurgeries are being projected for the future. "Robotics and remote visualization methods, supported by high-reliability, low-latency communications are needed to support applications such as telepresence surgery" (President's Information Technology Advisory Committee, 1999).

■ Applications for Education: Transforming the Way We Learn

Vision: Any individual can participate in on-line education programs regardless of geographic location, age, physical limitation, or personal schedule. Everyone can access repositories of educational materials, easily recalling past lessons, updating skills, or selecting from among different teaching methods in order to discover the most effective ways of learning. Educational programs can be customized to each individual's needs, so that the information revolution reaches everyone and personal digital libraries provide a mechanism for managing one's accumulated knowledge resources. Learning involves all our senses, to help focus each student's attention and better communicate educational material. (President's Information Technology Advisory Committee, 1999)

"Learning anytime, anywhere" will be a reality in the upcoming decade. Health care professionals and consumers will have access to a wealth of knowledge at their fingertips. Collaborative learning environments centered on the learner will become commonplace. Learners will engage in learning by participating in virtual environments. Learners will be able to use personal digital assistants or intelligent agents to help in acquiring updated knowledge. Faculty will serve as guides by filtering and focusing knowledge. They will serve as mentors for learners. Learning will not be limited to traditional higher educational structures. Learning corporations, already forming, will be major players in the production of knowledge.

Educational institutions will face dramatic changes (Denning, 1996; Skiba, 1997). Universities that generate content every day through course delivery will become involved in new functions related to content. Universities will be involved in the generation of content (production), packaging of content (programming), or the presentation of content (distribution) (Tsichritzis, 1999). Some universities will perform all three functions. Some may specialize in niche markets and focus on one of the functions. There are many scenarios projected for higher education; the one thing that is certain is that it will not be "business as usual." Telehealth applications that include an educational focus will certainly benefit from the transformation of the way we learn.

Applications for Research: Transforming How We Conduct Research

Vision: Research is conducted in virtual laboratories in which scientists and engineers can routinely perform their work without regard to physical location—interacting with colleagues, accessing instrumentation, sharing data and computational resources, and accessing information in digital libraries. All scientific and technical journals are available on-line, allowing readers to download equations and databases and manipulate variables to interactively explore the published research. (President's Information Technology Advisory Committee, 1999)

The process of conducting research will be greatly enhanced by technologies, and telehealth applications with a research focus will flourish in this virtual research environment. Lederberg and Uncapher (1989) first mentioned the use of these virtual research environments when they introduced the concept of a research collaboratory. The National Council of Research (1993) defined a collaboratory as a "center without walls in which the nation's researchers can perform research without regard to geographic location—interacting with colleagues, accessing instrumentation, sharing data and computational resources, and accessing information from digital libraries." There are numerous collaboratories already established, and growth of these will continue as data mining, visualization techniques, and knowledge repositories become more prevalent.

Challenges and Issues

If this transformation is to occur, the health care profession must tackle some key challenges and issues. These issues center on legal, ethical, and public policy arenas.

Legal Issues

The predominant legal issues concerning telehealth are licensure and liability and malpractice. During the 1995 legislative session, 19 states dealt with issues concerning telehealth (Waters and Shotwell, 1995). The following paragraphs will explore the practice implications of each of these issues.

Licensure

The lack of infrastructure for interstate licensure has been a key impediment to the growth of telehealth. Currently, each state has established practice acts for medical and allied health professionals that dictate the procedures for obtaining and renewing a license to practice within that state. In April 1996, the Federation of State Medical Boards proposed creation of a limited interstate license for teleconsulting physicians, which was rejected by the American Medical Association in June 1996. The issues contributing to the defeat of the measure included a concern that rural patients would leave their rural primary care provider for a specialist, the cost of telehealth equipment, and payment for provision of telehealth services (*Medical Economics*, 1997).

In February 1997, the Center for Telemedicine Law published a white paper concerning interstate licensure (*http://www.ctl.org/ctlwhite.html*). The key findings in this paper are summarized below:

- Telemedicine has the potential to substantially improve access to needed health care services and medical expertise.

- The basic standards to qualify to practice medicine in each state are, to a large extent, uniform.

- State requirements for "licensing by endorsement" are time-consuming, costly, and confusing.

- Several states have recently adopted legislation that addresses licensing requirements for interstate practice.

- State and federal policy-makers should examine strategies to encourage the adoption of uniform standards and administrative requirements for licensure coupled with local responsibility for monitoring and enforcement of the quality of physician services.

- Disciplinary activities and the enforcement of licensure laws are functions that can best be conducted by the states; and

■ Many of the issues related to the licensing of allied health professionals in an environment of increasing interstate activity are similar to those discussed in this report. (p. 1)

The United States Congress contracted with the Center for Telemedicine Law for a background paper concerning telehealth licensure issues in early 1997 (*http://www.ntia.doc.gov/reports/telemed/legal.htm*). Alternative approaches to licensure outlined in that report include consulting exceptions, endorsement, mutual recognition, reciprocity, registration, limited licensure, national licensure, and federal licensure. In the following paragraph, each approach is briefly defined, and implications for the current practice environment are identified.

Consulting exceptions are common to most states. They allow an out-of-state physician to provide services at the request of and in consultation with a referring physician. However, these exceptions were developed for rare occurrences and not expected to be used on a full-time basis, as they would be for telehealth. **Licensure by endorsement** is currently used to permit providers licensed in one state to apply for licensure in another state in which they would like to practice. Unfortunately, in operationalizing telehealth, this could require providers to apply for licensure in all 50 states. **Mutual recognition** is a licensure system used in Europe and Australia in which licensing bodies agree to accept the policies of the licensee's home state. This method would require agreement by the states on standardized rules and regulations governing health care across the states. **Reciprocity** is an approach that would allow states to grant practice privileges to a provider of another state without further credential review. This would require states to develop agreements with several other states. In a **registration** system, a provider is required to notify another state of intent to practice. The provider would be required to follow the rules of the state but not to meet the state's entrance requirements. **Limited licensure** is an option in which providers are required to obtain a license in every state in which they practice. The provider would have the option of applying for a limited license in subsequent states that would specify a limited scope of practice. An assumption of this approach is that application requirements would be less burdensome for a limited scope of practice. **National licensure** involves standardized requirements for licensure throughout the United States. This option would create a centralized administration for licensure resulting in lost revenue for states, questions regarding legal authority of the states, logistical chal-

lenges, and funding concerns. A final approach is **federal licensure** in which providers are issued one license by the federal government that would be valid throughout the United States. The system would be administered through federal agencies at the national, state, or local level.

The American Nurses Association (ANA) (1999b) recently proposed three models of interstate practice. Model 1, facilitation of physically providing nursing services across state boundaries requires that a model nurse practice act as the basis of licensure uniformity. A centralized disciplinary verification system would be maintained, and a current license would be required in each state. This essentially allows each state to maintain control but adds the dimension of a centralized database for disciplinary action. Model 2, facilitation of providing nursing services across state boundaries through the use of telehealth, requires a registration mechanism for those providing telehealth services. This model simplifies the registration process and places accountability to the board of nursing with the out-of-state provider. Model 3, facilitation of providing nursing services across state boundaries through the use of telehealth, defines the site of the provider as the basis for regulatory control. This model would require (1) expansion of state practice acts to define telehealth and (2) only one license for the provider.

The National Council of State Boards of Nursing has developed a mutual recognition model of licensure (Simpson, 1998). This would allow nurses licensed in their home state to practice in other states under their respective state's Nurse Practice Act. Nurses would remain accountable to their home state board of nursing (State Legislative Trends & Analysis, 1998).

The State Licensure Committee of the American Telemedicine Association (ATA) (1998) issued recommendations for a policy statement (*http://atmeda.org/news/policy.html*) that:

■ Preserves the right of each state to regulate medicine in traditional face-to-face physical setting

■ Preserves licensure authority at the state level

■ Avoids unnecessary restraints on interstate commerce

■ Ensures that all patients have access to the health care expertise necessary to protect and promote their health, regardless of the location of the provider

■ Advances telemedicine as a valuable service delivery strategy that can play a critical role in overcoming time and distance barriers that often limit access to quality health care.

The ATA report continues with proposed "rules of engagement" for telemedicine

- A telemedicine request originates from a physician who is fully licensed in the patient's state.
- The patient and requesting physician must have a real physician-patient relationship.
- The patient and requesting physician must have a real face-to-face encounter.
- The out-of-state physician using telemedicine must be fully licensed in the state in which the physician is located.
- The responsibility of medical care for the patient must remain with the requesting physician.

Liability and Malpractice

The second major legal issue that must be addressed with telehealth is liability and malpractice. "Currently, malpractice cases hinge on two legal questions: (1) whether a physician-patient relationship existed and (2) whether the physician breaches his or her duty of care" (Saltzman and Lammers, 1997, p. 24). Part of the challenge concerning telehealth and liability is that there is a lack of statutory and case law (Saltzman and Lammers, 1997; Physician's Insurers Association of America, 1998). In addition, since medical liability originates when there is injury due to a breach in the standard of care, the fact that the standard of care in telehealth has not been defined is another area of concern (Physician's Insurers Association of America, 1998). The American Nurses Association does not believe that telehealth will impact the scope of practice, however. "Scopes of practice should be driven by decisions about allowable services based on the profession's or legislature's obligation to ensure ethical and high quality service" (American Nurses Association, 1999a).

"During the discussion at the PIAA Telemedicine Colloquium, consensus emerged that the liability resulting from a telemedicine encounter between a physician and patient would likely be direct liability as opposed to vicarious (liability imposed upon a person even though he is not a party to the specific occurrence)" (Physician's Insurers Association of America, 1998, p. 13). Two liability issues that may require consideration for telehealth encounters include equipment malfunction and failure to use the technology. With regard to the former, clinicians may be at increased risk if equipment mal-

function leads to an adverse event. In addition, if telehealth permits high-quality care, it is possible that clinicians may be held liable for failure to deliver it.

One advantage of telehealth applications from a liability perspective is that use of the technology generates an electronic medical record. "The existence of a recorded copy of the actual consultation, rather than (or in addition to) a summary note in the patient record should have major implications" (Ostbye and Hurlen, 1997, p. 270). Not only will the provider have a complete record, but the interaction may be used for educational sessions as well.

The PIAA (1998 p. 19) developed risk management recommendations for providers engaged in telehealth applications. A summary of the recommendations is provided below.

- Become proficient with the technology.
- Ensure that the use of telemedicine is appropriate for the situation.
- Educate the patient regarding options and limitations in the use of telemedicine.
- Become familiar with referring physicians and their credentials.
- Inform your insurance carrier of the nature and scope of your telemedicine practice.
- If technology does not provide a clear assessment or if results are equivocal, see the patient in person or refer him/her for face-to-face or follow-up consultation.
- Make sure there are realistic expectations of all parties. This technology is not perfect or appropriate for all types of interactions.
- Clarify roles and responsibilities of all practitioners. Make sure the division of responsibilities is clear and complete.
- Make sure contractual issues are reviewed and clarified.
- Maintain an archive of each system in use.
- Make every attempt to personalize the telemedicine encounter.
- Document, document, document.

Ethical Issues

The predominant ethical issues concerning telehealth are privacy, confidentiality, and security. The following definitions have been set forth by the American Society for Testing and Materials Committee E31 on

Healthcare Informatics, Subcommittee E31.17 on Privacy, Confidentiality, and Access (1997):

Privacy: "the right of individuals to be left alone and to be protected against physical or psychological invasion or the misuse of their property. It includes freedom from intrusion or observation into one's private affairs, the right to maintain control over certain personal information, and the freedom to act without outside interference."

Confidentiality: The "status accorded to data or information indicating that it is sensitive for some reason, and therefore it needs to be protected against theft, disclosure, or improper use, or both, and must be disseminated only to authorized individuals or organizations with a need to know."

Data security: "The result of effective data protection measures; the sum of measures that safeguard data and computer programs from undesired occurrences and exposure to accidental or intentional access or disclosure to unauthorized persons, or a combination thereof; accidental or malicious alteration; unauthorized copying; or loss by theft or destruction by hardware failures, software deficiencies; operating mistakes; physical damage by fire, water, smoke, excessive temperature, electrical failure or sabotage; or a combination thereof. Data security exists when data are protected from accidental or intentional disclosure to unauthorized persons and from unauthorized or accidental alteration."

System security: "The totality of safeguards including hardware, software, personnel policies, information practice policies, disaster preparedness; and oversight of these components. Security protects both the system and the information contained within from unauthorized access from without and from misuse from within. Security enables the entity or system to protect the confidential information it stores from unauthorized access, disclosure, or misuse, thereby protecting the privacy of the individuals who are the subjects of the stored information."

Buckovich et al. (1999) conducted a comparative review and analysis of 28 independent draft principles on privacy, confidentiality, and security. Eleven consistent principles were identified.

1. Individuals have a right to the privacy and confidentiality of their health information.
2. Outside the doctor-patient relationship, health information that makes a person identifiable shall not be disclosed without prior patient informed consent and/or authorization.

3. All entities with exposure or access to individual health information shall have security/privacy/confidentiality policies, procedures, and regulations (including sanctions) in place that support adherence to these principles.

4. Individuals have a right to access in a timely manner their health information.

5. Individuals have a right to control the access and disclosure of their health information and to specify limitations on period of time and purpose of use.

6. Employers have a right to collect and maintain health information about employees allowable or otherwise deemed necessary to comply with state and federal statutes (e.g., ERISA, drug testing, workers' compensation). However, employers shall not use this information for job or other employee benefit discrimination.

7. All entities involved with health care information have a responsibility to educate themselves, their staff, and consumers on issues related to these principles.

8. Individuals have a right to amend and/or correct their health information.

9. Health information and/or medical records that make a person identifiable shall be maintained and transmitted in a secure environment.

10. An audit trail shall exist for medical records and be available to patients on request.

11. Support for these principles needs to be at the federal level.

Public Policy

The Western Governors Association (WGA) (1998) identified three key policy barriers to the growth of telehealth initiatives. Those three issues include infrastructure planning and development, telecommunications regulation, and lack of reimbursement for telehealth services. In addition, the recent National Telecommunications and Information Administration (1999) report highlights a persistent problem called the digital divide . . . Internet "have-nots."

The WGA discovered that state policy makers failed to consider telecommunication needs across various state activities, resulting in missed opportunities for cost-sharing and reducing redundancy in states' networks. They proposed "tighter integration of strategic planning efforts for telemedicine and telecommunications" (Western Governors Association, 1998, p. 2). In addition, they proposed inviting private sector telecommunications companies, equipment manufacturers, and medical service providers to discussions.

One of the greatest issues in the regulation of telecommunications concerns the ability of communities to obtain the types of services necessary at affordable rates. The Telecommunications Act of 1996 leveled the playing field by requiring discounted services for rural health providers. Unfortunately, this program has been off to a slow start, but individual states are beginning to dedicate support for state-operated networks to support telehealth (Western Governors Association, 1998).

The historical funding sources for development of telehealth applications rested largely with the National Aeronautics and Space Administration and the Department of Defense (Grigsby and Sanders, 1998). Currently, Medicare reimbursement is generally not available (with the exception of certain Health Professional Shortage Areas). The reason for this is that telehealth applications do not meet the Health Care Financing Administration requirement for in-person, face-to-face contact. There is active debate about whether the use of telehealth represents a change in process or a change in access to health care.

The digital divide is still a persistent public policy issue. For the last 5 years, data were collected to address the penetration of telephone and computers in consumer homes. These analyses were directed to examine the haves and the have-nots in the information age. Here are some of the highlights of the most recent report (National Telecommunications and Information Administration, 1999). The penetration rates have increased nationwide in terms of people entering into the information age. Telephone penetration has remained unchanged since the last study in 1995 and remains at a 93.8 percent penetration. Computer penetration has grown substantially with the following changes in penetration: PC ownership has increased 51.9 percent; modem ownership has increased 139.1 percent, and E-mail access has expanded by 397.1 percent (National Telecommunications and Information Administration, 1999). Despite these increases, there has been a widening in the gap between lower and higher income families. The "digital divide" between certain groups of Americans has increased between 1994 and 1997. According to the NTIA (1999) report, "Blacks and Hispanics now lag even further behind than Whites in their levels of PC-ownership and online access." Single female heads of households and rural poor, young house-

holds, and rural and central city minorities constitute the profile of the least connected group of Americans. Significant populations still remain unconnected and will be unable to take advantage of the numerous telehealth applications highlighted in this chapter. Telehealth applications, particularly interactive health communications, may help to reduce health disparities through their potential for promoting health, preventing disease, and supporting clinical care for all; however, those with health problems are least likely to have access (Eng et al., 1998). Thus, this is another public policy issue that needs to be tackled if telehealth applications are to provide the maximum benefits to all.

Conclusion

Without a doubt, telehealth applications will proliferate in the future. Health care professionals need to seize the opportunities made possible by advanced technologies and create powerful and human-centered telehealth applications. To start this process, health care professionals need to become actively involved in resolving challenges and shaping public policy.

References

American Nurses Association. (1999a). *Core Principles of Telehealth*. Washington, D.C.: American Nurses Publishing.

American Nurses Association. (1999b). *Interstate Practice Models*. Unpublished Draft Report. Washington, D.C.: American Nurses Publishing.

American Nurses Association. (1997). *Telehealth, A Tool for Nursing Practice. Nursing Trends & Issues*, 2(4), 1–7.

American Society for Testing and Materials Committee E-31 on Healthcare Informatics, Subcommittee E-31.17 on Privacy, Confidentiality, and Access. (1997). *Standard Guide for Confidentiality, Privacy, Access, and Data Security Principles for Health Information Including Computer-based Patient Records*. Philadelphia: ASTM (Designation E-1869-97).

American Telemedicine Association. (1998). ATA State Medical Licensure Committee Draft Report to ATA Board of Directors. *http://atmeda.org/news/policy.html*

Balas, E. A., Jaffrey, F., Kuperman, G. J., et al. (1997). Electronic communication with patients, evaluation of distance medicine technology. *The Journal of the American Medical Association*, 278(2), 152–159.

Barrell, J. (1997). Telemedicine, you can't do that at home. *Infusion*, 4(2), 29–35.

Baruch College-Harris Poll. (1998). *http://www.midiacentral.com/magazines/md/oldarchives/199704/1997042504.html*

Bell, G. (1997). The body electric. *Communications of the Association of Computing Machinery*, 40 (2), 31–32.

Billinghurst, M., and Starner, T. (1999). Wearable devices: New ways to manage information. *Computer, 32 (1)*, 57–64.

Birnbaum, J. (1997a). ACM: Speaker's Corner. *Communications of the Association of Computing Machinery, 40* (1), 19.

Birnbaum, J. (1997b). Pervasive information systems. *Communications of the Association of Computing Machinery, 40* (2), 40–41.

Bleich, M. R. (1998). Growth strategies to optimize the functions of telephonic nursing call centers. *Nursing Economics, 16*(4), 215–218.

Bloch, C. (1999). *Federal Telemedicine Activities and Internet Sites.* Potomac, MD: Bloch Consulting Group.

Borowitz, S. M., and Wyatt, J. C. (1998). The origin, content, and workload of e-mail consultations. *The Journal of the American Medical Association, 280*(15), 1321–1324.

Brennan, P., Caldwell, B., Moore, S., et al. (1998). Designing HeartCare, custom computerized home care for patients recovering from CABG surgery. In C. G. Chute (Ed.), *Proceedings of the American Medical Informatics Association Annual Symposium* (pp.381–385). Philadelphia: Hanley & Belfus, Inc.

Brennan, P., Moore, S., and Smyth, K. (1995). The effects of a special computer network on caregivers of persons with Alzheimer's disease. *Nursing Research, 44,* 166–172.

Brennan, P., and Ripich, S. (1994). Use of home-care computer network by persons with AIDS. *International Journal of Technology Assessment in Health Care, 10,* 258–272.

Brennan, P., Ripich, S., and Moore, S. (1991a). The use of home-based computers to support persons living with AIDS/ARC. *Journal of Community Health Nursing, 8*(1), 3–14.

Brennan, P., Moore, S., and Smyth, K. (1991b). ComputerLink: Electronic support for the home caregiver. *Advances in Nursing Science, 13*(4), 14–27.

Buckovich, S. A., Rippen, H. E., and Rozen, M. J. (1999). Driving toward guiding principles: A goal for privacy, confidentiality, and security of health information. *Journal of the American Medical Informatics Association, 6,* 122–133.

Business Week (1996). *The Information Appliance. Special Report.* June 24, 71–96.

Business Week (1999). *Beyond the PC. Special Report.* 79–83, 86–89.

Chatterjee, S., and Pawlowski, S. (1999). All-optical networks. *Communications of the Association of Computing Machinery, 42*(6), 75–83.

Clark, D. (1997). Up Front: Breaking the teraflops barrier. *Computer, 30*(2), 12–14.

Cochrane, P., Heatley, D., and Pearson, I. (1996). Computers and the Aged. *http://www.labs.bt.com/people/cochrap/*

Council on Competitiveness. (1996). Highway to Health, Transforming U.S. Health Care in the Information Age. *http://nii.nist.gov/pubs/coc_hghwy_to_hlth/chp2.html*

Crawford, D. (1997). Introduction to 50th anniversary issue. *Communications of the Association of Computing Machinery, 40*(2), 29.

Crump, W. J., Kotte, T. E., Perednia, D. A., and Sanders, J. H. (1997). Is telemedicine ready for prime time? *Patient Care, 31*(3), 64–87.

Denning, P., (1996). Business Designs for the new university. *EDUCOM Review, 31*(6), 20–30.

Denning, P., and Metcalfe, R. (1997). *Beyond Calculation: The Next Fifty Years of Computing.* New York: Springer-Verlag.

Diepgen, G., and Eysenbach, T. (1998). Responses to unsolicited patient e-mail request for medical advise on the World Wide Web. *The Journal of the American Medical Association, 280*(15), 1333–1335.

Eng, T., Maxfield, A., Patrick, K., et al. (1998). Access to health information and support (policy perspectives). *The Journal of the American Medical Association, 280*(15), 1371–137.

Farber, D. (1997). Communications technology and its impact by 2010. *Communications of the Association of Computing Machinery, 40*(2), 135–138.

Ferguson, T. (1998). Digital Doctoring—opportunities and challenges in electronic patient-physician communication (editorial). *The Journal of the American Medical Association, 280*(15), 1361–1362.

Fridsma, D., Ford, P., and Altman, R. (1994). A survey of patient access to electronic mail, attitudes, barriers, and opportunities. In J. Ozbolt (Ed.), *Proceeding of the Annual Symposium on Computer Applications in Medical Care* (pp. 15–19). Philadelphia: Henly & Belfus, Inc.

Gilder, G. (1991). Into the telecosm. *Harvard Business Review, 69*(2), 150–155.

Gilder, G. (1997). Interview with George Gilder on the Bandwidth of Plenty. *Internet Computing, 1*(1), 9–18.

Grisby, J., and Sanders, J. (1998). Telemedicine: Where it is and where it's going. *Annals of Internal Medicine, 129*(2), 123–127.

Gustafson, D., Wise, M., McTavish, F., et al. (1993). Development and pilot evaluation of a computer based support system for women with breast cancer. *Journal of Psychosocial Oncology, 11,*69–93.

Healtheon. (1999). Physician use of internet explodes. *Health Management Technology, 20*(i2), 8.

Institute of Medicine. (1996). *Telemedicine: A Guide to Assessing Telecommunications in Health Care.* Washington, D. C.: National Academy Press.

Japsen, B. (1998). House calls—Kansas hospital's experiment in home health telemedicine cuts costs, visits. *Modern Healthcare, 28*(12), 47.

Johnson, B., Wheeler, L., and Deuser, J. (1997). Kaiser Permanente medical center's pilot telehome health project. *Telemedicine Today, 8,*16–19.

Kane, B., and Sands, D. Z. (1998). AMIA Internet Working Group, Task Force on Guidelines for the Use of Clinic-Patient Electronic Mail: Guidelines for the clinical use of electronic mail with patients. *Journal of the American Medical Informatics Association, 5*(1), 104–111.

Kassirer, J. P. (1995). The next transformation in the delivery of health care. *The New England Journal of Medicine, 332*(1), 52–54.

Kinsella, A. (1998). *Home Healthcare, Wired & Ready for Telemedicine ... The second generation.* Sunriver, OR: Information for Tomorrow.

Klemm, P., Reppert, K., and Visich, L. (1998). A nontraditional cancer support group, the Internet. *Computers in Nursing, 16*(1), 31–36.

Lederberg, J., and Uncapher, K. (1989). *Towards a National Collaboratory.* New York: The Rockerfeller University.

Lindberg, D., and Humphreys, B. (1998). Medicine and health on the Internet, the good, the bad, and the ugly. *The Journal of the American Medical Association, 280*(15), 1303–1304.

Mahoney, D., Tarlow, B., and Sandaire, J. (1998). A computer-mediated intervention for Alzheimer's caregivers. *Computers in Nursing, 16*(4), 208–216.

Malloy, C. (1998). Managed care and ethical implications in telephone-based health services. *Advance Practice Nursing Quarterly 4*(2), 30–33.

Mandl, K., Kohane, I., and Brandt, A. (1998). Electronic patient-physician communication, problems and promise. *Annals of Internal Medicine, 129*(6), 495–500.

Mann, S. (1997). Wearable computing: A first step toward personal imaging. *Computer 30,*(2), 25–32.

Miller, N. (1998). Leadership roundtable. Success to telemedicine program catches eyes. *Nursing Economics, 16*(3), 137.

Moore, M., and Krowchuck, H. (1997). Parent line, nurse telephone intervention for parents and caregivers of children from birth through age 5. *Journal of the Society of Pediatric Nurses, 2*(4), 179–187.

Morris, T., Guard, J., Marine, S., et al. (1997). Approaching equity in consumer health information delivery, net wellness. *Journal of the American Medical Informatics Association 4*(1), 6–13.

Mosby. (1998). *Medical & Nursing Dictionary,* (5th ed.), (p. 895E). St. Louis, MO: Author.

National Council of Research. (1993). *National Collaboratories: Applying Information Technology for Scientific Research.* Washington, D. C.: National Academy Press.

National Science and Technology Council. (1996). *High Performance Computing and Communications: Advancing the Frontiers of Information Technology.* A Report by the Committee on Computing, Information and Communications.

National Telecommunications and Information Administration. (1999). Americans in the Information Age: Falling Through the Net. Falling Through the Net Series on the Telecommunications and Information Technology Gap in America. (3d report). *http://www.ntia.doc.gov/ntiahome/digitaldivide/*

Niles, S., Alemagno, S., and Stricklin, M. (1997). Healthy talk, a telecommunication model for health promotion. *CARING Magazine, 16*(7), 46–50.

Ostbye, T., and Hurlen, P. (1997). The electronic house call: Consequences of telemedicine consultations for physicians, patients, and society. *Archives of Family Medicine, 6*(3), 266–271.

Osheroff, J. (1997). Online health-related discussion groups, what we should know and do [editorial]. *Journal of General Internal Medicine, 12,* 511–512.

Physicians Insurers Association of America (1998). *Telemedicine: A Medical Liability White Paper.* Rockville, MD: Physicians Insurers Association of America.

Phipps, R., and Merisotis, J. (1999). *What's the Difference? A Review of Contemporary Research on the Effectiveness of Distance Learning in Higher Education.* Washington, D.C.: The Institute for Higher Education Policy.

President's Information Technology Advisory Committee. *Information Technology Research: Investing in our Future* (1999). Arlington, VA: National Coordination Office for Computing, Information and Communications.

Robinson, T., Patrick, K., Eng, T., and Gustafson, D. (1998). An evidence-based approach to interactive health communication, a challenge to medicine in the information age. *The Journal of the American Medical Association, 280*(14), 1264–1269.

Rothman, D. (1999). Nanotechnology: The hope or the hype. *Technology Review, 102*(2), 44–45.

Saffo, P. (1997). Sensors: The next wave of innovation. *Communications of the Association of Computing Machinery, 40*(2), 93–97.

Saltzman, K., and Lammars, K. (1997). Telemedicine: Where health care services meet technology. *Infusion, 4* (2), 23–26.

Schneiderman, B. (1997). Beyond hope and fear. *Communications of the Association of Computing Machinery, 40*(2), 59–62.

Schlachta, L. M., Pursley-Crotteau, S. (1997). Leveraging technology, telemedicine in disease management and implications for infusion services. *Infusion, 4*(2), 36–40.

Sharf, B. (1997). Communicating breast cancer on-line; Support and empowerment on the Internet. *Women and Health, 26,*65–84.

Shu, E., Mirmina, Z., Nyström, K. (1996). A telephone reassurance program for elderly home care clients after discharge. *Home Healthcare Nurse, 14*(3), 154–161.

Simpson, R. (1998). Long-distance nursing kindles multistate licensure debate. *Nursing Management, 29* (12), 8–9.

Skiba, D. (1997). Transforming nursing education to celebrate learning. *Nursing and Health Care Perspectives, 18*(3), 124–129,148.

Skiba, D., and Mirque, D. (1994). The electronic community, An alternative health care approach. In S. Grobe and E. S. P. Plutyer-Wenting (Eds.). *Nursing Informatics, An International Overview for Nursing in a Technological Era* (pp. 388–392). Amsterdam: Elsevier.

Sparks, S. (1992). Exploring electronic support groups. *American Journal of Nursing, 92*(12), 62–65.

Spielberg, A. R. (1998). On call and online, sociohistorical, legal, and ethical implications of e-mail for the patient-physician relationship. *Journal of the American Medical Association, 280*(15), 1353–1359.

State Legislative Trends & Analysis. (1998). *Special Report to the 1998 House of Delegates.* Submitted by the Department of State Government Relations and the Department of Political and Grassroots Programs. *http://www.nursingworld.org/gova/hod98/index.htm*

Telemedicine Editorial. (1997). Obstacles to telecomedicine's growth. *Medical Economics, 74*(23), 69.

Telemedicine Report to Congress. (1997). Legal Issues—Licensure and Telemedicine. *http://www.ntia.doc.gov/reports/telemed/legal.htm*

Tsichritzis, D. (1999). Reengineering the university. *Communications of the Association of Computing Machinery, 42*(6), 93–100.

Waters, R., and Shotwell, L. (1995). Physicians grapple with state statutes, liability concerns. *www.arentfox.com/telemed/state_1999.html*

Weinberg, N., Schmale, J., Uken, J., and Weasel, K. (1996). Online help, cancer patients participate in computer-mediated support group. *Health & Social Work, 21,*24–29.

Western Governors Association. (1998). *Telemedicine Action Update.* Denver, CO: Western Governors Association.

Widman, L. E., Tong, D. A. (1997). Requests for medical advise from patients and families to health care providers who publish on the World Wide Web. *Archives of Internal Medicine, 157*(2), 209–212.

Witherspoon, J., Johnston, S., and Wasem, C. (1994). *Rural TeleHealth, Telemedicine, Distance Education and Informatics for Rural Health Care.* Boulder, CO: Western Interstate Commission of Higher Education Publications.

Working Group on Biomedical Computing Advisory Committee to the Director of National Institutes of Health. Biomedical Information Science & Technology Initiative. *http://www.nih.gov/welcome/director/060399.htm*

PART **9**

Research
Applications

26

Computer Use in Nursing Research

Betty L. Chang

1. Identify general goals of quantitative and qualitative research.
2. Discuss the use of computer programs in each step of the research process.
3. Identify the most appropriate tasks for the use of computer applications in quantitative and qualitative research.
4. Identify precautions in the selection of software for data analysis.

KEY WORDS

research process
quantitative
qualitative
data collection
data management
analysis

This chapter describes the use of computers in the various stages of the research process. Focus is placed on considerations in the preparation of the research proposal, data collection, data coding, data analysis, and dissemination of results. Both quantitative and qualitative approaches to research are discussed and brief examples of research are provided at the end of the chapter.

For decades, computers have been used to aid researchers in performing various aspects of the research process. With the advent of microcomputers for word processing, performing bibliographic searches, and data analyses, computers have become an indispensable tool for all aspects of the research process from proposal preparation to the reporting of results. The most obvious tasks within the research process accomplished with the aid of computers are the bibliographic search, proposal preparation, data collection, data coding and analysis, and the dissemination of results. Because of the advancement in the implementation of clinical systems, acceptable terminology/vocabularies to support nursing assessment, interventions, and evaluation, computers are increasingly being used for clinical and patient care research. Although the research process itself remains a complex cognitive process, certain aspects can be aided

by computers. For example, various types of nursing research examining outcomes of nursing care and the effect of interventions would have been prohibitive in the past, but with the aid of computers large data sets can be examined qualitatively and quantitatively.

The objective of this chapter is to provide an overview of the stages involved in nursing research and describe how computers can aid this process. In particular, this chapter will focus on some of the considerations in the preparation of the research proposal and subsequent considerations in data collection, data coding, data analysis, and dissemination of results. The use of on-line bibliographic retrieval systems is described in detail in the next chapter.

Considerations in Proposal Preparation

The first task in the identification of a problem depends on the nurse's previous experience as well as philosophical and theoretical orientation. The nurse's experience may determine the clinical areas or practice of interest as well as the philosophical and theoretical orientation. One's philosophical orientation provides background for one's approach to the development of science and theory, the determination of research methodology, the types of analytical techniques, and interpretation of results. The results and conclusions may in turn contribute to nursing practice. Because these philosophical orientations determine the theoretical/conceptual frameworks as well as the design and analysis used, they will be briefly described as a group here. The research plan must include the design of the research and an analysis plan. The analysis must be congruent with the design of the research, the type of data, and the manner in which they are collected. For each topic presented in this chapter, quantitative approaches and methods will be described followed by qualitative approaches.

Quantitative Approaches

The group of research approaches imprecisely referred to as quantitative research is derived from the contemporary empiricism and logical positivism philosophical orientations (Weiss, 1995). Quantitative research is not a single entity, but rather a set of related research and activities that are bound together by precision in quantification. Contemporary views of empiricism in nursing research aim to improve nursing practice through an approach that examines multiple environmental and personal variables that may help explain situational and individual differences in response patterns. The requirements of a hypothetical-deductive approach are that empirical data (measurable evidence from particular events or experiences) are a logical consequence of, or correspond to, a specific theory and its related hypotheses. The hypothesis can be tested to support or refute theory selected *a priori*, or in advance.

Qualitative Approaches

The collection of different research traditions (e.g., phenomenology, hermeneutics) often referred to as qualitative has in common the view that reality consists of the meanings in a person's lived experience (Omery et al., 1995). As such, the development of knowledge through research must examine the nature and structure of one's lived experience. Although such an examination may not cover the universe of methods for knowledge development, it nevertheless is important in the study of nursing and the patient's experience and responses to health, illness, and treatments. In this approach, theory is not tested. Instead, perspectives and meanings from the subject's point of view are described and analyzed. New theory may or may not be generated.

In summary, philosophical approaches (from which methodology is derived) influence research but may often be unacknowledged in the research process of proposal preparation, data collection, data coding, and analysis. After identifying a research problem, researchers most often proceed through the remaining steps of the research, where computers play an important role.

Proposal Preparation: The Research Plan

One of the first steps in the research process is proposal preparation. Word-processing applications for microcomputers have become widely if not universally accepted as an overall aid in the clerical preparation of the research proposal. A variety of packages are available such as Microsoft Word (Microsoft Corporation, 2000) and WordPerfect (Corel Corporation, 2000). They provide a number of capabilities not only in processing words and making deletions and insertions possible, but also in formatting, change in formatting, spacing, and including tables and graphics within the proposal. They also provide assistance in developing a table of contents and checking spelling and some mechanical assistance in examining sentence structure.

References can either be typed in directly or be compiled in a bibliographic database that is compatible with a number of word-processing applications. Some examples of bibliographic applications are Reference Manager (Institute Information Systems, 1997), Procite (Niles Software, 1999a), and Endnote (Niles Software, 1999b). These reference/bibliographic applications can not only be programmed to conform to a large variety of reference styles, but offer other capabilities such as importing bibliographic citations from external sources, obtaining on-line bibliographic searches, customizing reference types, and citing references as you write.

Data Collection

Nurses may already be familiar with data collection. Patient monitoring, patient care documentation, and interview data are collected by nurses, although not always for research purposes. Data collection can take a number of forms depending on the type of research and variables of interest. Computers are used in data collection for surveys and questionnaires as well as to capture physiological and clinical nursing information in quantitative or descriptive patient care research. In terms of qualitative research requiring narrative content analysis, the computer can be used to record the observations, narrative statements of subjects, and memos of the researcher in initial word-processing applications for future coding. These narrative statements, like the quantitative surveys, can be either programmed for use in microcomputers or on the Internet's World Wide Web (WWW) so that subjects' responses can be entered directly into the computer.

Quantitative Data Collection

Questionnaires   Surveys and questionnaires, traditionally administered in paper and pencil forms, can be programmed into a computer application either in a microcomputer or on a Web site accessed through the Internet. The use of notebook microcomputers has gained popularity in recent years for allowing the user to enter the data directly into the computer program at the time of an interview with a subject. Responses to questions can be entered by the respondent or a surrogate directly into the computer or Web site through Internet access. The data from the Internet can then be downloaded for analysis.

Physiological Data   The collection of patient physiological parameters has long been used in physiological research. Some of these parameters can be measured directly from patient monitoring devices such as cardiac monitoring of heart rhythm, rate, and fluid or electrolytes. Measurements taken from spirometers and various types of imaging (e.g., neurological, cardiovascular, cellular) can also be entered directly from the patient into a computer program for analysis. Numerous measurements of intensity, amplitude, patterns, and shapes can be characterized by computer programs and used in research. For example, DNA damage can be measured by computer imaging of single cells following gel electrophoresis. Damaged DNA is drawn out of the cell nucleus during the procedure and appears as a comet when stained with fluorescent dye. Images are analyzed for the amount of DNA inside versus outside the densely stained nuclear region. Figure 26.1 presents an image of a single human sperm cell following single cell gel electrophoresis. The amount of DNA outside the dense nucleus is an indicator of double-stranded DNA breakage.

Nursing Care Data   The American Nurses Association (ANA) has supported the need to standardize nursing care terms for computer-based patient care systems. The clinical and economic importance of structured recording to represent nursing care was recognized by the acceptance of the Nursing Minimum Data Set (Werley et al., 1986). The American Nurses Association has accepted seven systems of terminology for the descrip-

tion of nursing practice: the North American Nursing Diagnosis Association (NANDA) taxonomy of nursing diagnosis, Georgetown Home Health Care Classification (McCormick et al., 1994; Saba, 1997; Zielstorff et al., 1995), Nursing Interventions Classification (Bulechek and McCloskey, 1997), Nursing Outcomes Classification (Daly et al., 1997), Patient Care Data Set (Ozbolt, 1999), Omaha Home Health Care (Martin and Norris, 1996), and the International Classification of Nursing Practice (Saba, 1997; Zielstorff at al., 1995). Other terminology that may encompass issues of major interest to nursing is the Minimum Data Set (MDS and MDS+) which is part of the Residence Assessment Inventory (RAI) used for the documentation of resident problems in nursing homes (Hansebo et al., 1999a, 1999b; Zulkowski, 1999).

Although none of the above has emerged as a de facto standard, a structured coding system is needed for the recording of patient care problems that are amenable to nursing actions, the actual nursing actions implemented in the care of patients, and the evaluation of the effectiveness of these actions. The use of structured terms across health care settings would provide for comparability of patient care using patient records.

Qualitative Data Collection

Patient care studies reported in the literature as having the subjects enter their own responses via a computer are studies on caregivers of persons with Alzheimer's and AIDS patients (Brennan and Ripich, 1994). Computers are not only able to record the subject's responses

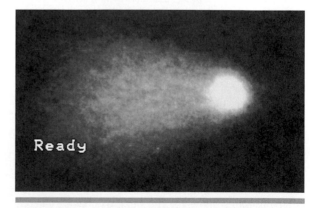

Figure 26.1
Physiologic imaging of a sperm cell.
(Courtesy Dr. Wendie Robbins, University of California Los Angeles School of Nursing, Los Angeles, CA.)

to the questions but also routinely record the number of minutes the subject was "on-line" and number of times they "logged-in." Simple electronic audiotaping is often used during interviews, whereby the interviews are entered into a word-processing program by clerical assistants in preparation for analysis.

The narrative statements entered into a word processor are stored for subsequent coding and sorting according to one's theoretical framework and categories that may emerge from the data as determined cognitively by the researcher. It is important to point out that for both quantitative and qualitative data, the computer application program is only a mechanical, clerical tool to aid the researcher in manipulating the data.

Data Coding

Quantitative Approaches

In quantitative studies, the data for the variables of interest are collected in a numerical form. These numerical values are entered into designated fields in the process of coding. Coding may be inherent in software programs for the physiologic data and many of the electronic surveys. The coding may be generated (by a computer program) from measurements directly obtained through imaging or physiological monitoring or entered into a computer by a patient or researcher from a printout or a questionnaire/survey into a database program. Most statistical programs contain data editors that permit the entry of data by a researcher as part of the statistical application. In such a situation, fields are designated, and numerical values can also be entered into the appropriate fields without the use of an extra program. Alternatively, initial coding can be entered into one of many general purpose data management programs such as Excel (Microsoft, 2000). The data management program used should be one that is compatible with common statistical packages so that the coded data can be analyzed by the researcher.

Care must be taken in coding and entering the data. The coding of data is a combination of cognitive decisions and mechanical clerical recording of responses in a numerical form. There are several ways of reviewing and "cleaning" the data prior to analyses. Some computer programs allow for the same data to be entered twice (preferably by different people to check for errors). One also must check for missing data and take them into consideration in the coding and analyses.

Reviewing data for values outside of those allowable is another way of examining the data for errors.

Qualitative Approaches

Historically, qualitative researchers have relied on narrative notes that may be often first audio-recorded then transcribed by a typist. Coding qualitative text-data was a time-consuming task, often involving thousands of pages of typewritten notes and the use of scissors and tape for the development of coding and categories. With the advent of computer packages, the mechanical aspects of the coding and sorting have been reduced. The researcher must decide on which text may be of interest and use a word-processing program to search for words, phrases, or other markers within a text file using any of a number of word-processing software packages. Some specific software packages developed for qualitative research coding and analysis interface directly with the most popular word-processing software packages. The application program Ethnograph (Seidel and Clark, 1984) was one of the first packages developed specifically for the purpose of managing some of the mechanical tasks of qualitative data analysis. Another qualitative package commonly used is NUD.IST (Non-numerical Unstructured Data Indexing Searching and Theorizing) (Gahan and Hannibal (1998); Richards and Richards, 1993). This program has been described by Richards and Richards (1993) as assisting the researcher to establish an index of data codes and seek relationships among the coding categories. The ease with which researchers can code and recode large amounts of data with the aid of computerized programs encourages the researcher to experiment with different ways of thinking about the data and recategorizing them. Retrieval of categories or elements of data is facilitated by computer storage.

In Ethnograph, the narrative text is first imported, and each line is numbered. The text is then "coded" by indicating segments that pertain to a particular code. Once the codes are entered, the Ethnograph program can be instructed to search the text (individually or across multiple cases) for specific coded segments. These segments are then generated as output and can be incorporated into a word-processing program or printed directly from Ethnograph for review. Figure 26.2 presents the result of a search for the codes "history" (history of the injury) and "signs" (signs and symptoms associated with injury) in one individual case. The results show that the code

```
SEARCH CODE: HISTORY, SIGNS

#-HISTORY
       :   As you reconstruct the history, when     24 -#ᵃ
       :   he fell -- this guy fell off the back    25  #
       :   of his truck.  The first thing that      26  #
$-SIGNS
       :   happened he had -- he had weakness or    27  #  -$ᵇ
       :   paralysis and numbness in both his       28  #   |
       :   legs.  Couldn't move for almost an       29  #   |
       :   hour.  And it began to come back.  And   30  #   |
       :   ever since that time he's had these --   31  #   |
       :   these weird sensations and pain --       32  #   |
       :   pain has gone from his legs.  Bladder    33  #   |
       :   and bowel disturbance.  Had a GU work-   34  #  -$
       :   up.  They can't document that he has a   35  #
       :   (------------).  I think he does.        36  #
       :   Impotence.  And I think he contused      37  #
       :   the spinal cord is what he did.          38 -#
a = # indicates the primary code in this segment "history".
b = $ indicates the secondary code in this segment "signs"; this code is also
    a sub-segment of the "history" segment.
```

Figure 26.2
Example of coding using Ethnograph.

"history" consists of a 15-line segment, while the code "signs" consists of an 8-line segment embedded within the "history" segment.

Data Analysis

Various types of quantitative and qualitative data analyses can be applied to nursing research such as quality improvement studies, intervention research, and outcomes research. A number of commercial software packages are available on microcomputers and on organizations' servers for use by everyone on the network. Some of the common ones are Statistical Package for Social Sciences (SPSS Inc., 1991), Statistical Analysis Services Institute (SAS Institute, 1999), Ethnograph (Seidel and Clark 1984; Seidel et al., 1994), and NUD.IST (Richards and Richards, 1993). Below is an overview of the methods used in quantitative and qualitative data analysis followed by three examples of data analyses used for different research questions.

Quantitative Analyses

Quantitative analysis is defined as "the building of models in which relations between conceptual elements of the inquiry are described quantitatively" (Behrens and Smith, 1996). There are myriad ways to consider data analysis. The presentation below is organized around the broad types of research of interest in nursing and general research goals or questions. The researcher may use different types of analyses depending on the goal of research. These goals may require different statistical examinations: descriptive/exploratory analyses, hypothesis testing, estimation of confidence intervals, model building through multivariate analysis, and structural equation model building. Various types of nursing research may contain a number of these goals. For example, to test a nursing intervention, one may first perform descriptive/exploratory analyses followed by a test of the hypotheses. Quality improvement, patient outcome, and survival analysis studies may likewise contain a number of different types of analyses depending on the specific research questions. The paragraphs below will first address some of the different types of analyses required by goals of the research. This description is followed by examples of types of nursing research that incorporate some of these types of analyses.

Exploratory Analysis   The researcher may first explore the data means, modes, distribution pattern, and standard deviations and examine graphic representations such as scatter plots or bar graphs. Tests of association or significant differences may be explored through chi-squares, correlations, and various univariate, bivariate, trivariate analyses and an examination of quartiles. The researcher can then easily identify patterns with respect to variables as well as groups of study subjects of interest. It is safe to say that well-known commercial statistical packages usually include programs for these analyses. Two of the most popular programs in use today are the Statistical Package for Social Sciences (SPSS Inc., 1999), and Statistical Analysis Services (SAS Institute, 1999).

During this analysis process, the researcher may recode or transform data by mathematically multiplying or dividing scores by certain log or factor values. New variables can also be created by combining several existing variables. These transformations or "re-expressions" allow the researcher to analyze the data in appropriate and interpretable scales (Behrens and Smith, 1996).

As part of exploratory analysis, simple and multiple regression analyses can be used to examine the relationship between selected variables and a dependent measure of interest. Certain models can be developed to determine which collection of variables provides the best prediction of the dependent measure. An example of a template taken from a commonly used program can be seen in Fig. 26.3.

The major commercial statistical programs also contain computer graphics systems for producing multidimensional plots, charts, maps, and other displays on screens and printers. A variety of patterns and colors can be used for these graphics to facilitate the reporting of results. Statistical computing is often done in the same environment as word processing and related applications such as graphics production. Many programs provide for graphic layouts and can be linked to spread sheet databases and word processors.

```
CONGESTIVE HEART FAILURE
MODEL  NCare = Rural, Urban, Hospsiz1, Hospsiz2, Hospsiz3, Char1, Char2, Char3, Char4
```

```
Model:  MODEL1
Dependent Variable:  NCare

Analysis of Variance

Parameter Estimates
```

Variable	DF	Parameter Estimate	Standard Error	T for Ho: Parameter= 0	Prob > |T|	Variable Label
INTERCEP	1	1.99	0.11	18.29	0.0001	Intercept
RURAL	1	-0.31	0.17	-1.77	0.08	RURAL
URBAN	1	-0.16	0.11	-1.50	0.14	URBAN
HOSPSIZ1	1	0.69	0.17	4.17	0.00	LESS THAN OR EQUAL TO 100 BEDS
HOSPSIZ2	1	0.25	0.13	1.89	0.06	101-200 HOSPITAL BEDS
HOSPSIZ3	1	0.22	0.11	1.92	0.06	201-400 HOSPITAL BEDS
CHAR1	1	0.21	0.13	1.60	0.11	EQUIPMENT
CHAR2	1	0.44	0.13	3.30	0.00	NURSE/PATIENT RATIO
CHAR3	1	0.52	0.13	3.84	0.00	AUTONOMY IN DECISION MAKING
CHAR4	1	0.12	0.13	0.92	0.36	LICENSED

Figure 26.3
Example of regression analysis.

Hypothesis Testing or Confirmatory Analyses

Hypothesis testing or confirmatory analyses are based on an interest in relationships and describing what would occur if a hypothesis were true. The analysis of data allows us to compare the actual outcomes with the hypothesized outcomes. Inherent in hypothesis testing is the probability (p value) of an event occurring given a certain relationship. These are conditional relationships based on the variables selected for study, and the typical mathematical tables and software for determining p values are accurate only insofar as the assumptions of the test are met (Behrens and Smith, 1996). Certain statistical concepts such as statistical power, type II error, selecting alpha values to balance type II errors, and sampling distribution are decisions that the researcher must make regardless of the type of computer software. These concepts are covered in greater detail in research methodology courses and are outside the scope of the present discussion.

Model Building

An application used for confirmatory hypothesis testing approach to multivariate analysis is structural equation modeling (SEM) (Byrne, 1984). Byrne describes this procedure as consisting of two aspects: (1) that the causal processes under study are represented by a series of structural (i.e., regression) equations, and (2) that these structural relations can be modeled pictorially to enable a clearer conceptualization of the theory under study. The model can be tested statistically in a simultaneous analysis of the entire system of variables to determine the extent to which it is consistent with the data. If goodness of fit is adequate, the model argues for the plausibility of postulated relationships among variables (Byrne, 1984). Most researchers may wish to consult a statistician to discuss the underlying assumptions of the data and plans for testing the model. Different types of modeling programs, such as LISREL (Joreskog and Sorbom, 1978) or EQS (Byrne, 1984), are commercially available. The researcher will identify latent (unobservable) variables of interest (e.g., emotions) and link them to those that are observable (direct measurement) and plan with the statistician to specify and examine the impact of one latent construct on another in the modeling of causal direction.

Meta-analysis

Meta-analysis is a technique that allows researchers to combine data across studies to achieve more focused estimates of population parameters and examine effects of a phenomenon or intervention across multiple studies. It uses the effect size as a common metric of study effectiveness and deals with the statistical problems inherent in using individual significance tests in a number of different studies. It weights study outcomes in proportion to their sample size and focuses on the size of the outcomes rather than on whether or not they are significant.

Although the computations can be done with the aid of a reliable commercial statistical package, the researcher needs to consider the following specific issues in performing the meta-analysis (Behrens and Smith, 1996): (1) justify which studies are comparable and which are not, (2) rely on knowledge of the substantive area to identify relevant study characteristics, (3) evaluate and account for differences in study quality, and (4) assess the generalizability of the results from fields with little empirical data. Each of these issues must be addressed with a critical review prior to performing the meta-analysis.

Meta-analysis offers a way to examine results of a number of quantitative research that meet meta-analysis researchers' criteria. Meta-analysis overcomes problems encountered in studies using different sample sizes and instruments. Behrens and colleagues remind us that it is important not simply to rely on the market power of a program. Even widely used programs may have extensive numeric errors. As a hedge against these difficulties, potential users should read software reviews provided by statistical journals such as *American Statistician* (Behrens and Smith, 1997).

In summary, the major theme of this section has been the plurality of traditions in quantitative research analysis. As computers free researchers from the hand analysis, researchers will have increased opportunities to focus on the philosophical, theoretical, and logical underpinnings of these approaches.

Qualitative Data Analysis

Qualitative research, like quantitative research, is not a single entity, but a set of related yet individual traditions, aims, and methods. Some individual traditions within qualitative research are ethnography, grounded theory, phenomenology, and hermeneutics. The distinguishing feature of qualitative research is that the goal is to understand the qualities or essence of phenomena and/or focus on the meaning of these events to the participants or respondents in the study. The forms of data are usually the words of the respondents or informants rather than numbers. Computerization is especially helpful to the researcher in handling large amounts of data.

Computer Application Programs   A number of general-purpose or specific software packages can be used in qualitative analysis: one package that can be used is a free text retrieval program such as that available in a word-processing program; another is any of a number of standard database management or indexing programs; a third is a program specifically developed for the purpose of qualitative analysis. Two of the commonly used special-purpose programs for qualitative analysis are Ethnograph (Seidel and Clark, 1984) and NUD.IST (Richards and Richards, 1993). In addition, logic-based systems that use "if-then" rules for representation of relationships and conceptual network systems are also available (Huberman and Miles, 1999).

General-Purpose Software   Word-processing programs in current use offer a number of features useful to the qualitative researcher. The ability to search for certain key words allows the researcher to tag the categories of interest. In addition, such features as cut and paste; linking texts; insertion of pictures, tables, and charts; and the inclusion of video and audio data enhance the application.

Data management programs (e.g., Excel) can be used to categorize data, link categories, and address a number of queries within categories, domains, or themes of interest. For example, the researcher can list all early adolescents who smoked more than one pack (of cigarettes) per day who gave birth to pre-term babies. These programs work better for discrete rather than unstructured texts.

Special-Purpose Software   As mentioned, some software have been developed for the specific purpose of analyzing qualitative data. Ethnograph is one such program, which is used after the data have been entered using a word-processing program and converted to an ASCII file. Each file can be designated by its context and identifying features with markers provided by the computer program. The researcher can have the program produce a file that numbers each line of the narrative data. From this line file, the researcher can begin to assign each line or paragraph a category. The researcher keeps track of the category definitions and is alert to dimensions that emerge. Recoding can be done to provide for inductive thinking and iterative comparisons. Through the use of a "search command," the computer program can be made to search for data segments by categories throughout the typed document.

Ethnograph provides a column format, permitting numbered lines in the first column and categorical notations in the second column. Using a command entered by a researcher, it can selectively or globally delete or replace coding categories and produce an output file containing sorted, cross-referenced coded segments from the original text data sets entered via a word-processing program. The split screen allows the researcher to view more than one file at a time, so is useful in constant comparison and contrasting of data. Researcher memos and theoretical notes written by the researcher during analysis can also be stored and retrieved with Ethnograph.

NUD.IST (Richards and Richards, 1993)   With this program, the researcher establishes an index of data codes and seeks relationships among the coding categories. NUD.IST uses a hierarchical tree structure to provide a graphic representation of the relationships between and among codes/categories. The ability of the NUD.IST program to search for co-occurring codes, identifying relationships among codes, helps the researcher to gain new insight from the data. Computer enhancements that build connections between categories of data may suggest relationships between concepts, but it is up to the researcher to establish the meaning and significance of the suggested relationships through intensive analysis (Taft, 1993).

Logic-Based Systems   These applications use rules for representation of hypotheses. Although some of the retrieval patterns are Boolean, such as looking for one code or another in combinations in a text, they may also search for positive and negative cases of a code (Huberman and Miles, 1999). The program may also be used to print out matrices if the researcher determines a set of codes for columns (e.g., ages), and another set for rows (e.g., categories of statements indicating a range of depression). Each cell in the matrix then will contain the text segments indexed by both the column and row codes for the cell (Huberman and Miles, 1999).

Conceptual Network Systems   A system known as concept diagrams, semantic nets, or conceptual networks is one in which information is represented in a graphic manner. The objects in one's conceptual system (e.g., age, experiences) are coded and represented by a box diagram (node). The objects are linked (by arcs) to other objects to show relationships. Like rule-based systems, semantic nets have been widely used in artificial intelligence work. In order to view the relationships of an object in the system, the researcher examines the node in the graph and follows the arcs to and from it

(Huberman and Miles, 1999). Semantic network applications may be useful in model building and providing a pictorial overview.

Data Analysis for Qualitative Data Qualitative data analyses often occur on an ongoing basis with data collection in a reflexive and iterative fashion. There is no clear demarcation of when data collection should end and analysis begin. The process of obtaining observations, interviews, and other data over a period of time results in a vast body of data that may be hundreds or thousands of pages of field notes and researcher memos. Although computer applications can aid considerably in organizing and sorting this massive data, the theoretical and analytical aspects of decision-making about concepts and themes must be made by the researcher.

As an example, some of the tasks the computer can facilitate in data analysis using grounded theory (one approach to qualitative research) are as follows. Once a researcher has determined which parts of the interviews and observations can be tagged as categories, certain properties or dimensions can be determined and coded. The researcher may engage in "constant comparison" to compare every incident that has been categorized by the same code and compare its meaning with other incidents similarly categorized. This process should continue until the researcher determines that the categories are internally consistent, fit with the data, and are saturated. Saturation is achieved when the researcher can find no more properties for a category and new data are redundant with the old (Behrens and Smith, 1996).

Strauss and Corbin (1990) suggest that, in the later stages of research, the researcher may engage in axial coding. In this stage, the research elaborates and explains key categories considering the conditions under which the event occurs, the processes that take place, and possible consequences. Glaser (1978) indicates that the researcher may engage in theoretical sampling, which is a deliberate search for episodes in incidents that enlarge the variances of properties and place boundaries around categories.

Uses and Caution Software programs for qualitative research save time for the researcher in terms of file management, reducing the manual labor of cutting, pasting, sorting, and manual filing. They may also encourage the researcher to examine the data from different perspectives, re-coding and reorganizing the data in different frameworks.

One must be mindful that qualitative analysis is a cognitive process, not a mechanical one. The essence of qualitative research is the meaning and interpretation of the data within context. Taft believes that there may be cause for concern when researchers assume the reality of the concepts identified and emphasize their frequency rather than their meaning (1993). The ability of software enhancements to generate quasi-frequency distributions and cross-tabulations may tend to further increase the investigator's confidence in believing such findings and relationships when in fact these may be an artifact of the way in which the data are manipulated. While computer programs facilitate coding, organization of data, and preparation of the data for interpretation, they cannot replace the thinking and decision-making that is at the heart of qualitative analysis. As in all research, the burden of analysis and interpretation rests on the researchers.

■ Dissemination of Results

While dissemination of results continues to occur by traditional means such as presentations at professional meetings and publication in journals and monographs, on-line reporting is becoming increasingly common. Some Web sites frequented by nurses are peer review journals such as *Online Journal of Nursing Informatics (http://www.cisnet.com/)* and selected nursing articles on various Web sites such as that of the American Nurses Association *(http://www.nursingworld.org)*. Nursing forums sponsored by various professional nursing organizations (e.g., *American Journal of Nursing*, Sigma Theta Tau, National League for Nursing) often allow participants to chat on-line with presenters or authors of certain articles on designated dates during scheduled times. Nearly all organizations have their own Web sites. Some examples are the Alzheimer's Disease Education and Referral Center *(http://www.alzheimers.org)*, American Heart Association *(http://www.americanheart.org)*, American Medical Informatics Association *(http://www.amia.org)*, and RAND Corporation *(http://www.rand.org)*. The Cochran Collection has numerous centers all over the world (e.g., for San Francisco, E-mail: *sfcc@sirius.com*; Canada: *http://hiru.mcmaster.ca/cochrane/centres/canadian/*, Dutch: *http://www.amc.uval.nl*, Italian: *http://www.areas.it*; Germany:*httpi://www.cochrane.de*; Providence, RI: *http://www.cochrane.org*). As with all publications, on-line as well as hardcopies, the information accessed must be evaluated by the users for their appropriateness for the purpose for which it was retrieved.

Reports to some agencies may be submitted on-line. In fact, there is a trend for all paper submissions to be accomplished on-line. For many agencies within the federal government, the grant application, submission, and reporting are all performed on-line.

Regardless of the method of submission and medium for publication, the published article may be incorporated into one or several on-line bibliographic retrieval systems. By means of bibliographic retrieval systems, a search may be made as described in Chap. 27, and the record may be retrieved either as a listing, listing with abstract, or in many cases listing with abstract and complete article.

Other means of dissemination for results of research such as clinical guidelines are through health agencies or health care facilities for utilization by health care professionals. These guidelines can often be integrated into a hospital's or health care facility's information system and evaluated after a period of use.

The foregoing has described the application of computers for both quantitative and qualitative research in the steps of the research process: proposal preparation, data collection, data coding and data analysis, and research dissemination. We turn next to a few examples of research in which some of the above-mentioned strategies or combinations thereof have been used in various types of research.

Examples of Research Studies

Some examples of quantitative nursing studies that use large hospital databases for research are provided by Maas (1997), Daly et al. (1997), Bernabei et al. (1994), and Johnson and Maas (1998). To study outcomes, a query question may be: When patients with a stratified validated diagnosis are treated by (item X), what are the differences in mortality, disability, subsequent symptoms, side effects, or costs? (Daly et al., 1997). The data for outcome analysis generally include patient demographic and/or hospital characteristics, antecedent variables, interventions (care or treatment variables), and outcomes (mortality, hospital readmission, changes in symptoms or status). Patients may be examined by groups or characteristics or by stratified sampling by a selected variable such as hospital size. Examples of variables used for outcome analysis may include the following:

Demographics: age, gender, ethnicity, or type of insurance.

Intervening variables: nursing assessments, reassessments, procedures, patient and family teaching.

Outcomes: may include   cost, length of stay, mortality, functional and mental status, status of

decubiti, anxiety, patient satisfaction, number of falls.

A number of large data sets are available for researchers who wish to conduct secondary data analyses. For example, national data sets such as the MDS for nursing homes, uniform hospital discharge data, or datasets from insurance companies or health care systems can be used (Hansebo et al., 1999; Zulkowski, 1999 Hansebo et al., 1999; Chang, et al., 1996).

Another example of a study using large databases is SAGE (Bernabei et al., 1994) (Systematic Assessment of Geriatric Drug Use via Epidemiology). The database is composed of (1) nursing home resident data collected with the MDS, (2) data on drugs used at the time of MDS assessment, (3) health services-related Medicare claims, (4) structural and staffing facility information from the OSCAR (On-line Survey Certification of Automated Records) archive, and (5) health market and county census data from the Area Resource File. After the linking and processing of the data, analyses were performed by using the statistical program SAS. Bernabei et al. (1994) found that over 10 percent of the facilities had special care units, indications of health deficiencies were present for more than two thirds of the facilities, and the proportion of physicians and nursing personnel were highly variable among the states studied (Kansas, Maine, Mississippi, New York, and South Dakota).

Research on patient treatments and outcomes can contribute to evidence-based research for developing clinical guidelines by the Agency for Healthcare Research and Quality (AHRQ) U.S. Preventive Services Task Force, the Canadian Task Force on the Periodic Health Examination, and the American College of Physicians (Atkins and DiGuiseppi, 1998). More recently, studies have been undertaken by the American Nurses Association (1996, 2000) in the examination of nurse staffing and patient outcome. Systematic reviews of research on specific conditions, recommended treatment, and outcomes were conducted in the development of these guides. Moreover, important contributions by personnel other than physicians (e.g., nurses) have not been well-documented in order for definitive recommendations to be made. Definitive trials have been completed for only a minority of preventive services (Atkins and DiGuiseppi, 1998) and clinical conditions. Given the time and expense of long-term trials, Atkins and DiGuiseppi (1998) recommend several alternatives for researchers. These methods include observational studies, linking single studies, and the use of meta-analysis.

Examples of Qualitative Research

An ethnograph was used by Smyer and Chang (1999) to describe a typology of caregivers who use respite care and the phases of its adoption. Using anthropological fieldwork methods, data were obtained directly from the caregivers during informal interviews, which were audiotaped, and from nontechnical literature (notes written by family members to the staff). Transcribed interviews were read for meaningful units and emerging themes (coherent ideas). Coding was performed in which data were read, separated into meaningful units, examined, compared, categorized, and conceptualized. Throughout the process, memos of initial thoughts regarding the interview were recorded in the margins and subsequently utilized in the coding analysis or interpretation of the data. The meaningful units and major broader categories of ideas (themes) were coded and compared and contrasted to detect similarities and differences among the caregivers. Themes and dimensions that arose from categories were identified and coded. Certain categories judged to be central to the study (e.g., type of respite) were related to other categories. Nursing notes, medical records, social work commentary, and hospital financial and admission records as well as notes left for staff before a respite care stay by caregivers were also analyzed. Nontechnical literature supplemented interviews and provided a cross-check on data.

Koopman and Schweitzer (1999) used a phenomenological qualitative research method to explore an individual's experience of having symptoms of multiple sclerosis (MS) for a period of time and then being told he/she had MS. Interviews were conducted with five purposefully selected participants. The process of data analysis highlighted common threads and patterns among informants in which four major themes emerged. The themes were: (a) whispered beginnings (listening for meanings and creating possible answers); (b) echoes of silence (worrying; wondering; waiting); (c) the spoken words (hearing the name of the diagnosis and telling others their story); and (d) creating voice (claiming the diagnosis and refocusing). These themes, derived from the patient's own words, facilitate the health care professionals' understanding of individuals experiencing early symptoms of MS.

Summary

This chapter has reviewed two of the loosely grouped philosophical orientations underlying approaches to research and the use of computers in various stages of the research process. We have also provided examples of some quantitative and qualitative studies that have utilized computers and various commercial application packages. Hopefully, the plurality of approaches derived from different philosophical orientations and the computer applications briefly described will be a beginning for further exploration for the reader. With the facilitation of the mechanical and clerical aspects of research by computers, the researcher will be freed to interpret new relationships and gain added insight never before available. The coming decade will offer yet undreamed of possibilities for nursing research.

References

American Nurses Association. (1996). *Nursing Quality Indicators: Definitions and Implications*. Washington, D. C.: American Nurses Association.

American Nurses Association. (1997). *Implementing Nursing's Report Card: A Study of RN Staffing, Length of Stay and Patient Outcome*. Washington, D. C.: American Nurses Association.

American Nurses Association (2000). *Nurse Staffing and Patient Outcomes in the Inpatient Hospital Setting*. Washington, D.C.: American Nurses Association.

Atkins, D., and DiGuiseppi, C.G . (1998). Broadening the evidence base for evidence-based guidelines. *American Journal of Preventive Medicine, 14*, 335–344.

Behrens, J. T., and Smith, M. L. (1996). Data and Data Analysis. In D. Berliner and R. Calsee (Eds.), *Handbook of Educational Psychology* (pp. 945–989). New York: MacMillan Library Reference.

Bernabei, R., Bambassi, G., Lapane, K., et al. (1994). Characteristics of the SAGE database: A new resource for research on outcomes in long-term care. *Journal of Gerontology: Medical Sciences, 54*, M25–M33.

Brennan, P. F., and Ripich, S. (1994). Use of a home-care computer network by persons with AIDS. *International Journal of Technology Assessment In Health Care, 10*, 258–272.

Bulechek, G. M., and McCloskey, J. (1997). All users of NIC encouraged to submit new interventions, suggest revisions. Iowa Intervention Project Research Team. *Image: The Journal of Nursing Scholarship, 1*, 10–20.

Byrne, B. M. (1984). *Structural Equation Modeling with EQS and EQS/Windows: Basic Concepts, Applications, and Programming*. Thousand Oaks, CA: Sage Publications.

Chang, B. L., Lee, J., Pearson, M., et al. (1996). *Where Are the Data. Outcome Measures and Care Delivery Systems*. Washington, D.C: AHCPR.

Corel Corporation. (2000). *Wordperfect 9 (2000)*. Ottawa, Ontario, Canada.

Daly, J. M., Maas, M. L., and Johnson, M. (1997). Nursing outcomes classification. An essential element in data sets for nursing and health care effectiveness. *Computers in Nursing, 15,* S82–S86.

Gahan, C., and Hannibal, M. (1998). *Doing qualitative Research using QSR NUD.IST.* Thousand Oaks, CA: SCOLARI Sage Publications Software.

Glaser, B. G. (1978). *Theoretical Sensitivity.* Mill Valley, CA: Sociological Press.

Hansebo, G., Kihlgren, M., and Ljunggren, G. (1999a). Review of nursing documentation in nursing home wards—changes after intervention for individualized care. *Journal of Advanced Nursing, 6,* 1462–73.

Hansebo, G., Kihlgren, M., Ljunggren, G., and Winbald, B. (1999b). Staff views on the Resident Assessment Instrument, RAI/MDS, in nursing homes, and the use of the Cognitive Performance Scale, CPS, in different levels of care in Stockholm, Sweden. *Journal of Advanced Nursing, 3,* 642–653.

Huberman, A. M., and Miles, M. B. (1999). Data management and analysis methods. In N. K. Denzin YSL (Ed.), *Handbook of Qualitative Research* (pp. 428–440). Thousand Oaks, CA: Sage Publications.

Institute Information Systems. (1997). *Reference Manager* (Version 8). Carlsbad, CA.

Johnson, M., and Maas, M. (1998). Implementing the Nursing Outcomes Classification in a practice setting. *Outcomes Management for Nursing Practice, 2,* 99–104.

Joreskog, K. G., and Sorbom, D. (1978). *LISREL IV's User's Guide.* Chicago, IL: National Educational Resources.

Koopman, W., and Schweitzer, A. (1999). The journey to multiple sclerosis: A qualitative study. *Journal of Neuroscience Nursing, 1,* 17–26.

Maas, M. L. (1997). Advancing nursing's accountability for outcomes. *Outcomes Management for Nursing Practice, 1,* 3–4.

Martin, K. S., and Norris, J. (1996). The Omaha System: A model for describing practice. *Holistic Nursing Practice, 11,* 75–83.

McCormick, K. A., Lang, N., Zielstorff, R., et al. (1994). Toward standard classification schemes for nursing language: Recommendations of the American Nurses Association Steering Committee on databases to support clinical nursing practice. *Journal of the American Medical Informatics Association, 1,* 421–427.

Microsoft Corporation. (2000). *Excel 97/2000.* Redmond, WA.

Microsoft Corporation. (2000). *Microsoft Word 97/2000.* Redmond, WA.

Niles Software Inc. (1999a). *ProCite* (Version 3.0). ISI ResearchSoft. Berkeley, CA.

Niles Software Inc. (1999b). *Endnote.* (Version 3.0). ISI ResearchSoft. Berkeley, CA.

Omery, A., C. E. Kasper, and G. G. Page (Eds.) (1995). *In Search of Nursing Science* (pp. 139–158). Thousand Oaks, CA: Sage Publications.

Ozbolt, J. G. (1999). *Testimony to the NCVHS Hearings on Medical Terminology and Code Development.* School of Nursing and Division of Biomedical Informatics, School of Medicine, Vanderbilt University.

Richards, L., and Richards, T. J. (1993). OSR NUD.IST. Victoria, Australia: Qualitative Solutions & Research Dty, Ltd.

Saba, V. K. (1997). Why the home health care classification is a recognized nursing nomenclature. *Computers in Nursing, 15,* S69–S76

SAS Institute. (1999). *Statistical Analysis System.* Cary, NC.

Seidel, J., and Clark, J. (1984). The Ethnograph: A computer program for the analysis of qualitative data. *Qualitative Sociology, 7*(12), 110–125.

Seidel, J., Friese, S., and Lenard, C. (1994). *Ethnograph* (Version 4.0) Amherst, MA: Qualis Research Associates.

Smyer, T., and Chang, B. L. (1999). A typology of consumers of institutional respite care. *Clinical Nursing Research, 1,* 26–50.

SPSS Inc. (1999). *Statistical Package for Social Sciences (SPSS).* Chicago.

Strauss, A, and Corbin, J.M . (1990). *Basics of Qualitative Research: Grounded Theory Procedures and Techniques.* Newbury Park, CA: Sage Publications.

Taft, L. B. (1993). Computer-assisted qualitative research. *Research in Nursing & Health, 16,* 379–383.

Weiss, S. J. (1995). Contemporary empiricism. In A. Omery, C. E. Kasper and G. G. Page (Eds.), *In Search of Nursing Science* (pp. 13–17). Thousand Oaks, CA: Sage Publications.

Werley, H. H., Lang, N. M., and Westlake, S. K. (1986). The Nursing Minimum Data Set Conference: Executive summary. *Journal of Professional Nursing, 2,* 217–224.

Zielstorff, R. D., Lang, N. M., Saba, V. K., et al. (1995). Toward a uniform language for nursing in the US: Work of the American Nurses Association Steering Committee on Databases to Support Clinical Practice. *Medinfo, 8,* pt. 2, 1362–1366.

Zulkowski, K. (1999). MDS+ Items not contained in the pressure ulcer RAP associated with pressure ulcer, prevalence in newly institutionalized elderly. *Ostomy/Wound Management, 1,* 24–33.

CHAPTER 27

Computerized Information Resources

Diane S. Pravikoff
June Levy

OBJECTIVES

1. Identify steps in choosing appropriate databases.
2. Identify steps in planning a computer search for information.
3. Identify sources of information for practicing nurses.
4. Identify the difference between essential and supportive computerized resources.

KEYWORDS

information retrieval
MEDLARS
CINAHL
unified medical language systems
World Wide Web
information resources
health reference databases

This chapter presents information about electronic resources that are easily available and accessible and can assist nurses in maintaining and enhancing their professional practice. These resources aid in maintaining currency with the published literature, developing a list of sources for practice, research and/or education, and collaborating with colleagues.

As is evidenced by earlier chapters, nurses use computers for many purposes. Most attention has been paid in the past to computerized patient records, acuity systems, and physician ordering systems, among others. However, one of the major purposes for which computers can be used is searching for information. Many information resources are available by computer, and the information retrieved from them can be used to accomplish different ends. In fact, just as the method in a research study should be determined by the question being asked, the information resources should be appropriate to the need. It is important that the nursing professional determine her/his exact requirements before searching for information. Planning the search will be stressed throughout this chapter.

To maintain their professional credibility nursing professionals must (1) maintain currency with the published literature; (2) develop and maintain a list of bibliographic and other sources on specific topics of interest for practice, research, and/or education; and (3) collaborate and network with colleagues regarding issues of professional practice. Electronic resources are available to meet each of these needs. This chapter addresses each of these requirements for professional credibility and will discuss both essential and supportive computerized resources available to meet them. *Essential* computerized resources are defined as those resources that are vital and necessary to the practitioner to accomplish the specific goal. In the case of maintaining currency, for example, these resources include bibliographic retrieval systems such as MEDLINE or the CINAHL database, current awareness, or review services and may be accessible in various formats: CD-ROM, Internet, or World Wide Web. *Supportive* computerized resources are those that are helpful and interesting and supply good information but are not necessarily essential for professional practice. In meeting the requirement of maintaining currency, supportive computerized resources include document delivery services, electronic publishers, and metasites on the World Wide Web. There are many resources available to meet each of the above requirements for professional credibility. For the purposes of this chapter, selective resources will be identified and discussed as examples of the types of information available. Web site URLs of the various resources will be included as well.

■ Maintaining Currency with the Published Literature

It is obvious that one of the most important obligations a nurse must meet is to maintain currency in her/his field of practice. With the extreme demands in the clinical environment—both in time and amount of work—nurses need easily accessible resources to answer practice-related questions and ensure that they are practicing with the latest and most research-based (evidence-based) information. Information is needed about current treatments, trends, medications, safety issues, business practices, and new health issues among other topics.

The purpose of the information retrieved from the sources listed below is to enable nurses to keep abreast of the latest and most research-based information in their selected field. Both quantity *and* quality must be considered.

When using an information resource, check that:

1. The resource covers the specialty/field needed

2. The primary journals and peripheral material in the field are included

3. The resource is updated regularly and is current

4. The resource covers the years needed

5. The resource covers material published in different countries and in different languages

6. There is some form of peer review, reference checking, or other means of evaluation

Essential Computerized Resources

Essential computerized resources for maintaining currency include bibliographic retrieval systems for the journal literature, current awareness services, and review services of the journal literature and currently published books. All of these assist the nurse in gathering the most current and credible information.

Bibliographic Retrieval Systems   One of the most useful resources for accessing information about current practice is the journal literature. While there may be delays between the writing and publishing of an article, this time period is seldom more than a few months. The best way to peruse this literature is through a bibliographic retrieval system, since there is far too much literature published to be able to read it all. Bibliographic retrieval systems also allow filtering and sorting of this vast amount of published material.

A bibliographic retrieval system database allows the nurse to retrieve a list of citations that give the bibliographic details of the material indexed, subject headings, and author abstracts when possible. The nurse can search these systems using subject headings or keywords on a particular topic—subject or keyword searching. Most bibliographic retrieval systems have controlled vocabulary, also known as a thesaurus or subject heading list, to make electronic subject searching much easier. For this reason, the vocabulary is geared toward the specific content of the database. These controlled vocabularies are made available on-line as part of the database. Keyword searching is necessary when there are no subject headings to cover the concepts being searched. The nurse can also search by specific fields including author, author affiliation, journal title, ISSN, grant name or number, or publication type. In bibliographic retrieval systems, most fields in the records are word-indexed and can be searched individually to retrieve specific information.

Previously available as print indexes, these systems are now available electronically on CD-ROM, through on-line services, or via the World Wide Web. To access them, the nurse requires a computer with a CD-ROM drive, a modem and/or Internet access.

Since each of these bibliographic retrieval systems has its own specific content, it is possible that a nurse may have to search several systems to retrieve a comprehensive list of citations on a particular topic. Lists with descriptions of appropriate bibliographic retrieval systems can be found on the World Wide Web, e.g., Networked Digital Resources by The University of Michigan (*http://henry.ugl.lib.umich.edu/libhome/digResources/ Health.html*), Database Descriptions by Dykes Library (*http://www.kumc.edu/service/dykes/TIPSHEET/*) and MEDLINEplus by the National Library of Medicine (NLM) (*http://medlineplus.nlm.nih.gov/medlineplus/ searchdatabases.html*).

The main bibliographic retrieval systems that should first be considered by nurses are: MEDLINE, the

CINAHL database, ERIC, PsycINFO, and the Social SciSearch database.

MEDLINE   The NLM's MEDLARS (Medical Literature Analysis and Retrieval System) system has over 40 on-line databases containing over 18 million references (MEDLARS) (Table 27.1). One of these, MEDLINE, covers 3,900 journals in 40 languages from 1966 to the present in the fields of medicine, nursing, preclinical sciences, health care systems, veterinary medicine, and dentistry (MEDLINE). The nursing subset in MEDLINE is drawn from the International Nursing Index (INI) and covers 328 nursing journals (International Nursing Index, 1998). The database is updated weekly on the World Wide Web and monthly on CD-ROM.

The NLM's databases use a controlled vocabulary (thesaurus), called MeSH (Medical Subject Headings) (*www.nim.nih.gov/databases/databases.html*). These index terms facilitate subject searching within the databases.

MEDLINE and the nursing subset are available free over the World Wide Web through the NLM's home page at *http://www.nlm.nih.gov*. There are two ways to search this database: PubMed and Internet Grateful Med (*www.nim.nih.gov/pubs/factsheets/medline.html*). The database is also available through the commercial vendors mentioned below. All of these options allow the nurse to search by subject, keyword, author, title, or a combination of these. An example of different searches with a display using the Cinahl Information Systems interface is shown in Figs. 27.1 and 27.2.

Loansome DOC allows the nurse to place an order for a copy of an article through the National Network of Library of Medicine (NN/LM), and for more than 200 journals there are links to the publishers' Web pages, where the full article can be viewed or requested for a fee (*www.nim.nih.gov/pubs/factsheets/medline.html*).

CINAHL   The CINAHL database, produced by Cinahl Information Systems, provides comprehensive coverage of the literature in nursing and allied health from 1982 to the present. It also covers chiropractic, podiatry, health promotion and education, health services administration, biomedicine, optometry, women's health, consumer health, and alternative therapy (*Cumulative Index to Nursing and Allied Health Literature*, 1998). Over 1,200 journals and books, pamphlets, dissertations, audiovisuals, software, and proceedings are indexed. Some journals covered are published in other countries. Full text for some critical paths, research instruments, practice acts and standards of practice, drugs, legal cases, patient education handouts, accreditation and clinical innovation documents, and Web site descriptions is available. It is updated monthly.

The CINAHL database also uses a controlled vocabulary for effective subject searching. The CINAHL *Subject Heading List* uses the National Library of Medicine's MeSH terms as the standard vocabulary for disease, drug, anatomical, and physiological concepts (*CINAHL 1999 Subject Heading List*, 1999). There are approximately 4,250 unique CINAHL terms for nursing and the allied health disciplines. Specific field searching and quality filters are available in the CINAHL database and are similar to those found in MEDLINE. An essential part of research papers is the list of references pointing to prior publications. Cited references from selected nursing and allied health journals are searchable in the CINAHL database.

This bibliographic retrieval system and the others mentioned below are available through commercial vendors on CD-ROM, through on-line services, or via the World Wide Web. Some of the main commercial vendors are Dialog Corporation, Ovid Technologies, SilverPlatter Information, Inc., OCLC (Online Computer Library Center, Inc.), EBSCO Publishing, and Aries Systems Corporation. It is possible to check on the Web sites of these commercial vendors which databases are available and if there are any new ones.

ERIC   The ERIC (Educational Resources Information Center) database is published by the United States Department of Education and contains more than 950,000 citations covering education-related literature. It covers virtually all types of print materials, published and unpublished, from 1966 to the present day. This database gives the nurse a more comprehensive coverage of education (research and practice) than any other bibliographic retrieval system. The database is updated monthly on the World Wide Web and quarterly on CD-ROM (About AskERIC). A controlled vocabulary, *Thesaurus of Eric Descriptors*, assists with computer searches of this database on the Internet through the World Wide Web, through Gopher, through the commercial vendors mentioned above, and through public networks. As with the other two bibliographic databases mentioned above, nurses are able to access all of the data in each record on ERIC by searching, using subject headings or keywords or by searching for a word(s) in a specific field (Barrett and Colby, 1995).

Table 27.1   A List of Major MEDLARS Databases

Database	Subject	Type
General Databases		
AIDSDRUGS	Substances being tested in AIDS-related clinical trials	Factual
AIDSLINE (AIDS information on-LINE)	AIDS and related topics	Bibliographic citations
AIDSTRIALS (AIDS clinical TRIALS)	Clinical trials of substances being tested for use against AIDS, HIV infection, and AIDS-related opportunistic diseases	Factual and referral
BIOETHICSLINE (BIOETHICS on-LINE)	Ethics and related public policy issues in health care and biomedical research	Bibliographic citations
ChemID (CHEMical IDentification)	Dictionary of chemicals	Factual
DIRLINE (Directory of Information Resources on-LINE)	Directory of organizations providing information services	Referral
HealthSTAR (Health Services, Technology, Administration, and Research)	Clinical (emphasizes the evaluation of patient outcomes and the effectiveness of procedures, programs, products, services, and processes) and nonclinical (emphasizes health care administration and planning) aspects of health care delivery; combines former HEALTH (Health Planning and Administration) and HSTAR (Health Service/Technology Assessment Research) databases	Bibliographic citations
HISTLINE (HISTory of medicine on-LINE)	History of medicine and related sciences	Bibliographic citations
HSPROJ (Health Services Research Projects in Progress)	Health services research including health technology assessment and the development and use of clinical practice guidelines	Research project descriptions
ILS (Integrated Library System)	Catalogs of books, audiovisuals, and journal articles held at National Library of medicine, as well as a list of health-related organizations	Bibliographic citations
MEDLINE (MEDlars on-LINE)	Biomedicine	Bibliographic citations
MeSH Vocabulary File	Thesaurus of biomedicine-related terms	Factual
OLDMEDLINE	Biomedicine	Bibliographic citations
POPLINE (POPulation information on-LINE)	Family planning, population law and policy, and primary health care, including maternal/child health in developing countries	Bibliographic citations
PREMEDLINE	Biomedicine	Bibliographic citations
SDILINE (Selective Dissemination of Information on-LINE)	Biomedicine	Bibliographic citations

Table 27.1   A List of Major MEDLARS Databases *(continued)*

Database	Subject	Type
SPACELINE	Space life sciences	Bibliographic citations
TOXLINE (TOXicology information on-LINE)	Toxicological, pharmacological, biochemical, and physiological effects of drugs and other chemicals	Bibliographic citations
TOXNET Databases: Toxicology data network		
CCRIS (Chemical Carcinogenesis Research Information Systems)	Chemical carcinogens, mutagens, tumor promoters, and tumor inhibitors	Factual
DART (Developmental and Reproductive Toxicology	Teratology. Developmental and reproductive toxicology	Bibliographic citations
EMIC and EMICBACK (Environmental Mutagen Information enter BACKfile)	Mutagenicity; genotoxicity	Bibliographic citations
ETICBACK (Environmental Teratology Information Center BACKfile)	Teratology. Developmental and reproductive toxicology	Bibliographic citations
GENE-TOX (GENEtic TOXicology	Chemicals tested for mutagenicity	Factual
HSDB (Hazardous Substances Data Bank)	Hazardous chemical toxic effects, environmental fate, safety, and handling	Factual
IRIS (Integrated Risk Information Systems)	Potentially toxic chemicals	Factual
RTECS (Registry of Toxic Effects of Chemical Substances)	Potentially toxic chemicals	Factual
TRI (Toxic chemical Release Inventory) series	Annual estimated releases of toxic chemical to the environment, amounts transferred to waste sites, and source reduction and recycling data	Numeric
TRIFACTS (Toxic chemical Release Inventory FACT Sheets)	Health, ecological effects, safety, and handling information for most of the chemicals listed in the TRI (Toxic chemical Release Inventory) files	Factual

Reproduced, with permission, from Fact Sheet NLM OnLine Databases and Databanks *(http://www.nih.gov/pubs/factsheets/online—databases.html)*.

PsycINFO   The PsycINFO database, produced by the American Psychological Association, provides access to psychologically relevant literature from journals, dissertations, reports, scholarly documents, books, and book chapters with more than 1.5 million references covering 1887 to the present. Updated monthly, most of the records have abstracts or content summaries from material published in over 45 countries (What is PsycINFO?). Using the *Thesaurus of Psychological Index Terms*, the nurse can search for specific concepts effectively. Keyword and specific field searching are also available (Walker, 1994).

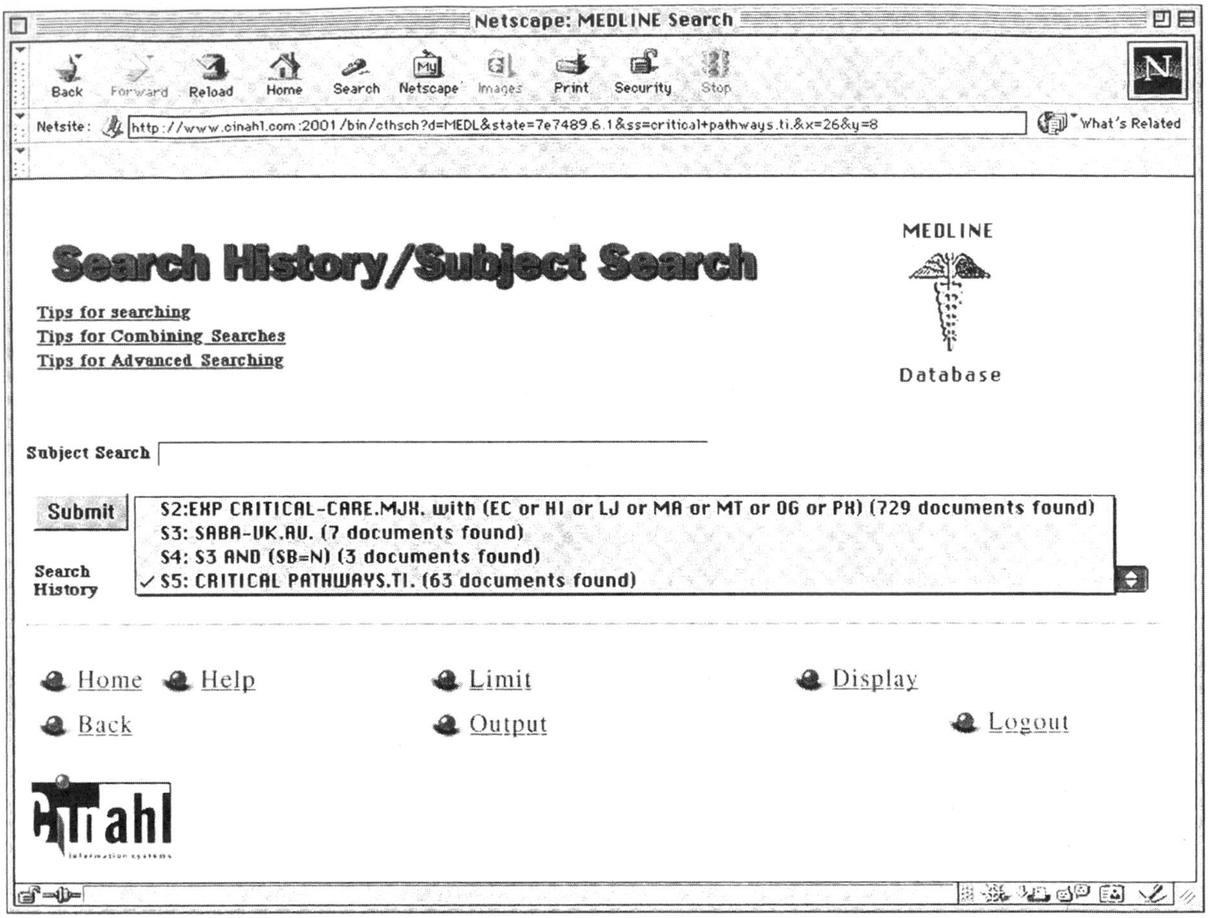

Figure 27.1
MEDLINE search.
(Courtesy Cinahl Information Systems.)

Social SciSearch Produced by the Institute for Scientific Information (ISI), the Social SciSearch database is an international multidisciplinary bibliographic retrieval system that covers 1,500 journals in the social, behavioral, and related sciences. Since the database contains all of the records published in the Social Sciences Citation Index, the nurse can search the cited references as in the citation index in the CINAHL database. The database covers 1972 to the present and is updated weekly (Social SciSearch).

A few other bibliographic retrieval systems to keep in mind are the NLM/NIH databases such as Health STAR, DIRLINE, CHID online (Combined Health Information database), CANCERLIT, AIDSLINE, the American Association of Retired Persons (AARP) database AgeLine, the Excerpta Medica database EMBASE, the National Technical Information Service NTIS database, and the Dissertation Abstracts database.

Current Awareness Services Most bibliographic retrieval systems are updated monthly or quarterly. Some are even updated weekly. In addition to the delay between writing and publishing the material that is indexed in the database, there is also a delay between the receipt of material, the indexing, and finally the inclusion of the citations for the indexed material in the database. To obtain access to more current material than that available in a bibliographic

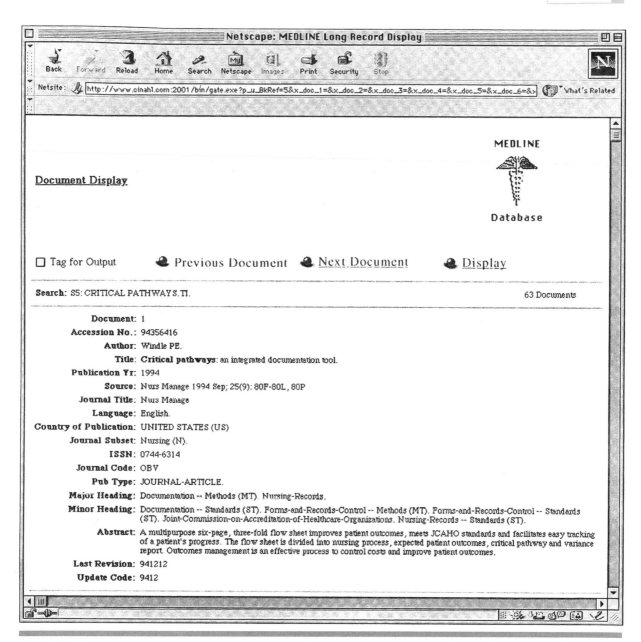

Figure 27.2
MEDLINE search result.
(Courtesy Cinahl Information Systems.)

database, the nurse should use a current awareness service.

Current awareness services are helpful when used in addition to bibliographic retrieval systems. These services provide access to tables of contents of journals and allow individuals to request articles of interest. They may include not only journal articles but also proceedings from conferences, workshops, symposia, and other meetings. Often, hospital or university librarians may provide these services as well.

Unlike the bibliographic databases, where subject searching using controlled vocabulary is available, only keyword searching for the subject, author, title, or journal is available in current awareness services or databases.

Some current awareness services or databases are Current Contents, Reference Update, UnCover, PREMEDLINE, and the CINAHL current awareness database.

Current Contents from ISI provides a current awareness service to over 7,000 journals and 2,000 recently published books and conference proceedings in the fields of science, social science, technology, and arts and humanities. Complete bibliographic information together with English language author abstracts and publisher names and addresses are provided (Current Contents).

Weekly issues covering 1,300 publications of Reference Update, also compiled by ISI, can be received via diskette or via the Internet. Reference Update uses the references provided in the ISI subscription service covering more than 60 disciplines, including pharmacology, medicine, cardiovascular systems, physiology, psychiatry, behavioral sciences, and public health (Reference Update).

UnCover, from the UnCover Company, is an on-line current awareness alerting service covering nearly 18,000 English language periodicals. Searching this database is free (About UnCover).

Added in August 1996, PREMEDLINE (one of the NLM's databases) provides basic citation information and abstracts daily. Once these citations have been indexed with MeSH terms, publication types, GenBank accession numbers, and other indexing data, they are added to MEDLINE and deleted from PREMEDLINE (MEDLINE).

The current awareness service offered by Cinahl Information Systems, publishers of the CINAHL database, is available on the CINAHL*direct* on-line service. This service is similar to that described above which contains citations of those articles received but not yet indexed with CINAHL subject headings from the CINAHL thesaurus. The fields that are keyword-searchable include the article title, author, and journal title. There is no charge to use this database. Similar to PREMEDLINE, the records, once indexed, are included in the CINAHL database and deleted from the current awareness database. An example from this database is shown in Figs. 27.3 and 27.4.

The second type of current awareness provided by Cinahl Information Systems is within the bibliographic database itself, where the searcher is able to choose from a group of 15 specific or special interest categories, which actually function as "virtual" databases. Possibilities include such areas as Advanced Nursing Practice, Case Management, Home Health Care, or Military/Uniformed Services. By selecting one of these categories, documents are retrieved that are either in specific journals in the field or have been selected by indexers as being of interest to those in that field. The results can be limited by any of the available limits on the database, e.g., publication type such as research, journal subset such as peer-reviewed, presence of full text, etc. A nurse with limited time can peruse the latest literature in one of these fields in this way (Figs. 27.5 and 27.6).

Review Services   Although the bibliographic retrieval systems and the current awareness services and databases act as filters to the ever-exploding literature, sometimes the information retrieved needs to be evaluated further to determine whether or not it is appropriate. For example, a monthly literature search might be done on a bibliographic and current awareness database and then a review service checked for commentaries on the sources retrieved. Supportive computerized resources that synthesize the literature (e.g., *Online Journal of Knowledge Synthesis in Nursing* published by Sigma Theta Tau International or the Cochrane Library Database of Systematic Reviews), review services such as Doody's Review Service, reviews noted in bibliographic databases, or review journals, such as *ONS Scan in Oncology, AAC Current Journal Review, ACP Journal Club*, etc., can be used to evaluate sources. Review services provide information to searchers about recently published books, journal articles, audiovisuals, and software. These reviews may also include ratings, opinions, or commentaries about the material.

Doody's Review Service, a service offered as a membership benefit to those belonging to Sigma Theta Tau and other nursing professional groups, develops a profile on its members and sends a weekly E-mail bulletin describing books that meet the parameters of the profile. The service currently contains over 65,000 print and electronic titles. The rating system used is a star system. The searcher can use author names, title, specialty, publisher, and keywords to find books of interest. The results show price, ISBN, and publisher as well as the rating. The information presented allows serious consideration of the book along with information to assist in making choices. Another Web site,

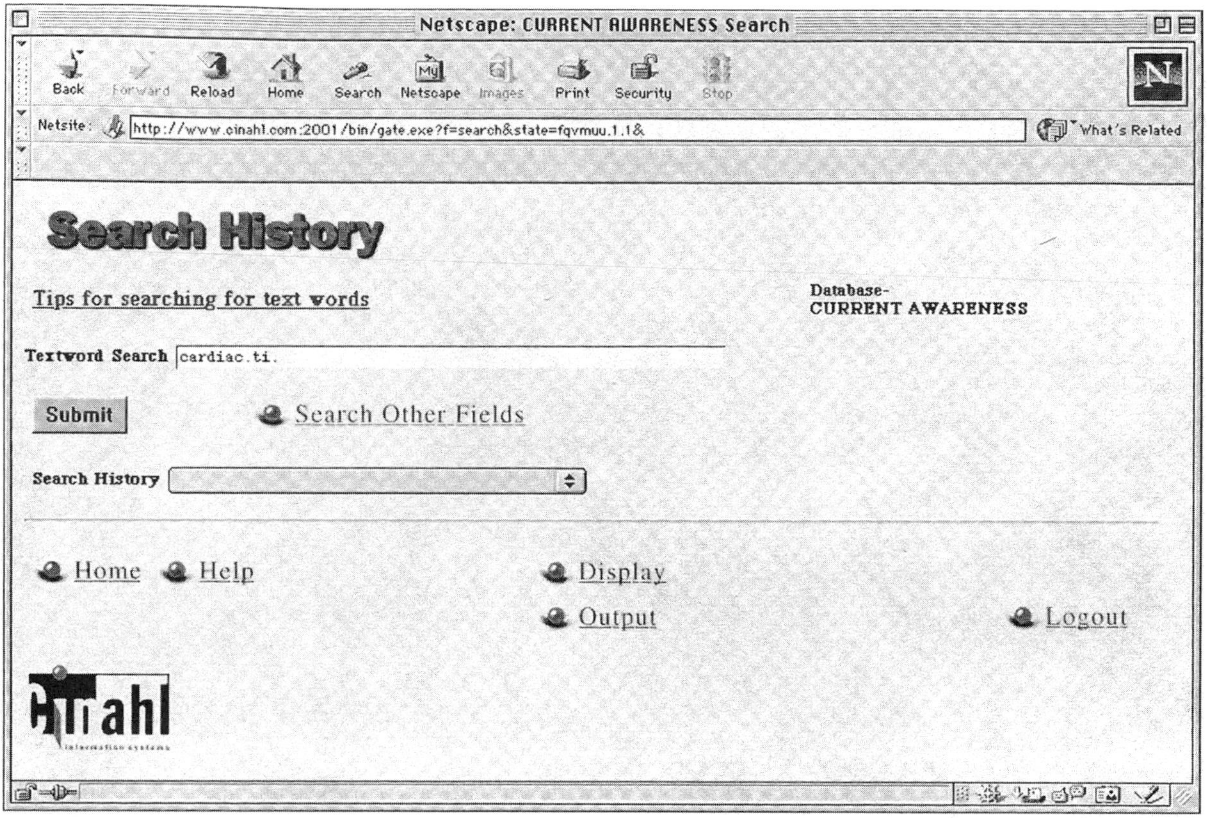

Figure 27.3
Current awareness search.
(Courtesy Cinahl Information Systems.)

http://www.nursingbooks.com, described as designed for nurses by nurses, allows for searching by keyword, author, and title. Tied to the Barnes and Noble Web site and search engine, the site categorizes books into various areas, including Care Plans, Caring for the Elderly, and Health Promotion and Prevention. Although reviews are not always present, the tables of contents for individual books, along with synopses, are included.

It is well-known, of course, that books are generally long in the development stage and are not as current as journal articles or documents on the World Wide Web. However, the *depth* of material presented in books must be considered. An in-depth discussion of *all* aspects of cardiac rehabilitation, for example, may be valuable in planning care and would probably not be examined in a journal article where space is a considera-

tion. Yet it would still be necessary for maintaining currency in the field.

Supportive Computerized Resources

Supportive computerized resources that assist the nurse in maintaining currency provide additional information and enhance the value of the essential computerized resources described above.

Document Delivery Services   Obtaining a bibliographic list of citations is only the first step in obtaining information on a particular topic. After carefully evaluating the citations, either from the title and/or the abstracts, or after using one of the review processes described above, the nurse will need to get the full text

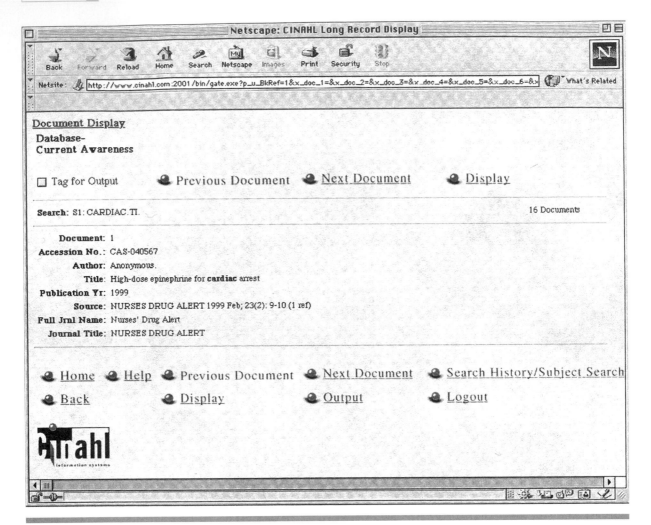

Figure 27.4
Current awareness search result.
(Courtesy Cinahl Information Systems.)

of the sources retrieved. A local library would be the first place to go to locate the items retrieved in a search. Publishers of journals or books, database vendors and providers (NLM, American Psychological Association, Ovid Technologies, EBSCO Publishing, UMI), and document delivery services (UnCover, ISI, Cinahl Information Systems) are secondary sources through which full text of items can be obtained for a fee. Fees differ depending on the service and the urgency of the request. Hard copy is usually sent via fax, mail, or electronic delivery (Stricker, 1998).

Electronic Publishers   Another resource option is publications, such as electronic journals, MMWR, etc., that are available on the World Wide Web. Sparks (1999) presents an excellent case for the importance of including electronically published information in a search for information. It offers several advantages over print material, including the speed of publishing, the comparatively small amount of space required for publishing, and the ease of availability of the documents. These advantages are important; however, because a document is published quickly does not necessarily

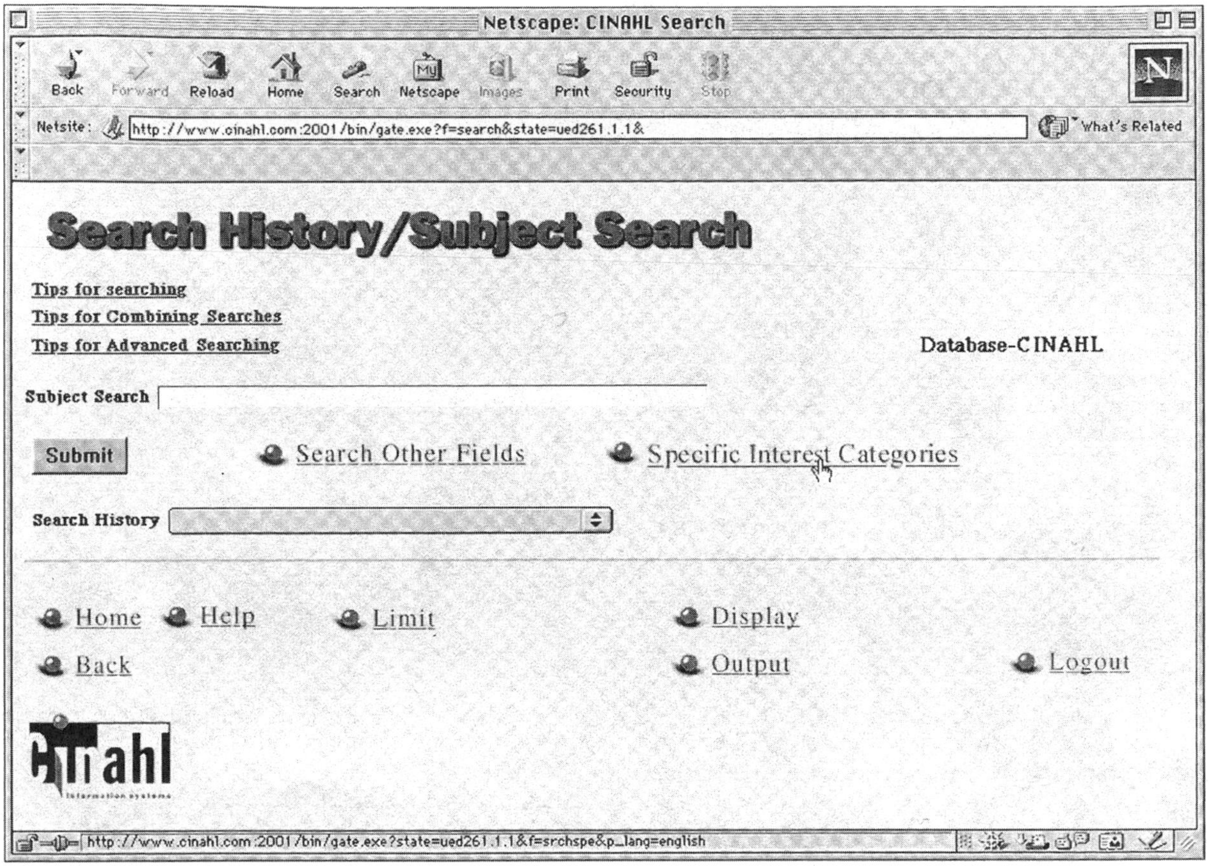

Figure 27.5
Specific interest group category initial screen on the CINAHL database.
(Courtesy Cinahl Information Systems.)

mean it is accurate. The credibility and accuracy of the source of electronically published material must always be considered. The criteria mentioned above along with additional criteria discussed later can be useful in evaluating this material. For a list of electronic publications consult Web sites such as the Virginia Commonwealth University's Web site at *http://views.vcu.edu*. Some of the main electronic-only nursing journals are *Online Journal of Knowledge Synthesis in Nursing*, published by Sigma Theta Tau; *Online Journal of Issues in Nursing*, published by Kent University School of Nursing in partnership with the American Nurses Association; *Online Journal of Clinical Innovations*, published by Cinahl Information Systems; *On-Line Journal of Nursing Informatics*, published in Penn-

sylvania; and *Australian Electronic Journal of Nursing Education*, published at Charles Stuart University in Australia. Other journals such as *Nursing Standard Online* have print counterparts but may have portions that are electronic-only.

Nursing publishers and organizations have their own Web sites, which give details about new publications, sometimes full text of some of the latest journal articles, official position statements of organizations, and/or practice guidelines. To identify the Web sites of nursing publishers and organizations, search Web site indexes such as Yahoo (*http://www.yahoo.com*) or browse Web site lists on Web sites such as that of the University of Buffalo Library (*http://ublib.buffalo.edu*) or the Worldwide Nurse Web site (*http://www.*

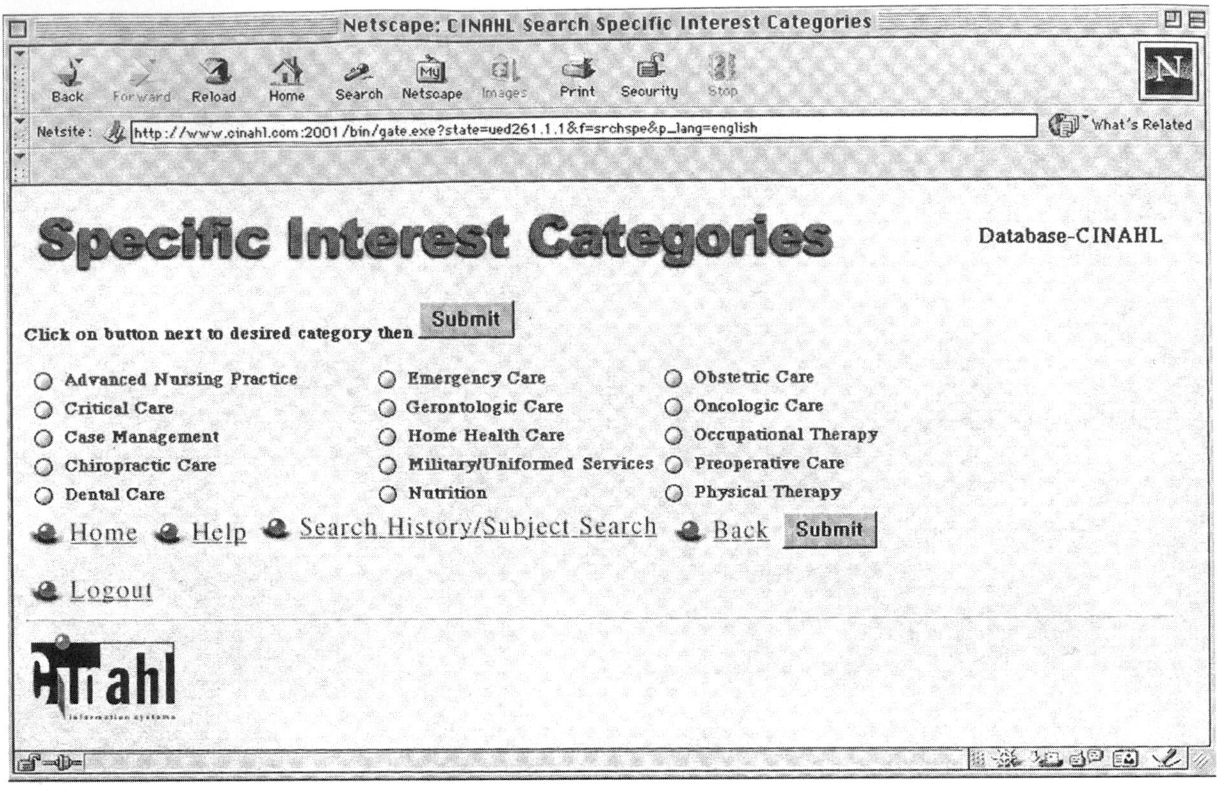

Figure 27.6
Available 1999 specific interest categories.
(Courtesy Cinahl Information Systems.)

wwnurse.com). On a Web site index such as Yahoo, do a general search for "nursing and publishers," "nursing and organizations," or "nursing and associations" or under the specific names of the publishers and organizations (e.g., Delmar, etc.).

Lippincott-Raven, Williams & Wilkins (*http://www.nursingcenter.com*) has placed the *American Journal of Nursing, Nursing Research, Computers in Nursing*, and *Journal of Nursing Administration*, among others, on their journals page with issues from January 1996 to the present. The site has search capability that allows keyword searching of the contents of the journals on the site. Many nursing organizations provide a significant amount of support to practicing nurses. Many publish journals and provide these as a member

benefit. They also provide access to the full text of their position statements and/or practicing guidelines. Some of these publications are the American Nurses Association's Web site NursingWorld (*http://www.nursingworld.org/*) and the Web sites of the American Academy of Nurse Practitioners (*http://www.aanp.org/*), American College of Nurse Practitioners (*http://www.nurse.org/acnp/*), the Association of Pediatric Oncology Nursing (*http://www.apon.org/*), and many, many others. Details regarding new publications and details regarding ordering items can be found on Web sites of most publishers.

Metasites on the World Wide Web　　Since there is so much information on the World Wide Web, identification and evaluation of Web sites is very important to determine which provide valid information. One of the ways to identify Web sites is to consult a metasite. There are several Web sites that can be classified as metasites concerning the same specific topic. The Hardin Meta Directory of Health Internet Sites, sponsored by the Hardin Library for the Health Sciences at the University of Iowa (*http://www.lib.uiowa.edu/hardin/md/*), is one of these as is National Information Center on Health Services Research and Health Care Technology (NICHSR) (*http://www.nlm.nih.gov/nichsr/hsrsites.html*), a government site. These sites basically function as lists of lists that provide links to other subject-specific Web sites.

Other sites function as metasites within their own Web site. CINAHL*Sources* on the Cinahl Web site contains an indexed selection of Web sites that are described both in terms of the organization and the contents of the Web site itself. These Web sites can also be reached directly from the table of contents page if the nurse has no need for the additional information presented in the description.

Once the Web sites have been identified, it is very important to evaluate them. The nurse should ask the following questions: (1) Who created the site? (2) Is the purpose and intention of the site clear? (3) Is the information accurate and current? (4) Is the site well-designed and stable? (Schloman, 1999).

There are also Web sites that can be used to evaluate other Web sites. OMNI (Organising Medical Networked Information) (*http://omni.ac.uk/seminars/seminar95/*) is a collaborative British effort to identify, select, evaluate, describe, and provide access to biomedical network resources. HON (Health on the Net Foundation) (*http://www.hon.ch/*), is an international initiative to promote effective Internet development and use in the areas of medicine and health. BioSites (*http://www.library. ucsf. edu/biosites/*) is a collaborative project of the Pacific Southwest Regional Medical Library (Durkin, 1997). Other Web sites that critically evaluate are Six Senses Seal of Approval (*http://www.sixsenses.com*); National Council Against Health Fraud (*http://www.ncahf.org*), a voluntary health agency that focuses on health fraud; and Quack Watch (*http:// www.quackwatch.com*), a member of the Consumer Federation of America (Schloman, 1999; Durkin, 1997). Additionally, Web sites providing information or discussions concerning specific diseases should be evaluated in this way (e.g., the Web sites of the American Diabetes Association (*http://www.diabetes.org/*) American Heart Association (*http://www.amhrt.org/*), and the Multiple Sclerosis Foundation (*http://www.msfacts.org/*).

Developing and Maintaining a List of Sources for Research/Practice/ Education

Essential Computerized Resources

The purpose of the information retrieved from these information resources is to enable nurses to answer specific questions that relate to research, practice, and/or education. For example:

- A staff nurse needs to find information to share with her/his colleagues on the nursing assessment of alcoholism.

- A nursing student has to finish a term paper and needs to find five nursing research studies on caring for a Hispanic patient with a myocardial infarction.

- A nurse manager needs to find research studies and anecdotal material showing the best way to prevent patient falls in her/his health facility.

Bibliographic Retrieval Systems   Resources essential in answering this type of question again include bibliographic databases as well as various Web sites. Once again, the resources need to be carefully evaluated for coverage and currency. Once a resource has been selected, the nurse breaks down her/his needs into a search statement such as, "I need information on the nursing assessment of alcoholism." The information on this topic would best be found in a bibliographic database. On such a database, the best method of searching is to do a subject search using controlled vocabulary (MeSH headings in MEDLINE, CINAHL subject headings in the CINAHL database, etc.).

SEARCH STRATEGIES   One of the most important aspects of searching the literature is formulating the exact strategy to obtain the information from a resource, whether from a bibliographic retrieval system or a Web site. There are six steps in planning the search strategy.

1. Plan the search strategy ahead of time.

2. Break down the search topic into components. To find information on the nursing assessment of alcoholism, remember to include synonyms or related terms. The components of the search would be alcoholism and nursing assessment. Sometimes the terms for the search will be subject headings in the database's subject heading list (often called a thesaurus); in other cases, they won't be (Fig. 27.7).

3. Check for terms in a subject heading list, if available. If the concept is new and there are no subject headings, a textword or keyword search is necessary. For example, before the term "critical paths" or "critical pathways" was added to MeSH or the CINAHL *Subject Heading List*, it was necessary to do a textword search for this concept. A search using the broad term "case management" would have retrieved many articles that would not necessarily discuss or include critical paths.

4. Select "operators," which are words used to connect different or synonymous components of the search.

The "and" operator, for example, makes the search narrower or more specific as the results of the search for two different terms will only result in records that include *both* terms as subject headings (Fig. 27.8) (Verhey et al., 1998).

The "or" operator can be used to connect synonymous or related terms, which broadens the search (Fig. 27.9).

The "not" operator can be used to exclude terms (Fig. 27.10).

5. Run the search.

6. View the results.

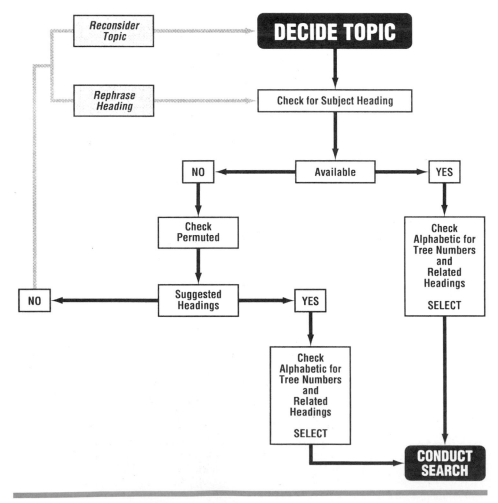

Figure 27.7
Strategy for a successful literature search.
(Courtesy Cinahl Information Systems.)

Practice Guidelines and Position Statements
Organization-specific practice guidelines, position statements, and standards of practice can often be accessed and obtained from the Web site of an individual's professional organization. These are extremely useful documents that present information on the scope of practice, qualifications, and education among other important details. Additionally, Cinahl Information Systems currently includes nurse practice acts as one of its publication types in the CINAHL database. These appear in full text and can be read on-line or printed.

Continuing Education and Computer-Assisted Learning   Many nurses do not have the time or money to attend conferences and workshops to keep abreast of the latest information in their specialties or to complete the necessary units or credits for continuing education for relicensure or recertification. The World Wide Web is a wonderful source for nurses that can be used to satisfy their requirements for continuing education (CE). The sites are easy to access, and there is no travel time or great expense involved (Plank, 1998). To identify CE Web sites visit Nursing Network Forum at *http://www.access.digex.net/~nurse/website.htm*, Alta Vista at *http://*

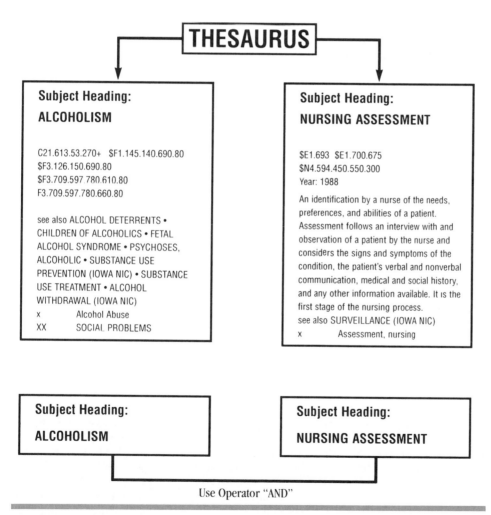

Figure 27.8
Subject headings using AND operator.
(Courtesy Cinahl Information Systems.)

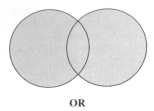

OR

Concept 1 "OR" Concept 2 = This means that only articles with *either* concept 1 and concept 2 are searched for.

Figure 27.9
Venn diagram OR.

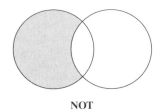

NOT

Concept 1 "NOT" Concept 2 = This means that only articles with both concept 1 that do not include concept 2 are searched for.

Figure 27.10
Venn diagram NOT.

www.altavista.com, Excite at *http://www.excite.com*, Magellan at *http://mckinley.com*, or Infoseek at *http://www.infoseek.com* (Plank, 1998). There are many nursing sites that offer on-line CE and CEU certificates: NurseOne at *http://www.nurseone.com*, Health Interactive at *http:// www.rnceus.com*, SpringNet CE Connection at *http:// www.springnet.com/ce.htm*, the Lippincott-Raven site at *http://www.nursingcenter.com/ continuing/*, and many others (Sullivan, 1997).

As mentioned at the beginning of this chapter, nurses use computers for many purposes. Computer-assisted instruction (CAI), computer-assisted learning (CAL), and interactive videodisc (IVD) provide easy learning experiences using a computer. The *Directory of Educational Software* by Christine Bolwell rates the various software programs and also identifies the method used in the software (e.g., tutorial, drill and practice, simulation, games, tests, etc.) (Hawley and Desborough, 1998). Ratings can also be found in nursing journals.

Supportive Computerized Resources

Topic-Related CD-ROMs   Supportive computerized resources that assist in practice, research, and education include computerized topic-related CD-ROMs that contain all types of health information including drug and treatment information, anatomy, and physiology. Specific products such as the *Merck Manual* or the *Physician's Desk Reference* are also available in various electronic formats. The National Library of Medicine's *Virtual Man and Virtual Woman*, the computer models of the human body, available on 23 CD-ROM discs, are excellent educational tools. The National Library of Medicine itself claims the "largest collection of medical knowledge in the world." The Cochrane Library's *Database of*

Systematic Reviews, available on-line and on CD-ROM, is another excellent source.

Web sites of particular interest in this category include the Nursing Theories Page (*http://www.ualberta. ca/~jrnorris/nt/theory.html*) and the Virginia Henderson Library and Research Registry (*http://www.stti. iupui. edu/library/*) as well as the Interagency Council on Information Resources for Nursing (ICIRN) and the Key Nursing Journals chart appearing on its Web site. ICIRN also prepares "Essential Nursing References" published biannually in *Nursing and Health Care Perspectives* (Allen et al., 1998).

 ### Collaboration and Networking Regarding Issues of Professional Practice

Nurses frequently gather information from their personal networks—either at the worksite or at professional meetings. The increased availability of computers makes contact with other professionals much easier, resulting in networking and collaboration possibilities heretofore impossible. Information retrieved by this method enables nurses to learn from their colleagues' experiences. When considering with whom to network, the specialty of the person should be evaluated along with experience, the material they have published in their field, and the research undertaken by the institution with which they are affiliated. Most of this information is not published and would be unavailable through traditional information resources.

Computerized resources for collaboration and networking vary in several technical details (e.g., their focus, the presence or absence of a moderator to monitor messages, the number of participants, and their level of interactivity).

Essential Computerized Resources

Electronic Mail and Listservs   An important fundamental computerized resource for collaboration and networking is electronic mail (E-mail), which is at the core of almost any electronic communication. Necessary components for E-mail are an Internet service provider (ISP) such as America OnLine or Earthlink and an E-mail software such as Eudora or those provided by Web browsers (NetScape or Internet Explorer). E-mail allows one-to-one communication between individuals and can provide immediate response to practice-related questions.

A second essential computerized resource for collaboration is an electronic discussion group or "listserv." Listservs allow individuals to subscribe free of charge and to read and respond to messages via E-mail. Since the messages are posted to all of the members, the listserv allows sharing and dissemination of information with colleagues. Some listservs have a closed membership for a specific group (e.g., librarians or specific nursing groups), and some are moderated. In a moderated group, an individual or group of individuals reads the messages prior to distribution to the group (Hayden, 1997). Subject-specific listservs include NURSENET (general nursing), Nrsing-L (nursing informatics), NrsingEd (education issues/faculty), and Nurseres (research). Specialty listservs are very helpful in increasing dialogue between individuals within the same specialty.

Supportive Computerized Resources

Electronic Bulletin Boards, Forums, Newsgroups, and Chat Rooms   Bulletin boards, forums, newsgroups, and chat rooms are examples of supportive computerized resources. Similar to a traditional bulletin board, the electronic version has an administrator who sends the discussion to various Web sites, where nurses visit to read and participate in the discussion (Hayden, 1997). This format for electronic networking has almost entirely been replaced by forums and newsgroups, which have become more and more sophisticated in their interactivity and design. The premise behind each of them is similar. An individual posts a message concerning a topic (known as a "thread") for others to read and respond to. Lippincott's Nursing Center (*http://www.nursingcenter.com*), for example, has many different forums under broad nursing categories such as roles, care settings, and areas of practice. Participants can respond to a previously posted thread

or begin a new one in any of these broad areas or the subtopics within them. Newsgroups operate in much the same way but have a tendency to be less focused. All of these resources are interactive but on a delayed basis. An individual may respond to a message immediately or wait several days. Chat rooms, on the other hand, are interactive in "real time." Conversations in chat rooms can be compared to telephone conversations—without the benefit of sound. Examples of chat rooms can be found at *http://virtualnurse.com/ICQPAGE/* or *http://www.nursingnet.org/*.

Each of these methods of collaboration and networking provides an option for nurses to use to contact and build relationships with other professionals concerning issues important to them.

Summary

While these three categories of information needs have been discussed as if they were independent of one another, a nurse might often find that she/he has needs that transcend all three categories or that fall under a different category each time, depending on the task. For example, a staff nurse may need to investigate the best methods to assess and manage pain. The process of retrieving appropriate information would be to first search for research studies and anecdotal material on the topic of pain management and pain measurement. This would involve a search for pain measurement or pain with therapy, drug therapy, and diagnosis using essential computerized resources such as bibliographic retrieval systems like MEDLINE or the CINAHL database.

Networking with other professionals facing the same task would be an additional step in this process. The nursing listservs mentioned above under "Collaboration and Networking Regarding Issues of Professional Practice" would be an important and essential resource, while E-mailing colleagues who are specialists in the field of pain would be a supportive resource. To locate specialists, a bibliographic retrieval system could be searched for research studies on pain measurement or management. The author affiliation field in the records retrieved would help track the institution with which the author is affiliated.

Making sure to keep current on any new material published on pain measurement and pain management, using current awareness services or Web sites, would also be vital in locating information on this topic. Bibliographic retrieval systems, already searched as an essential resource could be searched each month to assess what new material had been published on the topic. Supportive computerized resources might include a similar search for papers on the Cochrane Library's *Database of Systematic Reviews*, or consulting electronic publications such as *Online Journal of Knowledge Synthesis in Nursing* or *Online Journal of Clinical Innovations*. The articles in the latter journal, in fact, have corresponding summaries that are indexed and appear in full text on the CINAHL database, making them easily accessible in a traditional literature search to answer practice questions.

An important part of identifying and using these essential and supportive computerized resources is the evaluation of each of them to assess whether or not it is appropriate to locate the information needed. Therefore, the nurse must determine what she/he is looking for; identify the most appropriate resources to locate the information needed; and, using the criteria discussed throughout this chapter, evaluate the resources to assess if they are valid, current, and accurate.

Finally, it is important to realize that computerized information resources are like a "moving target" in that technology is changing so quickly that resources used today may be gone, unavailable, or outdated tomorrow. The use of bibliographic retrieval systems, search engines, and metasites encourages searching by *subject* or *concept*, which is the most reliable way to cope with the ever-changing nature of technology. This is vital to maintaining currency with the published literature, developing and maintaining a list of sources of topics of interest for practice, research, and/or education, and collaboration and networking with colleagues regarding issues of professional practice.

References

About AskERIC: Welcome to the AskERIC Service for Educators. *http://ericir.syr.edu/About*

About UnCover. The UnCover Company Home Page. *http://uncweb.carl.org/unchome.html*

Allen, M., Barry, R., Bick, D., et al. (1998). Essential nursing references. Interagency Council on Information Resources for Nursing. *Nursing and Health Care Perspectives, 19,* 230–237.

Barrett, L., and Colby, A. (1995). Eric's indexing and retrieval: 1995 update. In J. E. Houston (Ed.), *Thesaurus of ERIC descriptors* (13th Ed.) (pp. xiii–xvii). Phoenix, AZ: Oryx Press.

CINAHL 1999 Subject Heading List. (1999). Glendale, CA: Cinahl Information Systems.

Cumulative Index to Nursing & Allied Health Literature 43(part B). (1998). Glendale, CA: Cinahl Information Systems.

Current Contents. *http://www.isinet.com/products/cc/cc.html*

Durkin, C. (1997a). Accessing Internet—tips for hospital librarians. *National Network, 22*(2), 12–13.

Durkin, C. (1997b). Tracking and evaluating Web sites. *National Network, 21*(2), 8,11.

Hawley, P., and Desborough, K. (1998). The computer as tutor. *Canadian Nurse, 94*(4), 31–35.

Hayden, K. A. (1997) Internet tools and resources in continuing health education. *Journal of Continuing Education in the Health Professions, 17,* 121–127.

International Nursing Index. (1998). Hagerstown, MD: Lippincott Williams & Wilkins.

MEDLARS. *http://www.nlm.nih.gov/databases/medlars.html* MEDLINE *http://www.nlm.nih.gov/databases/medline.html*

Plank, R. K. (1998). Nursing on-line for continuing education credit. *The Journal of Continuing Education in Nursing, 29,* 165–172.

Reference Update. *http://www.isinet.com/products/ru/ru.html*

Schloman, B. F. (1999). Whom do you trust? Evaluating Internet health resources. *Online Journal of Issues in Nursing,* (January 28, 1999). *http://www.nursingworld.org/ojin/infocol/info_1.htm*

Social SciSearch online. *http://www.isinet.com/products/citation/citssci.html*

Sparks, S. M. (1999). Electronic publishing and nursing research. *Nursing Research, 48,* 50–54.

Stricker, U. D. (1998). Deliver Me: When subscribing is not an option. *Information Highways, 5*(4):20–25.

Sullivan, B. H. (1997). Linkages. *The Washington Nurse, 27*(3), 24.

Verhey, M. P., Levy, J. R., and Schmidt, R. (1998). *Information RN.* Glendale, CA: Cinahl Information Systems.

Walker, A. (1994). *Thesaurus of Psychological Index Terms* (7th Ed.). Washington, D. C.: American Psychological Association.

What is PsycINFO? *http://www.apa.org/psycinfo/whatis.html*

Recommended Reading

Ardito, S. C. (1998). The Internet: Beginning or end of organized information. *Searcher: the Magazine for Database Professionals, 6*(1), 52–57.

Benner, J. (1997). Nursing the Net. Researching health care topics on the Internet. *Nursing, 27*(9), 28–29.

Blythe, J., Royle, J. A., Oolup, P., et al. (1995). Linking the professional literature to nursing practice: Challenges and opportunities. *AAOHN Journal, 43*(6), 342–345.

Burnham, J., and Shearer, B. (1993). Comparison of CINAHL, EMBASE, and MEDLINE databases for the nurse researcher. *Medical Reference Services Quarterly, 12*(3), 45–57.

Farmer, J., and Richardson, A. (1998). The potential of the Internet: Improving access to information for nurses working in remote areas. *Bibliotheca Medica Canadiana, 19*(3), 95–97.

Glossbrenner, A., and Glossbrenner, E. (1997). *Search Engines for the World Wide Web.* New York: MIS Press.

Morris, D. H. (1996). Locating the information superhighway on-ramp: You can get there from where you are. *Journal of the American Dietetic Association, 96*(1), 14–16.

Putnam, N. C. (1998). Searching MEDLINE free on the Internet using the National Library of Medicine's PubMed. *Clinical Excellence for Nurse Practitioners, 2*(5), 314–316.

Sparks, S. M., and Rizzolo, M. A. (1998). World Wide Web search tools. *Image: the Journal of Nursing Scholarship, 30*(2), 167–171.

Tietze, M. F., and Huber, J. T. (1995). Electronic information retrieval in nursing. *Nursing Management, 26*(7), 36–37, 41–42.

Wright, K. B. (1996). Management, informatics, & technologies. The Internet and nursing: A vital link. *MEDSURG Nursing, 5*(3), 209–211, 203.

Yensen, J. (1998). Connecting points: Electronic nursing resources. Systematic, fast, comprehensive search strategies in nursing. *Computers in Nursing, 16*(1), 23–29.

PART 10

International Perspectives

28

Canada

Kathryn Hannah

OBJECTIVES

1. Describe nursing's role in information systems in Canada.
2. Identify major organizational structures that have led to standards in Canada.
3. Understand the organizational factors influencing information system development in Canada.
4. Describe the Canadian Nursing Components for Health Information Systems.

KEY WORDS

information systems
standards
hospital information systems
nursing minimum data set (NMDS)
public policy

Nursing's role in managing information in health service organizations and care facilities in Canada is similar to that in other developed countries. Of necessity, it is related to the role of nursing within the organization. In most hospitals, nurses manage both patient care and patient care units within the organization. Usually, nurse clinicians manage patient care, and nurse managers administer the patient care units within the organization. Therefore, for some time, nursing's role in the management of information has been considered to include both the information necessary to manage patient care using the nursing process and the information necessary for managing patient care units within the organization.

With regard to the nursing management of patient care, nursing practice is information-intensive. Nurses constantly handle enormous volumes of patient care information. In fact, nurses constantly process information mentally, manually, and electronically. Nurses have long been recognized as the interface between the patient and the health care organization. Like nurses in other countries, Canadian nurses integrate information from many diverse sources throughout the organization to provide patient care and to coordinate the patient's contact with health care services and facilities. In addition, they manage patient care information for purposes of providing nursing care to patients. There is also a long-standing tradition that nurses have the role of custodians of information on behalf of other caregivers and users of patient information. A seminal study in three New York hospitals found that registered nurses spend from 36 to 64 percent of their time on information handling, with those in administrative positions spending the most time (Jydstrup and Gross, 1966).

A major factor that influences nursing's role in managing patient care environments is the patient assignment methodology in use in the hospital or in individual patient care units (Hannah and Shamian, 1992). Each of these patient assignment methodologies requires a different nursing role in managing patient care information and consequently different information management skills for the nurses involved. Similarly, nursing's role in managing information for purposes of administering patient care units is influenced by the role of the nurse managers within the organization. Variations in decision-making, patient assignment, documentation protocols, and institutional governance style all affect nursing's role in information management for administrative purposes. However, the single most important element that determines nursing's role in information management for administrative purposes is the governance model in use in the hospital (Hannah and Shamian, 1992).

History of Health Information in Canada

In Canada, the Management Information System (MIS) Group evolved through a merger of the Management Information System Project and the National Hospital Productivity Improvement Program in 1989. The MIS Group developed data collection guidelines that focus primarily on financial and statistical data with limited capture of patient clinical data. Besides demographic data, the clinical data are limited to resource consumption data and data required for record abstracts. These clinical data are limited to physician-derived data. Thus, there are no clinical nursing data elements captured and stored based on the MIS guidelines.

The Hospital Medical Records Institute (HMRI) was founded in 1963 by the Ontario Hospital Association and Government of Ontario to develop a health care database. In 1977, the HMRI became an independent, federally chartered organization for the purpose of health care data management. The HMRI gathers data abstracted from patient hospital records and processes these data to provide information to health care providers, managers, and planners to aid in the delivery of health services (Youngblut, 1991). Since submission of abstracted medical record data to the HMRI was not mandated by all provincial health ministries, the HMRI database fell short of being a national database. The care items included in this data set were (and continue to be) limited to physician-derived data including most responsible diagnosis, primary diagnosis, secondary diagnosis, and procedures. Noteworthy, again, is the total absence of clinical nursing data.

The Canadian Institute for Health Information (CIHI) was established in 1993. It was a merger of the HMRI, the MIS Group, and two branches formerly within the federal departments of Health Canada and Statistics Canada. The Institute is an independent, not-for-profit organization mandated to coordinate the development and maintenance of comprehensive and integrated health information for Canada. CIHI is responsible for providing accurate and timely information in order to establish sound health policies, manage the Canadian health system effectively, and create public awareness of factors affecting good health.

In 1996, CIHI formed the Partnership for Health Informatics/Telematics to give leadership to shaping the national agenda for information and technology standards in health care. The goals of the Partnership are to:

■ Define and adopt emerging standards for health informatics and telematics in order to ensure the

evolution of a nonredundant, nonconflicting set of standards for Canada

■ Collaborate with other standards-setting organizations in Canada and internationally

■ Utilize the standards to enable the development of national, longitudinal electronic health records, accessible to health providers, researchers, and policy makers as well as health monitoring and surveillance agencies (Canadian Institute for Health Informatics, 1997).

One of the activities of a working group of the Partnership has been the development of the Canadian Classification of Health Interventions (CCI). The CCI differs from the classifications systems developed in the United States in that it is service provider- and service setting-neutral. This means that the same codes are intended to be applicable regardless of whether a physician, nurse, or respiratory technologist performed the intervention and whether the intervention was performed in an operating room, emergency department, clinic, or practitioner's office. Service provider and service setting information is captured as separate data elements in the "client" record.

Contextual Factors Influencing the Development of Health Information in Canada

Canadians have a unique health care system. One of the things that makes the Canadian health care system unique is the belief in health as a right—not as a privilege, or an economic commodity, but rather as a right for Canadians. This philosophy is reflected in the principles on which the provincial health systems in Canada are based, and it is legislated through the Canada Health Act by which all Canadian provinces abide. These principles include universality, portability, accessibility, comprehensiveness, and public administration. In addition, health is a provincial responsibility in Canada, not a federal one. Conformity on health matters between provinces is by mutual consent and agreement, not legislation.

Unfortunately, like other health care systems, in Canada the provincial health systems are presently in a box analogous to the room in which Alice in Wonderland found herself when she began to grow. The system is under enormous pressures, as depicted in Fig. 28.1. These factors are well described and documented elsewhere (Hannah, Ball, and Edwards, 1999; Hannah and Anderson, 1994).

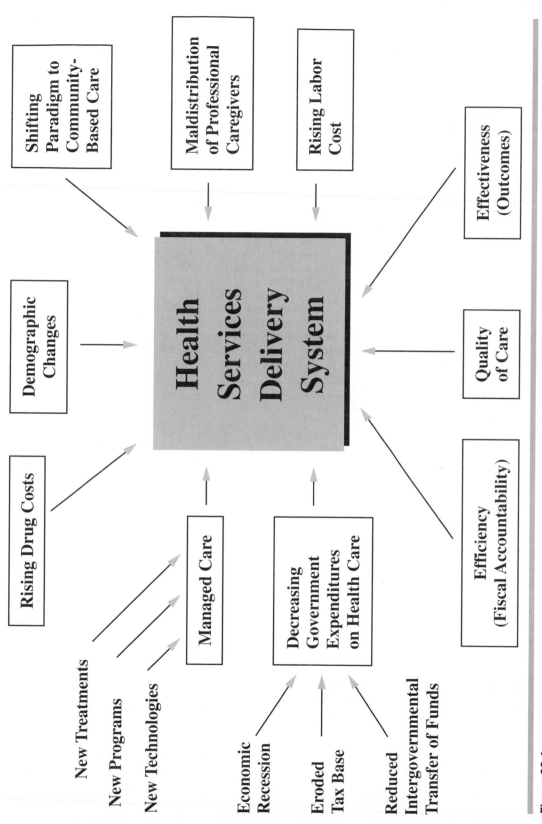

Figure 28.1
Pressures on the Canadian health services delivery system.

481

The overall picture is one in which the expenses and costs associated with health care are rising and the resources available to pay for health care in Canada have been reduced. Canadian nurses need to find ways to be more efficient and more effective and maximize the quality of care that is available to Canadians with the available resources. Strategies have been identified to provide enhanced information management to facilitate the management of our ever-diminishing health resources.

These are some of the factors that are influencing the drive towards the identification of essential data needs of nurses. In Canada, the information revolution has prompted initiatives by health care organizations to develop or acquire automated information systems focused on the utilization of data for the purposes of resource allocation, patient-specific costing, and outcomes of services. The information revolution has also been a driving force in the evolution of national health information through the formation of the Canadian Institute for Health Information.

During the 1990s, Canadian health care systems underwent profound reform initiated by action at the federal and provincial level in response to numerous reports and commissions (Epp, 1986; Angus, 1989; Wilk, 1991; Information Highway Advisory Council, 1995; Canadian Network for the Advancement of Research, Industry, and Education, 1996; Health Canada, 1997; National Forum on Health, 1997). Roles of health care providers and organizations were examined with a view to eliminating duplication of services and functions as well as providing efficient delivery of quality health care. New models of care delivery are emerging, such as "patient-focused care" and "hospitals without walls," directed at elimination of inefficiency in the structure and approach to health care. De-institutionalization of care and changes in the scope of medical practice are occurring. In addition, there is an increasing trend towards consumerism in which self-help groups, disease-specific groups, and other special interest groups expect to be involved in their own care. Another common outcome of the reviews most provinces conducted of their health care systems was recognition of information systems as a key enabler (and lack of quality information as a key barrier) to health sector reform.

The inevitable conclusion is that information and information management will become increasingly important in the future. Canadian nursing must ensure that information related to the nursing contribution to patient care is available in local and national data sets.

Thus, the data elements from which this information is derived must be collected and stored in a retrievable format.

Obstacles to Effective Nursing Management of Information in Canada

In Canadian hospitals, like most U.S. or European hospitals, the major obstacles to more effective nursing management of information are the sheer volume of information, the lack of access to modern information handling techniques and equipment, and the inadequate information management infrastructure. The volume of information that nurses manage on a daily basis, either for patient care purposes or organizational management purposes, is enormous and continuing to grow. Nurses continue to respond to this growth with incredible mental agility. However, human beings do have limits, and a major source of job dissatisfaction among Canadian nurses is information overload resulting in information-induced job stress.

Antiquated manual information systems and outdated information transfer facilities are information-redundant and labor-intensive processes, to say nothing of an inappropriate use of an expensive human resource. Modern information transfer and electronic communication systems allow rapid and accurate transfer of information along electronic communication networks.

Software and hardware for modern electronic communication networks are only two aspects of an information infrastructure. The other major aspect is lacking in most hospitals and health services organizations, i.e., the absence of appropriate infrastructure to facilitate information management. Infrastructure includes but is not limited to data management policies and procedures, methods for data stewardship and custodianship, user training, and information management support staff. Support staff are necessary to support nurses in analyzing and interpreting information appropriately.

Issues Related to Effective Nursing Management of Information

Primary among the nursing issues related to information management in Canada is the lack of adequate educational programs in information management techniques and strategies for nurse clinicians and nursing managers. At the time of writing, there are only a few preservice nursing education programs in Canada offering a course in modern information management techniques and strategies related to nursing. At a minimum, such a program must include advanced study of information management techniques and strategies such as information flow analysis and the use of spread sheets, databases, and word-processing packages. Ideally, such courses would also introduce concepts and provide hands-on experience related to the use of patient care information systems.

Another major issue is that nursing is frequently underrepresented in the selection and installation of patient care information systems and financial management systems in Canada. Regrettably, many senior nurse managers fail to recognize the importance of this activity and opt out of the process. They then complain when the systems do not meet the needs of nursing. Canadian senior nursing executives must recognize the importance of allocating staff and money to participate in the strategic planning process for information systems in their organizations. Other senior management personnel must also recognize the importance of nursing input into the strategic planning process for information systems. In any hospital, nurses are the single largest group of professionals using a patient care system, and nursing represents the largest part of the budget requiring financial management. Nursing, therefore, represents the single largest stakeholder group in Canada related to either a patient care information system or a financial information system.

Nurses have been involved in the management of nursing information since the initial systems for gathering minimum uniform health data, which can be traced back to systems devised by Florence Nightingale over a century ago (Verley, 1970). This early role in the management of nursing information began to change dramatically with the introduction of computers into health care and nursing environments. The role evolved as nurses became more involved in the selection and utilization of information systems. These developments have been well-documented elsewhere (Hannah et al., 1999) along with detailed information on the nursing responsibilities, roles, and contributions to the selection and implementation of information systems in health care organizations. The issues for nurses no longer relate to computers or management information systems, but rather information and information management. The computer and its associated software are merely tools to support nurses as they practice their profession. Far too much attention has been directed to the technology rather than its content. Current hospital information systems do little to assist nurses in their real

role, which is providing nursing care. Canadian nurses must be able to manage and process nursing data, information, and knowledge to support patient care delivery in diverse care delivery settings. In order to accomplish this goal, Canadian nurses are increasingly focusing on the contents (the data) contained in information systems instead of being distracted by the glamor and romance of the technology.

Unfortunately, despite Nightingale's early attempts to develop a nursing database, nurses in Canada have yet to reach consensus on the minimum set of data elements essential to the practice of nursing and the coding of those elements. In fact, at the present time in Canada, there are absolutely no nursing data elements that are collected and stored provincially or nationally for use in decision-making related to health policy or resource allocation. Nurses in Canada who have developed a heightened awareness of the importance of collection, storage, and retrieval of nursing data have recognized these data gaps. In 1990, attention began to be directed at initiating the process by which the nursing profession in Canada will begin to address the essential data needs of nurses in all practice settings in Canada (Canadian Nurses Association, 1990).

The patient discharge abstracts prepared by medical records departments across Canada currently contain no patient care delivery information. The abstracts therefore fail to acknowledge the contribution of nursing during the patient's stay in the hospital. This is important, because the abstracts are used by many agencies for a variety of purposes including funding allocation and policy-making. Presently, much valuable information is being lost. This information is important in determining the actual costs of hospitalization and the effectiveness of nursing care in achieving appropriate patient outcomes.

At a time when considerable emphasis is being placed on the development of a national health database in Canada, it is important that a minimum number of essential nursing elements be included in that database. In Canada, these nursing data elements are beginning to be referred to as the Nursing Components of Health Information (HI:NC). Such a set of data elements would be similar to the uniquely nursing elements included in the Nursing Minimum Data Set (NMDS), which has been tested in the United States. The nursing profession in Canada must provide the leadership in defining appropriate nursing data elements to be included in the national health database, specifically through the patient discharge abstract. In Canada, there is a need to extend the use of the concept of the Nursing Components of Health Information.

Thus, the salient issue in information management for nurses in Canada is identification of nursing data elements that are essential for collection and storage in a national health database. These data elements must reflect the data that nurses use to build information that is the foundation for clinical judgement and management decision-making in any setting where nursing is practiced. The remainder of this chapter will focus on the issue of defining those data elements that are essential to the practice of nursing.

Initiatives Directed at the Development of Nursing Components of Health Information for Use in Canada

In Canada, nurses are in the fortunate position of recognizing the need for nursing data elements at a time when the status of national health information is under review. The challenge for nurses is to capitalize on this timing and define those data elements required by nurses in Canada. To prevent nurses in Canada from losing control of nursing data, nurses must take a proactive stance and mobilize resources to ensure the development and implementation of a national health database that is congruent with the needs of nurses in all practice settings in Canada. Some initiatives intended to promote the vision, of a national health database becoming a reality in Canada, are in progress.

Prompted by the work of our U.S. colleagues on the NMDS, and in response to contextual factors influencing nursing in Canada, nurses in Canada have recognized the importance of the collection and storage of essential data elements (Canadian Nurses Association, 1990). Initiatives are currently under way directed at building awareness and consensus regarding the definition and coding of these essential data elements. Among these initiatives are strategic plans for the development of nursing components of health information for use in Canada.

In the Canadian province of Alberta, the Alberta Association of Registered Nurses (AARN) showed that it recognized the importance of the development of an NMDS through initiatives that included:

1. Establishing the definition of an NMDS as a priority in the 1991–92 year.
2. Submission of a resolution to the Canadian Nurses Association (CNA) in June 1990 calling for a national consensus conference "to develop in Canada a standardized format (Nursing Minimum Data Set) for purposes of ensuring entry, accessibility, and retrievability of nursing data."

This resolution was adopted for action by the CNA in 1990.

At the Canadian national level, the CNA responded to the AARN's NMDS resolution by organizing an invitational conference, with national representation. The focus of the conference was the discussion of the content for and issues related to the development of an NMDS. This was the first conference in Canada devoted solely to the discussion of this important topic. The Nursing Minimum Data Set Conference was held in Alberta in October 1992. This NMDS conference, a historic event, culminated in the development of recommendations to provide direction for the development of a Canadian nursing minimum data set. Among these recommendations were proposed data elements to be considered for inclusion as nursing components of a national health database in Canada. As well, a number of strategies were proposed that may be undertaken to achieve consensus on nursing data elements to be included in a national health database.

The data elements displayed in Table 28.1 were proposed for addition to the HMRI database as an initial step towards creating a cross-sectoral, multidisciplinary, longitudinal national health database in Canada (Canadian Nurses Association, 1993).

The nursing care items endorsed are comparable with those included in the U.S. NMDS; however, considerable discussion ensued over the labeling of two of the nursing care elements (Werley, 1988a). "Client status" was accepted as the label that represents the phenomena addressed by nurses that are commonly labeled "nursing diagnosis" by nurses in the U.S. Client status is client-focused and conceptually broader, since it is situationally dictated and thus more representative of nursing settings and populations; as well, it reflects a wellness approach. Client outcomes was accepted as the label for nursing outcomes again to emphasize the client focus. Data elements proposed for inclusion in the service items category include those items in the national data set and two nursing-specific items: unique nurse identifier and principal nurse provider. These nursing data elements will enable the unique nursing contributions to client well-being to be tracked.

The strategies proposed for the achievement of consensus among Canadian nurses on nursing data elements for inclusion in a Canadian data set for health information are well-documented in the proceedings of the conference (Canadian Nurses Association, 1993).

Table 28.1 Canadian Institute for Health Information (CIHI) Health Information Data Elements and Proposed Nursing Components

Care Items
Medical diagnosis
(Most responsible, primary, secondary)
Procedure and dates
Client status*
Nursing interventions*
Nursing intensity*
Client outcomes*

Patient Demographics
Health care number
Date of birth and age
Sex
Weight
(Newborns and infants 28 days or less)
Postal code
Race/ethnicity*
Unique geographical location*
Unique lifetime identifier*

Service Items
Province/institution number/chart number
Most responsible consultant
Admission date and hour
Institution from
Admission category
Admit by ambulance
Discharge date and hour
Length of stay
Institution to alive/death code
Responsibility for payment
Main patient service
Unique nurse identifier*
Principal nurse provider*

*Proposed Nursing Components of Health Information (HI:NC) elements

Continued commitment from the CNA is integral to the success of this professional issue.

At the 1993 CNA Biennial Meeting a resolution was passed resulting in a change in the name to Health Information: Nursing Components. This name is intended to reflect the importance of the nursing data elements being incorporated into a national health information data set rather than being created as a stand-alone data set. As well, this new name is congruent with the focus of the Canadian national health data set; a focus that emphasizes the client and the client's needs and outcomes as opposed to the individual health care disciplines. To that end, the National Nursing Informatics Initiative of the Canadian Nurses Association (1999) includes three independent related projects/groups:

1. **Health Information: Nursing Components (HI:NC) Working Group.** This group dates back to 1990, when CNA adopted a resolution to convene a national consensus conference to develop an NMDS. In 1993, the term NMDS was changed to HI:NC to reflect nursing components as part of a broader, multidisciplinary health information database. In 1997, CNA established the HI:NC Working Group of CNA composed of representatives of all provincial nursing associations and a representative from the Nursing Informatics Special Interest Group (NISIG), an interest group of the Canadian Organization for the Advancement of Computers in Health (COACH). This working group developed a workbook, *Nursing and Health Information: Towards Consensus on Nursing Care Elements,* and achieved consensus on three essential nursing care data elements (client status, nursing intervention, and client outcomes) to include in health information systems. The HI:NC Working Group is in the process of developing an integrated lobby strategy to seek policy initiatives such as adoption by information systems software developers; funding for additional testing and research; broad-based consensus and support for HI:NC within nursing communities and front-line nurses; and support from nursing leaders for action on HI:NC. Strategies involve meetings with key stakeholders, letters, conference presentations, published articles, etc.

2. **National Nursing Informatics Project (NNIP).** In 1998, an NNIP steering committee was formed to address the broad issue of promoting acceptance and use of information technologies as basic tools for information management and exchange in

nursing. Representatives are from five key nursing organizations, including the Association of Chief Executive Nurses, CNA, Canadian Association of University Schools of Nursing (CAUSN), Registered Nurses Association of British Columbia (RNABC), and the NISIG of COACH. A working committee was established to undertake a National Nursing Informatics Project, which has four goals:

- Develop consensus on a definition of nursing informatics for Canada.

- Recommend nursing informatics (NI) competencies for entry-level nurses and specialists, managers, educators, and researchers.

- Identify curriculum implications and strategies for both basic and continuing nursing education.Determine priorities for implementing national nursing informatics education strategies.

As an initial step in developing nursing informatics education strategies, the NNIP steering committee has developed a discussion paper to elicit feedback from stakeholders in national nursing organizations, educational institutions, and nursing employers. The working group has developed and circulated (May 31, 1999) a draft discussion paper and feedback questionnaire for content and format review before distributing widely for feedback. The discussion paper addresses six key areas:

- Definition of NI

- Proposed taxonomy of NI competencies

- Current opportunities for NI education

- Key support factors in developing NI education

- Key barriers in developing NI education

- Developing a national NI education plan

3. **Staff Advisory Group: Nursing Informatics**
   In 1999, a Staff Advisor Group: Nursing Informatics was formed as a national lobby strategy to advise CNA staff on general policy directions related to nursing and health informatics. Representatives were already involved in CIHI committee work. Duties include:

- Informing CNA of potential policy issues

- HI:NC follow-up

- Coordinating with HI:NC working group

- participating in national consultations related to health informatics, e.g., CMA's Health Information Privacy Code, Cochrane Collaborating

Centre, Canadian Advisory Committee to ISO's Technical Committee on Health Informatics

Discussions have focused on clarifying CNA's role in CIHI partnership and what outcome CNA expects. Generally, CNA recognizes the need for clinical nursing data for future decision-making and the need to assume a leadership role with national groups like CIHI.

As nurses in Canada embark on the development of the nursing components of health information, several issues germane to the development of minimum data sets emerge. The first need is to ensure that data are available, reliable, valid, and comparable. It is also important to define the scope of the data set to ensure that only those essential data elements are collected and to avoid proliferation of data. Further, attention must be directed at the coordination and linkage of data. There are three aspects of data linkage that demand attention. First, the hardware must have the capability of supporting database linkage. Second, the content must be developed in a manner that lends itself to integration. Finally, the ethics of data linkage with respect to patient information, including security confidentiality and privacy of data, must be addressed (Hannah, 1991).

Once the nursing components of health information are established, three issues emerge: first, promoting the concept to ensure widespread use; second, educating the users to ensure the quality of the data that are collected; and finally, establishing mechanisms for review and revision of the data elements.

Implications of the Nursing Components of Health Information

In the absence of a system for the collection, storage, and retrieval of nursing data elements, it is evident that much valuable information is being lost. In Canada, as in other countries, this information is important to demonstrate the contribution nursing makes to the care of the patient and to demonstrate the cost-effectiveness of nursing care (Werley, 1988b; Werley and Zorn, 1988; Werley, Devine, and Zorn, 1991). As we move away from nursing-specific models of patient care delivery to models that focus on the patient, emphasizing collaboration of disciplines, health care providers with multiple skills, standardization of care, and streamlining of documentation through charting by exception, it is imperative that nurses be able to articulate what is and is not nursing's role. Further, nurses will be asked to demonstrate nursing's contribution to patient care in terms of outcome criteria that are objective and measurable. Nurses require nursing data to identify outcomes of nursing care, defend resource allocation to nursing, and justify new roles for nursing in the health care delivery system (Gallant, 1988; McPhillips, 1988; Werley et al., 1991). Similarly, nurses need to understand and value nursing data so that in the selection and implementation of information systems for their organizations, nurse administrators insist that they or their designate play a major role and that nursing data needs are incorporated into the selection and implementation criteria.

While on the one hand nurses must preserve a professional nursing identity, Canadian nurses must balance this against professional ghettoization. The collection and storage of essential nursing data elements that are not integrated as components of a national data set will serve to ghettoize nursing, especially in a socialized health case system such as Canada's. This is dangerous at a time when significant emphasis is being placed on multidisciplinary collaboration, patient-focused care, and patient outcomes. In Canada, contributions to the only national health database are voluntary rather than legislated, and the elements are established by consensus rather than by legislation. In view of priorities in Canadian health care as well as the culture of negotiation and consensus, the nursing participation in the determination of the integrated data elements could not be more clear.

Nurse clinicians need to know what nursing elements are essential for archival purposes so that nursing documentation is inclusive of these elements. With the move toward standardization of care through the use of care maps, it is essential that outcomes of nursing care be determined and included in the care maps. As health care organizations embrace the concept of charting by exception in an effort to decrease the valuable hours spent by health care workers in documentation, nurses must be sure that those tools that outline the inherent patient care delivered are not devoid of nursing's contribution to patient care, for in the absence of data that reflect nursing activities there is no archival record of what nurses do, what difference nursing care makes, or why nurses are required. At times of fiscal restraint, objective nursing data are required to substantiate the role of nurses and the nurse: patient ratios required in the clinical setting.

Nurse researchers need a database of essential data elements to facilitate the identification of trends related to the data elements for specific patient groups, institutions, or regions and to assess variables on multiple levels including institutional, local, regional, and national (Werley, 1988b; Werley and Zorn, 1988; Werley et al., 1991). The collection and storage of essential nursing data elements will facilitate the advancement of nursing as a research-based discipline. Nurse educators need these essential nursing data elements to develop nursing knowledge for use in educating nurses and to facilitate the definition of the scope of nursing practice (McCloskey, 1988).

Finally, the definition of nursing components of health information is essential to influence health policy decision-making. Historically, health policy has been created in the absence of nursing data. At a time when Canada is in the midst of profound health care reform, it is essential that nurses demonstrate the central role of nursing services in the restructuring of the health care delivery system.

 ## Summary

It is clear that a priority for nursing in Canada is the identification of the nursing components of health information, those essential nursing data elements that must be collected, stored, and retrieved from a national health information database. Nursing leaders must respond to the challenge to identify those data essential for the management of patient care and patient care units. The nursing components of health information have the potential to provide nurses with the data required to build information for use in reshaping nursing, as a profession prepared to respond to the health needs of Canadians in the 21st century. However, the window of opportunity to have nursing data elements included in a national data set is narrowing. Nurses must ensure that the vision of nursing components in the Canadian national health information system becomes a reality for nursing in Canada.

 ## References

Angus, D. E. (1989). *Review of Significant Health Care Commissions and Task Forces*. Ottawa: Canadian Nurses Association.

Canadian Institute for Health Informatics (CIHI). (1997). *Partnership for Health Informatics/Telematics*. Ottawa.

Canadian Network for the Advancement of Research, Industry, and Education (CANARIE). (1996). *Towards a Canadian Health Iway: Vision, Opportunities, and Future Steps*. Ottawa: (CANARIE).

Canadian Nurses Association. (1990). Report of the resolutions committee. Unpublished report.

Canadian Nurses Association. (1993). *Papers from the Nursing Minimum Data Set Conference.* Ottawa.

Canadian Nurses Association (1999). http://*www.cna-nurses.ca*

Epp, J. (1986). *Achieving Health for All: A Framework for Health Promotion.* Ottawa: Health and Welfare Canada.

Gallant, B. J. (1988). Data requirements for the nursing minimum data set as seen by nurse administrators. In H. H. Werley and N. M. Lang (Eds.), *Identification of the Nursing Minimum Data Set* (pp. 165–176). New York: Springer.

Hannah, K. J. (1991). The need for health data linkage hospital/institutional needs: a nursing statement. In *Hospital Medical Records Institute, Papers and Recommendations from the National Workshop on Health Care Data Linkage* (pp. 17–18). Don Mills: Hospital Medical Records Institute.

Hannah, K. J., and Anderson, B. (1994). Management of nursing information. In J. Hibbert and M. Kyle (Eds.), *Canadian Nursing Management.* Toronto: Saunders.

Hannah, K. J., Ball M.J., and Edwards, M.J.A. (1999). *Introduction to Nursing Informatics* (2nd ed.). New York: Springer-Verlag.

Hannah, K. J., and Shamian, J. (1992). Integrating a nursing professional practice model and nursing informatics in a collective bargaining environment. *Nursing Clinics of North America.* Philadelphia: W. B. Saunders.

Health Canada. (1997). Health and the information highway (news release). Ottawa: Health Canada.

Information Highway Advisory Council. (1995) *Final Report of the Information Highway Advisory Council.* Ottawa: Industry.

Jydstrup, R.A., and Gross, M.J. (Winter 1966). Cost of information handling in hospitals: Rochester region. *Health Services Research, 1,* 235–271.

McCloskey, J. C. (1988). The nursing minimum data set: Benefits and implications for nurse educators. In *National League for Nursing, Perspectives in Nursing 1987–1989* (pp. 119–126). New York: National League for Nursing.

McPhillips, R. (1988). Essential elements for the nursing minimum data set as seen by federal officials. In H. H. Werley and N. M. Lang (Eds.), *Identification of the Nursing Minimum Data Set* (pp. 233–238). New York: Springer.

National Forum on Health. (1997). *Canada Health Action: Building on the Legacy.* Ottawa: Health Canada.

Verley, H. (1970). *Florence Nightingale at Harley Street.* London: Dent & Sons.

Werley, H. H. (1988a). Introduction to the nursing minimum data set and its development. In H. H. Werley and N. M. Lang (Eds.), *Identification of the Nursing Minimum Data Set* (pp. 1–15). New York: Springer.

Werley, H. H. (1988b). Research directions. In H. H. Werley and N. M. Lang (Eds.), *Identification of the Nursing Minimum Data Set* (pp. 427–431). New York: Springer.

Werley, H. H., and Zorn, C. R. (1988). The nursing minimum data set: Benefits and implications. In *National League for Nursing, Perspectives in Nursing—1987–1989* (pp. 105–114). New York: National League for Nursing.

Werley, H. H., Devine, E. C., Zorn, C. R., et al. (1991). The nursing minimum data set: Abstraction tool for standardized, comparable, essential data. *American Journal of Public Health, 81,* 421–426.

Wilk, M. B. (1991). *Health Information for Canada 1991: Report of the National Task Force on Health Information.* Ottawa: National Health Information Council.

Youngblut, R. (1991). Hospital Medical Records Institute (HMRI). *National Health Information Council, 2* (1), 10.

CHAPTER **29**

Europe

Ulla Gerdin
Elly Pluyter-Wenting
William T. F. Goossen
Marianne Tallberg

OBJECTIVES

1. Describe the development of nursing terminology in Europe.
2. Describe components of standards in electronic patient records.
3. Describe the European learning package for nursing informatics.

KEY WORDS

information systems
standards
hospital information systems
culture
public policy

This chapter concentrates on nursing informatics in Europe and research and development in the areas of terminology, patient record systems, and education. It provides an overview of European projects on nursing informatics and ongoing standardization work. This chapter includes the following:

- Major European projects on nursing informatics
- Current use and development of nursing terminologies in Europe
- Standardization work
- Electronic patient records
- A European curriculum and courseware for nursing informatics

Major European Projects on Nursing Informatics

The European Commission (EC) is a major driving force and funder of development of health care informatics. Projects funded by EC are all cross-cultural. Each project involves more than three countries, health care professional users, educators, and administrators. Researchers and vendors are also represented. English is the working language in all projects.

Prioritized projects today and in the years to come concern the structure of the patient record, communication of patient data, terminology, education, and security. At present, there are four projects involving nursing and run by nurses: Nightingale, Telenurse ID, WiseCare, and Action. Some of these projects have impact outside Europe; e.g., the alpha version of the International Classification for Nursing Practice (ICNP) from the International Council of Nurses in Geneva has its origin in the Telenurse project.

Telenurse ID

Telenurse ID *(http://www.telenurse.net)* will produce two exploitable items in the area of information technology (IT) products. These include an assortment of integrated nursing subsets of electronic patient records, produced by leading suppliers and validated by a large number of committed users. The other item is the proposal for an improved beta version of the International Classification of Nursing Practice (ICNP). The alpha version was created by the Telenurse project with permission of the International Council of Nurses (ICN). The purpose of the ICNP is to serve as a unifying framework for electronic documentation of nursing care in Europe, including members of the European Union, as well as Central Eastern European countries.

WISECARE

The Workflow Information Systems for European Nursing Care (WISECARE) project *(http://www.echo.lu/telematics/health/wisecare.html)* is a joint activity of the European Oncology Nursing Society, several European universities, software companies, and consultants. Its goal is to use electronic patient records for clinical and resource management information with a focus on patient outcomes. Advanced information and communication technology is used to collect and process data on oncology nursing care and to feed back information to participating wards and the oncology nursing associations.

ACTION

The Assisting Carers Using Telematics Interventions to Meet Older Person's Needs Project (ACTION) *(http://www.echo.lu.telematics/disabl/action.html)* is a nursing-led collaborative venture involving several universities, family carers as users, and local health care organizations at all levels. The goal of the ACTION project is to enhance independence, autonomy, and quality of life for elderly people and family carers by the application of information and communication technology. The project demonstrates that through a combination of familiar technologies, such as television, and by carefully applying additional information and communication technologies, on-line effective care information and direct communication between family carers and professional carers has become a reality.

 ## Current Use and Development of Nursing Terminologies in Europe

A common denominator for nursing terminology in Europe is the nursing process and its structure. Recent decades have witnessed several initiatives and pluralism in development and implementation. The use of defined terminologies is currently widespread and appreciated by nurses all over Europe. Differences in language, culture, and health care systems result in great variances in the development. For example, in England and the Netherlands, the purpose of the terminology development is the improvement of clinical documentation. English nurses use the Clinical Codes and Dutch nurses are beginning to use the International Classification of Impairments, Disabilities, and Handicaps (ICIDH; in its new version, ICIDH-2, called the International Classification of Impairments, Activities, and Participation),

(http://www.who.int/msa/mnh/ems/icidh/introduction.htm). On the contrary, the Belgian nursing minimum data set is meant to bridge the gap between clinical information and the national health system.

Hoy (1997) identified several different purposes for the use of terminologies. He argues that it is necessary to work with more than one terminology system. He distinguishes between the following purposes for comparable nursing information:

- Clinical
- Clinical documentation
- Quality assurance
- Managerial
- Epidemiological
- Policy-making

The higher the level of aggregation, he argues, the more structure and abstraction is necessary for the nursing terminology and information.

A European Standard for Nursing Concepts

The European standardization organization (CEN) *(http://www.cent251.org)* endorses the development of a "system of concepts to support nursing." The aim of this standard is the definition of a system of concepts and semantic categories. This work produces standard definitions for categories relating to patient-oriented nursing care and the relationship of these concepts to each other. The concepts shall focus on basic principles of nursing, including—but not limited to—patients' perception, nurses' definition of the diagnosis, intervention, describing outcome, etc. As a consequence, it will permit a harmonized construction, maintenance, and use of relevant classifications and nomenclatures. The recommended system of concepts will be formalized into a model in harmony with the work on a concept system to support continuity of care (CEN, 1999).

Association for Common European Nursing Diagnoses, Interventions, and Outcomes

During the early 1990s, a need to develop a culturally sensitive nursing terminology in Europe was recognized; this terminology should reflect the diversity of all different European countries. European nurses need a common terminology to be able to share and compare information and to ensure that nursing is visible in local, national, and European policy. The Association for Common European Nursing Diagnoses, Interventions, and Outcomes (ACENDIO) was established in Brussels in 1995. ACENDIO provides a network across Europe for nurses interested in the development of a common nursing terminology. The focus of ACENDIO is to:

- Identify terms and categories for nursing diagnoses, interventions, and outcomes
- Validate and standardize these materials throughout Europe
- Translate materials where necessary
- Cooperate in the development of the ICNP as a unifying framework for nursing classifications
- Ensure comparability and compatibility with classifications, standards, and databases in Europe

European Trials and Use of the International Classification for Nursing Practice

The initiative taken by ICN to develop an ICNP for worldwide use has created a variety of activities throughout Europe. To be able to test ICNP, the alpha version has been translated into Danish, Greek, Icelandic, Finnish, Italian, Dutch/Flemish, French, Portuguese, Swedish, and German. Trials are performed in nearly all of these countries.

Additional activities include ensuring compatibility with existing classifications from the World Health Organization (WHO) and CEN/TC251. A future goal is to establish an international framework and a database that incorporates the ICNP, the nursing minimum data set, a nursing resource data set, and regulatory information.

National Examples of Terminology Systems and Ongoing Terminology Work

Nursing Minimum Data Sets and Workload (Patient) Classifications
Terminologies referred to here are the Minimale Verpleegkundige Gegevens (MVG), Résumé Infirmier Minimum (RIM), Minimale Psychiatrische Gegevens (MPG) in Belgium, and The Netherlands Nursing Minimum Data Set (NMDSN).

Since 1988, all Belgian general hospitals are required by law to collect nursing intervention data four times a year. MVG/RIM is a nursing minimum data set, with 23 well-defined nursing interventions used in the Belgian national health statistics for policy-making and partly for funding of nursing care. Other purposes include clinical epidemiology, resource planning, and quality assurance (Sermeus and Delesie, 1997). In addition, a minimum data set for Belgian psychiatric hospitals has recently been established. This is a multidisciplinary data set that includes patient problems and nursing care (Hermans, 1996).

A validation of the Belgian MVG terminology has been performed in Finland. It shows that the NMDS has a wider usability in Europe. It is hoped that this research will have a positive effect on the really wide variety of terminologies in patient classification. Seppälä (1992) showed that there are at least 33 different patient classification systems used in Europe.

The NMDSN currently includes 24 nursing diagnoses, 32 nursing interventions, and 4 nursing outcomes. Future changes in this NMDSN can be expected and will be in line with continuous work on the national nursing classifications.

Many Swiss hospitals and nursing homes use standardized nomenclature when they measure nursing workload with tools having their own vocabularies like LEP (Leistungs Erfassung in der Pflege), PRN (Projet de Recherché en Nursing), or PLAISIR (Planification Informatisée des Soins Infirmiers Requis). In Switzerland, a new law has deeply affected recent developments in health care reform. New rules for statistics, including nursing care, have been introduced, and a Swiss NMDS is under way. The work is being led by a coalition of cantonal and federal authorities together with the Swiss Nurses Association. A first range of results was planned for early 1999.

Nomenclatures and Classification Systems Denmark is developing the Health Care Sector Classifications System (SKS), a multidisciplinary classification of which nursing classifications are a part. The nursing intervention classification was released for use in 1996 and the work with nursing diagnoses and assessment classification is ongoing (Madsen and Burgaard, 1997).

Sweden has developed a national terminology database to support electronic patient record systems. The Nurses Association is working together with all other health care disciplines on the development of a common terminology database on defined concepts and their relations. The VIPS model and terminology—a Swedish model for nursing systematic documentation—was developed using empirical and theoretical studies as well as empirical testing. The model is based on the nursing process, and it holds key words on two levels. Experience has shown that the key words have good content validity in different areas of nursing care. The

VIPS is used today in patient record systems both in Finland and Sweden. Today, the nurses in these sites have access to huge sources of nursing data (Ehrenberg, et al., 1997). A nomenclature of nursing interventions, based on observations and recordings of nurse-patient interactions, was developed in Finland in 1992 (Halttunen, 1992). Iceland has developed its own health record system (SAGA), which includes a local terminology for nursing care.

The Clinical Codes (former Read Codes/Thesaurus) are today a coded standard nomenclature of health care terms—Crown-copyrighted in the United Kingdom (UK). It was in the beginning a purely medical nomenclature, but soon its creator, Dr. James Read, understood the necessity of an enlargement to include nursing and other professions allied to medicine. The nursing projects, like the medical and allied health projects, were directed from the National Health Centre for Coding and Classification. It co-worked with the nursing profession's established Strategic Advisory Group for Nursing Information in the UK. The aim of the project was to produce an agreed upon, systematically arranged thesaurus of nursing, midwifery, and health visiting terms. Six working groups representing different nursing main areas were set up, and even more nurses from subspecialities were involved in expanding and refining terms. This way, the nursing community was actively involved in establishing its own standard. The terms were collected from the nursing literature, patient records, spoken communications, etc. The project started officially in 1993 and was finished in 1995. The Codes, which exist as a dictionary in computer files and not in book form, enable a complete patient record to be coded and stored in a computer system. The codes are cross-referenced to and compatible with other standard medical coding systems, such as, for example, ICD 10.

In the Netherlands, the official classification for nursing diagnoses is in its first test phase. The work is based on the ICIDH and has been rearranged for use as terminology for nursing diagnoses (Ten Napel, 1996). The ICIDH has been chosen for reasons of multidisciplinary collaboration and (future) use of integrated electronic health records. Preliminary work for nursing interventions has been done. Because of the great amount of confusion concerning nursing outcomes, a Delphi study to clarify this issue is under way (van der Bruggen and Groen, 1997). There is no work on a nursing outcome classification available yet, although some nursing outcomes indicators have been included in the NMDSN.

The North American Nursing Diagnoses Association and the Nursing Intervention Classification Used in Europe.   Translations of the North American Nursing Diagnoses Association (NANDA) and Nursing Intervention Classification (NIC) are available in Germany. The need for unified nursing terminology is recognized in Switzerland as well (Van Gele, 1996). NANDA and NIC materials are tested in several hospitals and units in the German-speaking part of Switzerland.

In France, the nursing documentation is according to the nursing process. NANDA is translated for nursing diagnoses, and a free text style is used to document nursing actions and nursing outcomes. An example of NANDA use is the work with Nurse International Diagnosis (NID) of NANDA-validated diagnoses by AFEDI-FRANCE. In Italy, there is no officially acknowledged terminology system. The most commonly used terminology refers to NANDA diagnostic taxonomy and its derivatives. Scales to identify nursing diagnoses (e.g., bedsores risk, coma scale, and dependency for activities of daily living [ADL] are used in different settings).

The picture in Portugal is distinct for different parts of the country. On the mainland, the implementation of the nursing process is not very common. In Madeira, an autonomous region, NANDA nursing diagnosis and Carpenito's Collaborative Problems have been used at the hospital at Funchal. Madeira plans to test the ICNP as a Telenurse-ID Sponsoring Partner. At Porto, the University, together with hospitals and community settings are developing a computerized patient record system that includes ICNP terminology.

Standardization Work

The European standardization organization for Medical Telematics (CEN/TC 251) (1999) was established in 1991. "CEN/TC 251 is supported by the European Commission DGIII (Industry), Healthcare authorities, suppliers of IT-solutions and Users to develop standards that enable compatibility and interoperability between independent systems in healthcare." Today, four committees share the responsibilities to develop standards for information models, a system of concepts and terminology, technology for interoperable communication, and security. All European countries are members of CEN. Nursing is represented in several of the projects (e.g., system of concepts to support continuity of care, electronic health care record communication—extended architecture, and systems of concepts for nursing).

Electronic Patient Records
necessities for EPR ①

Health care information systems need unified and controlled terminologies to be able to communicate with other systems. Health care information systems also require a common basic architecture to allow communication of context. The third prerequisite for communication is security and access control. Health care professionals (e.g., almoners, dieticians, dentists, nurses, occupational therapists, physiotherapists, physicians, and speech therapists), recording in the same patient record, using the same terminologies, and analyzing patient data from a holistic viewpoint, are those who set the arena and the patient record platform.

From the user's point of view, the electronic patient record should have functionality that supports:

- Day-to-day activities in patient care
- Communication of patient data
- Long-term storage
- Follow-ups and statistics

A Multi-Professional Approach

Each profession has its own recording needs and traditionally its own terminology. Table 29.1 describes the content on the top level of a multiprofessional process-oriented patient record. All professions follow the same layout and process, but the number of headings and hierarchical levels in the documentation differs between professional categories. The goal is to have one patient-one record, common terminologies, and architecture. The work has started, but it will take years before the patient record to a full extent can be said to be multiprofessional.

Patient Record Architecture

It must be possible to communicate information in a patient record to another electronic patient record system without losing quality in content or context. This is possible only if the communicating systems have the architecture of information in common. The standardized patient record system architecture is described with respect to content, data elements, and logic structure.

The European standard for electronic patient record architecture (CEN, 1999) structures the record data elements in record items and record item complexes.

A patient record can include a number of different types of record items and record item complexes. Each record item and record item complex has a set of attributes and should be uniquely identified. Tables 29.2 through 29.5 show the attributes. The attributes described here meet European ethical and legal demands for patient records. A common list of possible types must be available in every patient record system.

Table 29.1 Description of Top Level Content in a Multiprofessional Patient Record

Profession	Assessment	Problem Identification	Goal	Intervention	Outcome
All	Patient administrative data	Patient examination			
All	Social history	Patient examination	Social needs	Social goals	Social rehabilitation	Measures of outcome
Physician	Medical history	Patient examination	Medical diagnosis	Medical goals	Medical treatment	Measures of outcome
Nurse	Nursing history	Patient examination	Nursing diagnosis or nursing problem	Nursing goals	Nursing care	Measures of outcome
Physiotherapist	Functional state of health history	Patient examination	Problem identification	Functional goals		Measures of outcome
Occupational therapist	Activity history	Patient examination	Problem identification	Rehabilitation goals		Measures of outcome

Courtesy Swedish Institute for Health Services Development, Spri Print 361,1998.

Table 29.2   A Record Item Type Is Defined by the Values and/or References of Its Attributes

| Record Item Type | Attributes | | |
	Requirements	Comments	Examples
ID of record item type	Compulsory	Unique	Unique ID of vital signs
Name of record item type	Compulsory	Familiar to the professions	Vital signs
Version no.	Compulsory	Attributes can be added or disclosed	
Status	Compulsory	Valid or not valid	
Type of content	Compulsory	Form and classification, reference to terminology server	Value, free text National or local term standards
Terminology	Optional	Reference to terminology	
Presentation	Optional	Form	

Courtesy Swedish Institute for Health Services Development, Spri Print 361,1998.

Table 29.3   A Record Item Is Defined by the Values and/or References of Its Attributes

| Record Item Type | Attributes | | |
	Requirements	Comments	Examples
ID of record item type	Compulsory	Reference to current record item type	Unique ID of vital signs
ID of record item	Compulsory	Unique	Unique ID of blood pressure
Version no.	Optional	Attributes can be added or disclosed	
Status	Compulsory	Valid or not valid	
Content	Compulsory		130/70

Courtesy Swedish Institute for Health Services Development, Spri Print 361,1998.

The key element in the standard is the record item. It represents independent information, e.g., the recorded value of a blood pressure or free text under a keyword such as patient status and nursing diagnoses.

The record item complex links record items together and gives them the context to which they belong. A patient record always includes at least one record item and one record item complex. Record item complexes can also be linked together. The patient record itself should be seen as a record item complex; other examples are different views of patient data.

 A European Curriculum and Courseware for Nursing Infromatics

Aim and Set-Up

In 1995, the European Commission decided that nurses should become adequately educated in the field of telecommunication and information technology. It was recognized that the nursing profession is the largest profession in the health care providers group and that nurses play a key role in health care communication.

Table 29.4   A Record Item Complex Type Is Defined by the Values and/or References of Its Attributes

| Record Item Type | Attributes | | |
	Requirements	Comments	Examples
ID of record item complex type	Compulsory	Unique	Unique ID of admission notes
Name of record item complex type	Compulsory	Familiar to the professions	Admission notes
Category	Compulsory	Unique	
Version no.	Compulsory	Attributes can be added or disclosed	
Status	Compulsory	Valid or not valid	
Authorization parameters default	Compulsory	Reference to classification for authorization	Access control
Responsible for content	Compulsory	Reference to resource database	List of nurses
Recorder	Compulsory	Reference to resource database	List of nurses
Time of recording	Compulsory	Form	
List of included record item, -complex types ID	Compulsory	At least one	

Courtesy Swedish Institute for Health Services Development, Spri Print 361,1998.

Table 29.5   A Record Item Complex Is Defined by the Values and/or References of Its Attributes

| Record Item Type | Attributes | | |
	Requirements	Comments	Examples
ID of record item complex type	Compulsory		Unique ID of admission notes
ID of record item complex	Compulsory	Unique	Unique ID of patient status
Name of record item complex	Compulsory	Familiar to the professions	Patient status
Version no.	Compulsory	Attributes can be added or disclosed	
Status	Compulsory	Valid or not valid	
Authorization parameters, current	Compulsory	Reference to authorization control database	
Patient ID	Compulsory	Unique, reference to patient database	ID, name and address
Responsible for content	Compulsory	Reference to resource database	List of nurses
Recorder	Compulsory	Reference to resource database	List of nurses
Time of recording	Compulsory	Form	
Verification of content	Compulsory	Reference to resource database	Signature
Time of verifying	Compulsory	Form	
List of included record item, -complex types ID	Compulsory	At least one	

Courtesy Swedish Institute for Health Services Development, Spri Print 361,1998

Under the leadership of the university of Athens and with substantial financial support of the EC, a project was defined. The purpose was to develop a specific nursing informatics curriculum and accompanying courseware that could be incorporated in the present nursing curricula in the different countries of Europe, as well as standing on its own. The project, called Nightingale *(http://asklipios.dn.uoa.gr/nightingale)*, was initiated and led by the University of Athens. The aim was to develop a curriculum in the multidisciplinary field of nursing informatics within 3 years. The curriculum should fit into all levels of nursing education and training at various sites across Europe. The following six countries took an active part in the development work: Greece, The Netherlands, Belgium, United Kingdom, Denmark, and Portugal.

In order to educate nurses for the telematics era, a European base was found essential to assure that the results could be broadly used throughout Europe. The work had to be user-driven to reach a European consensus. Nightingale established a Users and Policymakers Group, with representatives from 13 European countries. The participants of this group were selected IMIA-NI and EFMI WG5 (Special Interest Group on Nursing Informatics of the International Medical Informatics Association and the European Federation of Medical Informatics, respectively) European members. The members of the User and Policymaker Group represented their countries as experts in the area of Nursing Informatics and brought relevant national networks to Nightingale. Another party taking part in the development was the industry in the field of CD-ROM technology and hospital information systems.

A special peer group was appointed with experts from Australia, North America, and Europe. Close cooperation was established with another European project, the IT EDUCTRA project. This project's task was to develop education and teaching material for health informatics.

Curriculum and Multimedia Courseware

Table 29.6 shows the content of the curriculum as a whole. It is divided into three distinctive domains: Building Nursing Knowledge, Informatics, and Organizational Impact. More than 15 different topics for system modules were identified.

The User and Policymaker Group focused on the concept of nursing informatics as related to the role of nurses in the health care process. The following definition of nursing informatics was adopted:

Nursing Informatics is the multidisciplinary scientific endeavour of analysing, formalising and modelling how nurses collect and manage data, process data into information and knowledge, make knowledge based decisions and inferences for patient care, and use this empirical and experimental knowledge in order to broaden the scope and enhance the quality of their professional practice. The scientific methods central to nursing are focussed on:

- using a discourse about motives for computerised systems
- analyzing, formalizing and modelling nursing information processing and nursing knowledge for all components of nursing practice: clinical practice, management, education and research
- investigating determinants, conditions, elements, models and processes in order to design, and implement as well as test the effectiveness and efficiency of computerized information, (tele-) communication and network systems for nursing practice, and
- studying the effects of these systems on nursing practice (Goossen, 1996)

Nurses must be made aware of the fact that management of information is an important part of the nursing role in the care process. Nightingale stated that on one hand nursing data are essential in the primary process of care delivery and on the other hand nursing data should not be considered isolated but instead related to all the information on a patient. Consequently, nursing information is an integral part of the electronic patient record.

Different Types of Courseware   A large number of nursing teachers were part of the Nightingale test sites. Multimedia courseware was developed. The following material and facilities are now available:

- Package of 200 transparencies
- Nightingale lexicon on CD-ROM
- World Wide Web site
- Interactive training material on CD-ROM
- Textbook in nursing informatics

Validation of Transparencies   The Nightingale transparency package is based on the content of the curriculum. It has been tested and evaluated by teachers and students in a number of different European countries. The package showed good acceptance by both groups, but since some areas were not sufficiently

Table 29.6.   Curriculum Content Is Divided into Three Domains: Building Nursing Knowledge, Informatics, and Organizational Impact

Building Knowledge

Introduction into nursing (basic principles of informatics in relation to nursing)

■ Nursing process: terminology, classification, codification, data sources

■ Transferring data into information

■ Linking nursing diagnosis to cognitive skills

■ Patient education

Nursing Informatics

■ Health informatics

■ General introduction to health

■ Computer literacy and hands on experience

■ Information tools

■ Support systems

■ Data protection and confidentiality: general principles, security, legal and ethical issues, privacy, and legislation

■ Data analysis methods: bio-statistics, (data collection, analysis, interpretation), simulation, mathematical modeling (physiology, nursing), mental modeling, and cognitive decision-making

■ Electronic patient record: hospital/community information support systems; electronic patient record, principles (content, structure, database model, etc.); telecommunication and networking; patient documentation; nursing information system

Organizational impact

■ General introduction on the impact of informatics on organizations

■ General introduction to health care systems

■ Ergonomic aspects and user interfaces: data input; data presentation; human-computer interaction; integrated system; standardization

■ Class interconnectivity

■ Social impact of informatics

---

covered, the package was extended from 125 to 200 pieces. The transparencies have been or will be translated into more than 10 languages.

Lexicon on CD-ROM   The Nightingale Lexicon includes the meta terminology for nursing informatics. It was developed by using corresponding work of CEN/TC251 and ICNP.

Interactive Courseware Material on CD-ROM   It was decided at an early point of the development that an interactive program focusing on the use of an electronic patient record should be developed. The material gives the student the opportunity of two threads: either follow a patient from admission to discharge, or learn by a more structured, lecture-based approach.

Both threads take the student to practical situations in a hospital, with and without an electronic patient record system.

The program allows cross-referencing from one point to another. It clearly shows the positive effect on courseware for nursing informatics when it is based on daily practice in health care. The program combines "close to home" information and feelings together with theoretical abstract parts.

Textbook   To guide teachers and students through the theoretical part of the courseware, a textbook of more than 500 pages was written by well-known experts in the field of nursing informatics. The book was edited by John Mantas and Arie Hasman (in press).

Perspective and Implementation

Dissemination of information about the Nightingale curriculum and courseware material to European nursing schools and universities took place during 1999. The European Commission endorsed this work and also implementation of the Nightingale curriculum in the institutions of the participating countries.

Summary

It is obvious that the diversity of developments in the different European countries brings several different approaches to the development of terminology systems and electronic patient records. The formalization of nursing terminology becomes stricter when the level of aggregation is higher. The level of aggregation is dependent on the purpose, which on its own is dependent again on the particular situation in each country. Although the ICNP was first launched in Europe and the EC funded its development, the national terminology systems are not always compatible. ACENDIO works further on this issue to eventually standardize nursing care terminology in Europe. One option for future work in the area of terminology includes further development of enumerative work, possibly leading to endless lists of terms. The ICIDH can be seen as an example for such an approach. Another option is a multi-axial classification system that allows free combinations of a rather limited but expressive set of terms. This adheres to the CEN work. However, this approach requires highly skilled classification and content specialists and further explicit limitations of meaningless combinations (Hardiker and Rector, 1998). A third option is to choose a very limited set of items such as in the minimum data sets. However, these have limited value for clinical care for the individual because their scope is too broad. Choices in this area are heavily dependent on the national situation in the different countries.

It should be possible to transfer health care information between information systems, and after the transfer the content as well as the context should remain. The European standardization effort describes the patient record structure in two main types of elements, record items and record item complexes, in order to achieve this.

The European Commission decided that nurses should become adequately educated in the field of telecommunication and information technology. It was recognized that the nursing profession is the largest profession in the health care providers group and that nurses play a key role in health care communication. A specific nursing informatics curriculum and accompanying courseware was developed that could be incorporated in the present nursing curricula in the different countries of Europe.

References

CEN. (1999). CEN/TC251 prENV 12265,1995, Electronic healthcare record architecture. (EHCRA) and CEN/TC251 Short strategy study: "Systems of concepts for nursing: a strategy for progress."

Ehrenberg, A., Ehnfors, M., and Thorell-Ekstrand, I. (1997). The Vips model—Implementation and validity in different areas of nursing care. In U. Gerdin, M. Tallberg, and P. Wainwright (Eds.), *Nursing Informatics: The Impact of Nursing Knowledge on Health Care Informatics* (pp. 408–410). Amsterdam: IOS Press.

Goossen, W. T. F. (1996). Nursing information management and processing: A framework and definition for systems analysis, design and evaluation. *International Journal of Biomedical Computing, 40,* 187–195.

Halttunen, A. (1992). The nomenclature of nursing interventions—A national project in Finland. In K. C. Lun, P. Degoulet, and T. E. Piemme et al. (Eds.), *Medinfo 92* (pp. 993–995). Amsterdam: North Holland.

Hardiker, N. R., and Rector, A. L. (1998). Modeling nursing terminology using the GRAIL representation language. *Journal of the American Medical Informatics Association, 5*(1),120–128.

Hermans, H. (1996). *Nieuwsbrief over Ziekenhuis Registratie Systemen,* no. 14. Brussels: Ministry of Health.

Hoy, D. (1997). Managing expectations: Users, requirements and the international classification for nursing practice. In R.A. Mortensen (Ed.), *ICNP in Europe: Telenurse* (pp. 207–215). Amsterdam: IOS Press.

Madsen, I., and Burgaard, S.A.J. (1997). The Danish national health classification system—nursing interventions classification: A part of a common Danish health care classification. In U. Gerdin, M. Tallberg, and P. Wainwright (Eds.), *Nursing Informatics: The Impact of Nursing Knowledge on Health Care Informatics* (pp. 32–36) Amsterdam: IOS Press.

Seppälä, A. (1992). *Suomessa käytössä olevia hoitoisuusluokituksia.* Helsinki: Helsingin yliopistollinen keskussairaala.

Sermeus, W., and Delesie, L. (1997). Development of a presentation tool for nursing data. In R. A. Mortensen (Ed.), *ICNP in Europe: Telenurse* (pp. 167–176). Amsterdam: IOS Press.

Ten Napel, H., (1996). Ontwerp WCC-standaard Classificatie van Diagnostische Termen voor de Verpleegkunde. Zoetermeer, WCC Vaste Commissie voor classificaties en definities.

van der Bruggen, H., and Groen, M. (1997). Patient outcome. Naar definiering en classificering van resultaten van verpleegkundige zorg. *Verpleegkunde, 12*(2)68–81.

Van Gele, P. (1996). Ist eine Standardisierung und Klassifizierung der Pflegetatigkeit notwendig? PCS News (May 23, pp. 29, 30–36).

CHAPTER **30**

Pacific Rim

Evelyn J.S. Hovenga
Robyn Carr
Michelle Honey
Lucy Westbrooke

OBJECTIVES:

1. Describe the development of nursing informatics in some Pacific Rim countries.
2. Identify historical milestones, changes, and trends influencing nurses to embrace informatics.
3. Discuss nursing informatics leadership, international links, education, research, and their impact upon the development of nursing informatics as a nursing discipline or specialty.

KEY WORDS:

information systems
standards
hospital information systems
public policy

The evolution of nursing informatics has varied in each of the Pacific Rim countries. The adoption of informatics usually began as a vision by one or more individuals. Such people used any number of opportunities plus their leadership skills to promote and disseminate the use of information technologies to support nurses in all areas of nursing practice. This occurred in health care, educational, and government organizations, as well as within the information technology industry and via any number of new and existing professional organizations. Events external to the nursing profession frequently became the catalyst stimulating some type of activity by nurses towards the adoption of informatics. International and multidisciplinary links have assisted these beginnings and its progression. Australia, New Zealand, and Hong Kong have made considerable progress since the early 1980s in this regard, although much remains to be done. Nurses in a number of other countries in this region have only just begun or have yet to learn about nursing informatics.

The Asia Pacific Medical Informatics Association (APAMI) was formed in 1993 as a regional group of the International Medical Informatics Association. APAMI has helped launch national health care informatics asso-ciations in Malaysia, Indonesia, and the Philippines and has generated awareness about the field in India, Pakistan, Sri Lanka, and Fiji. Other member nations are Australia, Hong Kong, Japan, Korea, New Zealand, the People's Republic of China, Singapore, Taiwan, and Thailand. Nurses in these countries who are interested in promoting informatics to their profession need to link up with this network.

Evidence suggests that many nurses continue to have some difficulty in embracing these technologies to support their practice (Ho and Horenga, 1999; Wiltshire and Moser, 2000). Furthermore, it continues to be a challenge for nurses to obtain appropriate education in informatics both during their initial nurse education and as a component of post-nurse registration specialist courses. Notwithstanding these conditions, an increase in computer use by practicing nurses in Australia and New Zealand is creating an awareness of the opportunities and gains to health care resulting from an increase in the use of computers, information, and telecommunication technologies. Thus, nurses in all health environments are becoming more dependent on electronic information.

This chapter aims to provide an overview of these historical events, primarily from Australia and New

Zealand, and to highlight critical success factors for the benefit of those who have yet to embark on such a journey. The chapter concludes by summarizing significant events and examining their impact on the evolution of nursing informatics in this region.

 ## Health Informatics in New Zealand

New Zealand's total population is under 4 million. These people are predominantly found in the urban areas, with the greater Auckland area having over a third of the total population. There are currently 107,778 registered nurses, of whom 46,000 are practicing, and 9,988 of these are situated in the Auckland area. Thus, Auckland by default becomes the hub of the drive for greater health informatics awareness. Nursing Informatics New Zealand (NINZ) identifies with and supports the International Medical Informatics Association—Nursing Informatics (IMIA-NI) definition of nursing informatics:

> Nursing informatics is the integration of nursing, its information, and information management with information processing and communication technologies, to support the health of people world wide.

Figure 30.1 describes the major influences of nursing informatics in New Zealand. Each item shown is summarized in more detail below.

The hub labeled "Informatics Influences" represents information collection, since this is seen as central to nursing, informatics, and health care. The other entities identified are significant players in New Zealand's health care system, which influences nursing informatics and its development. Health care in New Zealand is chiefly funded by the government, through the Ministry of Health to the centralized Health Funding Authority (HFA). Overall, the funding of health care in New Zealand is driven by business requirements, where information is used as the basis for cost-effective quality care, given limited resources. The HFA encourages a competitive environment for the providers of health care who contract, for never-sufficient resources, to supply a range of health care services. Health care is available for all resident New Zealanders via this national system. The cost of every consultation with the general practitioner is subsidized by the government and is free for children under 6 years of age. Tertiary care is almost totally publicly funded, and there is an impression in New Zealand that if you have an accident or are acutely sick, then good quality public hospital care will be available. There is, however, competition between private and public health care in the primary and secondary arena. Elective surgery is now more often provided in the private sector, although it may be funded by the public sector, as the public hospitals struggle to cope with long waiting lists and beds full of acutely ill and injured people.

The government also controls health care provision and funding through agencies such as the Accident Compensation Corporation (ACC). The ACC provides a range of health benefits and subsidies to assist individuals in the event of an accident. The establishment of the ACC has virtually eliminated suing for compensation in the event of an accident covered by the ACC. Information is collated about the nature and costs associated with accidents. ACC funding is provided through a levy on employers and employees. However, abuse of ACC services has resulted in the system becoming unable to cope financially. Recent legislation has seen the emergence of private health schemes offering ACC type care.

All prescription-related medicines are regulated by the government through Pharmac. Subsidies are available on a range of medicines, although only a few options within each drug classification may be subsidized by Pharmac. The public can purchase an increasing number of over-the-counter remedies, and there is an increasing need for drug information. There is a move to change legislation to allow New Zealand registered nurses to prescribe a range of prescription medicines. Debates are currently taking place regarding this issue. Nurses require ready, easy access to current information about drugs and associated material.

Government

The Ministry of Health is interested in information collection, and much of this occurs through the auspices of the New Zealand Health Information Service (NZHIS). This body controls the national database, which holds registration for 95% of New Zealanders. The NZHIS database uses a unique identifier, which is now assigned at birth, and is designed to follow the individual through each health care event in his/her life. The unique identifier is called the National Health Index number, or the NHI. The NHI allows easier tracking of information through health care episodes.

The National Minimum Dataset (NMDS) is a single integrated collection of health data, developed in consultation with health sector representatives and required at the national level for policy formulation, performance monitoring, evaluation, and research. These data

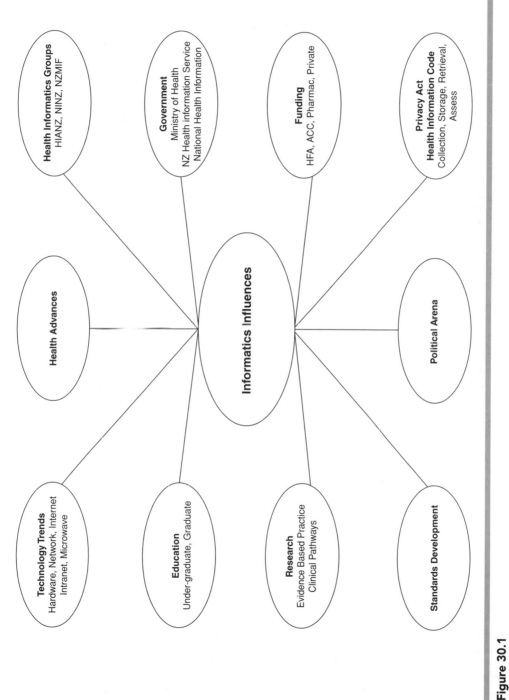

Figure 30.1
Major influences of nursing Informatics in New Zealand.

are to be reported by all hospitals, including private hospitals. Statutory requirements govern the reporting of certain diseases such as cancer, tuberculosis, and other communicable diseases.

All information collection, storage, access, and retrieval in New Zealand is governed by the Privacy Act (1993) and the Health Information Code (1994) and subsequent amendments. This act is one of the most comprehensive pieces of privacy legislation anywhere in the world.

New Zealand Health Informatics Groups

There are a number of informatics interest groups in New Zealand, each with a slightly different focus. The longest established group, founded in 1989, is the Health Information Association of New Zealand (HIANZ). Their members tend to be involved with medical records and medical libraries. NINZ was formed in 1991. The New Zealand Health Informatics Foundation (NZHIF) was founded in 1994. The members of NZHIF tend to represent industry, medical practitioners, and government bodies. Initiatives between the three informatics groups have commenced to find ways of working collaboratively. Early discussions investigating the possibility of formalizing this by the formation of an umbrella health informatics group has been seen as a positive and sensible move by all concerned.

New Zealand at Present

The status of nurses' use of computers in patient care depends on the facility. Computer use in high-dependency areas, such as intensive care, is greater, and it correlates with the urgency of information need. In lower-dependency areas, computer use by nurses is limited. Few hospitals have electronic records and care plans. There is a mix of the traditional paper records and some innovative use of electronic systems. Examples include nurses designing their own data collection screens using a tree structure consistent with Windows technology and clinicians identifying data that they wish to collect and enter electronically into the hospital patient system. The clinical record is attached to the patient file, which is a small start to an electronic patient record.

The provision of health care in the community is a growth area, and there are systems being developed that provide ease of use and the portability required. As an example, the Royal NZ Plunket Society Inc., the main provider of well child health service for the chil-

dren under 5 years of age and their families, has introduced a national database, as a registry of all of their clients. The 29 area offices around the country use the Internet to connect to the centralized database. Work is in progress to introduce hand-held computers for Plunket nurses to enter their event data and to again use the Internet to send the data back to the main repository.

Another community-based example is in the mental health field. Community mental health workers in one pilot program were supplied with notebook computers, and their communication and coordination of service within the team all occurred electronically. Despite some initial resistance, the legibility and improved documentation did enhance the collaboration between team members.

Language and Terminology

There is no standard use of a nursing vocabulary in New Zealand, although there is much interest in how this might be achieved, especially across primary and secondary care. There are New Zealand representatives actively involved in a number of international initiatives towards this end.

Administrative information systems in the health sector are basically using two methods to classify patients. Secondary care facilities were using International Classification of Diseases (ICD) 9 codes and have recently moved to ICD 10, while primary providers, primarily general practitioners, are using READ Codes. The coding is generally done by clerical staff in secondary care and either by the general practitioner or by clerical staff within primary care.

Acuity and Rostering

There are two areas of nursing management that have constantly been presented as suited to technological solutions. Information systems that deal with acuity or level of need/amount of dependency on nursing service have had several forms within New Zealand. There appears to be no single preferred method of assessing this, and there are variations found depending on the type of care being provided and the organizational culture.

Rostering or scheduling of nurses faces a similar situation with a range of systems in use: some totally electronic, while others remain either manual or a mix. The systems that appear to be most well-accepted are those linked to other aspects of administration, such as unit budgets, acuity, and payroll. The obvious advantages in time-saving, cost-tracking, and greater efficiency for nurse managers are recognized.

Trends in New Zealand Health Care

One of the current trends is integrated care. This has political implications. It is being examined as a means to provide better service between primary, secondary, and tertiary health sectors. The NHI is seen as pivotal to plans for integrated care, although privacy issues and working in a cooperative manner within a competitive funding environment are also barriers.

Another move is towards collaboration between health providers. Consultation across health disciplines and the use of interdisciplinary and multidisciplinary teams to provide a wider range of health services are being encouraged. The use of a single client health record within an organization is common, and each health professional involved with the care of the individual documents on a shared chart. At this stage, these remain predominantly paper records. Some general practitioners maintain an electronic health record within their practice. Some trials have commenced looking at smart card technology, and discussions have started to examine the concepts and issues behind a client-held record. The preference at this early stage seems to be towards a cumulative health record collected over the lifetime of the individual.

These changes to the way nurses work with other health professionals lead to the inference of the reduced need of nursing informatics as a separate interest group. Instead, we may see the development of health informatics as a stronger identity with a range of health professionals working together towards a common interest.

Health Informatics in Australia

Australia is a federation of eight states and territories. It has a population of 16–17 million. Approximately 71 percent of all its households are located in inner and outer urban and provincial areas, mostly near cities on the coast. The history of the formation of medical, health, and nursing informatics groups reflects the difficulties experienced as a consequence of a federal system of government and vast distances between population centers.

Australia has had a representative to IMIA's Working Group 8 (WG8) (now NI sig) since 1984. Nurses were the second group of health professionals to organize themselves to promote informatics; the general practitioners were first, beginning in the late 1970s. Nursing Informatics is now a special interest group of the Health

Informatics Society of Australia (HISA), which came into existence in 1993. It has been a long and torturous path to reach this position.

Historical Developments

Nursing informatics in Australia began with the Royal Australian Nursing Federation (now ANF) in 1984 with the production of a position paper, on "Computerised Patient Data and Nursing Information Systems" (Royal Australian Nursing Federation, 1984) based on an earlier discussion paper (Jenkins, 1984). Secondly, the Seventh National Conference of the College of Nursing, Australia (now Royal College of Nursing Australia) held in Melbourne in May 1985 had as its theme "Information Processing—Challenges and Choices for Nurses." Clare Ashton from the United Kingdom, who at that time chaired the British Computer Society Nursing Specialist Group and who was a member of the IMIA's WG8, was the invited guest speaker. Other prominent speakers were Evelyn Hovenga, who was Australia's IMIA WG8 representative; Gillian Biscoe, a W. K. Kellogg Australian Nursing Fellow then studying at the University of California, San Francisco; and Hazel Labka, who had been awarded a short-term W. K Kellogg Australian Nursing Fellowship to undertake an investigative study of the application of computers to the educative, administrative, and clinical fields of nursing. This inspired a small group of midwives, including Joan Edgecumbe, who is now the Executive Officer of the Health Informatics Society, Australia. At a meeting of members of the Midwives Association in October 1985, this small group decided to call a general meeting of nurses interested in computer use. This took place in November that year and was attended by about 70 nurses who agreed to establish the Nursing Computer Group. A regular newsletter documenting their activities was produced. This group continued to flourish and hosted the Fourth International Symposium on Nursing Use of Computers and Information Science in Melbourne in 1991. Also, in October 1986, the Royal Australian Nursing Federation adopted a position statement on "Computerisation in Health Services—Implications for Nursing."

In 1978, the Royal College of General Practitioners held its first computer conference, and in 1979 this college promulgated a computer policy, which was reaffirmed in 1988. It formed a national computer committee in 1986 following the establishment of several state-based medical computing interest groups. The RACGP Standards for Computerised Medical Records Systems were released in 1988. In 1987, this college established the position of Computer Fellow in conjunction with Monash University's Department of Community Medicine.

In South Australia, the Royal Adelaide Hospital Nurses Education Fund sponsored a National Nursing Conference to celebrate their 150 Jubilee in July 1986. The theme was "From Lamp to Light Pen—Computers in Nursing." One of their guest speakers was Professor Kathryn Hannah, who represented Canada in IMIA's WG8, was its Vice Chair, and had chaired the second international symposium on nursing use of computers and information science, held in Calgary in 1985. Dr. Hannah was the inaugural visiting fellow at the Royal Adelaide Hospital and also spoke at a seminar held in Melbourne organized by the Lincoln Institute of Health Science (now Latrobe University). Three members of the Victorian Nursing Computer Group were at this conference and networked with nurses from other states. At that time, it was discovered that the Royal Australian Nursing Federation's Queensland branch had established a nursing computer special interest group a little later than the Victorians. They had 20 to 30 members. Western Australia had a 2-year-old group, and other states were in the process of organizing themselves. As a result of this meeting, these groups began to exchange information about their activities.

Prior to 1986, there were other health professionals with an interest in informatics who regularly attended a variety of international conferences. At the Medinfo '86 symposium held in Washington, D.C., around 20 Australians met and decided to form a network with the aim of promoting health informatics among health professionals. They met again at Medinfo '89 in Singapore. As a result of these discussions, other groups were also formed in several states over the years that followed. In the meantime, the Australian Computer Society (ACS), Inc. was the organization that represented Australia to IMIA.

By late 1989, initiatives were taken in Western Australia to form an Australian Medical Informatics Association (AMIA) with state-based branches. In early 1990, 16 health informatics enthusiasts representing interests in academia, anaesthesia, artificial intelligence research, the Australian Computer Society, dentistry, general practice, library services, medical coding and terminology, medical records, system design, nursing, pathology, research, and government met in South Australia and established the Australian Health Informatics Association (SA) Inc. This group published Health Informatics News and Technology (HINT), six issues per annum. In Queensland, an informal group of health pro-

fessionals had organized regular educational meetings throughout 1990. In early July 1991, this became the Australian Health Informatics Association (Qld). Early 1991 also saw the establishment of a Health Informatics group in New South Wales (HIANSW). Their first meeting was attended by 36 people representing a wide range of health professionals including nurses as well as computer scientists, software developers, and hardware vendors. This group also produced a regular newsletter titled "CHIP—Computers in Health Information Processing." At that time, the inaugural meeting of the AMIA (Victorian Branch) was also held.

A postconference meeting of nurses from all states and territories was held in Melbourne following the international nursing informatics symposium in April 1991 to discuss the formation of a National Nursing Informatics group. Everyone agreed to work together, but the formalization of a new national organization was problematic due to differences between the state-based groups regarding affiliations with other professional nursing organizations. Subsequently, the Nursing Computer Group Victoria changed its name to Nursing Informatics Australia, launched a new look magazine, and established a secretariat with the symposium proceeds. One representative from each state-based group was appointed to form the Australian Nursing Informatics Council (ANIC) in 1992 to facilitate networking and ongoing discussions to unite the groups into one national organization.

By late 1991, AMIA had affiliated with the ACS to become that organization's medical informatics special interest group and had organized a one-day health track at the ACS annual conference held in Adelaide that year. This was seen as an opportunity for members of the many disparate groups to meet and discuss the possibility of forming one national organization. This special meeting was attended by around 40 people who were duly informed that AMIA's newly established board had adopted a constitution the day prior to the meeting. All present were invited to join AMIA, but according to the constitution membership was restricted to people with a degree. This meant that many nurses, i.e., all those with a hospital nursing certificate or a diploma would be excluded as a consequence. There was also a debate about the name, since many of those present preferred the term "health" to "medical." The meeting closed with these issues unresolved. Some time later advice was received that nurses would be welcomed by AMIA.

Another attempt at uniting the groups was made early 1992 at the first HIANSW conference held in Laura, New South Wales to discuss how to best work together and how health (medical) informatics should be represented at IMIA. By that time, there were 23 distinct groups and a further four individuals who represented Australia in some way internationally. All were invited to participate in these discussions. This resulted in a resolution to:

1. Form a National Council of Health Informatics Groups.
2. Combine three newsletters/journals, CHIP, HINT, and Nursing Informatics Australia, into one national and multidisciplinary magazine with a national editorial board. The first issue of *Informatics in Healthcare Australia* came out in May 1992.

Another meeting called by AMIA was held later that year in Melbourne. This led to a discussion paper summarizing deliberations, and a scenario for the development of one new national organization to represent the field of health informatics in Australia was presented. The paper was widely circulated to members of all groups for feedback. Meanwhile, ANIC initiated the idea to organize a national conference in 1993. Several groups supported this idea, and since NIA was the only organization with the necessary funds, this group managed this inaugural conference. A special meeting of representatives from interested groups, facilitated by Dr. Ian Graham, who was the Director, Centre for Health Informatics at the Austin Hospital, was held in Sydney in early 1993 with the objective of finalizing this issue. This meeting produced a draft Constitution for HISA, reflecting an agreed set of principles. This was presented to potential HISA members at its inaugural general meeting held in conjunction with the inaugural Health Informatics Conference (HIC '93), and they voted for its adoption. Conference profits were then used to fund the further development of the constitution and incorporation. This was finally achieved in mid-1994.

Nursing Informatics in Hong Kong

Hong Kong nurses established NURSINFO (HK) Ltd. in 1991, and this organization has enjoyed a consistent increase in membership. They have as their motto "Nursing Informatics for Excellence in Patient Care." They organize regular educational activities, use a communication network, produce a regular newsletter, and are actively involved with the Hong Kong Society of Medical Informatics and the Hong Kong Computer Society. Together they participate in the organization of trade exhibits and regular conferences. The Hong Kong Hospital Authority is responsible for over 40 hospitals

and over 50 specialist clinics that are part of a large multisite, multiprotocol intelligent data network to provide seamless data communications throughout. Implementation began in 1993. By 1997, an integrated patient administration system and a pharmaceutical supplies system had been implemented in 43 hospitals. Hospitals with an excess of 1,000 beds each had a clinical management system that included laboratory information and results, a medication order entry system, and an outpatient appointment booking system, and they were working on the development of integrated patient documentation. Their aim is to provide a longitudinal patient record documenting the care and services provided by multidisciplinary health care teams.

Standards Development

In 1995, NINZ produced standards for nursing informatics guidelines covering accountability, confidentiality, health and safety, the essence of nursing, professional development, and resource management principles for which standards and associated dependencies were identified. These were shared with the international nursing informatics community, and feedback was sought to guide their further refinement.

In New Zealand, the Ministry of Health both separately and through the New Zealand Health Information Service is working with interested health providers and informatics groups, including NINZ, towards the establishment and refinement of health information standards. The New Zealand work in progress is cognizant of the Australian and international standards and is not seeking to recreate standards. The Standards Association of New Zealand controls the formal process for the acceptance and publication of standards. A number of standards are issued jointly as both Australian and New Zealand standards. There is close collaboration between Standards New Zealand and the Standards Australia IT/14 Health Informatics committee. Standards Australia were persuaded to establish a health informatics committee in 1992. It now has several active technical subcommittees and works closely with other similar groups. Nurses are represented via the Royal College of Nursing and Central Queensland University. The focus in Australia has been in the area of standards development to facilitate data interchange to first of all support all types of E-commerce and now to support the interchange of clinical data. This is putting a greater emphasis on the need for a standard architectural structure for patient records and terminologies.

Australian Government Initiatives

The Australian House of Representatives Standing Committee on Family and Community held an enquiry into Health Information Management and Telemedicine and published its report "Health on Line" in late 1997. Many of their findings and recommendations are now guiding health informatics and telehealth government initiatives. Among these was a National Health IT Standards Workshop as one step in a 3-year initiative aimed at facilitating the shift to increased interoperability of information systems in the health sector. Information technology (IT) in health is seen as the key to providing the means of achieving better integration of care, for enabling services to be focused on the consumer, and for reducing duplication of waste. The results of this workshop were then considered by the Standards Australia Health Informatics committee (SA IT/14) as the basis for developing a workplan for standards development. This was done in concert with the workplan being developed by the newly established International Standards Organisation Technical Committee Health Informatics (ISO TC 215), which is chaired by the SA IT/14 project manager.

The Australian Institute for Health and Welfare (AIH&W) provides research and statistical support to the commonwealth, states, and territories. In 1993, all public health authorities, the Australian Bureau of Statistics, and the AIH&W signed an agreement to improve the quality of and cooperation in the development of national health information. This now provides the national infrastructure needed to provide high quality health data. It includes the National Health Data Dictionary of established data definitions and data standards, the National Health Data Collection and Reporting Guidelines, national minimum standard edits, and data policy guidelines. Implementation is supported by the Australian Health Ministers' Advisory Council (AHMAC), who have established a National Health Information Management Group, a National Health Informatics Council, and a National Telehealth Committee. The latter became the Australian New Zealand Telehealth Committee in 1996 *(http://www. telehealth.org.au/)*.

Telehealth is an area that is developing very rapidly around the country. A 1998 status report listed well over 70 telehealth programs and projects with applications in a range of specialty areas. This is increasing almost daily as the nation's telecommunications infrastructure is improving as a result of significant funding through the Commonwealth's Regional Telecommunications Infrastructure Fund and its "Networking the Nation" project. Also, the National Office for the National Information Economy (NOIE) is the Australian government body responsible for developing strategies to address the key issues arising from the convergence of the information economy, information technology, and telecommunications *(http://www.noie.gov.au/)*.

The Collaborative Health Informatics Centre (CHIC) Ltd. is an independent (but funded for 3 years by the Commonwealth Government Department of Industry, Science, and Resources) not-for-profit company initially established by the Queensland state government in 1996. This state government continues to provide additional funding *(http://www.chic.org.au/)*. Its mission is "to facilitate collaboration between health care providers and IT&T suppliers to improve health outcomes." It acts as a clearing house for the collection and dissemination of information about the Australian informatics industry. To a large extent, its activities overlap with those performed by HISA; the difference is that they have considerable financial resources, whereas HISA, as a professional organization obtains its income from membership fees, conference profits, and industry sponsorship.

There was a tendency to focus on the collection of hospital data. This changed in 1998 with the launch of a comprehensive program of national data collection in general practice and the release of version 1.0 of the National Community Services Data Dictionary and other related publications. The AIH&W has developed the National Health Information Knowledgebase, an Internet-based interactive electronic storage site for national health metadata. It includes a powerful query tool and is regarded as a world benchmark in data/metadata registries (NHWI, 1998) *(http://www.aihw.gov.au.)*

During the 1980s, work began in collaboration with Professor Fetter from Yale University to develop patient classification systems to describe the case-mix serviced by health care organizations. Since 1992, the Australian National Diagnosis Related Group (AN-DRG) standard has been in use first for the purpose of monitoring and comparison of hospital activity and later for costing and funding purposes. This system relies on data obtained from individual patient records, including the ICD codes. A number of case-mix systems are in use to suit a variety of patient populations. Nurses use these for clinical path development and to cost nursing services.

Research

Health-related information has a number of uses. Apart from the direct use of information in the care of clients, there is a growing awareness of the need for timely and accurate data for research. Two specific areas that are currently gaining more attention within nursing informatics are clinical pathways and evidence-based practice. Work in these areas is fledgling, but nurses are looking to international colleagues to keep abreast of developments. Australia now has a few Ph.D. students who are conducting research in areas of nursing informatics. Some are now publishing quality papers (Chu and Cesnik, 1998; Ribbons, 1998a-c), and all are very much involved in promoting IT applications to support nursing practice and education. HISA organizes an annual conference, where between 40 and 60 papers are presented each year. These plus the papers published in its magazine are indexed in CINAHL. Collectively, these provide a good overview of progress in health informatics in Australia. Health Informatics does not exist as a research category for the major government research funding organizations such as the Australian Research Council or the National Health & Medical Research Council, which makes it difficult to obtain research funds from these organizations. NINZ, and more recently the NINZ together with NZHIF, organize national conferences on health informatics every second year. These have provided an excellent forum for the sharing of implementation and associated research from around the country.

Education

In New Zealand, nursing informatics has been recognized as significant by the Ministries of Health and Education since the early 1990s. A national Guidelines for Teaching Nursing Informatics curriculum was introduced into the undergraduate preparation of nurses programs in 1991. The extent of those being implemented has varied between schools of nursing, depending mostly on resources (of interested staff, hospitals where information systems are in use for live examples, and classroom facilities like computer suites for teaching). In 1998, the University of Otago, in conjunction with Wellington Medical School, offered for the first time a Diploma in Health Informatics. There was considerable interest from a range of health professionals from around the country. Nursing informatics as a postgraduate specialist subject has not yet been recognized or developed by any of the schools of nursing.

In the New Zealand clinical field, most of the training for computer use is the responsibility of the employer. This has the advantage of being relevant to the specific needs of the area of practice. It also permits ongoing training to be more easily and conveniently provided on site. The disadvantage associated with training provided by the employer is that the training covers what the employer thinks the staff need to know. It tends to ignore the larger conceptual areas that have the potential to encourage staff to consider what else they want to know and look at possibilities beyond those currently supplied. Despite this, there are sufficient nurses actively seeking further education and training in the area of health informatics. This is evidenced in the increasing number of nurses involved with the training, implementation, and support of information systems in all areas of health care.

The first Australian experiences of nurses using computers were compiled into an edited text by Graham MacKay and Anita Griffin in 1989. The first Australian textbook on health informatics was published in 1996 (Hovenga et al., 1996). Much of nursing informatics education was provided by nursing computer/informatics groups via study days, seminars, and conferences during the 1980s and 1990s. The Lincoln Institute of Health Sciences (now Latrobe University) provided registered nurses undertaking postregistration degrees with opportunities to include computer studies in their course as early as 1979. Central Queensland University introduced nurses to computers in 1989 with a strong commitment to a computer-assisted–managed learning project (Zelmer et al., 1991). A 1990 survey of all tertiary nursing programs in Australia found that 27 percent (10 out of 37 respondents) had more than 5 years' experience of teaching computing to nurses, and 73 percent (27) included computing within their nursing programs most frequently as a core unit (Hancock and Henderson, 1991). There has been little progress since then. Informatics education for nurses in Australia varies considerably from one university to another (Hovenga et al., 1999). Most have one person attempting the impossible, often in environments where fellow nurse academics have little or no knowledge of informatics. In some instances, there is active resistance to its introduction.

One exception is Monash University, where there are several academics interested in and using IT to support nurse education. Thus, informatics is integrated into their undergraduate nursing program to some extent, although the only undergraduate informatics unit offered is not core to the degree. A certificate course in health informatics has been offered since 1999. Most universities offer one unit of study within their undergraduate nursing pre- and postregistration programs as an elective. The only other postgraduate program available in Australia is a Graduate Diploma and Master degree in Health Administration and Information Systems, which has been offered since 1992 by Central Queensland University. Some of these graduates are now pursuing Ph.D. studies, others are actively engaged in promoting the use of IT in the workplace, and many work in hospital-based nursing informatics positions.

 ## Technology Trends

Technology continues to increase in capability and complexity. Although the cost for individual items of technology decreases, our demands for this technology, and therefore our overall spending, increase. Health care in New Zealand is moving towards consolidating high-tech medical care in fewer but better-equipped health care facilities to provide both quality and cost-effective care. The enormous changes in the technology nurses use to support client care, are seen most in the intensive care unit and in the care of premature babies. Nurses need to be prepared to work alongside and utilize technology to best care for clients. Health care organizations are now looking to implement clinical information systems and electronic patient records.

 ## Summary

It is clearly evident that the professional health, medical, and nursing organizations play a major role in the awareness-raising, education, and dissemination of knowledge about the field of health informatics. This is becoming increasingly complex with the proliferation of government initiatives spanning multiple government departments. This is a reflection of the multidisciplinary nature of health informatics. Nurses, as the largest group of health professionals, have a major role to play. This requires a sound knowledge about the many stakeholders so that nurses can play a role in coordinating their efforts to ultimately benefit the health care consumer, our patients, communities, and society as a whole.

 ## References

Chu, S., and Cesnik, B. (1998). Improving clinical pathway design: Lessons learned from a computerised prototype. *International Journal of Medical Informatics, 51*, 1–11.

Hancock, H. A., and Henderson, A. M. (1991). Of Floppy Disks and Feminism. In: E. Hovenga, K. Hannah, K. McCormick, and J. Ronald (Eds.), *Nursing Informatics '91 Proceedings of the Fourth International Conference on Nursing Use of Computers and Information Science.* Melbourne: Springer-Verlag.

Ho, M. K., and Hovenga, E. J. S. (1999). What do nurses have to say about information technology in their workplace? In J. Walker, S. Wheaton, M. Wise, and K. Stark (Eds.), *HIC 99 Handbook of Abstracts.* Full paper on CD-ROM of proceedings, HISA, Melbourne, Australia.

Hovenga, E. J. S., Kidd, M., and Cesnik B. (1996). *Health Informatics, An overview.* South Melbourne: Churchill Livingstone.

Hovenga, E. J. S., Luck, J., Plummer, A., and Ho, M. (1999). *An Australian Survey of Informatics Education in Health, Medical and Nursing Programs* (research in progress).

Jenkins, E. (1984). *ANF Professional Officer.* Correspondence to the author.

MacKay, G., and Griffin, A. (1989). *Nurses Using Computers: Australian Experiences.* Armidale, New South Wales: A.C.A.E Publications.

NHWI News International recognition for the Knowledgebase. (1998). *AIH&W Newsletter*, No.14, December 1998, p. 3.

Ribbons R. M. (1998a). Practical applications in nurse education. *Nurse Education Today, 18*, 413–418.

Ribbons R. M. (1998b). The use of computers as cognitive tools to facilitate higher order thinking skills in nurse education. *Computers in Nursing, 16*, (4), 223–228.

Ribbons R. M. (1998c). Guidelines for developing interactive multimedia: Applications in nurse education. *Computers in Nursing, 16*, (2), 109–114.

Royal Australian Nurses Federation. (1984). *Computerised Patient Data and Nursing Information Systems: Some Considerations.* Melbourne, Australia.

Wiltshire, V., and Moser, C. (2000). Research into the attitudes of nurses to computers in progress at Central Queensland University, Rockhampton, Australia.

Zelmer, A. C., Lynn, B., McLees, M. A., and Zelmer, A. E. (1991). A Progress Report on the Use of CAL/CML in a Three Year Pre-Registration Diploma Program. In: E. Hovenga, K. Hannah, K. McCormick, and J. Ronald. (Eds.), *Nursing Informatics '91; Proceedings of the Fourth International Conference on Nursing Use of Computers and Information Science.* Melbourne; Springer-Verlag.

31

South America

Heimar F. Marin
Daniel Sigulem

OBJECTIVES

1. Discuss nursing informatics development in South America.
2. Identify the use of information technology in clinical practice.
2. Describe educational perspectives and distance learning.
4. Discuss standards initiatives.

KEY WORDS

nursing informatics
distance education
clinical informatics
computer research
PAHO
DIS-UNIFESP
Latin American informatics
NIEn/UNIFESP
BIREME Library
LILACS
vocabulary
standardization
ICNP-Brazilian version

Nursing Informatics in South America has been based much more on the activities of individuals than on a policy established by governments or by national efforts. However, the use of technological resources has been a visible tendency in nursing education, practice, research, and administration. The growth of information technology in Latin America and the Caribbean has been consistently the world's highest since 1985 (Pan America Health Association/World Health Organization, 1998). Consequently, the use of technology in nursing sectors of activities followed the evolution of technology use in the region.

Nurses are using computer resources to improve patient care and communication. At the present time, computers are considered an important tool to help nurses take care of patients and to organize nursing service and nursing education.

The objective of this chapter is to present an overview of the development of nursing informatics in South America, identifying some initiatives in clinical practice, education, and research, including discussion on the current development and trends of computer system applications to support the nursing profession.

 ## Background

Nursing has been identified around the world as an emerging profession for more than 100 years. The professional evolution has been a continuous process influenced by science and technology. Furthermore, technology has been the driving force to further nursing development. Nurses are the primary users of technology in health care. Historically, nurses are used to facing challenges, adapting new tools into the practice to improve their performance, and creating new models to enhance patient care. Technology can be a tool to help nurses face further challenges and discover how to use its resources to innovate and maybe to redesign their way of taking care of people (Marin, 1996).

The beginning of a new century represents not only an opportunity to face different challenges and to develop new objectives and good solutions for future needs but also the time to identify strategies to achieve resolution of these specific issues in order to emphasize the nursing profession and nursing's contribution to the health of the population.

Technology is causing significant modification of human activities and, consequently, of the way we learn and work. Traditional methods of teaching, managing, and practicing a profession do not support the requirements of modern life anymore.

As a tool, computers have been recognized as an important resource to support many activities. Their importance is widely recognized in the storage, retrieval, and analysis of information. It is also common knowledge that information is the key element to make a decision in the health care area. In addition, there is evidence that an explosion in the quantity of information available is occurring; scientific knowledge doubles every 2 years (Zielstorff et al., 1993).

The more specific information there is to support clinical decisions, the better care that can be delivered to the patient. The quality of care is related to the scope of knowledge and information that health providers can access on which to base their clinical decision-making processes. Technology plays an important role in facilitating access to the information. Gradually, each country is becoming more aware of the possibilities to apply technology resources to dynamize activities in taking care of clients/patients.

Implementation of health informatics technology in South America should be built around a comprehensive patient-oriented model, where all providers can be supported by the system and where the information is shared across geographic frontiers. The Pan American Health Organization (PAHO) has published guidelines and protocols to orient the development and deployment of information technology in Latin America and the Caribbean (Pan America Health Association/World Health Organization, 1998). However, the development of these systems continues to be an isolated initiative based on the financial and organizational ability of each country or state in the region.

At the same time, it is important to emphasize that Latin America and the Caribbean region rank third in information technology expenditure. A study performed by the Pan America Health Organization/World Health Organization (WHO) showed that the Information Society Index, based on the use of information, computer, and social infrastructure, is evolving rapidly. Although expenditures represent 5 percent of the world total, the growth of information technology in Latin America and the Caribbean has been consistently the highest since 1985 (Pan America Health Association/World Health Association, 1997).

 ## Nursing Informatics and the Electronic Health Record

In South American countries, as in any other countries in the world, the initial motivation to develop computer systems in the health care area was driven by financial and administrative concerns. The hospital sector can be considered the area better served by information systems. According to PAHO (1998), countries like Brazil, Mexico, Argentina, Colombia, Chile, and Paraguay have computer systems in 31 to 50 percent of their hospitals.

Many of these countries initiated their computerization experiences around 1985. In Argentina, Belgrano Hospital was one of the pioneers in introducing computerized systems. It is a public hospital that created its own system, a local network connecting about 18 working areas. The hospital information system has programs such as Pharmacy, Personnel Department, Emergency Service, Admission and Discharge Office, Laboratory, and others (Rodas et al., 1995). As a general tendency, there is no specific program for nursing documentation, where clinical data can be processed. However, general patient data that are also used for nursing administration are included in the whole system as specific elements.

In Brazil, many initiatives to implement hospital information systems began around 1980. Hospitals have been working to design their own systems in order to attend to specific needs and policies. The initial systems were also designed to support finance and administrative issues, and many hospitals still have just those computer application programs available. More recently, systems addressing patient care have been implemented to support all providers, including nursing documentation, in order to facilitate control and to better record the quality of care to the client. Examples of these systems can be found in cities like Porto Alegre, Brasília, Rio de Janeiro, São Paulo, and many others. In addition to Brazil, Chile, Venezuela, and Argentina are also developing or updating their systems according to an electronic patient record model.

Many additional initiatives are spread throughout the Latin American countries. It can be observed that the use of the computer as an instrument to support nurses' activities in taking care of patients still needs a lot of investment of human and material resources. Clinical systems based on the nursing process are not common in these countries. Most of the computer systems implemented are intended to control administrative data.

Information systems in use do not attend to the specific nature of nursing practice and its information processing requirements, although frequently nurses are responsible for data entry of modules such as drugs, pharmacy request, bed control, and patient admission.

Another issue to be considered is that when hospital information systems are being developed, the resources needed for nursing options are insufficient. The major interest is still the financial and administrative control. Programs to support the nursing process continue to be isolated initiatives and have had little impact.

Otherwise, nurses are becoming more involved with the design, implementation, and evaluation of hospital information systems. Vendors and developers recognize that the success of a computer system requires nursing input and collaboration. Safran et al. (1989) demonstrated that when providing patient care, nurses use a computerized hospital information system more often than any other group of health care professionals.

In addition, as an open and evolving market, international developers are making investments to sell and implement computer systems in South America. At the present time, South America represents the most promising market in the world for technology.

Even so, it is necessary to emphasize that the inclusion of nursings' elements of practice in the patient record is the responsibility of nurses. They need to be involved with the programmers, vendors, and developers to drive the profession. Taking care of patients is what nurses know how to do. Therefore, it is essential to assure that all information required to perform nursing care is present in the health information systems.

At a time when the tendency is toward a computer-based patient record, it is mandatory that nurses be able to identify what kind of nursing data and information will constitute nursing knowledge. Nurses cannot stand by and wait for vendors and developers to adapt technology to nursing practice.

It is necessary to identify what kind of technological resources can be used to improve nurses' performance. There are many options for each area of application, and the selection must be done considering the existing organizational, technological, and local requirements.

Distance Learning and the Educational Perspectives in Nursing Informatics

Technology is transforming not only nursing practice but also nursing training and the education models. With the introduction of computers in the health care area, nurses became primary users, responsible for data input. Consequently, they had to become computer-literate in order to utilize computer technology in an efficient manner. To meet educational and training needs, nursing schools and hospitals initiated programs to prepare nurses to use computers.

In the educational process, computers can be used for instruction and evaluation. Continuing education programs of health care institutes are including this subject for discussion to provide skills for nurses using computers to enhance their performance. In addition to teaching how to use computer applications, course instructors are also considering the use of computers to teach nursing content.

Computer applications in nursing education are also changing nursing education from a passive teaching to an active learning process. Computers allow students to work at the time that best meets their specific needs. Usually, the programs are very interactive and easy-to-use and offer immediate feedback about students' performance.

Furthermore, computer technology is providing students who live in distant regions, who have difficulties in accessing the main educational centers, the opportunity to improve their personal knowledge base. There has been a trend toward distance learning program development in South America. A contributing factor to the development and success of these programs is the distance between countries and cities due to the geographic characteristics of South America.

One pioneer program was developed by the Departamento de Informática em Saúde at the Universidade Federal de São Paulo (DIS-UNIFESP), Brazil. Since 1995, a group of experts in education and computer science have been studying different methodologies and models to make courses available through the Internet. At the present time, they are offering courses comprising different models, such as an electronic book that has the ability to integrate text, sound, and image simultaneously. They are also developing an interactive program that incorporates problem-based learning processes.

The DIS-UNIFESP first offered an Internet long-distance specialization course in nutrition in the public health area. Since then, courses in ophthalmology, orthopedics, and cardiology have also been made available, and the most recent initiative is a course in sexual education for teenagers (Sigulem, 1997). The experience of DIS-UNIFESP has been shared with other universities, and at the present time, countries like Argentina, Mexico, Chile, and Venezuela are also making available long-distance courses in health care.

Formal education in nursing informatics such as a specific nursing informatics specialization course is also being provided. The Núcleo de Informática em Enfermagem at the Universidade Federal de São Paulo (NIEn/UNIFESP) was the first center to offer the specialization degree in South America. NIEn/UNIFESP also provides, since 1989, the nursing informatics discipline in its graduate and undergraduate nursing programs.

Considering that education is a life-long process and an empowering force that enables an individual to achieve higher goals, these educational programs are certainly the best direction to the next millennium.

Research in Nursing Informatics

Nursing is an information-dependent profession in which computers can be used to explore and discover new knowledge. Moreover, computers can be used to redesign a body of nursing knowledge accordingly to the new models of practice presented by modern society.

South American countries are developing different research projects to explore the use of computers not only to conduct nursing research using statistical software, spread sheets, databases, and word processing, but also and more importantly to identify the implications of computer resources in nursing clinical practice, administration, and teaching.

Access to health care literature is provided by consulting the available bibliographic databases. Using World Wide Web resources, one can have access to the BIREME Library (Centro Latino Americano e do Caribe de Informação em Ciências da Saúde), which is the central library of the Federal University of São Paulo. Its origin dates back 1965–1967, offering services such as bibliographic searches and supplies and selective dissemination of information.

Since its foundation, BIREME has incorporated a series of databases such as LILACS, which is the first and main database, a trilingual Spanish-English-Portuguese system with approximately 3,000 highly selective standard medical periodicals (Estevéz, 1995). Also, BIREME provides access to the CINAHL (Cumulative Index to Nursing and Allied Health Literature) and MEDLINE (Medical Literature Analyses and Retrieval System On Line).

The communication technology has facilitated scientific research, providing high quality information searches at a low cost. Use of the Internet is becoming even more widespread throughout South America. Almost all educational centers provide Internet resources to students and professors. However, if this access is not provided, one can easily find a commercial provider.

In the past 3 years, there has been a brisk growth of Internet connectivity in South America as measured by the number of hosts. By January 1997, 164,051 hosts were registered under the geographic domain with more than 2 million users. For instance, by this time, Brazil had registered approximately 7,500 hosts, Mexico 3,000, and Argentina 1,000. However, this figure does not reflect the real total number of hosts because organizational domain hosts were not included (Pan America Health Organization/World Health Organization, 1998). Recent changes in telecommunications reform, accompanied by competition, cheaper rates, and better service, are also arriving, especially in Brazil, Argentina, Chile, and Peru.

Included in this investigation of computer use in nursing practice are some computer programs being developed for use in patient and nursing education. One of the focal points has been the use of computers to teach nursing and health content. As an example, the Nursing Informatics Group at the Federal University of São Paulo developed an educational system in prenatal hygiene to be used as a tool to teach pregnant women. This system received the award of best poster presentation at the Nursing Informatics World Conference in Stockholm, 1997. Systems like this one have been considered a subject of research in many South American countries as a way to enhance patient education.

In fact, research has been the most productive sector in nursing informatics. Several research projects are being conducted exploring different applications of computers in nursing care and nursing education. One of these research projects was developed utilizing artificial intelligence resources to design a decision support system in prenatal care to identify risk factors during pregnancy (Marin, 1994). Another example is the Multilit program, which is a computer program to investigate the incidence of renal lithiasis in Brazil, collecting standardized information during the patient assessment. The system allows identification of the national morbidity in lithiasis (Sigulem, 1997).

A practical example is the ADTP project, which is a decision support system in tuberculosis. This system was also pioneered by DIS-UNIFESP, and it was implemented in 1997 in Recife, a city located in the northeast region of Brazil. The main objective is to reduce the prevalence of this disease in the city, helping providers to attend patients and to control the treatment.

The most recent initiative is related to the use of telematics resources. DIS-UNIFESP is developing a multidisciplinary project in telematics to be implemented in a slum community located in São Paulo. The objective is to make available to the people who live in that community access to health care 24 hours a day. Nurses and physicians from the Universidade Federal de São Paulo will be connected to a small center constructed in the neighborhood, where another nurse will be attending the clients and use the telematics resources to help him/her in the diagnoses and interventions.

Vocabulary for Nursing Practice

Sharing and communicating information is essential to make decisions and to be able to deliver care. Exchange of information requires the communicating parties to agree on a communicating channel, an exchange protocol, and a common language The language includes an alphabet, words, phrases, and symbols that express and assign meaning, understood by all users (Pan America Health Association/World Health Organization, 1997).

Computerization has pushed nurses to adopt protocols to document and communicate patient care. The use of common language becomes more critical and even more demanding to accomplish in the computerization era. Sometimes standardization is criticized because of its inflexibility. However, standardization allows the promotion of the development of a nursing information system to communicate the nature of nursing and to expand nursing knowledge (McCloskey and Bulechek, 1994).

In relation to the nursing profession, the use of vocabulary has been considered from different perspectives. Clark (1995) pointed out that "communicating among ourselves has always been important but communicating with other people about nursing has acquired a new urgency since we are forced to recognize that the value of nursing is no longer apparent to those who have the power to influence our practice." Other issues to be considered are reimbursement policies, cost containment, and technological development in recent years.

However, it is nurses' responsibility to decide not only what kind of data are important to describe the contribution of nurses in the health care process and to assure continuous care, but also to decide how these data could be described. What kind of language will be useful to support the several different activities performed by nurses? In fact, the use of vocabulary in nursing must assure both communication among the nurses and communication between nurses and the other providers responsible for patient care.

Clark (1995) also emphasized that "it is a cruel paradox that while we know that nursing is universal because the human needs that it exists to meet are

universal," at the present time there are no empirical means of comparing nursing practice across countries or even across clinical settings or client groups within a country. Using a common vocabulary would allow nurses to compare practices and costs, to analyze the content of the nursing process, and to verify how the current information supports the continuous care.

The importance of using standard terminology to describe nursing care in order to facilitate data retrieval and analysis is recognized by South American nurses. Efforts have been made in this area, and now different clinical vocabularies are available. However, building a vocabulary that standardizes the clinical nomenclature for use in clinical practice and that fulfills all requirements is a challenge.

The North American Nursing Diagnoses Association (NANDA) taxonomy is the taxonomy most used by nurses to document nursing diagnoses in practice. In Brazil, it was introduced around 1990 due to the initiatives of nursing professors from the Universidade Federal da Paraíba, a state located in the northeast region of Brazil (Farias et al., 1990). It is necessary to observe that NANDA taxonomy was the only one translated into the Portuguese language until 1997. Consequently, many nurses in the country know just NANDA and have been trying to adapt the NANDA list of diagnoses to their practice even though the terms are very abstract, not intuitive, and unfamiliar to the Brazilian culture.

In 1990, the International Council of Nurses (ICN) initiated a long-term project to develop an International Classification for Nursing Practice (ICNP) with the objective to establish a common language about nursing practice to be used for describing nursing care for people in a variety of settings (Mortensen, 1996). Years later, some nursing associations in South America, stimulated by the International Council of Nurses also initiated a project to develop a classification for nurses in community care. This project, the "Classification for Nursing Practice in Collective Care," is supported by ICN and the Kellogg Foundation.

The ICN recommended that the research project should be elaborated in order to investigate the community nursing care in Latin America. Consequently, since 1995, Brazil, Chile, Colombia, and Mexico have conducted national projects that will be integrated into the ICNP.

In Brazil, the dissemination of the ICNP started around 1996, when NIEn/UNIFESP became a sponsoring partner in the Telenurse Consortium, a project led by Randi Mortensen, Director of the Danish Institute for Health and Nursing Research. According to this

partnership, NIEn/UNIFESP responsibilities were to
translate the ICNP alpha version into the Brazilian
Portuguese language, to make a field test of the ICNP
alpha version in order to identify possible matches to
the local terms in the patient record, and also to implement it in an electronic patient record.

The paper and electronic forms of the ICNP Brazilian version *(http://www.epm.br/enf/nien/cipe)* have
been available since September 1997. The content was
presented during the Nursing Informatics Conference in
October 1997. The field test was performed at the São
Paulo Hospital, a teaching hospital at the Universidade
Federal de São Paulo. This preliminary study found that
the nurses are using just a few terms of those available
in the ICNP alpha version. Although the ICNP alpha
version can be used to document nursing phenomena
and interventions, it still demands a more intensive
process of dissemination among Brazilian nurses, and
more efforts must be made in order to facilitate the
practice implementation (Marin, 1999). Recently,
NIEn/UNIFESP started a new project to translate and
test the Home Health Care Classification (HHCC) system developed by Saba (1992). Home care is an evolving area in Brazil and demands specific terminology to
document nursing care.

It would be much more productive and easy to use a
standard vocabulary if South American nurses developed
a national database of nursing terminology and used this
database to establish mutual relations of the local terms
with standard vocabulary developed by ICN, NANDA,
Nursing Intervention Classification (NIC), Nursing-
Sensitive Outcomes Classification (NOC), HHCC, and
others. Using national and regional terms could facilitate
the documentation of nursing care and could be more
intuitive for nurses in their daily practice, respecting their
local culture.

The most frequently used vocabularies may not necessarily be the best ones, but they may reflect the demands
of insurance companies and other payers. Although there
are quantitative differences in terms of breadth of coverage and internal representational structure, no clinical
vocabulary has been elected so far as the ultimate solution for clinical documentation automated retrieval and
rapid communication. Several obstacles have yet to be
passed before nursing communities embrace a standardized vocabulary that proves useful in a variety of tasks
and settings: regional, national, and international (Marin
and Machado, 1996).

The task is a challenge, and continuous studies must
be done to reach the equilibrium that will facilitate nursing practice documentation around the world.

Summary

Besides innovations and several applications distributed among the countries, telecommunication is still a
demanding area in South America. Countries recognize
that progress in the telecommunication sector is essential to the establishment of health informatics and to
ensure the global competitiveness of their economies
(Pan America Health Association/World Health Organization, 1998).

Nursing informatics as an integrated part of health
care follows the progress that has been made in the whole
sector of health informatics. Because of the wide variety
among countries and even inside larger countries, the
development of nursing informatics is conducted on a
case-by-case basis, taking into consideration the specific
requirements of each region. Furthermore, the development and deployment of nursing informatics is dependent
upon national priorities and human capabilities.

This situation represents a great opportunity for
nursing. The future is exciting, because with technological advances nurses have the chance to drive their own
destinies. Adapting technological resources to their practice will help nurses to see emerging trends in the healthcare field as challenges and unique opportunities for
career growth. There are new roles, new areas, and new
jobs demanding experts. Nurses can be consultants, software designers, managers, entrepreneurs, and more.
Opportunities are wide open for those who have decided
to incorporate information technology into their daily
practice in the process of taking care of patients.

References

Clark, J. (1995). An International Classification for
Nursing Practice (ICNP). In S.B. Henry, W.L. Holzemer,
M. Tallberg, and S.J. Grobe (Eds.), *Informatics:
The Infrastructure for Quality Assessment and
Improvement in Nursing* (pp. 25–31). San Francisco,
CA: University of California Nursing Press.

Estevéz, C., and Sosa-Iudicissa, M. (1995). BIREME,
The Latin American Health Information Center in
São Paulo, Brazil. In M. Sosa-Iudicissa, J. Levett, J.S.
Mandil, and P.F. Beales (Eds.), *Health, Information
Society and Developing Countries* (p. 63–66). The
Netherlands: IOS Press.

Farias, J. et al. (1990). *Diagnóstico de Enfermagem:uma
Abordagem Coneceitual e Prática*. João Pessoa: Santa
Marta, 160 pages.

Marin, H. F. (1994). *Sistema de Apoio à decisão em
assistência pré-natal normal*. São Paulo; UNIFESP.

Marin, H. F. (1996).Nursing informatics applications.
In N. Oliveri, M. Sosa-Iudicissa, and C. Gamboa

(Eds.), *Internet, Telematics and Health* (p. 265). The Netherlands: IOS Press.

Marin, H.F. (1999). Translating and testing ICNP in Brazil. In R. A. Mortensen, (Ed.), *ICNP and Telematic Applications for Nurses in Europe* (pp. 254–257). Amsterdam: IOS Press.

Marin, H. F., and Machado, L. O. (1996). Introduction to clinical vocabularies: What does the clinician need to know? Proceedings. *The Eight National Conference on Clinical Computing in Patient Care: Capturing the Clinical Encounter. Proceedings.* Boston.

McCloskey, J. C., and Bulechek, G.M. (1994) Standardizing the language for nursing treatments: An overview of the issues. *Nursing Outlook*, 42, 56.

Mortensen, R. (1996). *The International Classification for Nursing Practice ICNP With TELENURSE Introduction.* Copenhagen: Danish Institute for Health and Nursing Research.

Pan America Health Association/World Health Organization. (1997). *Health Technology Linking the Americas. Moving Towards a Vision: Implementing and Using Information Systems and Technology to Improve Health and Healthcare in Latin America and the Caribbean.* Washington, D.C.: Series Health Services Information Systems.

Pan America Health Association/World Health Organization. (1998). *Information Systems and Information Technology in Health: Challenges and Solutions for Latin America and the Caribbean.* Health Services Information Systems Program. Division of Health Systems and Services Development. Washington, DC, 1998.

Rodas, E., Morici, P., Daveggio, S. et al. (1995). Computerized systems in the Belgrano Hospital and the promotion of self-governing groups. In M. Sosa-Iudicissa, J. Levett, and S. Mandil et al., *Health, Information Society and Developing Countries* (pp. 67–76). The Netherlands; IOS Press.

Saba, V. K. (1992) Home Health Care Classification (HHCC) of nursing diagnoses and interventions. *Caring* 11, 50–57.

Safran, C., Slack, W. V, and Bleich, H. (1989) Role of computing in patient care in two hospitals. *MD Computing, 6,* 141–148.

Sigulem, D. (1997) *Um novo paradigma de aprendizado na prática médica da UNIFESP/EPM.* São Paulo: (1995). UNIFESP.

Zielstorff, R. D., Hudgings, C. I., and Grobe, S. J. (1993). *Next-Generation Nursing Information Systems: Essential Characteristics for Professional Practice.* Washington, D. C.: American Nurses Association.

PART **11**

The Future of Informatics

32

Future Directions

Kathleen A. McCormick

OBJECTIVES

1. Describe a future vision of nursing informatics in the new millennium.
2. Identify the key components of continuous speech recognition systems.
3. Describe the uses of data warehouses and knowledge repositories.
4. Define genomic informatics and describe some uses of it in health care in the future.
5. Understand how genomic informatics will require the integration of data from many clinical, medical, environmental, and knowledge sources.

KEY WORDS

continuous speech recognition
voice
data warehouses
knowledge repositories
genomic informatics
bioinformatics
computational biology

The chapters of this new edition include content related to many future directions. Authors have developed entire chapters describing telehealth, data mining, decision supports for health providers and consumers, and the Internet. In this chapter, the aim is to synthesize them into a vision of what health care might have for information system supports in the year 2020. Also, this chapter will describe some new information systems that have not been described in the book. Beginning with a practitioner scenario (Mason, 1994), this chapter will describe how the new voice technologies, knowledge repositories or clearinghouses, and genomic information systems might be used in the future.

A Millennium Scenario

The nurse practitioner is in her car and is on the way to work. As usual, she turns on the radio to get the road report, what roads to avoid and the estimated time of arrival if she goes the usual route. After turning off the radio, the practitioner turns to her portable computer and TELLS the computer to log on to her server at the office. She TELLS the computer to open E-mail. The computer scans the messages and finds one that is marked urgent. The computer INFORMS her that she has an E-mail message from the administrative coordinator that one of her patients is not feeling well and would like to come in to the office today. The practitioner TELLS the computer to REPLY that she has an opening at 11:00 A.M. and SENDS the message back to the administrative coordinator. The rest of the ride to work is routine, responding to about 20 to 30 messages that have come in prior to arrival at work. There was one important new policy that the hospital/clinic had circulated. She TOLD the computer to print it, file it, and store it in a subdirectory on work-related new policies.

Upon arriving at work, the administrative assistant has printed out a listing of all current orders, critical pathways, treatments needed, patients who need to be seen, those who need documentation dictated, what orders need to be considered today, what orders from yesterday need to be changed, and what considerations she needs to make regarding a patient with post-operative complications. Another urgent E-mail has arrived, and the practitioner TELLS the computer to open it. It is a video from a patient who is at home with a child with fever and congestion and has transmitted a view of the ears from a home otoscope connected to the computer, a snapshot of the throat, and a quick scan culture of the throat. Obviously, the clinician makes the diagnosis of otitis media without effusion on the clinical record. The computer searches the patient's history and the evidence and reports back to the clinician that this is the fifth occurrence of otitis with this 4-year-old child in the past 6 months. Was there a decibel hearing loss? The practitioner orders an audiogram for the child, which it transmits to the consultant, and sends a command to the scheduler system to make an appointment. The practitioner orders the child an antibiotic and sends it to the nearest drugstore to the family's zip code (53774), and the E-mail program sends a message to the parent saying that an appointment has been made for a hearing test and why and informing the parent of the medications at the drugstore. The patient's insurance company is billed for the transaction electronically. When the mother sees the new urgent E-mail message, she opens it and it also prints out the complications, indications, and side effects of the antibiotic. The new occurrence of the otitis media is transferred to the FAMILY HEALTH SYSTEM, where all of the documentation has resided since the children were born. It includes all immunizations, encounters with clinicians, treatments, and complications. The information is also carried by each family member on their SMART CARD, since they travel between several states to work.

Then the practitioner begins updating his/her orders; she TELLS the computer to order from the pharmacy an antibiotic for a patient who has a new fever. The computer suggests several antibiotics that are known to be effective for the type of bacteria that the patient has and the cost differential of different drugs.

The practitioner continues to SEE recommendations, MAKE DECISIONS, and TELL the computer what to order.

At 10:50 A.M. prior to the patient's arrival in the clinic, a picture of the patient and all previous encounters and recommendations are shown on the screen. The practitioner refreshes his/her memory that this was the 40-year-old woman who is pregnant for the first time. When the patient enters, the practitioner can visually see that the patient has gained 10 to 15 pounds. Asking her about her symptoms, the practitioner repeats those symptoms out loud in the front of the patient. The computer SEARCHES the knowledge repository and returns with recommended actions. Since the patient is also having headaches, the computer prompts the clinician to

rule out preeclampsia. The practitioner puts an armband around the patient, and a blood pressure is taken and TRANSMITTED to the computer. . . . 210/110 mmHg. The computer also indicates the prevalence of abnormalities on chromosome 7 with women with preeclampsia. The practitioner writes an order for an amniocentesis, ultrasound, and genetic testing of the mother for the obesity gene and the fetus for chromosomal abnormalities. The orders are transmitted to the appropriate clinics, and the mother leaves with schedules for the tests.

Much later that day, after seeing 32 new patients, the practitioner sees another urgent E-mail message. Because an emergency case has just come into the clinic, she puts it into STORE and FORWARD to home.

Upon arriving at home, the clinician opens her E-mail and the urgent message that she did not have time to look at during the day. She tells the computer to open it. In it is the ultrasound of the pregnant women's baby, the results of amniocentesis, and a genotyping of mother and child. The mother has preeclampsia and a genetic abnormality on chromosome 7, consistent with obesity and preeclampsia in women. She is given an appointment in the genetic engineering clinic to reverse this condition.

Unfortunately, there are noted alterations on several genes in the fetus. The practitioner asks, "Wasn't this the mother who did her dissertation in Sweden during Chernobyl and ate reindeer meat?" The practitioner orders a search of the environmental repository on the mother and determines that between certain significant years, the mother was in fact in Chernobyl.

The decision support system suggests that the mother test the child for chromosomal aberrations. The order is written . . .

This scenario could go on, but it is meant only to point out some of the new technologies that were described in this book, such as the use of the Internet for communication between clinician and patient/consumer, voice/continuous speech recognition, wireless computing, portable, and handheld devices, consumer involvement in decisions, telehealth, large data warehouses and repositories, clinician decision support systems, thin client computing, data mining, and genomic informatics.

The concepts of voice, data warehouses and repositories, and genomic informatics will be highlighted in this chapter. The other concepts were described in previous chapters. This chapter looks to the future of the integration of many systems described in this book, to a unified health record, the availability of knowledge repositories, and the forces of genetics on the new information system needs.

Voice/Continuous Speech Recognition

Continuous speech recognition is defined as "the method by which natural or conventional speech is recorded, and phoneme recognition is used to recognize streams of speech sounds" (Clark, 1998). Phonemes are the basic units of speech sounds, the "atoms" of speech. A dictionary contains the various symbols for each phoneme; these symbols describe how the words should be pronounced. Phonemes are made up of vowels and consonants, and each will produce different waveforms. Continuous speech recognition systems are composed of three subsystems (Zafar et al, 1999):

Input: an input, such as a microphone, acts as a signal transducer, converting sounds spoken by the clinician into electrical signals.

Digitizer: a digitizer, such as a sound card, digitizes the electrical signal. This signal is sampled at various rates, between 6,000 and 20,000 samples per second, which creates a series of decimal numbers proportional to the intensity of the sound at each point.

Software: the speech engine software serves as a transcriptionist, converting data into text words.

Figure 32.1 is a picture of the digitized sounds in the spoken words "FREE SPEECH." (from Zafar et al., 1999).

Speech recognition involves two stages. (1) The speech recognition system distinguishes the waveforms generated from the phonemes. (2) The pattern recognition component identifies the phonemes and maps these into words. Then the digitized signal is partitioned into spaced units of 10 to 20 milliseconds, called frames. In Fig. 32.1, the dark bands correspond to the frequencies for vowels. The dips in the frequencies are usually from consonants. The dashed arrows correspond to "noise." Thus, the signal is converted into a power spectrum consisting of vowels, consonants, and noise. The features are then extracted into a set of 15 to 20 numbers that best represent a frame and are insensitive to background noise.

Next, in order to convert the digitized signal input into words, the boundaries of the phonemes must be identified. A rapid change in amplitude is usually the set point. The next stage classifies each segment as a particular phoneme. Algorithms such as hidden Markov models (HMMS) often are used to identify these occurrences of phonemes. To identify what the phoneme represented within the boundary, the waveform of the segment is analyzed. A speech engine inspects the segment and

characterizes what the waveform might mean, a kind of phonetic waveform software.

The final step in the process is recognition mapping of phonetic sequences into words. This step requires the integration of a phonetic dictionary, listing the phonetic spelling of all words used by the user, and a language model of probabilities of how the words will be used in a sequence. For example, the phonetic dictionary alone could not discriminate the f in the word "free" from the ph in "phone" or the gh in "tough." The software also has to discern that there is no e in "straight," but it carries the same phoneme as weight. Language models also have to consider separating the types of words in the phrases: "two pills for two days" from the patient waiting "too long" to get back "to the clinic."

Areas where continuous speech recognition has been piloted successfully include stationary environments such as in pathology and radiology (Rosenthal et al., 1998; Nakatsu and Suzuki, 1995). In those quiet environments, the clinicians are sitting and dictating their findings. Recent uses in primary care are demonstrating benefits in medical health care (Zaphar, 1999).

To date, there are dictionaries to transcribe medications, surgical specialties, family practice, and most medical specialties. Nursing must be prepared with dictionaries of terms in order to have continuous speech recognition available in their practices in the future. The nursing profession must also be prepared to ask the right questions of vendors when evaluating new speech recognition systems. Basic questions are:

1. Does it come with a dictionary of nursing terms?
2. How accurate is the system?
3. How long does it take to train the system to the user's voice?
4. Will the user have to retrain the system if he/she has a cold?
5. How well does the system track pauses or background noise?
6. Will I be able to use the system at my bedside, for E-mail, in my office, on the mainframe?
7. Can the system run in a network environment?

Data Warehouses or Knowledge Repositories

Where will clinicians go in the new millennium to find the best evidence, basic science, policies, quality indicators, and tools to measure and evaluate outcomes of care? This section describes an Internet repository of

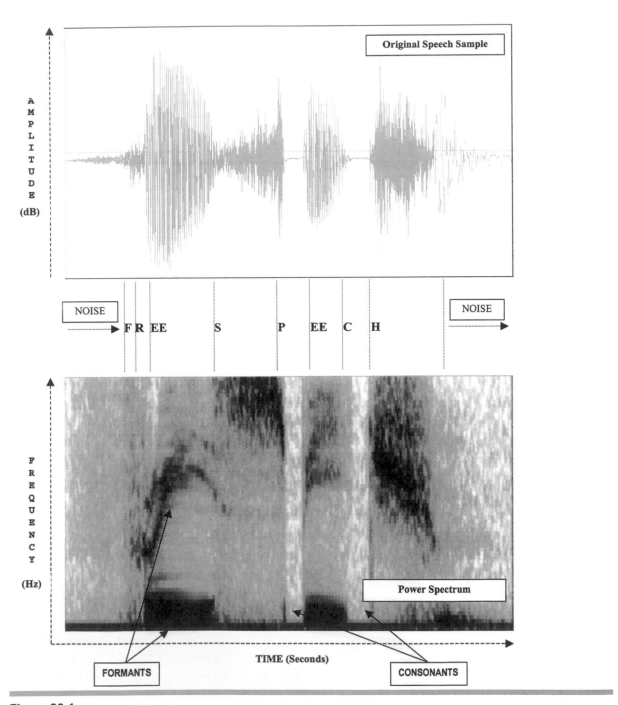

Figure 32.1
Digitized sounds of spoken words.
(Reproduced, with permission, from Zaphar et al., 1999).

information and the integration of databases from disparate sources into data warehouses that will be available to clinicians universally and from all practice environments. Models of data warehouses or repositories should reside in a National Health Care Knowledge Base (Greenes and Lorenzi, 1998). Models of this repository currently exist in such resources as C-GAP from the National Cancer Institute.

What is C-GAP?

C-GAP is located on the Web at *http://www.ncbi.nlm. nih.gov/ncicgap/*. C-GAP stands for Cancer Genome Anatomy Project. C-GAP was developed to unite the newest technologies, along with cost-effective and high-throughput capabilities, to identify all of the genes responsible for the establishment and growth of cancer. The challenge is coordination of these previously developed resources to be exploited by researchers and cancer specialists to determine which candidate genes investigators will spend time on and what new tools will be required to facilitate their discovery.

The intention of C-GAP is to have the genetic sequence data, microarray data, normal tissue, pathological tissue, MRI and PET scan images, and literature linked for particular cancer sites, e.g., breast, prostate, and leukemia. In that way, the clinicians can access the database for all of their questions in the diagnosis, prevention, and treatment of cancer.

The developer of C-GAP, Dr. Robert Strausberg stated that "Important in cancer discovery is the identification of the multiple genetic factors involved in tumor development" (Strausberg et al., 1997). Important in cancer discovery is the identification of these multiple genetic factors involved in tumor development, and the ability to determine which gene candidate is worthy of further investigation. Hundreds of candidate genes may be linked at some point in time to the progressive nature of tumor development. However, the task of deciding which are essential to spend time and energy on will ultimately be made by the investigating scientist. Improving the scientist's ability to more accurately and efficiently identify which candidate genes would make good therapeutics will be a fundamental step for the advancement of scientific cancer discovery. However, searching the raw databases is now taking approximately 90 percent of investigator's time.

Analysis of thousands of expressed genes will provide insight into novel gene discovery, clinical, prevention, and cancer control research. With the use of information technology tools, substantial opportunities exist for improving the ability to quickly and efficiently identify genetic anomalies. These tools will be critical in advancing the automation and interpretation of the ever-increasing data pool of sequence information.

What Other Data Repositories Will Be Needed?

The current clinical environment has produced data silos, or unorganized and uncoordinated data sources. Accessing them is inefficient, time-consuming, and costly. Coordination of biomedical data, clinical data, or educational information will require storage knowledge content, tools like data mining for knowledge management, and methods to move data from one source to another through common messaging standards and infrastructures.

The National Guidelines Clearinghouse *(http://www. ngc.gov)* is one such repository that was developed by the Agency for Healthcare Research and Quality (AHRQ). This clearinghouse includes all of the evidence or clinical practice guidelines being developed by the government and private sector professional organizations. If these guidelines were linked to clinical databases, clinical protocols used locally in practice, libraries of literature, and clinicians' desktops, then feedback on use of the guidelines could be transmitted back to the guideline developers on the appropriate utilization of the content.

The informatics resources need to consider the validity and reliability of the content, the version control (when was material updated?), a maintenance schedule, and how the content was changed in local uses. The content has to be evidence-based; consistent with medical and nursing terminology for measuring quality, outcomes, and costs; and capable of being inserted into clinical and medical information systems. Another important informatics resource will be the use of data mining tools to search for relevant knowledge related to the clinical conditions that the patient has. Intelligent agents need to bring the health practitioner updates daily, weekly, or monthly when changes have occurred in the data warehouse for the clinical conditions of patients. For example, nurses who deal with patients with Alzheimer's disease would like to know on a regular basis new genetic, environmental, clinical evidence, and treatment reports that have entered the knowledge repository. Alerts to one's personal E-mail will be possible during the new millennium.

When multiple users are linked to knowledge warehouses or repositories, collaborative work can be ongoing and dynamic (Kouzos et al., 1996). Information is not "owned" by an investigator or clinician. The "science of health care" is available to all. The uniqueness is the ability of the user to integrate the information into decision supports to evaluate its effectiveness and impact on outcomes of patient care and costs of care. The information is on a "just in time" basis of need for the clinician (Greenes and Lorenzi, 1998). Information is available when the clinician needs it, when he/she is with the patient, or when he/she aggregates data for review of quality information.

Genomic Informatics

Genomics is the science of genes and their functions. This new research field is helping us to better understand the molecular functions leading to disease and the interplay of genetics and chromosomal aberrations from the environment. The science of health care through genes, their interactions, their mutations, aging, and their relationship between normal body functions and disease is growing. Through an understanding of the normal functions of the different genes in humans (expressed in DNA sequences), their modes of expression (through RNA translation processes), and their functions in protein, scientists are now able to determine normal functions of control, prevention, embryogenesis, development, growth, reproduction, metabolism, aging, and responses to the environment. Through malfunctions in the normal function, diseases are expressed in various organisms. Thus, disease can be studied at a molecular level. For inherited and infectious diseases, the study of genomes allows the analysis of pathogenic agents and potential treatment options. Genetic diseases occur frequently in humans; single-gene defects occur in at least 1 in 100 individuals, chromosomal disorders in at least 1 in 150 newborns, and multifactorial diseases with a genetic component in 1 of 10 individuals (Rindfleisch and Brutlag, 1998).

Areas of genomics requiring bioinformatics support are listed in Table 32.1. These areas were described by others (Strausberg et al., 1997). They focus on the new molecular discoveries and point to areas of new growth in bioinformatics. This list does not include the need for integration with other databases that will be discussed later or the needs for text analysis and data mining, applying cluster analysis to databases.

The New Genetic Opportunity

Because of consistent funding and research discovery over the past 20 years, the National Institutes of Health have made significant progress in identifying and understanding the disruptions in basic cell processes

that occur in disease. With this discovery, it has become apparent that the way to prevent, detect, diagnose, and treat many diseases is to identify the genes involved in the pathophysiology. Discovery has also led to the recognition that genetic diseases can result from genetic heredity and chromosomal alterations that could have occurred as a result of lifestyle, environment, or a combination of factors. Variations in how diseases express themselves in individual people may also result from responses to hormones, diet, exposure to carcinogens, infectious groups, or yet undiscovered causes.

Disease Screening, Detection, and Diagnosis

Relatively expensive biosensors based on nanoscale ion channel switches have gone into commercial production (MHSS 2020, 1996). They allow detection of a wide range of diseases within minutes from a small sample of blood, saliva, or tissue. Biosensors will decrease the need for large laboratory analysis and extensive testing. Gene chips for analyzing distinctive patterns of genes active in different diseases will soon sweep aside traditional disease categories, replacing the former technologies with more powerful, complex ones consisting of families of genetically defined subtypes of disease. These new chips produce 64,000 data elements per patient. When subjected to different chemicals or hormones, one patient description may comprise millions of data elements. The data repositories to store these data, and integrate them with imaging data or pathological slides have created the need for enormous databases, expert algorithms to cluster information, integration with other data sets, and text mining and retrieval capabilities. As the gene chips reach reasonable costs, extensive genetic profiling and/or genotyping will be possible for more citizens.

Treatment and Prevention

With better detection and diagnosis will come an ability to customize care with therapeutic selections based on precisely diagnosed disease tailored to individual biochemistry or clusters of patients who are manifesting similar patterns of genetic aberrations. Drug discovery and the developmental process will be accelerated and fundamentally redesigned in response to this specificity. Biotechnology and genomics will produce new generations of treatments. Gene therapy will revolutionize the history of diseases such as cancer, heart disease, arthritis, diabetes, Alzheimer's, and others (National Cancer Institute, 2000). The inventions of the next century will

Table 32.1   Areas of Genomics Requiring Bioinformatic Development

Molecular Level
▪ DNA chip technology
▪ Gene expression analysis
▪ Assessing changes in genomic DNA
▪ DNA array assembly
▪ Identifying cellular proteins
▪ Structure-based functional genomics
▪ Protein networks (protein-protein interactions)

Database Level
▪ Registries/repositories
▪ Text indexing and retrieval
▪ Algorithm development, data mining
▪ Integration of molecular, clinical, medical, publication, and epidemiological databases
▪ Integration of disparate databases hosting genetic sequencing or protein sequence data

Strausberg, R., Dahl, C.A., and Klausner, R.D., 1997.

be comparable in their impact to past changes such as the introduction of the microscope, anesthesia, oxygen, vaccines, antibiotics, and chemotherapy.

Biochemically based nanocomputers and bioelectronic computers will be developed in time for solving complex combinatorial problems or recognizing patterns in complex genetic profile images. There is much to be discovered in what we know from previous patterns of disease. Through surveillance, diseases have been monitored for incidence, survival, risk factors, and death among populations. Different kinds of data have been collected on populations to identify environmental effects, to identify geographic areas with higher than average rates of disease (especially cancer), to study patterns and outcomes of care, and to identify risk groups for research and public health intervention programs.

Single Gene versus Complex Genetic Diseases

It is becoming apparent that many types of diseases are not single genetic diseases but instead result from combined, small effects of many genes and the interactions of the genes with the environment, hormones, diet, virus exposure, and other causes. Important in most major disease discovery is identifying the multiple genes involved by detecting variations in a gene's sequence for disease-associated genes. A polymorphism can have

functional significance in the body if it gives rise to a protein variant or it influences the expression of a particular gene. The information from polymorphisms allows scientists to map a disease-related gene, which is an important step in cloning a gene and identifying the protein that the gene encodes.

Informatics Requirements in the Genomic Environment

New techniques in molecular genetics, combined with robust statistical and epidemiological approaches, will be required to discover gene-environment interactions and their influence on disease. By correlating the individual molecular response of the gene with the environmental response, susceptibility to environment and lifestyle will become better understood. This effort will require access to a population-based repository of biological specimens. Beyond human studies, technologies will have to be developed to validate mouse models of disease-related genetics.

With the expansion of information at the molecular level, chromosomal aberrations are being uncovered in large volumes. Databases of chromosomal aberrations will be needed to store the information. Integration between chromosomal databases and epidemiology, clinical trials, and surveillance data will be required.

These registries will require the integration of cytogenetic and physical maps of the genome for more precise analysis of chromosomal aberrations. Imaging agents and technologies will need to be incorporated into current tool sets for this level of chromosomal aberrations.

Information systems will be required to collect, store, analyze, and integrate molecular data with epidemiological and clinical data. New algorithms, pattern analysis, and heuristics will be required to study the interaction between genes and individual genetic variations, results from clinical trials, and the environmental influences on disease prevention, risk, diagnosis, and treatment. This research process involves collecting massive amounts of data from several genes and multiple possible alterations in each gene. Data on these gene alterations could be correlated with the outcomes of clinical trials and drug intervention studies. The nature of clinical trial research as we know it today will be very different.

This integration requires dynamic information infrastructures linking data from several disparate databases. It also requires the application of security measures to assure protection of the data for scientific discovery. Integration of information within genetic bibliographic databases will be required for scientists and clinicians to find information in larger and larger pools of genome sequence data, publications, and clinical trial results. Natural language processing tools, knowledge discovery systems, and expert retrieval and browser tools will become more important. The scientist and clinician will require knowledge robots to search, retrieve, and synthesize information in a timely manner and in presentable formats.

Networks of genetic clinical trial research are being initiated. The integration of information from clinical trials in sites in different geographic locations needs an underlying architecture, standards for transmission, and format to be sent. These data in turn require integration with large collaborative studies of disease susceptibility from environmental and other exposures. The linking of clinical trials with disease genetic networks need appropriate integration.

Centralized and accessible repositories will be required to link information from molecular studies, to clinical trials to the surveillance to epidemiological information. These repositories will be centers that contain secure, protected genetic information for research purposes. The registries that result from integrated information need to have controlled access, security, and advanced retrieval and browser tools.

Repositories of information will have to be developed to exchange information related to all levels of genomics.

 ## Summary

This chapter took a peek into the future in three major areas: continuous speech recognition, data warehouses and repositories, and genomic informatics. It also integrated concepts that were described in detail in several of the new chapters of this book to show the use of these tools, such as data mining, in the new genomic environment. There are many new ways that diseases will be prevented, diagnosed, and treated in the new millennium. This chapter is meant to stimulate the thinking of nursing students at the baccalaureate and graduate levels to consider the role that informatics will play in the search for diagnostic causes and treatment answers. It is possible that the concepts in this chapter will be realized at the beginning of the new millennium more quickly than one could predict, and we have not even begun to predict the information system applications in health care at the middle and end of the new millennium.

It promises to be an interesting future. Hopefully, the nurses of the new millennium will be prepared for the challenges.

 ## References

Clark, H. (1998). Continuous speech recognition: What you should know. *Journal of American Health Informatics Management Association, 69*(9), 68–69.

Greenes, R. A., and Lorenzi, N. M. (1998). Audacious goals for health and biomedical informatics in the new millennium. *Journal of the American Medical Informatics Association, 5,* 395–400.

Kouzes, R. T., Myers, J. D., and Wulf, W. A. (1996). Collaboratories: Doing science on the Internet. *Computer, August,* 40–6.

Mason, D. H. (1994). Scenario-based planning: decision model for the learning organization. *Planning Review, 22,* 6–11.

MHSS 2020. (1996). Envisioning tomorrow to focus today's resources. A report to the Surgeon Generals of the DoD.

Nakatsu, R., and Suzuku, Y. (1995). What does voice-processing technology support today? *Proceedings of the National Academy of Sciences USA, 92,* 10023–30.

National Cancer Institute. *The Nation's Investment in Cancer Research : A Budget Proposal for Fiscal Year 2000.*

Rindfleisch, R. C., and Brutlag, D. L. (1998). Directions for clinical research and genomic research into the next decades. *Journal of the American Medical Informatics Association, 5,* 404–411.

Rosenthal, D. I., Chew, S. S., Dupuy, D. E., et al. (1998). Computer-based speech recognition as a replacement for medical transcription. *American Journal of Roentgenology, 170,* 23–5.

Strausberg, R.L., Dahl, C. A. and Klausner, R. D. (1997, April 15). New opportunities for uncovering the molecular basis of cancer. *Nature Genetics* (Supplement), 415–416.

Zaphar, A., Overhage, M. A., and McDonald, C. J. (1999). Continuous speech recognition for clinicians. *Journal of the American Medical Informatics Association, 6,* 195–204.

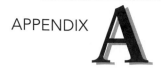
Home Health Care Classification (HHCC) System

Two Terminologies: HHCC of Nursing Diagnoses and HHCC of Nursing Interventions with 20 Care Components

Virginia K. Saba

A complete description of the HHCC of Nursing Diagnoses and Nursing Interventions with the 20 Care Components including their definitions are available on the Internet

Internet Address:

http://www.dml.georgetown.edu/research/hhcc

Table A.1 Home Health Care Classification—20 Nursing Components: Alphabetic Index and Codes

A	ACTIVITY COMPONENT
B	BOWEL ELIMINATION COMPONENT
C	CARDIAC COMPONENT
D	COGNITIVE COMPONENT
E	COPING COMPONENT
F	FLUID VOLUME COMPONENT
G	HEALTH BEHAVIOR COMPONENT
H	MEDICATION COMPONENT
I	METABOLIC COMPONENT
J	NUTRITIONAL COMPONENT
K	PHYSICAL REGULATION COMPONENT
L	RESPIRATORY COMPONENT
M	ROLE RELATIONSHIP COMPONENT
N	SAFETY COMPONENT
O	SELF-CARE COMPONENT
P	SELF-CONCEPT COMPONENT
Q	SENSORY COMPONENT
R	SKIN INTEGRITY COMPONENT
S	TISSUE PERFUSION COMPONENT
T	URINARY ELIMINATION COMPONENT

Home Health Care Classification of Nursing Diagnoses with Expected/Actual Outcomes and Coding Structure

The coding structure for HHCC of Nursing Diagnoses and Expected Outcomes/Goals is shown. The coding structure consists of five alphanumeric characters.

Home Health Care Component:	1st alpha code A–T
Nursing Diagnosis Major Category:	2nd/3rd digit: 01–50
Nursing Diagnosis Subcategory:	4th decimal digit: 1–9
Discharge Status/Goal:	5th digit: 1–3
	(Use only one)

(1 = Improved, 2 = Stabilized, 3 = Deteriorated)

Table A.2   Home Health Care Classification of Nursing Diagnoses and Coding Scheme: 50 Major Categories and 95 Subcategories

A   **ACTIVITY COMPONENT**

- 01   Activity Alteration
  - 01.1   Activity Intolerance
  - 01.2   Activity Intolerance Risk
  - 01.3   Diversional Activity Deficit
  - 01.4   Fatigue
  - 01.5   Physical Mobility Impairment
  - 01.6   Sleep Pattern Disturbance
- 02   Musculoskeletal Alteration

B   **BOWEL ELIMINATION COMPONENT**

- 03   Bowel Elimination Alteration
  - 03.1   Bowel Incontinence
  - 03.2   Colonic Constipation
  - 03.3   Diarrhea
  - 03.4   Fecal Impaction
  - 03.5   Perceived Constipation
  - 03.6   Unspecified Constipation
- 04   Gastrointestinal Alteration

C   **CARDIAC COMPONENT**

- 05   Cardiac Output Alteration
- 06   Cardiovascular Alteration
  - 06.1   Blood Pressure Alteration

D   **COGNITIVE COMPONENT**

- 07   Cerebral Alteration
- 08   Knowledge Deficit
  - 08.1   Knowledge Deficit of Diagnostic Test
  - 08.2   Knowledge Deficit of Dietary Regimen
  - 08.3   Knowledge Deficit of Disease Process
  - 08.4   Knowledge Deficit of Fluid Volume
  - 08.5   Knowledge Deficit of Medication Regimen
  - 08.6   Knowledge Deficit of Safety Precautions
  - 08.7   Knowledge Deficit of Therapeutic Regimen
- 09   Thought Processes Alteration

E   **COPING COMPONENT**

- 10   Dying Process
- 11   Family Coping Impairment
  - 11.1   Compromised Family Coping
  - 11.2   Disabled Family Coping
- 12   Individual Coping Impairment
  - 12.1   Adjustment Impairment
  - 12.2   Decisional Conflict
  - 12.3   Defensive Coping
  - 12.4   Denial
- 13   Post-Trauma Response
  - 13.1   Rape Trauma Syndrome
- 14   Spiritual State Alteration
  - 14.1   Spiritual Distress

F   **FLUID VOLUME COMPONENT**

- 15   Fluid Volume Alteration
  - 15.1   Fluid Volume Deficit
  - 15.2   Fluid Volume Deficit Risk
  - 15.3   Fluid Volume Excess
  - 15.4   Fluid Volume Excess Risk

G   **HEALTH BEHAVIOR COMPONENT**

- 16   Growth and Development Alteration
- 17   Health Maintenance Alteration
- 18   Health Seeking Behavior Alteration
- 19   Home Maintenance Alteration
- 20   Noncompliance
  - 20.1   Noncompliance of Diagnostic Test
  - 20.2   Noncompliance of Dietary Regimen
  - 20.3   Noncompliance of Fluid Volume
  - 20.4   Noncompliance of Medication Regimen
  - 20.5   Noncompliance of Safety Precautions
  - 20.6   Noncompliance of Therapeutic Regimen

H   **MEDICATION COMPONENT**

- 21   Medication Risk
  - 21.1   Polypharmacy

I   **METABOLIC COMPONENT**

- 22   Endocrine Alteration
- 23   Immunologic Alteration
  - 23.1   Protection Alteration

J   **NUTRITIONAL COMPONENT**

- 24   Nutrition Alteration
  - 24.1   Body Nutrition Deficit
  - 24.2   Body Nutrition Deficit Risk
  - 24.3   Body Nutrition Excess
  - 24.4   Body Nutrition Excess Risk

K   **PHYSICAL REGULATION COMPONENT**

- 25   Physical Regulation Alteration
  - 25.1   Dysreflexia
  - 25.2   Hyperthermia
  - 25.3   Hypothermia
  - 25.4   Thermoregulation Impairment
  - 25.5   Infection Risk
  - 25.6   Infection Unspecified

L   **RESPIRATORY COMPONENT**

- 26   Respiration Alteration
  - 26.1   Airway Clearance Impairment
  - 26.2   Breathing Pattern Impairment
  - 26.3   Gas Exchange Impairment

M   **ROLE RELATIONSHIP COMPONENT**

- 27   Role Performance Alteration
  - 27.1   Parental Role Conflict
  - 27.2   Parenting Alteration
  - 27.3   Sexual Dysfunction
- 28   Communication Impairment

28.1   Verbal Impairment
29   Family Processes Alteration
30   Grieving
    30.1   Anticipatory Grieving
    30.2   Dysfunctional Grieving
31   Sexuality Patterns Alteration
32   Socialization Alteration
    32.1   Social Interaction Alteration
    32.2   Social Isolation

N   SAFETY COMPONENT

33   Injury Risk
    33.1   Aspiration Risk
    33.2   Disuse Syndrome
    33.3   Poisoning Risk
    33.4   Suffocation Risk
    33.5   Trauma Risk

34   Violence Risk

O   SELF-CARE COMPONENT

35   Bathing/Hygiene Deficit
36   Dressing/Grooming Deficit
37   Feeding Deficit
    37.1   Breastfeeding Impairment
    37.2   Swallowing Impairment
38   Self Care Deficit
    38.1   Activities of Daily Living (ADLs) Alteration
    38.2   Instrumental Activities of Daily Living (IADLs) Alteration
39   Toileting Deficit

P   SELF-CONCEPT COMPONENT

40   Anxiety
41   Fear
42   Meaningfulness Alteration
    42.1   Hopelessness
    42.2   Powerlessness
43   Self-Concept Alteration

43.1   Body Image Disturbance
43.2   Personal Identity Disturbance
43.3   Chronic Low Self-Esteem Disturbance
43.4   Situational Self-Esteem Disturbance

Q   SENSORY COMPONENT

44   Sensory Perceptual Alteration
    44.1   Auditory Alteration
    44.2   Gustatory Alteration
    44.3   Kinesthetic Alteration
    44.4   Olfactory Alteration
    44.5   Tactile Alteration
    44.6   Unilateral Neglect
    44.7   Visual Alteration
45   Comfort Alteration
    45.1   Acute Pain
    45.2   Chronic Pain
    45.3   Unspecified Pain

R   SKIN INTEGRITY COMPONENT

46   Skin Integrity Alteration
    46.1   Oral Mucous Membranes Impairment
    46.2   Skin Integrity Impairment
    46.3   Skin Integrity Impairment Risk
    46.4   Skin Incision
47   Peripheral Alteration

S   TISSUE PERFUSION COMPONENT

48   Tissue Perfusion Alteration

T   URINARY ELIMINATION COMPONENT

49   Urinary Elimination Alteration
    49.1   Functional Urinary Incontinence
    49.2   Reflex Urinary Incontinence
    49.3   Stress Urinary Incontinence
    49.4   Total Urinary Incontinence
    49.5   Urge Urinary Incontinence
    49.6   Urinary Retention
50   Renal Alteration

Adapted, with permission, from NANDA: *Taxonomy I: Revised 1990.* Reprinted with permission of V. K. Saba.

Home Health Care Classification of Nursing Interventions with Type Intervention Action and Coding Structure

The coding structure for HHCC of Nursing Interventions and Type Intervention Action is shown. The coding structure consists of five alphanumeric characters.

- Home Health Care
  Component: 1st Alpha Code A–T
- Nursing Intervention
  Major Category: 2nd/3rd Digit: 01–60
- Nursing Intervention
  Subcategory: 4th Decimal Digit: 1–9
- Type Intervention Action: 5th Digit: 1–4 (Use all that apply) (1 = Assess, 2 = Care, 3 = Teach, 4 = Manage)

Table A.3   Home Health Care Classification of Nursing Diagnoses and Coding Scheme: 60 Major Categories and 100 Subcategories

A   ACTIVE COMPONENT

01   Activity Care
    01.1   Cardiac Rehabilitation
    01.2   Energy Conservation

02   Fracture Care
    02.1   Cast Care
    02.2   Immobilizer Care

03   Mobility Therapy
    03.1   Ambulation Therapy
    03.2   Assistive Device Therapy
    03.3   Transfer Care

04   Sleep Pattern Control

05   Rehabilitation Care
    05.1   Range of Motion
    05.2   Rehabilitation Exercise

B   BOWEL ELIMINATION COMPONENT

06   Bowel Care
    06.1   Bowel Training
    06.2   Disimpaction
    06.3   Enema

07   Ostomy Care
    07.1   Ostomy Irrigation

C   CARDIAC COMPONENT

08   Cardiac Care

09   Pacemaker Care

D   COGNITIVE COMPONENT

10   Behavior Care

11   Reality Orientation

E   COPING COMPONENT

12   Counseling Service
    12.1   Coping Support
    12.2   Stress Control

13   Emotional Support
    13.1   Spiritual Comfort

14   Terminal Care
    14.1   Bereavement Support
    14.2   Dying/Death Measures
    14.3   Funeral Arrangements

F   FLUID VOLUME COMPONENT

15   Fluid Therapy
    15.1   Hydration Status
    15.2   Intake/Output

16   Infusion Care
    16.1   Intravenous Care
    16.2   Venous Catheter Care

G   HEALTH BEHAVIOR COMPONENT

17   Community Special Programs
    17.1   Adult Day Center
    17.2   Hospice
    17.3   Meals-on-Wheels
    17.4   Other Community Special Program

18   Compliance Care
    18.1   Compliance with Diet
    18.2   Compliance with Fluid Volume
    18.3   Compliance with Medical Regime
    18.4   Compliance with Medication Regime
    18.5   Compliance with Safety Precautions
    18.6   Compliance with Therapeutic Regime

19   Nursing Contact
    19.1   Bill of Rights
    19.2   Nursing Care Coordination
    19.3   Nursing Status Report

20   Physician Contact
    20.1   Medical Regime Orders
    20.2   Physician Status Report

21   Professional/Ancillary Services
    21.1   Home Health Aide Service
    21.2   Medical Social Worker Service
    21.3   Nurse Specialist Service
    21.4   Occupational Therapist Service
    21.5   Physical Therapist Service
    21.6   Speech Therapist Service
    21.7   Other Ancillary Service
    21.8   Other Professional Service

H   MEDICATION COMPONENT

22   Chemotherapy Care

23   Injection Administration
    23.1   Insulin Injection
    23.2   Vitamin B12 Injection

24   Medication Administration
    24.1   Medication Actions
    24.2   Medication Prefill Preparation
    24.3   Medication Side Effects

25   Radiation Therapy Care

I   METABOLIC COMPONENT

26   Allergic Reaction Care
27   Diabetic Care

J   NUTRITIONAL COMPONENT

28   Gastrostomy/Nasogastric Tube Care
    28.1   Gastrostomy/Nasogastric Tube Insertion
    28.2   Gastrostomy/Nasogastric Tube Irrigation

29   Nutrition Care
    29.1   Enteral/Parenteral Feeding

29.2   Feeding Technique
29.3   Regular Diet
29.4   Special Diet

K   PHYSICAL REGULATION COMPONENT

30   Infection Control
   30.1   Universal Precautions
31   Physical Health Care
   31.1   Health History
   31.2   Health Promotion
   31.3   Physical Examination
   31.4   Physical Measurements
32   Specimen Analysis
   32.1   Blood Specimen Analysis
   32.2   Stool Specimen Analysis
   32.3   Urine Specimen Analysis
   32.4   Other Specimen Analysis
33   Vital Signs
   33.1   Blood Pressure
   33.2   Temperature
   33.3   Pulse
   33.4   Respiration
34   Weight Control

L   RESPIRATORY COMPONENT

35   Oxygen Therapy Care
36   Respiratory Care
   36.1   Breathing Exercises
   36.2   Chest Physiotherapy
   36.3   Inhalation Therapy
   36.4   Ventilator Care
37   Tracheostomy Care

M   ROLE RELATIONSHIP COMPONENT

38   Communicative Care
39   Psychosocial Analysis
   39.1   Home Situation Analysis
   39.2   Interpersonal Dynamics Analysis

N   SAFETY COMPONENT

40   Abuse Control
41   Emergency Care
42   Safety Precautions
   42.1   Environmental Safety
   42.2   Equipment Safety
   42.3   Individual Safety

O   SELF-CARE COMPONENT

43   Personal Care
   43.1   Activities of Daily Living (ADLs)
   43.2   Instrumental Activities of Daily Living (IADLs)
44   Bedbound Care
   44.1   Positioning Therapy

P   SELF-CONCEPT COMPONENT

45   Mental Health Care
   45.1   Mental Health History
   45.2   Mental Health Promotion
   45.3   Mental Health Screening
   45.4   Mental Health Treatment
46   Violence Control

Q   SENSORY COMPONENT

47   Pain Control
48   Comfort Care
49   Ear Care
   49.1   Hearing Aid Care
   49.2   Wax Removal
50   Eye Care
   50.1   Cataract Care

R   SKIN INTEGRITY COMPONENT

51   Decubitus Care
   51.1   Decubitus Stage 1
   51.2   Decubitus Stage 2
   51.3   Decubitus Stage 3
   51.4   Decubitus Stage 4
52   Edema Control
53   Mouth Care
   53.1   Denture Care
54   Skin Care
   54.1   Skin Breakdown Control
55   Wound Care
   55.1   Drainage Tube Care
   55.2   Dressing Change
   55.3   Incision Care

S   TISSUE PERFUSION COMPONENT

56   Foot Care
57   Perineal Care

T   URINARY ELIMINATION COMPONENT

58   Bladder Care
   58.1   Bladder Instillation
   58.2   Bladder Training
59   Dialysis Care
60   Urinary Catheter Care
   60.1   Urinary Catheter Insertion
   60.2   Urinary Catheter Irrigation

Reprinted with permission, courtesy of Saba.

KEY WORDS

Numbers for the chapters in which these key words appear follow in parentheses.

analysis (26)
analytical techniques (20)
bioinformatics (32)
BIREME Library (31)
CINAHL (27)
clinical decision support systems (14)
clinical informatics (31)
clinical information system (13)
cognition (23)
communication (7)
community health services (16, 17)
computational biology (32)
computer communication networks (21)
computer literacy (2)
computer literacy (23)
computer research (31)
computer science (1, 3, 4, 5, 6, 9, 20)
computer systems (2)
computer-assisted decision-making (1)
computing methodologies (23)
concept representation (12)
confidentiality (9)
consumer (21)
consumer health (22)
consumer-driven education (24)
continuous speech recognition (32)
creation of Web pages (7)
critical care (15)
critical pathways (14)
culture (28)
curriculum (1, 23)
data collection (26)
data management (26)
data mining (20)
data processing (5)
data warehouses (32)
decision support (22)

decision theory (22)
distance education (1, 24, 31)
distance learning (24)
DIS-UNIFESP (31)
electronic health record (11)
evaluation of Web resources (7)
faculty development (23)
genomic informatics (32)
guidelines (19)
health care (19)
health education (21)
health policy (8)
health reference databases (27)
health services administration (19)
HIPAA (10)
home care (16)
home health care (16)
hospital information systems (13, 15, 18, 28, 29, 30)
ICNP-Brazilian version (31)
informatics (11, 23)
information management systems (13)
information resources (27)
information retrieval (27)
information science (13)
information systems (1, 2, 3, 4, 5, 6, 8, 9, 13, 14, 15, 16, 17, 18, 19, 20, 21, 23, 25, 28, 29, 30)
information technology (23)
integrated advances (13)
integrated information systems (15)
Internet (1, 2, 7, 21, 25)
Internet courses (24)
knowledge discovery in databases (KDD) (20)
knowledge management (20)
knowledge repositories (32)
Latin American informatics (31)
learning interactively (24)
legislation and jurisprudence (10)

INDEX

ISBN 0-07-134900-6

90000

9 780071 349000